Early-stage Lung Cancer

Xiangpeng Zheng • Ming Li • Guozhen Zhang
Editors

Early-stage Lung Cancer

Screening and Management

人民軍醫出版社
PEOPLE'S MILITARY MEDICAL PRESS

Springer

Editors
Xiangpeng Zheng
Fudan University Huadong Hospital
Shanghai
China

Ming Li
Fudan University Huadong Hospital
Shanghai
China

Guozhen Zhang
Fudan University Huadong Hospital
Shanghai
China

ISBN 978-981-10-7595-7 ISBN 978-981-10-7596-4 (eBook)
https://doi.org/10.1007/978-981-10-7596-4
The print edition is not for sale in China Mainland. Customers from China Mainland please order the print book from: People's Military Medical Press.

Library of Congress Control Number: 2017964010

Printed on acid-free paper

This Springer imprint is published by Springer Nature
The registered company is Springer Nature Singapore Pte Ltd.
The registered company address is: 152 Beach Road, #21-01/04 Gateway East, Singapore 189721, Singapore

To our families and patients

Foreword

Lung cancer is one of the most common malignant tumors in China. Per cancer statistics published by the National Cancer Registry Center, over 600,000 new cases of lung cancer had been registered by 2010, with death resulting in half a million of them. China is undoubtedly confronting an extremely grim situation with respect to lung cancer in terms of absolute patient numbers, incidence, and mortality. In contrast to the descending trend in more developed Western countries, both the incidence and mortality of lung cancer are still increasing and have not yet peaked in China, and this growth is partly due to the accelerating industrialization, continuing urbanization, and changing lifestyles. Current statistics have revealed that more than half of lung cancers were diagnosed at the advanced or late stage, leading to poor treatment outcomes and imposing unaffordable economic burdens on both patients and national healthcare systems. Thus, quality of life and life expectancy are compromised, and the overall survival of Chinese lung cancer patients lags behind that of patients in more developed countries.

One of the key issues necessary for improving lung cancer treatment is the need to promote diagnosis and medical intervention. Early detection, early diagnosis, and early initiation of medical intervention have been universally accepted as comprising the fundamental principles in the management of lung cancer. However, since capabilities in diagnosis and medical decision-making vary between clinicians, the implementation of these principles varies, as well. In this aspect, Fudan University Huadong Hospital has invested enormous efforts and resources to this cause, making remarkable achievements nationally. The following examples are good representations of these endeavors.

First, to the best of our knowledge, Huadong Hospital is the first tertiary hospital nationwide to conduct low-dose CT (LDCT) screening for lung cancer. Thanks to that initiative, many subcentimeter lung cancers have been detected and surgically cured, gradually shifting the paradigm of lung cancer screening from traditional chest radiography to LDCT. The direct benefits of such a paradigm shift include satisfactory treatment outcomes and life expectancy that is not compromised.

Second, teamwork matters. About a decade ago, to manage the increasingly frequent detection of small pulmonary nodules along with the clinical application of multidetector-row CT (M.D.CT), the hospital launched its first multidisciplinary team (M.D.T) initiative, joined by experts from the Departments of Radiology, Pathology, Thoracic Surgery, and Radiation Oncology. The effort was led by Professor Guozhen Zhang, the radiologist nationally known as "God's eyes," and it eventually evolved into the Lung Nodule Diagnosis and Treatment Center (LN-DTC). At the center, patients receive one-stop comprehensive medical services, from the diagnosis and treatment of physical diseases to mental and emotional support. The central tenet of Dr. Zhang's medical practice is "reading the film, reading the patient." Inspired by the successful operation and fulfillment of the goals of the center, many hospitals established their own M.D.Ts, which has undoubtedly improved the treatment of lung cancer in China.

Third and most importantly, the development of the center can be attributed to the continuous dedication, unceasing innovation, the unwavering pursuit of medical knowledge, and the honing of skills of each member. To further improve the treatment outcome and prognosis of lung cancer, Dr. Zhang proposed the "EAST" principle for the management of SLCs: Early detection, Accurate diagnosis, minimally invasive Surgery, and Teamwork for precise biopsy. Recently, the center accurately diagnosed a lung cancer measuring 4 mm with surgical biopsy. Dr. Zhang observed the differences in biological behavior between SLCs and conventional mass-like lung cancers and was the first to propose the "CT angiogram of tumor angiogenesis (CTA-TA)" as the differentiating imaging technique, and this subsequently became the well-known CTA-TA sign. Today, tumor angiogenesis-centered images post-processing have been the cornerstone of the radiological assessment of SLCs, and as a result, the preoperative diagnostic accuracy of SLCs, especially adenocarcinoma in situ (AIS) and minimally invasive adenocarcinoma (MIA), has dramatically increased. In 2014 alone, more than 300 cases of very early-stage SLCs (stages 0 and I) were diagnosed with an accuracy of 95%. Moreover, to facilitate postoperative pathological examination, a technique called CT-guided fine-needle puncturing (CT-FNP) was developed to assist with the localization of lesions in re-aerated lung specimens. For those patients who are deemed unsuitable for surgical treatment, multiple nonsurgical ablative approaches have been developed, including stereotactic ablative radiotherapy (SABR) and radiofrequency ablation (RFA).

Regardless of the controversies over the management of SLCs, Dr. Zhang and his team invested enormous resources in the research and pushed the diagnostic and surgical limit of SLCs down to 4 mm, lower than the international standard. Most SLCs detected in the center undergo surgical treatment via video-assisted thoracoscopic surgery (VATS), and often no further treatment is required. The strategy of using surgery alone without adjuvant treatment appears to benefit patients in terms of quality of life and benefits society from a health economics perspective. "Innovation, Excellence" is the spirit of Huadong Hospital, and this sentiment is perfectly reflected in the achievements of the center, which have been reported by numerous media including China Central Television, Sina News, and Jifang Daily.

"Be compassionate to patients, be superior in medicine." This is the tenet Dr. Zhang has consistently pursued in his 50-year medical practice. Today, as always, he stands on the frontline in the battle against lung cancer, leading the wave of cancer research, mentoring young physicians, and educating students.

Written with the intention to share Dr. Zhang's valuable experience and research on lung cancer, as well as an interim report of the LN-DTC, this book focuses on the key pressing issues in lung cancer and its management, with an emphasis on submillimeter micronodular pulmonary nodules. The book also discusses advancements on anatomy, pathology, imaging, and treatment-related lung cancer management. We strongly believe that this book will be a significant addition to the literature that exists on lung cancer management in China and worldwide.

We humbly compose this foreword with deep admiration for Dr. Zhang's lifelong dedication to lung cancer research and appreciation on the twelfth anniversary of the center. We wish that every patient suffering from lung cancer could benefit in some way from Dr. Zhang's contributions to the field.

Zhuowei Yu, M.D.
Shanghai Hospital Association, Shanghai, China
Fudan University Huadong Hospital, Shanghai, China
Fudan University, Shanghai, China
Shanghai Institute of Geriatric Medicine, Shanghai, China
Chinese Association of Geriatric Research, Beijing, China
Shanghai Association of Rehabilitation Medicine, Shanghai, China
Division of Geriatrics, Shanghai Medical Association, Shanghai, China

Wen Gao, M.D.
Executive Board of Shanghai Medical Association, Shanghai, China,
Fudan University, Shanghai, China
Chinese College of Thoracic Surgeons, Shanghai, China
Fudan University Huadong Hospital, Shanghai, China
Chinese Society for Tuberculosis, Chinese Medical Association, Beijing, China
Chinese Society for Thoracic and Cardiovascular Surgery, Beijing, China

August 28, 2017

Overview

At the time when low-dose computed tomography (CT) began to prevail over conventional radiography for lung cancer screening, the detection of subcentimeter pulmonary nodules began to increase dramatically. In this context, this book discusses major issues and advancements in the diagnosis and treatment of incidentally detected, subcentimeter lung cancer (SLC). Dr. Guozhen Zhang, distinguished professor in radiology, proposed the "EAST" principle for the management of SLCs: Early detection, Accurate diagnosis, minimally invasive Surgery, and Teamwork for precise biopsy. The EAST principle is thoroughly expanded upon throughout the book. In Part I, experts from pathology and radiology comprehensively review the state-of-the-art advancements in the screening and evaluation of SLCs, and the cross-sectional anatomy of the lung and post-processing techniques of CT imaging are updated. Part II focuses on the imaging features, differential diagnosis, and radiologic-pathologic correlations of SLCs in the categories of pGGN, mGGN, and solid nodules, in compliance with the Guidelines on Lung Cancer Screening from the National Comprehensive Cancer Network (NCCN). Most importantly, the characteristic CT sign for SLC diagnosis and differentiation, the CT angiogram of tumor angiogenesis (CTA-TA sign), or the "neo-vessel mobilization and intercommunication" phenomenon—discovered and coined by Dr. Zhang—is extensively discussed. Part III briefly introduces the therapeutic management strategies for SLCs, including surgical and nonsurgical approaches, e.g., stereotactic ablative radiation therapy (SABR) and radiofrequency ablation (RFA). Finally, to highlight the applicability of subjects addressed in the previous chapters, authors have meticulously prepared 50 clinical cases of benign and malignant pulmonary nodules with in-depth discussion and experts' comments for a self-test for readers, with the goal of furthering understanding of the imaging and the management strategies for SLCs.

Preface

The Lung Nodule Diagnosis and Treatment Center Team. Front row (*seated*): Dr. Zhuowei Yu (*right*); Dr. Guozhen Zhang (*left*). Back row (*standing*): Dr. Xiangpeng Zheng (*right*); Dr. Ming Li (*middle*); Dr. Fanzhen Lv (*left*)

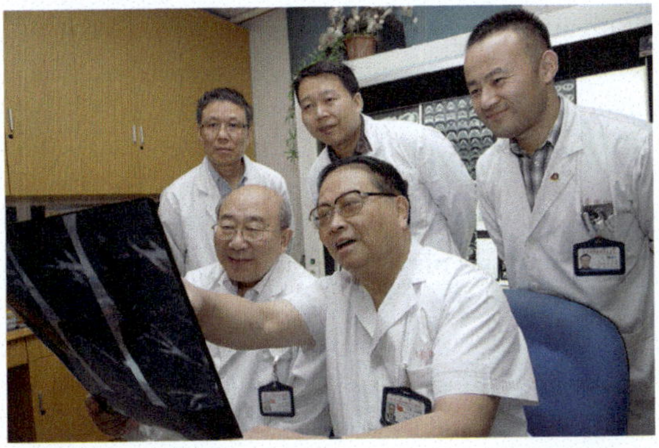

The Twelfth Anniversary of the Zhang Guozhen CT Consultation Center (CCC) and Lung Nodule Diagnosis and Treatment Center (LN-DTC) at Fudan University Huadong Hospital.

Lung cancer screening in high-risk populations is a pivotal measure for the early detection and management of this malignancy. Over the past decade, the screening approach has gradually evolved from conventional chest radiography to low-dose CT. With increasing employment of low-dose CT for screening, the number of incidentally detected micronodular lesions spiked. The accurate assessment and proper management of pulmonary micronodules are critical measures for patients' longevity and quality of life. Mounting evidence has shown that timely surgical removal of micronodular lung cancer via video-assisted thoracoscopic surgery (VATS) has dramatically improved the prognosis.

With strong support from the hospital administration, the Zhang Guozhen CT Consultation Center was established in 2005 as China's first imaging clinic. This center provided patients with comprehensive imaging consultation, a pattern that connects radiologists face-to-face with patients, and has won great acclaim for its improved diagnostic accuracy.

Under the leadership of the hospital president, Dr. Yu Zhuowei, the Zhang Guozhen Center on the Diagnosis and Treatment of Pulmonary Micronodules was established based on the CT Consultation Center and was joined by experts from the Departments of Thoracic Surgery and Radiation Oncology in 2013, to confront the challenge to medical communities from the increasing incidence of pulmonary micronodular lesions. In the new center, multidisciplinary medical teams offer patients one-stop medical services from diagnosis to treatment, which is consistent with international standards of cancer management, with the characteristics of individualized treatment to benefit patients to the furthest extent possible.

Based on thousands of micronodular lung cancer cases over the past decade, we propose an "EAST" principle for the management of SLCs that includes Early detection of subcentimeter nodules, Accurate diagnosis of lung cancers at stages 0/I, prompt Surgical removal of SLCs, and Teamwork for the pre-/postoperative localization of nodules for pathological assessment, with the goal of detecting and eradicating lung cancer at stages 0/I. Obviously, the challenge is massive. However, considering the astonishing 10-year survival of nearly 100% and the tremendous savings on social healthcare payments due to unnecessary adjuvant chemotherapy or radiotherapy, any endeavors to deal with such challenges are worthwhile. We have established systemic and reliable strategies in the diagnosis and treatment of SLCs, represented by the CT angiogram of tumor angiogenesis (CTA-TA) and the CT-guided fine-needle puncturing (CT-FNP) technique. Using these strategies, the center has achieved diagnostic accuracy in SLCs of above 95%.

During consultations and teaching in the past years, we noticed a lack of consensus in the clinic-radiologic-pathologic relationship, imaging techniques, and the management strategies for micronodular lung cancer, particularly adenocarcinoma in situ (AIS). Diagnostic standards and skills vary among physicians, hospitals, and regions, causing false-positive or false-negative diagnoses that subsequently mistakenly guide further medical intervention. This is one of the major reasons for a poor prognosis. Today, thanks to advancements in imaging techniques, the proportion of AIS in lung cancer has increased to above 30% from less than 5% in the 1980s, changing the profile of lung cancer. Therefore, it is extremely important to expand the research on diagnosis and treatment of very early-stage lung cancer for all parties involved in the management of this disease. Unfortunately, there is a lack of systematic materials such as books, training courses, or symposiums focusing on imaging assessment and management strategies for micronodular lung cancer. Hence, we decided to edit this book based on our previous work, emphasizing practicability.

In Part I, experts from pathology and radiology comprehensively review the state-of-the-art advancements of SLC in individual research fields, and information on the cross-sectional anatomy of the lung and post-processing techniques of CT imaging is updated. Part II focuses on the imaging features, differential diagnosis, and radiologic-pathologic correlations of SLCs, which are divided into three categories, namely, pGGN, mGGN, and solid nodules, in compliance with the Guidelines on Lung Cancer Screening from the National Comprehensive Cancer Network (NCCN). Most importantly, the characteristic CT sign for SLC diagnosis and differentiation, CT angiogram of tumor angiogenesis (CTA-TA) (discovered and coined by Dr. Zhang), is extensively discussed. Part III briefly introduces the therapeutic management strategies for SLCs, including surgical and nonsurgical approaches, e.g., stereotactic ablative radiation therapy (SABR) and radiofrequency ablation (RFA). Finally, to highlight the applicability of these subjects, the authors have meticulously prepared 50 clinical cases of pathologically proven benign and malignant pulmonary nodules with in-depth discussion and experts' comments for a self-test for readers, with the goal of furthering their understanding of imaging and the management strategies for SLCs.

Again, without the continuing support from the hospital, the center would not have been successful; without the establishment of the center, this book would not have come about. Therefore, on the twelfth anniversary of the Zhang Guozhen Center, the publication of this book is not simply a summary of past work but also an opportunity to express our deep gratitude for the hospital's support. The hospital president, Dr. Yu, graciously reviewed the book manuscript and provided numerous valuable comments; in addition, he composed the foreword with the general secretary, Dr. Gao. We are greatly appreciative.

We also owe a debt of thanks to our colleagues from the Departments of Radiology and Pathology; collaborators from Tongji University Pulmonary Hospital, Shanghai Jiao Tong University Chest Hospital, and Fudan University Zhongshan Hospital and Huashan Hospital; and publishing editors from People's Military Medical Press and Springer. Additionally, we are grateful for the inclusion of Mr. Yang Zhen's detailed delicate cartoons. And last but not least, we thank our families for their understanding and support.

Shanghai, China Guozhen Zhang, M.D.
Shanghai, China Xiangpeng Zheng, M.D., Ph.D.
Shanghai, China Ming Li, M.D.
August 28, 2017

Contents

Contributors

Qunhui Chen, M.D. Department of Radiology, Shanghai Jiaotong University, Shanghai Chest Hospital, Shanghai, China

Wen Gao, M.D. Department of Thoracic Surgery, Fudan University Huadong Hospital, Shanghai, China

Xiaojun Ge, M.D. Department of Radiology, Fudan University Huadong Hospital, Shanghai, China

Yihui Guan, M.D. Department of Nuclear Medicine, Fudan University Huashan Hospital, Shanghai, China

Fei Hu, M.D. Department of Radiology, Fudan University Huadong Hospital, Shanghai, China

Yanqing Hua, M.D. Department of Radiology, Fudan University Huadong Hospital, Shanghai, China

Yuxin Jiao, M.D. Department of Radiation Oncology, Fudan University Huadong Hospital, Shanghai, China

Xiu Jin, B.Sc. Department of Radiology, Fudan University Huadong Hospital, Shanghai, China

Cheng Li, B.Sc. Department of Radiology, Fudan University Huadong Hospital, Shanghai, China

Hailiang Li, M.D. Department of Interventional Radiology, Zhengzhou University Cancer Hospital, Zhengzhou, China

Ming Li, M.D. Department of Radiology and LN-DTC, Fudan University Huadong Hospital, Shanghai, China

Na Li, M.D. Department of Pathology, Shanghai Jiaotong University, Shanghai Chest Hospital, Shanghai, China

Haiquan Liu, M.D. Department of Radiology, Fudan University Huadong Hospital, Shanghai, China

Fanzhen Lv, M.D. Department of Thoracic Surgery and LN-DTC, Fudan University Huadong Hospital, Shanghai, China

Dingbiao Mao, M.D. Department of Radiology, Fudan University Huadong Hospital, Shanghai, China

Xudong Ni, M.D. Department of Internal Medicine, Fudan University Zhongshan Hospital, Shanghai, China

Jianjian Qiu, M.S. Department of Radiation Oncology, Fudan University Huadong Hospital, Shanghai, China

Yanping Ren, M.D. Department of Radiation Oncology, Fudan University Huadong Hospital, Shanghai, China

Gang Shen, B.Sc. Department of Radiology, Fudan University Huadong Hospital, Shanghai, China

Zi Tan, M.D. Department of Radiation Oncology, Fudan University Huadong Hospital, Shanghai, China

Ping Tang, M.D. Department of Radiology, Fudan University Huadong Hospital, Shanghai, China

Weilan Wu, M.D. Department of Radiology, Fudan University Huadong Hospital, Shanghai, China

Li Xiao, M.D. Department of Pathology, Fudan University Huadong Hospital, Shanghai, China

Dawei Yang, M.D. Department of Internal Medicine, Fudan University Zhongshan Hospital, Shanghai, China

Jianding Ye, M.D. Department of Radiology, Shanghai Jiaotong University, Shanghai Chest Hospital, Shanghai, China

Yulei Yin, M.D. Department of Pathology, Fudan University Huadong Hospital, Shanghai, China

Lingming Yu, M.D. Department of Radiology, Shanghai Jiaotong University, Shanghai Chest Hospital, Shanghai, China

Zhuowei Yu, M.D. Department of Internal Medicine and LN-DTC, Fudan University Huadong Hospital, Shanghai, China

Guozhen Zhang, M.D. Department of Radiology and LN-DTC, Fudan University Huadong Hospital, Shanghai, China

Huibiao Zhang, M.D. Department of Thoracic Surgery, Fudan University Huadong Hospital, Shanghai, China

Huilin Zhang, M.D. Department of Thoracic Surgery, Fudan University Huadong Hospital, Shanghai, China

Jie Zhang, M.D. Department of Pathology, Shanghai Jiaotong University, Shanghai Chest Hospital, Shanghai, China

Lin Zheng, M.D. Department of Interventional Radiology, Zhengzhou University Cancer Hospital, Zhengzhou, China

Xiangpeng Zheng, M.D., Ph.D. Department of Radiation Oncology and LN-DTC, Fudan University Huadong Hospital, Shanghai, China

Feng Zhu, M.D. Department of Radiology, Fudan University Huadong Hospital, Shanghai, China

Lei Zhu, M.D. Department of Pathology, Shanghai Jiaotong University, Shanghai Chest Hospital, Shanghai, China

Xiaohua Zhu, M.D. Department of Radiology, Shanghai Tongji University, Shanghai Pulmonary Hospital, Shanghai, China

Abbreviations

AAH	Atypical adenomatous hyperplasia
ACCP	American College of Chest Physician
AIS	Adenocarcinoma in situ
BAC	Bronchioloalveolar carcinoma
BED	Biologically effective dose
CPR	Curved planar reformation
CT	Computed tomography
CTA-TA	CT angiogram of tumor angiogenesis
EGFR	Epidermal growth factor receptor
GGN	Ground-glass nodule
GGO	Ground-glass opacity
HRCT	High-resolution CT
IAC	Invasive adenocarcinoma
LDCT	Low-dose CT
LLL	Left lower lobe
LPA	Lepidic predominant adenocarcinoma
LUL	Left upper lobe
M.D.CT	Multidetector CT
mGGN	Mixed ground-glass nodule
MIA	Minimally invasive adenocarcinoma
MIP	Maximum intensity projection
mMPLC	Metachronous multiple primary lung cancer
MPLC	Multiple primary lung cancer
MPR	Multiplanar reformation
MRI	Magnetic resonance imaging
NCCN	National Comprehensive Cancer Network
NSCLC	Non-small cell lung cancer
pGGN	Pure ground-glass nodule
psGGN	Part-solid ground-glass nodule
RFA	Radiofrequency ablation
RLL	Right lower lobe

RML	Right middle lobe
RTOG	Radiation Therapy Oncology Group
RUL	Right upper lobe
SABR	Stereotactic ablative radiotherapy
SBRT	Stereotactic body radiation therapy
SCLC	Small cell lung cancer
SLC	Subcentimeter lung cancer
sMPLC	Synchronous multiple primary lung cancer
SPN	Solitary pulmonary nodule
SSD	Shaded surface display
ssGGN	Semisolid ground-glass nodule
VATS	Video-assisted thoracoscopic surgery
VC	Vascular convergence sign
VDT	Volume doubling time
VEGFR	Vascular endothelial growth factor
VR	Volume rendering

Part I
Advances in Lung Cancer Screening and Diagnosis

Chapter 1
Advances in the Pathology of Lung Adenocarcinoma

Na Li, Jie Zhang, and Ming Li

1.1 The Historical Overview of Early-Stage Lung Adenocarcinoma

According to current pathology criteria, the early lung adenocarcinoma consists of adenocarcinoma in situ (AIS) and minimally invasive adenocarcinoma (MIA). It has been accepted that the progression of the majority of lung adenocarcinomas follows a stepwise process starting from atypical adenomatous hyperplasia (AAH) to AIS to MIA and finally to invasive adenocarcinoma. Hereunto, AAH and AIS are defined as preinvasive lesions representing a continuous lineage of intraepithelial neoplasia in alveolar structures.

In the 1960s, the concept of atypical alveolar hyperplasia or bronchioloalveolar hyperplasia was proposed. For decades, various terms have been adopted to describe such lesions, including atypical alveolar cuboidal cell hyperplasia, alveolar hyperplasia, atypical alveolar hyperplasia, atypical bronchioloalveolar hyperplasia, and bronchioloalveolar adenoma. Since the early 1990s, researchers proposed that this lesion may be the precursor lesion of lung adenocarcinoma and the initial stage of the development from adenoma to bronchioloalveolar adenocarcinoma and invasive adenocarcinoma. Studies using flow cytometry provided the evidence supporting that AAH is a neoplastic hyperplasia, like well-differentiated minute papillary adenocarcinoma, and concluded that AAH might be an adenoma or a well-differentiated adenocarcinoma. Autopsy data revealed that pulmonary AAH occurred in 2% of young healthy individuals and 23.2% of elderly patients with lung tumors. Also, AAH has a predisposition to appear adjacent to pre-existing invasive adenocarcinoma.

N. Li • J. Zhang (✉)
Department of Pathology, Shanghai Jiaotong University, Shanghai Chest Hospital, Shanghai, China

M. Li
Department of Radiology, Fudan University Huadong Hospital, Shanghai, China

X. Zheng et al. (eds.), *Early-stage Lung Cancer*,
https://doi.org/10.1007/978-981-10-7596-4_1

Thus, it is speculated that AAH could probably be the early event during the process from adenoma to adenocarcinoma. Subsequently, a large number of molecular biology studies, including the mutation of K-ras and EGFR, the polymorphism of K-ras, the expression of p53, and the lack of alleles, methylation, and overexpression of telomerase, confirmed the close relationship between AAH and lung adenocarcinoma from the cellular or genetic levels. In 1999, the WHO histopathologic classification officially introduced the concept of AAH with the definition of a preinvasive lesion of lung adenocarcinoma, which was applied in the consecutive 2004 WHO classification.

The current concept of AIS is modified from previous bronchioloalveolar adenocarcinoma (BAC). With regard to BAC, Masayuki Noguchi, a Japanese pathologist, conducted a pioneering work. In 1995, Noguchi et al. published a study report on the analysis of resected peripheral lung adenocarcinomas less than 2 cm from 276 cases [1]. By histological examination, small adenocarcinomas were grouped into six distinctive structural patterns: Noguchi types A, B, C, D, E, and F. These characteristic appearances were well correlated with the macroscopic features of the tumors and differences in their clinical behavior.

Histologically, type A BACs are well-differentiated localized diseases. Tumors are solitary, usually larger than 1 cm in greatest dimension with indistinct boundaries. Alveolar architectures remain intact but alveolar lining cells are replaced with minimal or mild thickening of the alveolar septa. Type A tumors are distinguishable from AAHs (or adenomas) by increased cellularity and cell atypia. Individual tumor cells resemble Clara cells, type II pneumocytes, or goblet cells. Fibrotic foci in the tumors are absent. Type B BACs have foci of alveolar structural collapse on the basis of type A diseases. Thus, except the fibrotic foci due to alveolar collapse, the overall microscopic appearance of type B is similar to that of type A, showing a replacement growth pattern and indistinct boundaries. Unique pleural indentation due to alveolar collapse is often detected.

The major feature of type C diseases is foci of active fibroblastic proliferation within localized lesions. Within the lesion, numerous fibroblasts with large nuclei are seen. And endothelial cells actively proliferate to generate neovasculatures. However, in the foci of alveolar collapse, active fibroblasts are absent, distinct from type B. Those tumor cells located in the fibroblastic foci have larger and more atypical nuclei than those in the peripheral region. In the periphery, tumor cells gradually replace pre-existing alveolar lining cells. Pleural indentation is a common finding. In some cases, it is difficult to distinguish type C from type B macroscopically.

Type D BACs are poorly differentiated adenocarcinoma with clear boundaries between cancer tissues and the noncancerous parenchyma. The tumor shows largely solid growth, with minor components of papillary and tubular growth, which makes it somehow resemble large cell carcinoma. Type E diseases, tubular adenocarcinoma, consist of acinar, tubular, and cribriform architecture, presumptively originating from or differentiating toward bronchial gland cells. Tumor cells with a signet ring appearance may be observed. The tumor boundary is always distinct. Type F diseases are papillary adenocarcinoma with a compressive growth pattern. Tumors grow in an expansive and destructive pattern, instead of replacing the alveolar lining cells as in other types. Thus, they have clear margins and usually are diagnosed as well-differentiated papillary adenocarcinomas, made up of tall columnar cells of the bronchial surface epithelial type.

The pathological classification has implications on clinical prognosis. The 5-year survival rate for types A and B was approximately 100% in comparison to 74.8% for type C, similar to the prognosis for small-sized pulmonary adenocarcinoma. Type C is viewed as an advanced carcinoma, evolving from type A or B in consistency with the concept of a multistep progression of pulmonary adenocarcinoma. In contrast, types D, E, and F are non-replacement-type adenocarcinomas with a worse prognosis than replacement-type adenocarcinomas (types A, B, and C). A stepwise progression has not been observed in these types, which implies a de novo pathogenesis for them. For those tumors classified as type C, D, E, or F, pulmonary lobectomy with lymph node dissection is the standard of care. If a tumor is type A or B, however, extensive lymph node dissection may be omitted. In the 1999 WHO classification system, Noguchi types A and B were designated as bronchioloalveolar carcinoma, and the 2004 WHO classification maintains the designation.

In 2011, IASLC/ATS/ERS proposed a multidisciplinary classification of lung adenocarcinoma on the basis of WHO classification system. According to the 2011 classification, pulmonary adenocarcinomas were grouped into three categories: preinvasive lesion, MIA, and invasive adenocarcinoma. Preinvasive lesions include AAH and AIS. Invasive adenocarcinoma could have multiple presentations, including lepidic, acinar, papillary, micropapillary, and solid with mucin production predominant. In addition, invasive adenocarcinoma had four variants, invasive mucinous adenocarcinoma, colloid adenocarcinoma, fetal adenocarcinoma, and enteric adenocarcinoma. For the first time, AIS and MIA were divided into three subtypes, non-mucinous, mucinous, and mixed (non-mucinous/mucinous). A comparative analysis between Noguchi classification and the 2011 classification indicates that type A is corresponding to classic AIS, type B to AIS with complex architecture, some of type C to MIA, and invasive adenocarcinoma covers types D, E, and F. The 2011 multidisciplinary classification system has been widely accepted in the clinical practice and studies of pulmonary adenocarcinoma.

1.2 The Pathological Features and Evolution of Early-Stage Adenocarcinoma

Past decades witnessed a dramatic increase in the incidence of lung adenocarcinoma, which has prevailed over squamous cell carcinoma as the most common histological subtype of lung carcinoma. In 2015, a total of 8292 lung cancers were surgically resected in Shanghai Chest Hospital. Among them, the percentage of lung adenocarcinoma was 62.86% (5212 cases). In the same year, the international multidisciplinary classification of lung adenocarcinoma was published in the Journal of Thoracic Oncology (JTO) as a collaborative effort of numerous experts from multiple organizations, including the International Association for the Study of Lung Cancer (IASLC), American Thoracic Society (ATS), and European Respiratory Society (ERS). The 2011 IASLC/ATS/ERS multidisciplinary lung adenocarcinoma classification (hereinafter referred to as "2011 classification") revised the conventional histopathologic classification which had been formulated exclusively by pathologists and without the participation of other professionals [2]. The 2011 classification solicited advice and comments from multidisciplinary panel members, including thoracic medical and surgical oncologists, pulmonologists, radiologists, molecular biologists, and pathologists as well. The purpose is to provide an integrated classification system on the basis of comprehensive advancement of lung adenocarcinoma from every aspect. Moreover, the 2011 classification is expected to reflect mounting evidence of prognostic and predictive researches and to guide the clinical management of lung adenocarcinoma. The majority of the 2011 classification was adopted by the 2015 World Health Organization (WHO) Classification of Tumors of the Lung, Pleura, Thymus and Heart with minor modifications (Table 1.1).

With the extensive adoption of 2011 classification in clinical practice, pathologists are required to update their knowledge to keep abreast of the trend in lung adenocarcinoma. During this course, there may have issues and uncertainty of applying the new system to the pathological diagnosis of early lung adenocarcinoma (including adenocarcinoma in situ and minimally invasive adenocarcinoma), which would be discussed from four aspects in the following sections.

Table 1.1 IASLC/ATS/ERS classification of lung adenocarcinoma (2011)

Preinvasive lesions
Atypical adenomatous hyperplasia (AAH)
Adenocarcinoma in situ (AIS)
Non-mucinous
Mucinous
Mixed
Minimally invasive adenocarcinoma (MIA)
Non-mucinous
Mucinous
Mixed
Invasive adenocarcinoma (IA)
Lepidic predominant
Acinar predominant
Papillary predominant
Micropapillary predominant
Solid predominant with mucin production
Variants of invasive adenocarcinoma
Invasive mucinous adenocarcinoma
Colloid adenocarcinoma
Fetal adenocarcinoma
Enteric adenocarcinoma

1.2.1 *Why Is the Term "Bronchioloalveolar Carcinoma, BAC" Abandoned?*

One of the major updates in the 2011 classification and the 2015 WHO classification is the discontinuation of "bronchioloalveolar carcinoma, BAC" and the induction of "adenocarcinoma in situ." By definition, the neoplastic cells in AIS lesions grow along pre-existing alveolar septa (lepidic growth) without stromal, lymphovascular, pleural, or alveolar space invasion. As known, most of the invasive adenocarcinomas develop from AAH, AIS, and MIA. In this dynamic evolution, especially in the early steps (AAH, AIS, and MIA), neoplastic cells grow in a lepidic pattern. In the past, adenocarcinomas with lepidic growth were diagnosed as BAC. With advancements in lung adenocarcinoma, lepidic growth can be observed in multiple subgroups with distinct prognosis (for instance, adenocarcinoma with a pure lepidic pattern, lepidic predominant invasive adenocarcinoma, and other subtypes of predominant invasive adenocarcinoma comprised of a lepidic pattern). According to the statistics reported in the 2004 WHO classification, the prevalence of BAC among lung adenocarcinomas is about 4%, but it could be as high as 22% according to some literature due to the heterogeneity of diagnostic criteria. The fluctuation in prevalence causes confusion not only in clinical practices and basic researches but also in tumor epidemiology. Therefore, in the 2011 classification, the panel recommended discontinuing the use of the term BAC but regrouping subtypes of BAC on the basis of histopathologic features, clinical presentations, and prognosis using more specific terms. Accordingly, AIS is introduced to describe localized, small (≤3 cm) adenocarcinoma with a growth restricted to neoplastic cells along pre-existing alveolar structures without collateral invasion. Tumors that meet criteria for AIS have formerly been classified as BAC by the criteria of the 1999 and 2004 WHO classifications and type A and type B adenocarcinoma by the 1995 Noguchi classification system.

1.2.2 *The Preinvasive Lesion: AAH and AIS*

In 2011 classification, AAH and AIS are classified as preinvasive lesions. AAH is a localized, small, usually 0.5 cm or less (Fig. 1.1a, b) proliferation of mildly to moderately atypical type II pneumocytes and/or Clara cells lining intact alveolar walls and occasionally respiratory bronchioles. Tumor cells could be rounded, cuboidal, low columnar, or "peg" cells with round to oval nuclei. Gaps are usually seen between cells (Fig. 1.1c). Intranuclear inclusions are frequent in neoplastic cells. These mitoses are extremely rare. There is a continuum of morphologic changes between AAH and AIS. A spectrum of cellularity and histological atypia occurs in AAH. The distinction between more cellular and atypical AAH and AIS can be difficult in histology and impossible in cytology. Radiologically, AAH characteristically presents as a faint, pure ground-glass nodule (GGN), usually measuring 5 mm

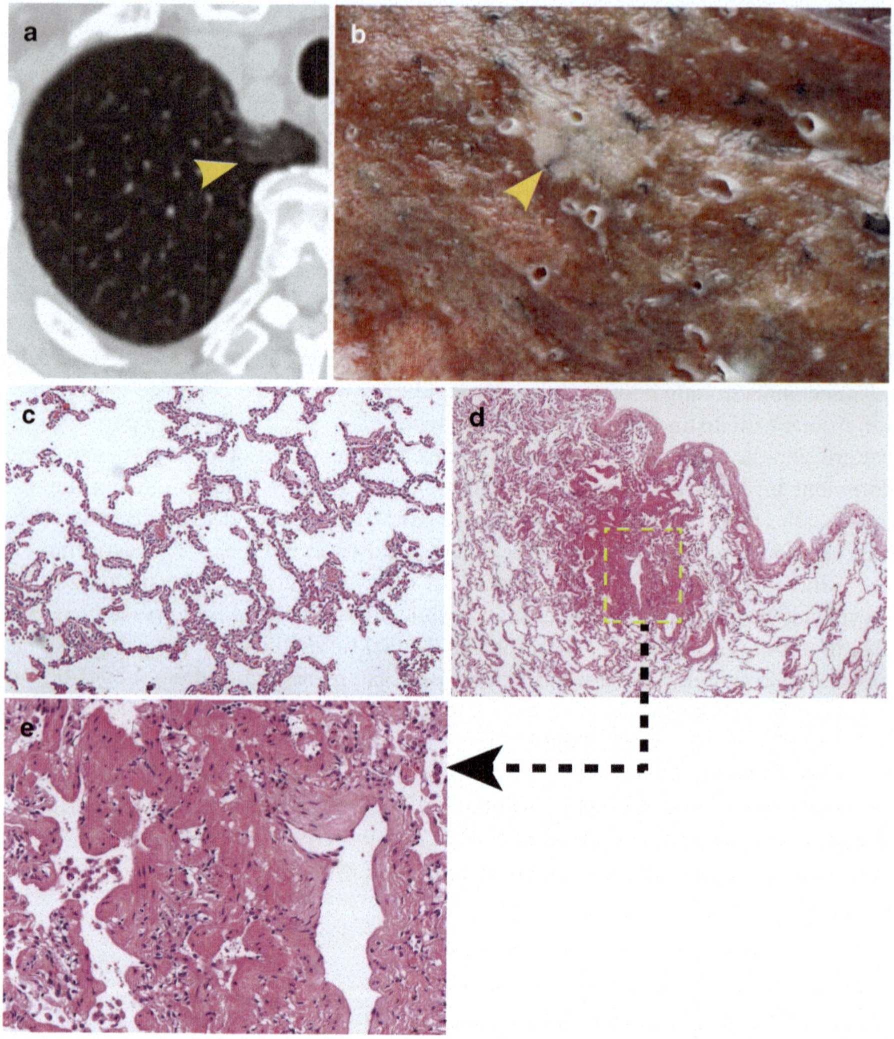

Fig. 1.1 Atypical adenomatous hyperplasia. (**a**) AAH appears as a pure GGN (arrowhead) in thin-sliced CT. (**b**) In resected specimens, AAH is a localized lesion, usually less than 5 mm in diameter with poorly defined margin (arrowhead). (**c**) Mildly widened septa and gaps between neoplastic cells are frequently seen in AAH lesions. (**d**) Regression is occasionally observed within AAH due to fibrotic replacement and collapse of alveolar structures. (**e**) Enlarged view of the region marked with a yellow box in D

or less in diameter but up to 12 mm reported in a minority of cases. AAH can be solitary or multiple with a predisposition to distribution along the subpleural area in lungs. To be noted, AAH belongs to the precancerous lesion, and not all AAH lesions would develop into AIS. Some AAH lesions may regress and disappear due to apoptosis of atypically neoplastic cells (Fig. 1.1d, e), indicative of the reversibility of AAH. Collapse and deformation of alveolar septa may be seen due to cellular loss. Some have classified AAH into low- and high-grade subtypes. However, the grading is not recommended according to the 2011 classification.

The concept of AIS in lung adenocarcinoma was put forward in the 2011 lung adenocarcinoma classification. By definition, AIS (one of the lesions formerly known as BAC) is a localized small (≤3 cm, Fig. 1.2c–e) adenocarcinoma with growth restricted to neoplastic cells along pre-existing alveolar structures (lepidic growth), lacking stromal, lymphovascular, or pleural invasion. Papillary or micropapillary patterns and intra-alveolar tumor cells are absent, no spread through air spaces. Septal widening with sclerosis/elastosis is common, particularly in non-mucinous AIS. Radiologically, AIS presents typically as a pure GGN. The pure GGN of AIS usually appears at thin-section CT as slightly higher attenuation than the very faint GGN of AAH. However, sometimes it appears as a part-solid nodule (Fig. 1.2a). AIS can be divided into two subtypes, non-mucinous and mucinous. Most of the AIS is non-mucinous. Mucinous AIS is extremely uncommon and usually appears solid radiologically. Histologically, no evidence of invasion is seen in AIS lesions (Fig. 1.3).

1.2.3 Minimally Invasive Adenocarcinoma

Adenocarcinomas containing lepidic grow pattern are not exclusively found in AIS. Minimally invasive adenocarcinoma (MIA) is introduced to describe those adenocarcinomas with lepidic growth pattern and minimal invasion in the 2011 classification and 2015 WHO classification. By definition, MIA is a small, solitary adenocarcinoma (≤3 cm), with a predominantly lepidic pattern and ≤5 mm invasion in greatest dimension in any one focus. The major difference between AIS and MIA is the existence of minimal or regional invasive components in the latter, and if the invasion exceeds 5 mm, invasive adenocarcinoma (IAC), lepidic predominant adenocarcinoma (LPA) in specific, should be diagnosed instead of MIA. Thus, the existence and extension of invasive component are of significance for the differentiation of AIS, MIA, and IAC. To be noted, MIA diagnosis is excluded if the tumor contains necrosis; invades lymphatics, blood vessels, and pleura; or spreads through air spaces.

The invasive component to be measured in MIA is defined as follows: (1) histological subtypes other than a lepidic pattern (i.e., acinar, papillary, micropapillary, and/or solid) or (2) tumor cells infiltrating myofibroblastic stroma. If there are multiple foci of invasion or the size of invasion is difficult to measure, recent data suggest that an estimate of invasive size can be made by multiplying the total percentage of the invasive (nonlepidic) components by the total tumor size.

Similar to AIS, MIA can be divided into mucinous and non-mucinous subtypes. Most of MIA is non-mucinous, and mucinous MIA is rare. MIA is variable in its imaging presentation and is not fully described yet, but a provisional description of the non-mucinous type at thin-section CT is a part-solid nodule consisting of a predominant ground-glass component and a small central solid component measuring 5 mm or less.

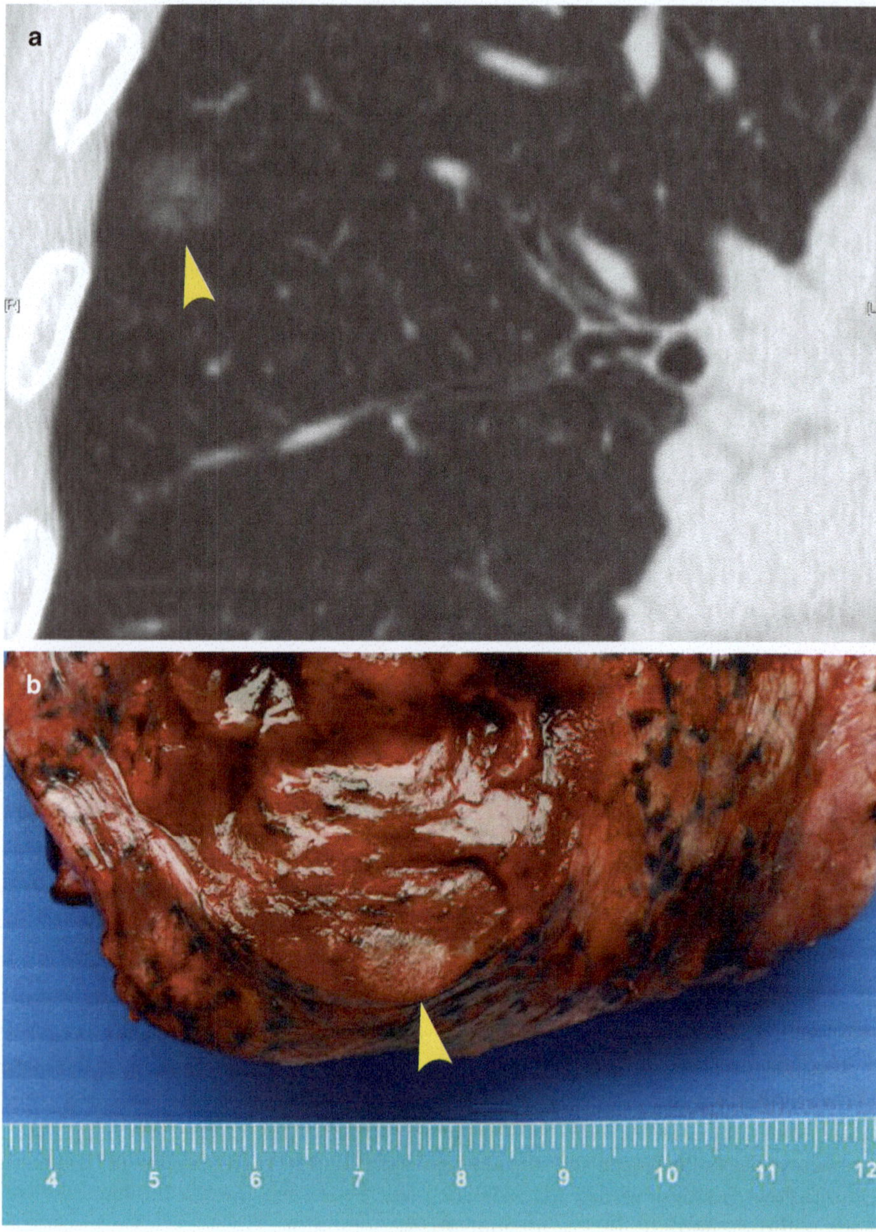

Fig. 1.2 Adenocarcinoma in situ. (**a**) The majority of AIS (arrowhead) appear as pure GGNs with slightly higher attenuation than AAHs. (**b**) AIS (arrowhead) has higher density than AAH in resected specimens and is usually less than 2 cm

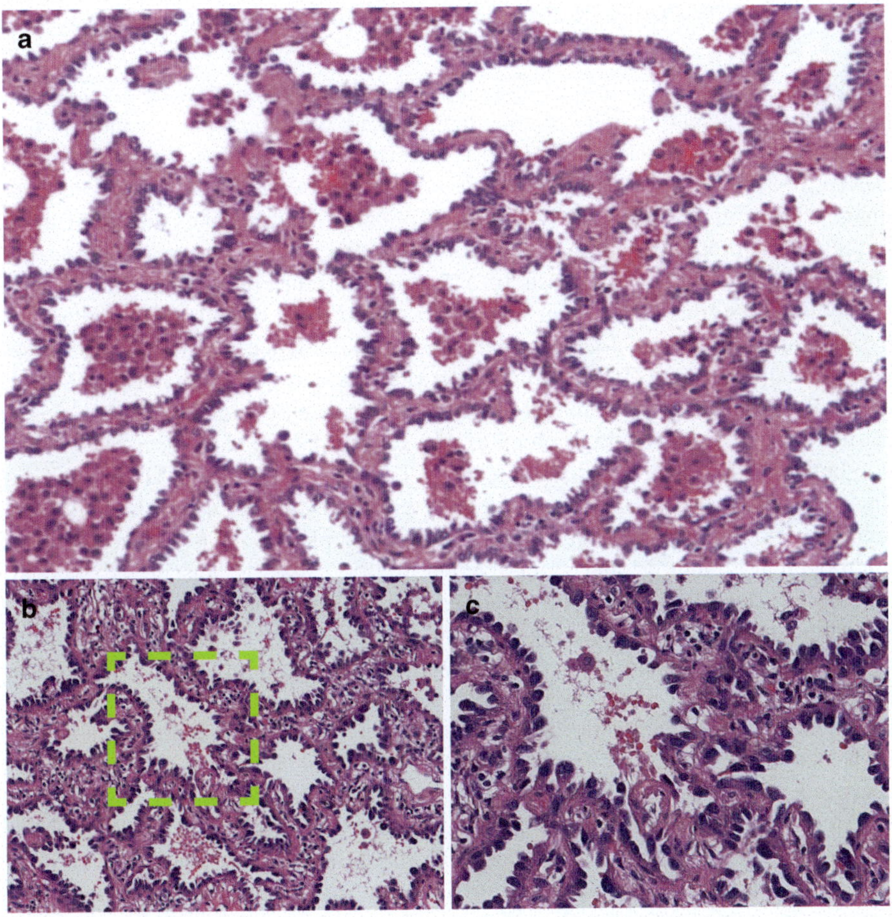

Fig. 1.3 The initial stage of AIS. (**a**) The neoplastic cells of AIS grow along pre-existing alveolar architectures without evident intercellular gaps. (**b**) Alveolar tension increases due to an intense alignment of neoplastic cells in highly proliferative AIS. (**c**) Enlarged view of the region marked with a yellow box in B

The theoretical basis of the 2011 classification and 2015 WHO classification is the recognition of the multistep evolution in lung adenocarcinoma. Currently, it has been widely accepted that the progression of the majority of lung adenocarcinoma follows a stepwise process starting from AAH to AIS, to MIA, to invasive adenocarcinoma. Of course, an exception exists. Some adenocarcinomas could be invasive adenocarcinoma at the very beginning by skipping earlier steps (AAH, AIS, and MIA). In comparison to those with classical developmental steps, these tumors tend to be highly aggressive in biological behavior, and lymph node metastasis in the lungs and/or mediastinum may occur at the diagnosis.

1.2.4 The Evolution of Early Lung Adenocarcinoma

Since AIS is viewed as the starting point in the development of lung adenocarcinoma, prompt detection and accurate diagnosis are of clinical significance. In the 2011 classification and 2015 WHO classification, the histopathologic diagnostic criteria of AIS have been elaborated in accompany with typical morphological images, but clinical practice is way too complicated, which makes the application of the criteria more difficult than expected. Hereby, I try to share my experience in clinical observation and diagnosis of AIS using current criteria. AIS can remain stable for a long time or grow very slowly for an extended period of time (reflected by a remarkable volume-doubling time). In clinical practice, we have an AIS case with annual low-dose CT follow-up for 10 years, which was ultimately surgically resected and pathologically confirmed with no evidence of invasion. The histological features and cellular morphology of AIS vary with time. An alternative transition between progression and regression has been observed within AIS lesions. In the initial phase of AIS, abnormal neoplastic cells grow along pre-existing alveolar architectures, lacking stromal, lymphovascular, or pleural invasion. Papillary or micropapillary patterns and intra-alveolar tumor cells are absent. No spread through air spaces is seen. Septal widening with sclerosis/elastosis is common, but no stromal invasion (Fig. 1.4a). Due to focal proliferative hyperactivity, the density of part of AIS lesion increases gradually with accumulation of atypical hyperplastic tumor cells. More than half of AIS diseases remain indolent for an extended period of time. The neoplastic cells may proliferate very slowly or maintain a constant size or even regress. As time passes by, cellular amount may drop due to apoptosis of neoplastic cells along the alveolar septa. Consequently, alveolar tension reduces and architectural intactness cannot be maintained, causing alveolar collapse and formation of fibrous scars. This process could repeatedly occur, ultimately leading to fibrous scar foci (Fig. 1.4b–d). Still, AIS is a malignant disease process, the majority of which will gradually progress, and varying amount of atypical cells could be found within the fibrotic scar foci. These cells are anaplastic with an appearance of tuft or papillary morphology. Gradually, they may acquire invasive biological behavior, infiltrate the stroma, and form the early microinvasive colony (Fig. 1.4e, f).

Once the microinvasion appears, the invasive progress could gain acceleration. The invasion expands and encroaches on adjacent tissues, including fibrotic scars. And the disease progresses to LPA and other subtypes of invasive adenocarcinoma.

Of note, during disease progression, pathological heterogeneity is evident within lesions. Indolent cells, regressing cells, and proliferating cells may coexist, resulting in the characteristic polymorphism in histopathologic examinations, accounting for the difficulty in diagnosis and interobserver discrepancy (Fig. 1.5).

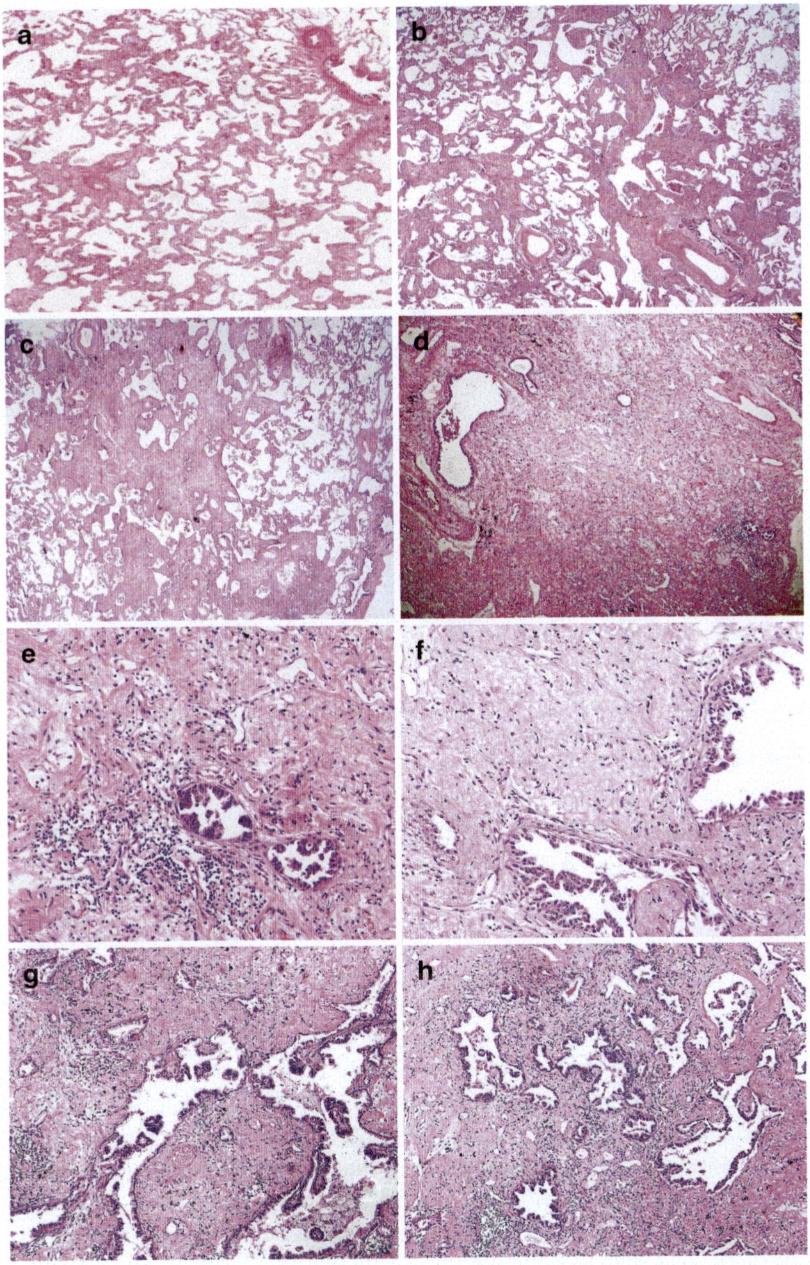

Fig. 1.4 The progression of AIS. (**a**) The morphologic feature of AIS in the initial stage. (**b**) As the tumor remains, fibrotic hyperplasia occurs. (**c**) Alveolar collapse, fibrotic proliferation within septa, and fibrotic scar are seen. (**d**) Variable sizes of fibrotic scars occur within the lesion. (**e**) Atypical glands are observed in fibrotic areas. (**f**) AISĐMIA. Invasive tumor cells grow in the peripheral area of the fibrotic scar (**g**) AISĐMIA. Tumor cells invade the fibrotic scar from the peripheral to the central area. (**h**) AISĐMIA. Fibrotic scars are gradually replaced by invasive adenocarcinoma

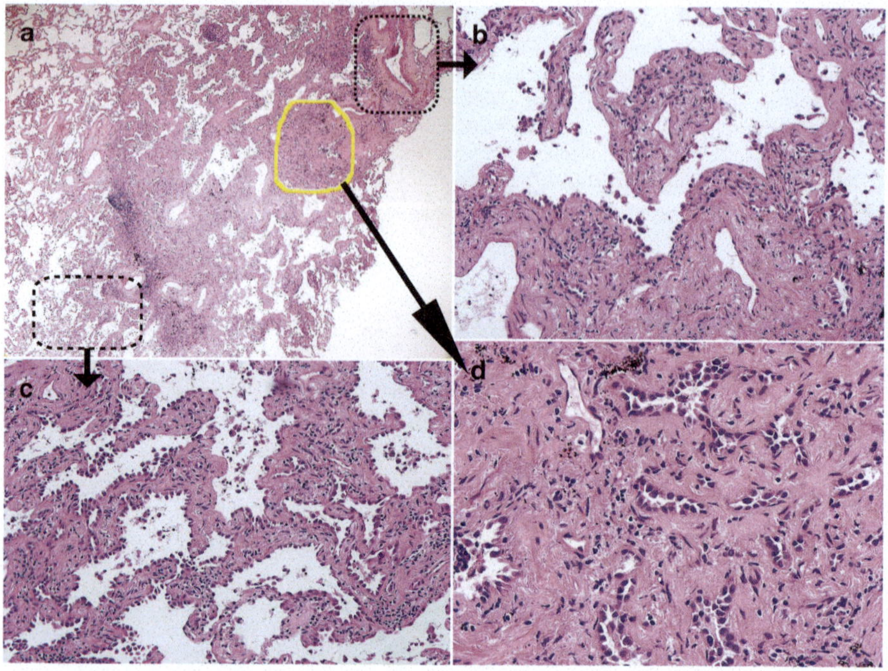

Fig. 1.5 The heterogeneity in AIS. (**a**) Polymorphism of the histopathologic change in AIS. (**b**) The alveoli with AIS are compressed due to fibrotic hyperplasia. (**c**) The typical histopathologic appearance in AIS. (**d**) Alveolar dilation and reduced epithelium are observed

1.3 The Essentials in Pathological Diagnosis of Early-Stage Adenocarcinoma

The current classification of lung adenocarcinoma was a collaborative accomplishment from multidisciplinary experts. Remarkably, it reflects recent advances in various frontiers of lung cancer research from biology to clinical practice. In contrast to the tradition that the pathological diagnosis was merely based on gross and microscopic examination of tissue samples, the new classification system puts more emphasis on multidisciplinary techniques and platforms beyond traditional histopathologic approaches. For instance, it is important to consult the high-resolution CT images in cases with suspicion of lung cancer, particularly small-sized early-stage lung adenocarcinoma. In recent years, radiology plays a more important role in the diagnosis of early-stage lung cancer with the development of thin-section high-resolution CT scanning technology. CT imaging provides excellent resolutions in many aspects, including size, density, morphology, and the border of the pulmonary nodules. AAH is the earliest preinvasive lesion, with characteristic CT features of less than 5 mm in diameter, pure ground-glass nodular opacity with few solid components. Most non-mucinous AIS present as pure ground-glass nodules and occasionally mixed ground-glass nodules, while mucinous AIS frequently are solid nodules. The majority of non-mucinous MIAs are part-solid nodules with the mixture of ground-glass and solid components. Invasive adenocarcinoma could be solid nodules and may also present as part-solid nodules. In comparison to a limited field of view in the pathological examination, lung CT could provide a full view of lesions and has the capability to discern solid and/or ground-glass components within lesions. Thus, CT imaging could guide precise sampling of resected specimens with an emphasis on areas with high probability of malignancy, such as areas with solid components.

However, CT imaging has its intrinsic limitations as a diagnostic modality in early-stage lung adenocarcinoma. Information derived from CT imaging is anatomical and no less than the millimeter in size, making it impossible to reflect microscopically architectural polymorphism along with the evolution of the tumor and the interaction with the surrounding tissues. For an accurate pathological diagnosis of AAH, the following aspects should be cautioned.

Firstly, nonneoplastic alveolar epithelial hyperplasia, including reactive hyperplasia of alveolar epithelial cells and bronchial epithelial cell metaplasia, should be distinguished from AAH. Reactive hyperplasia of alveolar epithelial cells often occurs in inflammatory and fibrotic lesions. Frequently, an evident injury history, such as pneumonia or acute lung injury, is present. AAH is less likely related to pulmonary inflammation or fibrosis. Unlike focal lesions seen in AAH, reactive alveolar epithelial hyperplasia is diffused with poor-defined margins. The morphology of proliferating cells is rarely atypical. Occasionally, a single, large bizarre cell appears in the background of inflammation, often suggesting inflammation rather than tumorigenesis. The reactive epithelial proliferation of alveoli may have a similar appearance to AAH under the low magnification, but the high magnification reveals these proliferating cells are ciliated bronchial epithelial cells, distinct from AAH. Overall, the criteria for the pathological diagnosis of AAH should include alveolar epithelial cell dysplasia, none or few alveolar macrophages and other inflammatory cells, the absence of pulmonary interstitial inflammation, and corresponding histological changes.

Secondly, it is critical to differentiate AAH from AIS. The differentiation of AAH and AIS mainly depends on three aspects: (1) the maximum diameter of AAH is usually less than 5 mm, rarely more than 8 mm (Fig. 1.1a); (2) the cells of AAH are not continuously arranged along the alveolar wall, while the tumor cells of AIS are usually continuous (Fig. 1.1b); and (3) AAH always shows a pure GGO (Fig. 1.2a) in CT imaging. Actually, AAH and AIS often belong to a continuous process and could appear simultaneously within the same lesion. If this happens, a diagnosis of AIS is appropriate when the tumor size is more than 5 mm. The differentiation of AIS from AAH is of clinical relevance, but both diseases are categorized as preinvasive lesions, and the clinical management is same. In some cases, it is challenging for pathologists to confidently differentiate AAH from AIS, which fortunately has no impact on the following management and prognosis.

Due to the subtle discrepancy between AIS and AAH/MIA, the accurate diagnosis of AIS is challenging and also the fundamental step of learning pathological diagnosis of lung adenocarcinoma. The diagnosis of MIA requires familiarity of diagnostic criteria of AIS. The histopathologic diagnosis of classic AIS is not difficult. Considering that the occurrence and development of AIS in vivo may exist for a long duration, lesions in AIS are often associated with complicated histological changes. For a case suspicious of AIS with complicated structural changes, a comprehensive analysis with caution is required with a particular emphasis on the following aspects.

Firstly, carefully examine the histological structure of the lesion and alveoli possibly involved. One of the main concerns is whether the alveolar structure is maintained. Proliferating tumor cells in AIS grow along the existing alveolar walls and do not disturb the intactness of alveolar walls. If alveolar structural deformation occurs, it probably indicates structural destruction from stromal invasion (Fig. 1.6a). Invasive adenocarcinoma has some characteristic pathological features, including complex glandular structures and papillary structures with fibrovascular cores (Fig. 1.6a).

Secondly, evaluate the arrangement and density of tumor cells. Tumor cells in AIS usually grow along alveolar walls without obvious gaps between cells. Cell density is moderate in most regions. It is rare that tumor cells are overpopulated,

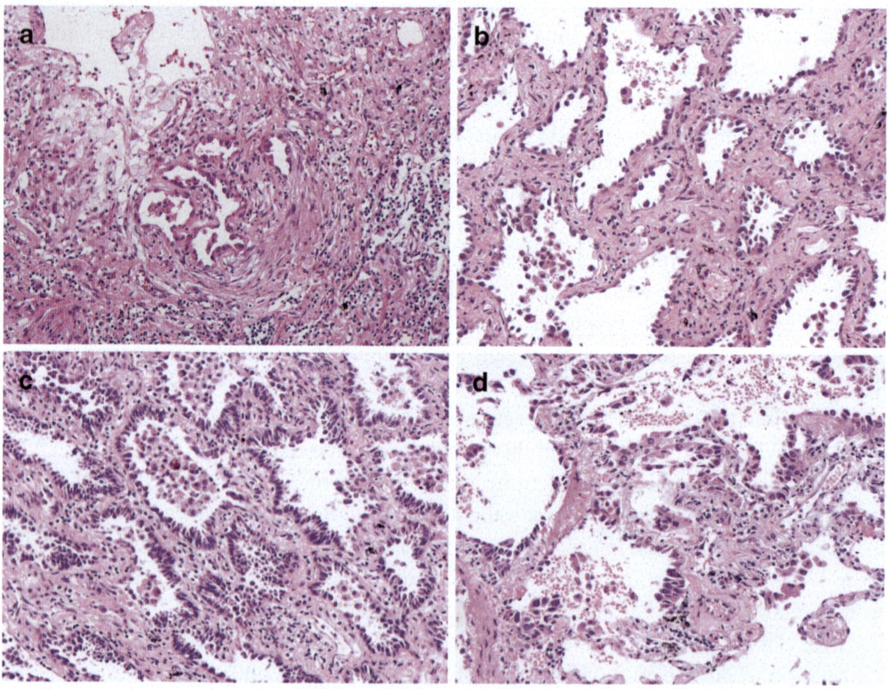

Fig. 1.6 The alignment and density of tumor cells. (**a**) Alveolar structure is destroyed and reconstructed due to the invasion of tumor cells. (**b**) AIS. Cell density increases due to stromal hyperplasia and alveolar shrinkage. (**c**) Invasive adenocarcinoma. Tumor cell density is higher than in AIS. Tumor cells continue proliferating in an uncontrollable manner resulting in a crowded and overlapped appearance. (**d**) Invasive adenocarcinoma. Dysplastic tumor cells grow into alveolar spaces in clusters

overlapped, or protruding into the cavity. Of note, focal density increment is frequently observed within AIS lesions partly due to pulmonary stromal hyperplasia and/or alveolar shrinkage following extrusion (Fig. 1.6b). In contrast, a significant increase in cell density is a frequent phenomenon in invasive adenocarcinoma. Hyperactive tumor cells are overlapped and congested, with remarkable alveolar extruding and stromal invasion. As a result, the alveolar tension significantly increases (Fig. 1.6c, d).

Thirdly, cautiously observe morphological features of tumor cells, including the size of tumor cells and the shape of the nuclear, chromatin, and nucleoli. If the size of tumor cells is larger than normal columnar epithelial cells, invasive adenocarcinoma is suggested (Fig. 1.7a, b). Peg cells of AIS have dark-stained nucleoli and often protrude into alveolar space. Intranuclear inclusions are commonly seen, but mitosis rarely occurs (Fig. 1.7c, d). In invasive adenocarcinoma, the nuclei of tumor cells are large and hypochromatic, and visible nucleoli or the nuclear chromatin is coarse (Fig. 1.7e).

Fourthly, pay close attention to the relationship between tumor cells and stroma. It is mandatory to discriminate the phenomenon of pseudo-infiltration and invasion (Fig. 1.8a). The pseudo-infiltration is due to reduced proliferative activity of tumor cells which causes insufficient tumor cells along the alveolar walls. As a result, the tension of involved alveolar walls is compromised. In fibrotic tissue hyperplasia, the alveolar septa are compressed. Distinguishing pseudo-infiltration from invasion is difficult. Two points may be helpful and should be kept in mind in such circumstance: (1) there exist desmoplastic changes within the tumor (Fig. 1.8b); (2) tumor cell morphology should be carefully examined. As seen in peg cells of AIS, the nuclei of alveolar epithelial cells with pseudo-infiltration are often dark-stained and have no mitotic figures (Fig. 1.8c). However, cells within the invasive areas have larger and vesicular nuclei, and coarse chromatin and nucleoli may be seen (Fig. 1.8d).

In the 2011 classification, AIS does not contain any papillary growth pattern, which means that once a papillary pattern is observed within a neoplastic lesion, AIS should be excluded and papillary adenocarcinoma is indicated. Unfortunately, the classification failed to give detailed clues for distinguishing the papillary pattern from the lepidic pattern commonly seen in AIS.

In the circumstance of intraoperative pathological diagnosis of AIS, we have established several rules in our department.

1. Since AIS has various morphological manifestations and it is not easy to identify whether the tumor invades stromal tissues based on frozen sections and then is very challenging to distinguish AIS from MIA or acinar adenocarcinoma, we do not recommend the use of the term AIS in most intraoperative pathological consultation. The pathologists with limited experience are advised to make a descriptive diagnosis with two options: alveolar and/or bronchial epithelial dysplasia with undefined stromal invasion which needs confirmation on the paraffin sections or adenocarcinoma with lepidic pattern and invasion which need to be confirmed on the paraffin sections. AIS may be diagnosed on frozen sections, unless the lesion appears as a pure ground-glass nodule in CT imaging.

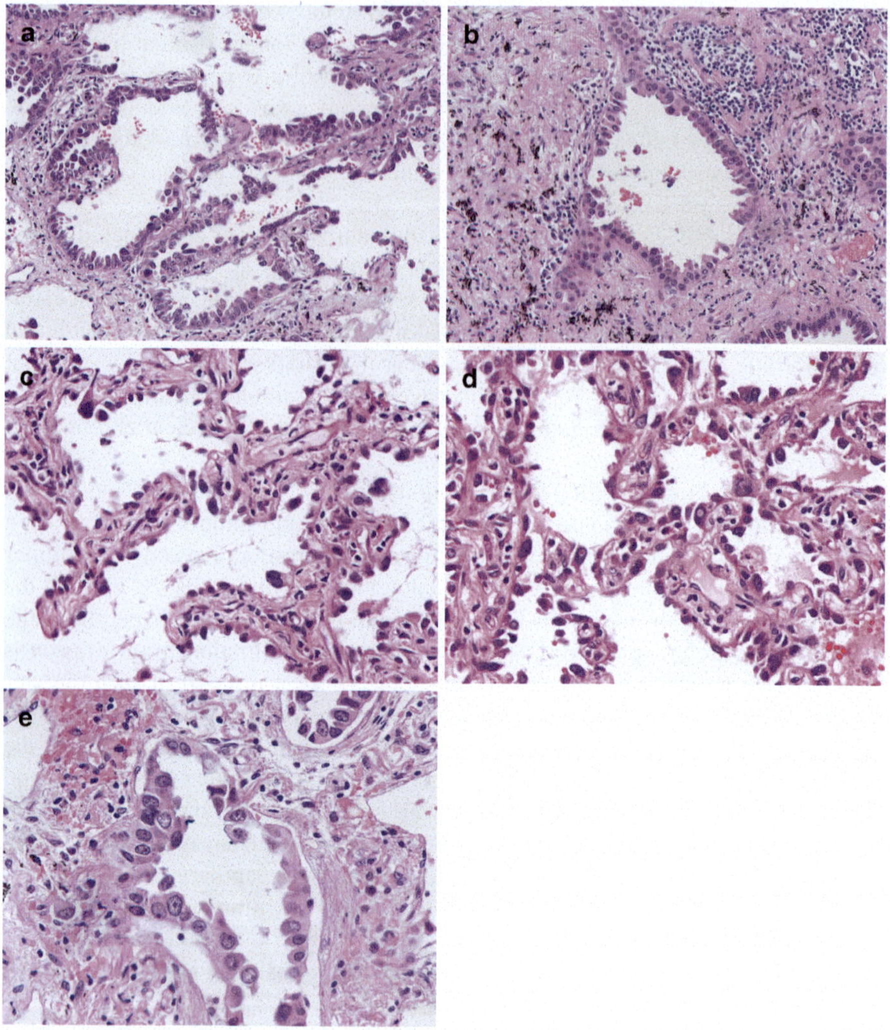

Fig. 1.7 The morphology of tumor cells. (**a**) Invasive adenocarcinoma. Tumor cells are crowded, clustered, or piled. (**b**) Invasive adenocarcinoma. The size of tumor cells is larger than normal columnar epithelium of bronchioles. (**c**) AIS. The tumor has moderate cell density and dark-stained nucleus. (**d**) AIS. Intranuclear inclusions can be frequently observed. (**e**) Invasive adenocarcinoma. Tumor cells have big nucleus, and the nuclei are vesicular with prominent nucleoli

2. The main tumor tissues should be reserved for paraffin-embedded sections to avoid the dilemma that the diagnosis from frozen sections is equivocal, but insufficient tissue is left for formalin-fixed and paraffin-embedded (FFPE) protocol.
3. Minimally invasive lesions could be found around fibrous scars if the tumor has developed for years.
4. The definitive diagnosis of AIS should be based on sufficient sampling and serial sections to exclude any potential invasive lesion (preferably in combination with CT

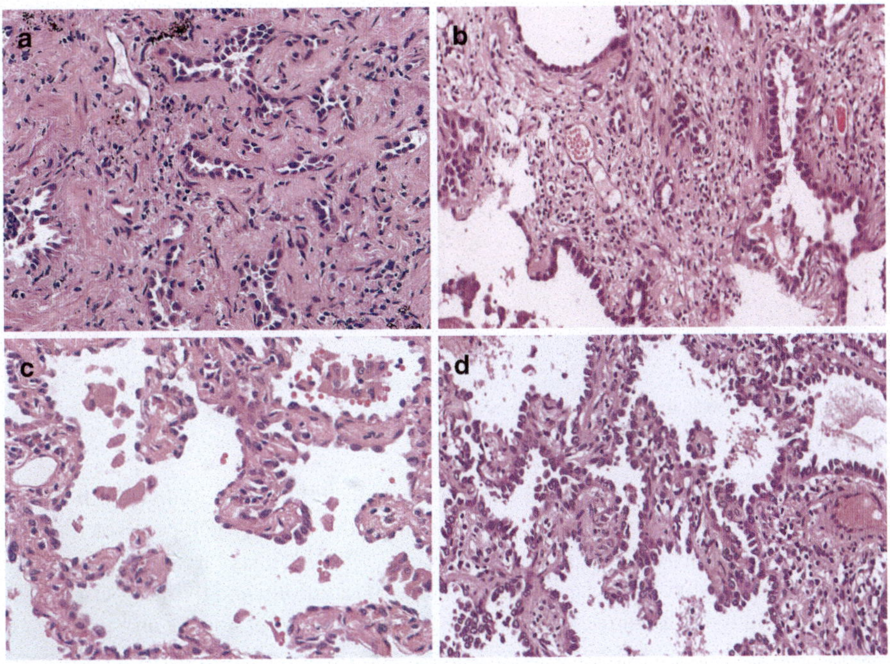

Fig. 1.8 Pseudo-infiltration and invasive adenocarcinoma. (**a**) Pseudo-infiltration. Tumor cells are compressed due to the interstitial and alveolar fibrosis. (**b**) Invasive adenocarcinoma. Neoplastic glands expand and invade alveolar interstitium. (**c**) AIS. Papillary alveolar septum hyperplasia and tumor cells are loosely aligned. (**d**) Papillary adenocarcinoma. Tumor cells are overlapped with a dysplastic nucleus

imaging). Tumor heterogeneity is seen in most AIS diseases. Fibrotic scars with varying size accumulate during the development and evolution of tumors due to the alveolar atrophy and/or organization of alveolar septa. If fibrotic changes are positive on frozen sections but negative on FFPE sections, double check of frozen sections with reference of CT imaging of the lesions is required (Fig. 1.9a, b) [3].

In the diagnosis of MIA, two key points merit emphasis among the diagnostic criteria: (1) the presence of invasion to lymphatics, blood vessels, and/or pleura or tumor necrosis favors invasive adenocarcinoma rather than MIA; (2) the invasive area in MIA is no more than 5 mm. However, if the majority of a tumor is occupied with an invasive component, invasive adenocarcinoma should be diagnosed, regardless of the size of the invasive area. Some small-sized micropapillary invasive adenocarcinomas have aggressive biological behavior and are prone to distant metastasis, which is uncommon in MIA.

LPA is exclusively used for non-mucinous invasive adenocarcinoma with predominantly lepidic growth. But MIA may be either mucinous or non-mucinous. Furthermore, the lepidic pattern may be seen in intrapulmonary metastatic tumors which should be distinguished from primary lung cancer. The lepidic pattern should be recognized as a part of invasive adenocarcinoma if it is not predominant.

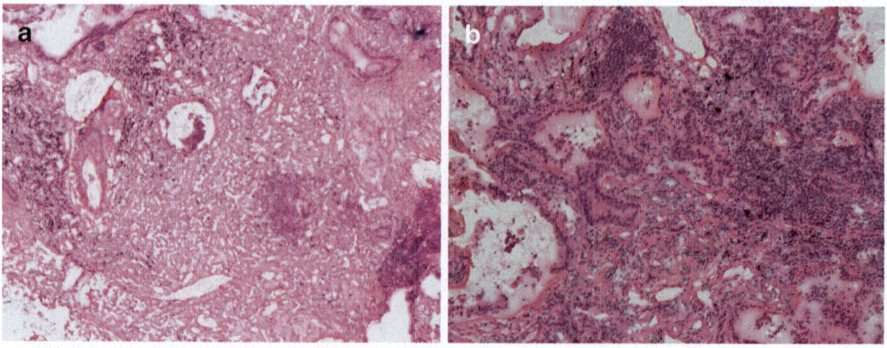

Fig. 1.9 The heterogeneity in AIS. (**a**) Initial examination of frozen sections showed only fibrous scar and residual bronchioles. (**b**) A repeated sampling of frozen sections revealed tumor cells around the fibrous scar

The 2011 classification is established by multidisciplinary specialists, indicating that pathologists should analyze tumors with multidisciplinary perspectives to generate a comprehensive and precise diagnosis. Pathologists are advised to be interactive with their colleagues in departments of radiology and thoracic surgery to understand imaging features of GGO, pGGO, mGGO, solid nodule and part-solid nodule, etc. and related clinical significance. The radiological imaging could provide a full view of the nodular disease, including anatomical location, size, density, and relationship to adjacent tissues. This information is valuable in guiding pathologists to sample tumor specimens as well as assisting pathologists to differentiate different diseases, such as AAH, AIS, and MIA. In conclusion, the 2011 classification of lung adenocarcinoma reflects multidisciplinary consensus with more clinical relevance in prognosis than any previous classification systems.

1.4 Advances in Molecular Biology of Micronodular Lung Cancer

The tumorigenesis and development of lung cancer are a complicated process, in which multiple genes and multistep progression are involved. The key event of tumorigenesis is nonfatal DNA damage caused by a variety of environmental and genetic carcinogenic factors in a synergistic or sequential manner. It has been reported that activation of oncogenes, inactivation of tumor suppressor genes, molecular alterations in genes associated with DNA repair and apoptosis regulation, as well as abnormal regulation of transcription of microRNA may result in aberrant gene expression level, thus promoting the malignant transition of healthy cells. Over the years, genomics and molecular biology have been developed at a remarkable pace, preliminarily shedding light on the etiology of lung cancer and related underlying molecular mechanisms. More than 20,000 mutations have been identified in the genomes of lung adenocarcinoma patients. Despite efforts to identify predictive markers of malignant transformation from early lung neoplasm to advanced lung cancer, genetic and molecular alterations behind such malignant transformation remain poorly understood. A considerable proportion of patients with incidentally detected early-stage lung cancers via low-dose CT lung cancer screening program or annual healthcare examination have no specific clinical symptoms. On the other hand, a limited amount of tumor sample limits complicated analysis (such as genome sequencing for gene mutations) beyond routine histological and/or immunohistochemical examination [4].

AAH has been regarded as the first histological step in a morphologic continuum culminating in the malignant adenocarcinoma, while AIS is the second preinvasive lesion, representing the stage between AAH and invasive adenocarcinoma. This section briefly reviewed potential driver genes related to the early progression of lung adenocarcinoma.

1.4.1 Epidermal Growth Factor Receptor Family

The epidermal growth factor receptor (EGFR, also designated ErbB) family contains four members, HER1 (erbB1, EGFR), HER2 (erbB2, NEU), HER3 (erbB3), and HER4 (erbB4). Each ErbB receptor consists of an extracellular ligand-binding region, a single transmembrane domain, and an intracellular tyrosine kinase domain. Upon binding with its epidermal growth factor (EGF) ligand, EGFR undergoes dimerization and its tyrosine kinase activity is activated by the autophosphorylation of tyrosine kinase domain. The activation of EGFR will further initiate several signal transduction cascades, such as PI3K/AKT/mTOR, ras/raf/MAPK, and JAK/STAT, and transmit extracellular signals into cell nucleus. EGFR has been proven as one of the driver genes in the tumorigenesis of lung cancer, and the genetic alterations could be mutations or amplifications, which more frequently occurred in lung adenocarcinoma. Also, growing body of evidence supports that EGFR gene mutations are early events in the development of lung adenocarcinoma. Asian patients with AAH are reported to have a variable incidence of EGFR gene mutations, ranging from 3 to 44%, higher than Caucasians. Additionally, in cases of bronchioloalveolar carcinoma (BAC, partly replaced by AIS in the 2011 classification), EGFR mutation varies from 10.8 to 85.7%, indicating that activation of EGFR may play a contributing role in the early developmental process of lung adenocarcinoma by conferring cancer cells with capabilities of anti-apoptosis and persistent proliferation.

Utilizing targeted next-generation sequencing (NGS) on multifocal AAHs, AISs, and MIAs, researchers have observed various genetic drivers within the same tumor, indicating that clonal expansion could be one of the early biological events in tumorigenesis. Moreover, EGFR, KRAS, and TP53 mutations have been identified as indicators of malignant transition.

1.4.2 Ras

The Ras (rat sarcoma) oncogene family consists of three genes, H-ras, N-ras, and K-ras, which are located on chromosome 1, 11, and 12, respectively. K-ras encodes a 21 kDa protein (p21). Typically, upon activation of EGFR signaling pathway, wild-type Ras protein is bound to GDP to form Ras-GDP complex in an inactive state. Once stimulated by upstream signal and guanine nucleotide exchange factor (GEF), GDP will be replaced by GTP to form active Ras-GTP complex which activates downstream signaling pathway, subsequently promoting cell proliferation through the Ras-dependent kinase cascade. The activation state of Ras is regulated by GTPase-activating protein (GAP). Upon the regulation of GAP, GTP in GTP-Ras complex is hydrolyzed to GDP, which turns the complex back to its inactive Ras-GDP complex. Oncogenic mutants of Ras have impaired intrinsic GTP activities due to loss sensitivity to GAP regulation, resulting in a persistently active Ras-GTP state and ultimately malignant biological behaviors such as hyperproliferation and tumorigenesis. Moreover, Ras could activate PI3K/AKT/mTOR signaling pathway, which is associated with cell proliferation, growth, differentiation, adhesion, and migration.

Point mutation is one of the major genetic events during the activation of Ras gene. H-ras and N-ras mutations are sporadic in lung cancer, while K-ras mutations are reported to be present in 25–40% of lung adenocarcinoma patients, with mutations dominantly occurring in codons 12 and 13 of exon 2 and codon 61 of exon 3. K-ras mutations are more prevalent in Caucasians, males, and smokers than Asians, females, and nonsmokers. In a study, K-ras mutation was found in 39% of AAHs, 42% of adenocarcinomas, and none in non-adenocarcinomas, suggesting that similar to EGFR mutations, K-ras mutation has functional roles in the initiating stage of lung carcinogenesis. This has been further confirmed by recent NGS studies of AAH, AIS, and MIA.

1.4.3 p53

p53, an important tumor suppressor gene located on chromosome 17p13, encodes a nucleophosmin of 53 KD, which plays a critical role in maintenance of genome stability. As well known, G1/S is an important cell cycle checkpoint, and the cell cycle arrest caused by DNA damages at G1/S is p53 dependent. In the physiological state, p53 protein remains at a constant but low level that has limited impacts on cell survival. The activation of p53 mediated by DNA damages stimulates transcription activity of multiple genes, including P21, Mdm2, and Bax. P21 is one of the cyclin-dependent kinase inhibitors that inhibit CDK activity and cell cycling and prevent damaged DNA from replication. Mdm2 can negatively regulate p53 by binding to p53 protein and inhibiting its transcription factor activity as well as facilitating the ubiquitination and resultant degradation of p53. Overexpression of Mdm2 may be another underlying mechanism behind uncontrolled cell growth in addition to p53 mutation. When cells are severely damaged, p53 will activate a number of apoptosis-related genes (such as Bax, Fas, and relevant genes in oxidative stress pathway) to induce cell death.

p53 is one of the most commonly mutated genes in lung cancer. The missense mutation of p53 leads to a conformational change in the DNA-binding domain and inhibits its activity. The analysis of p53 in 65 lesions of AAH, early BAC, and overt BAC showed that the expression level of p53 protein positively correlated with differentiation grade of tumor cells, suggesting that p53 protein expression has certain roles in the progression of BAC. In another study, 4 (8%) of 50 micronodular lung adenocarcinomas (less than 1 cm in diameter) harbored p53 mutations. The incidence of p53 gene mutation in very early stage of lung adenocarcinoma has been reported to be in a range of 6–36%. And the incidence increases with diseases advancing, indicating that mutation or overexpression of p53 may be involved in not only the tumorigenesis but also the maintenance and development of lung adenocarcinoma.

1.4.4 Rb

Retinoblastoma (Rb), the first tumor suppressor gene described in lung cancer, belongs to the cell cycle regulation factor family. As an essential protein in p16INK4a-cyclin D1-CDK4-Rb signaling pathway, Rb inhibits gene transcription involved in G1/S transition by binding with members of E2F transcription factor family to arrest cell cycle in G1 phase. Genetic alterations in cyclin D1, CDK4, and cell cycle-dependent kinase inhibitor P16 (CDKN2A) cause inactivation of p16INK4a-cyclin D1-CDK4-Rb signaling pathway, which is an early event in the tumorigenesis and development of lung cancer. In 50% of AAH and 70% of AIS, the expression of Rb was detected via immunohistochemistry (IHC). p16INK4a could be activated by homozygous deletion, methylation, and gene mutation. Gene amplification or other mechanisms can upregulate expression of cyclin D1 in AAH at a higher amplitude than in BAC and invasive adenocarcinoma.

1.4.5 Anaplastic Lymphoma Kinase

Anaplastic lymphoma kinase (ALK) was first identified in anaplastic large-cell lymphoma (ALCL). Rearrangements of ALK occur in a subset of lung cancers and result in echinoderm microtubule-associated protein-like 4-ALK (EML4-ALK) fusion gene, commonly due to an inversion in chromosome 2p with intron 13 of

EML4 fused to intron 19 of ALK (ALK [inv (2) (p21; p23)]). Variants of EML4-ALK fusions are identified based on the length of EML4, in which exons 1–13 of EML4 joining to exons 20–29 of ALK are most commonly observed. Continuous activation of EML4-ALK kinase leads to increased cell proliferation and inhibition of apoptosis due to activation of signaling pathways such as PI3K/AKT, JAK3/STAT3, and RAS/RAF/MAPK1.

ALK rearrangements occur in approximately 4% of unselected NSCLC patients with a predominance in younger and nonsmoking patients with adenocarcinomas. Unlike EGFR or p53, ALK is less likely to be detected in AAH and AIS, suggesting that ALK could be a biomarker of advanced lung cancer instead of early-stage diseases.

1.4.6 ROS1

Proto-oncogene tyrosine-protein kinase (ROS1), which encodes a transmembrane tyrosine kinase receptor, is located on chromosome 6p22. Unfortunately, very little is currently known about the roles of wild-type ROS1, and ligands of this receptor have not yet been identified. ROS1 shares high sequence homology with insulin receptor family and the kinase domain of ALK. The primary activation mechanism of ROS1 is chromosomal rearrangement, and the fusion partners of ROS1 contain FIG, KDELR2, TPM3, SDC4, LRIG3, EZR, SLC34A2, and CD74. However, the carcinogenic mechanism of these fusion proteins is still unknown. The downstream signaling cascades include PI3K/AKT/mTOR, STAT3, and RAS/MAPK/ERK.

ROS1 rearrangements are recognized in various cancers, including lung cancer, malignant glioma, bile duct carcinoma, and gastric carcinoma. The incidence in NSCLC patients is estimated to be 1–2%. Similar to ALK rearrangements, ROS1 rearrangements are more frequent in young, never-smoking Asian patients with lung adenocarcinoma. In a study of 1139 lung adenocarcinoma patients in China, fusion gene detection was performed. No ROS fusion was found in AIS and MIA diseases, indicating that ROS1 rearrangement is not an initiating molecular event but more likely involved in the progression of advanced lung adenocarcinoma.

1.4.7 RET

Located on chromosome 10q11.2, RET encodes a transmembrane tyrosine kinase receptor responsible for the migration and differentiation of neural crest-derived neuroblasts. It has been demonstrated that genetic alterations in RET gene are critical for thyroid papillary carcinoma and medullary thyroid carcinoma. RET rearrangements have been found in some patients with lung cancer, with exons 12–20 of the functional kinase domain fused with kinesin family 5B (KIF5B) gene. KIF5B-RET fusions are mutually exclusive of other driver mutations such as EGFR, KRAS, and ALK and have been found in 1–2% of lung adenocarcinoma patients by massively parallel signature sequencing (MPSS). In a large-scale screening study of 1139 lung adenocarcinoma patients, RET fusions were not found in either AIS or MIA, suggesting it is a late event during lung adenocarcinoma development.

Multiple molecules interact and form a complicated network in cells. The tumorigenesis and development of lung cancer are the results of multiple gene mutations. Loss-of-function mutations in one gene may lead to mutations of another gene, thus generating different subclones within tumors. Some of the subclonal cell population inherits the ability of invasion, thus promoting tumor progression. Genetic alterations with fundamental roles in the early development of lung adenocarcinoma are not yet fully understood. Thus more studies are needed. The development and utilization of second and third generation of sequencing technology would facilitate the understanding of the underlying molecular mechanism in early-stage lung cancer.

1.5 CT-Guided Fine-Needle Localization of Subcentimeter Nodules in Re-Aerated Lung Specimens

1.5.1 The Background for Development of CT-Guided Fine-Needle Localization of Subcentimeter Nodules in Resected and Re-Aerated Lung Specimens

In 2011, the International Association for the Study of Lung Cancer, the American Thoracic Society, and the European Respiratory Society proposed a new classification for lung adenocarcinomas. The new classification system fully affirmed the role of preoperative computed tomography (CT) examinations in the diagnosis of early-stage lung cancer. The data provided by studies using the new classification system indicate that patients with adenocarcinoma in situ (AIS) and minimally invasive adenocarcinoma (MIA) are expected to have 100% or nearly 100% disease-specific survival following complete resections. With the rapid development of multidetector spiral CT (MDCT) and video-assisted thoracoscopic surgery (VATS), not only small pulmonary nodules can be detected clearly, but also more and more patients with small nodules that are highly suspicious of lung cancer can be cured with minimally invasive surgery. Atypical adenomatous hyperplasia (AAH), AIS, and MIA often present as pure ground-glass nodules (pGGNs) or mixed ground-glass nodules (mGGNs) containing small amounts of solid elements on CT images; the diameter of such nodules is often less than 10 mm, and early intervention can improve the prognosis of patients with these lesions. However, due to the small size and low density, many of small nodules (especially those micronodules less than 10 mm) can be extremely difficult to be accurately positioned during surgery and in surgically resected specimens, posing a severe challenge to both thoracic surgeons and pathologists.

In addition, it is much more challenging for pathologists to localize all lesions when two or more GGNs are present in the same lobe. Due to biological behavioral heterogeneity, different lesions may be at different developmental stages even in the same lobe. For instance, some lesions may be IAC, but others may remain in earlier stages of MIA, AIS, and/or AAH. Behavioral heterogeneity could be the consequence of genetic heterogeneity. And numerous studies have reported that lung cancer is highly heterogeneous in comparison to other malignancies. Therefore, pathological examination of a single nodular lesion may not adequately represent the rest of nodules particularly in the circumstance of synchronous multiple primary lung cancers (SMPLC), which requests conducting pathological examinations on each suspicious lesion.

For precise localization and pathological examination of every single nodule suspicious of malignancy in CT imaging, we developed the methodology of CT-guided fine-needle localization of ground-glass nodules in re-aerated lung specimens [5]. As pulmonary tissues with nodule(s) are removed from the lungs, the whole bunch of specimens are much like a soft tissue without gas, and the natural air-soft tissue contrast between lung tissues and the lesions reduces or even disappeared, causing difficulty in finding lesions especially those pure ground-glass nodules. Restoring the natural contrast by re-aerating resected specimens could solve the problem, at least partly.

1.5.2 *The Procedure of CT-Guided Fine-Needle Localization of Ground-Glass Nodules in Re-Aerated Lung Specimens*

Surgical specimens are sent to the CT examination room immediately after resection, without washing, fixation, or incision. An inflatable aerator is used to inflate the lung specimens. The air outlet of an electric pump is connected to a rubber tube, and the end of the rubber tube is connected to a clinical infusion needle. The needle is inserted into the bronchi of the resected specimens, and the specimen is aerated after ensuring that no leak is detected. There are metal clips for sealing the notch in the specimens resected by VATS. As well re-aerated, the specimens are placed on the examination couch with position adjustment to match its in vivo shape in the chest according to the metal clips and marks by thoracic surgeons. Then a low-dose CT scan is performed on the well-aerated specimens. Images are real-time reviewed to identify nodules. As nodules are localized, fine needles are inserted by nodules with reference to CT positioning laser lines as does CT-guided biopsy. If nodules are not found in CT images due to inadequate contrast, the specimens should be scanned again after inflation with more air; this process should be repeated until nodular lesions are detected. Once an accurate location of a lesion is obtained in the specimen, with reference to preoperative CT images, a fine needle is inserted by the lesion to mark its location. As soon as all nodular lesions are localized with CT guidance, the specimens are delivered to the pathology department with the fine needle left in place (Fig. 1.10).

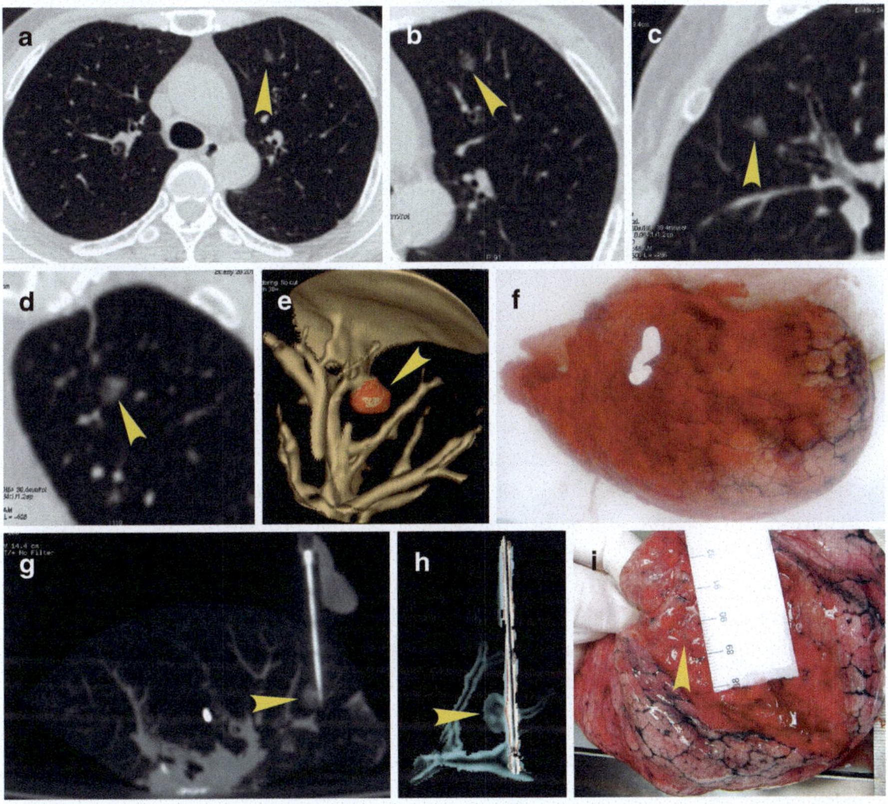

Fig. 1.10 CT-guided fine-needle localization of ground-glass nodules in re-aerated lung specimens. (**a–e**) CT image shows a mixed ground-glass nodule in the left upper lobe (arrowhead), and a fine vessel passed through the nodule. Preoperative CT examination diagnosis of the nodule was AIS. Left upper lobectomy was performed to remove the nodule. Since the lesion was very small, surgical specimens were sent to CT examination room for re-localization. The specimen was re-aerated to restore its physiological shape. As the specimen was well re-aerated (**f**), CT scanning was performed. When the nodular lesion was identified in CT images, the fine needle was inserted to mark its position (arrowhead, **g**). Three-dimensional reformatted image confirmed the relationship between the needle and the nodule (arrowhead, **h**). Then, the specimen was delivered to pathology department for sampling (arrowhead, **i**)

1.5.3 *Discussion Related to CT-Guided Localization of Pulmonary Nodules Ex Vivo*

With increasing application of low-dose CT for lung cancer screening, incidentally detected ground-glass nodules in otherwise healthy patients grow faster in amount and get smaller in size. The percentage of malignant lesions in persistent GGNs is higher than in solid nodules. Both AIS and AAH lesions are classified as preinvasive lesions in the 2011 classification with favorable 5-year survival. AIS and MIA lesions are generally very small and often appear as ground-glass opacities on CT images, which could possibly be omitted in conventional chest radiography. With the development of MDCT technologies and understanding of the characteristics of early-stage lung cancer, the accurate preoperative diagnosis rate for these small lung lesions is continually improving. Furthermore, the risk of surgical resection has been reduced with advances in surgical techniques, especially VATS. However, due to a small volume and low density, many of these lesions can be extremely difficult to be accurately positioned during surgery and in resected specimens.

Preoperative localization techniques allow a surgeon to locate focal lesions quickly and accurately during the operation and reduce potential intraoperative injuries. Preoperative CT-guided hook-wire positioning is one of these techniques. However, this technique has several drawbacks:

1. Preoperative CT-guided percutaneous fine-needle puncture can be traumatic and may cause complications, including hemorrhage, pneumothorax, hemothorax, and tumor spreading or implantation.
2. The positions of the hooks in pulmonary tissues could change, affecting the accuracy of resection and sampling of the specimens following the operation.
3. When lung nodules suspicious of malignancy are particularly small in size (e.g., less than 10 mm) or low in density, it can be extremely difficult for pathologists to accurately identify the location of the lesions in postoperative specimens, which may require sectioning and microscopic examination of the entire portion of resected pulmonary tissues where the lesion may exist.

Indeed, the rapid and accurate localization of lesions can dramatically shorten the anesthesia time, and the accurate localization of lesions facilitates accurate histopathologic diagnosis.

In contrast to preoperative localization, CT-guided localization of pulmonary nodules using re-aerated resected specimens is an ex vivo procedure, allowing for better access and higher-quality CT images. This highly accurate method of lesion positioning technique also allows efficient fine-needle localization of surgical specimens and avoids excessive damage to patients. In addition, it is suitable for resected specimens from thoracotomy and thoracoscopic surgeries. This procedure is highly dependent on the airway integrity of the surgical specimens, requiring thoracic surgeons to protect specimens as much as possible. In case of wedge resections, the surgical incision should be stitched carefully; if leaks are observed during the inflation process, these must be immediately repaired to avoid inflation failure. As the surgical specimens are kept under constant, moderate mechanical aeration during CT scanning, air leakage may be avoided.

In conclusion, CT-guided localization of lesions in surgical specimens using fine needles under constant, moderate mechanical aeration allows for rapid and accurate localization of lesions, thereby decreasing the occurrence of complications in patients if receiving preoperative localization procedures. It is particularly useful for localization and accuracy diagnosis of small ground-glass pulmonary nodules and multiple nodules in the resected pulmonary tissues.

References

1. Noguchi M, Morikawa A, Kawasaki M, Matsuno Y, Yamada T, Hirohashi S, Kondo H, Shimosato Y. Small adenocarcinoma of the lung. Histologic characteristics and prognosis. Cancer. 1995;75(12):2844–52.
2. Travis WD, Brambilla E, Noguchi M, Nicholson AG, Geisinger KR, Yatabe Y, Beer DG, Powell CA, Riely GJ, Van Schil PE, Garg K, Austin JH, Asamura H, Rusch VW, Hirsch FR, Scagliotti G, Mitsudomi T, Huber RM, Ishikawa Y, Jett J, Sanchez-Cespedes M, Sculier JP, Takahashi T, Tsuboi M, Vansteenkiste J, Wistuba I, Yang PC, Aberle D, Brambilla C, Flieder D, Franklin W, Gazdar A, Gould M, Hasleton P, Henderson D, Johnson B, Johnson D, Kerr K, Kuriyama K, Lee JS, Miller VA, Petersen I, Roggli V, Rosell R, Saijo N, Thunnissen E, Tsao M, Yankelewitz D. International association for the study of lung cancer/American thoracic society/European respiratory society international multidisciplinary classification of lung adenocarcinoma. J Thorac Oncol. 2011;6(2):244–85. https://doi.org/10.1097/JTO.0b013e318206a221.
3. He P, Yao G, Guan Y, Lin Y, He J. Diagnosis of lung adenocarcinoma in situ and minimally invasive adenocarcinoma from intraoperative frozen sections: an analysis of 136 cases. J Clin Pathol. 2016;69(12):1076–80. https://doi.org/10.1136/jclinpath-2016-203619.
4. The Cancer Genome Atlas Research Network. Comprehensive molecular profiling of lung adenocarcinoma. Nature. 2014;511(7511):543–50. https://doi.org/10.1038/nature13385.
5. Li M, Shen G, Gao F, Zheng X, Hua Y, Xiao L. CT-guided fine-needle localization of ground-glass nodules in re-aerated lung specimens: localization of solitary small nodules or multiple nodules within the same lobe. Diagn Interv Radiol. 2015;21(5):391–6. https://doi.org/10.5152/dir.2015.14516.

Suggested Readings

1. Bueno R, Hughes E, Wagner S, Gutin AS, Lanchbury JS, Zheng Y, Archer MA, Gustafson C, Jones JT, Rushton K, Saam J, Kim E, Barberis M, Wistuba I, Wenstrup RJ, Wallace WA, Hartman AR, Harrison DJ. Validation of a molecular and pathological model for five-year mortality risk in patients with early stage lung adenocarcinoma. J Thorac Oncol. 2015;10(1):67–73. https://doi.org/10.1097/jto.0000000000000365.
2. Burotto M, Thomas A, Subramaniam D, Giaccone G, Rajan A. Biomarkers in early-stage non-small-cell lung cancer: current concepts and future directions. J Thorac Oncol. 2014;9(11):1609–17. https://doi.org/10.1097/jto.0000000000000302.
3. Clement-Duchene C, Alla F, Gauchotte G, Marie B, Carnin C, Menard O, Vignaud JM, Martinet Y. Is there a relationship between the presence of lung mucosa preinvasive lesions and lung cancer incidence? Influence of tobacco consumption. Lung Cancer. 2014;84(2):134–8. https://doi.org/10.1016/j.lungcan.2014.02.003.

4. Cooper WA, Lam DC, O'Toole SA, Minna JD. Molecular biology of lung cancer. J Thorac Dis. 2013;5(Suppl 5):S479–90. https://doi.org/10.3978/j.issn.2072-1439.2013.08.03.
5. Eguchi T, Kadota K, Park BJ, Travis WD, Jones DR, Adusumilli PS. The new IASLC-ATS-ERS lung adenocarcinoma classification: what the surgeon should know. Semin Thorac Cardiovasc Surg. 2014;26(3):210–22. https://doi.org/10.1053/j.semtcvs.2014.09.002.
6. Gu B, Burt BM, Merritt RE, Stephanie S, Nair V, Hoang CD, Shrager JB. A dominant adenocarcinoma with multifocal ground glass lesions does not behave as advanced disease. Ann Thorac Surg. 2013;96(2):411–8. https://doi.org/10.1016/j.athoracsur.2013.04.048.
7. Henschke CI, Yankelevitz DF, Mirtcheva R, McGuinness G, McCauley D, Miettinen OS. CT screening for lung cancer: frequency and significance of part-solid and nonsolid nodules. AJR Am J Roentgenol. 2002;178(5):1053–7. https://doi.org/10.2214/ajr.178.5.1781053.
8. Izumchenko E, Chang X, Brait M, Fertig E, Kagohara LT, Bedi A, Marchionni L, Agrawal N, Ravi R, Jones S, Hoque MO, Westra WH, Sidransky D. Targeted sequencing reveals clonal genetic changes in the progression of early lung neoplasms and paired circulating DNA. Nat Commun. 2015;6:8258. https://doi.org/10.1038/ncomms9258.
9. Kadota K, Sima CS, Arcila ME, Hedvat C, Kris MG, Jones DR, Adusumilli PS, Travis WD. KRAS mutation is a significant prognostic factor in early-stage lung adenocarcinoma. Am J Surg Pathol. 2016;40(12):1579–90. https://doi.org/10.1097/pas.0000000000000744.
10. Kobayashi Y, Mitsudomi T, Sakao Y, Yatabe Y. Genetic features of pulmonary adenocarcinoma presenting with ground-glass nodules: the differences between nodules with and without growth. Ann Oncol. 2015;26(1):156–61. https://doi.org/10.1093/annonc/mdu505.
11. Lee NK, Park CM, Kang CH, Jeon YK, Choo JY, Lee HJ, Goo JM. CT-guided percutaneous transthoracic localization of pulmonary nodules prior to video-assisted thoracoscopic surgery using barium suspension. Korean J Radiol. 2012;13(6):694–701. https://doi.org/10.3348/kjr.2012.13.6.694.
12. Lee SM, Park CM, Goo JM, Lee HJ, Wi JY, Kang CH. Invasive pulmonary adenocarcinomas versus preinvasive lesions appearing as ground-glass nodules: differentiation by using CT features. Radiology. 2013;268(1):265–73. https://doi.org/10.1148/radiol.13120949.
13. Li W, Wang Y, He X, Li G, Wang S, Xu L, Yuan Z. Combination of CT-guided hookwire localization and video-assisted thoracoscopic surgery for pulmonary nodular lesions: analysis of 103 patients. Oncol Lett. 2012;4(4):824–8. https://doi.org/10.3892/ol.2012.800.
14. Morales-Oyarvide V, Mino-Kenudson M. Tumor islands and spread through air spaces: distinct patterns of invasion in lung adenocarcinoma. Pathol Int. 2016;66(1):1–7. https://doi.org/10.1111/pin.12368.
15. Pan Y, Zhang Y, Li Y, Hu H, Wang L, Li H, Wang R, Ye T, Luo X, Zhang Y, Li B, Cai D, Shen L, Sun Y, Chen H. ALK, ROS1 and RET fusions in 1139 lung adenocarcinomas: a comprehensive study of common and fusion pattern-specific clinicopathologic, histologic and cytologic features. Lung Cancer. 2014;84(2):121–6. https://doi.org/10.1016/j.lungcan.2014.02.007.
16. Trejo Bittar HE, Incharoen P, Althouse AD, Dacic S. Accuracy of the IASLC/ATS/ERS histological subtyping of stage I lung adenocarcinoma on intraoperative frozen sections. Mod Pathol. 2015;28(8):1058–63. https://doi.org/10.1038/modpathol.2015.71.
17. Weichert W, Warth A. Early lung cancer with lepidic pattern: adenocarcinoma in situ, minimally invasive adenocarcinoma, and lepidic predominant adenocarcinoma. Curr Opin Pulm Med. 2014;20(4):309–16. https://doi.org/10.1097/mcp.0000000000000065.
18. Yeh YC, Kadota K, Nitadori J, Sima CS, Rizk NP, Jones DR, Travis WD, Adusumilli PS. International Association for the Study of Lung Cancer/American Thoracic Society/European Respiratory Society classification predicts occult lymph node metastasis in clinically mediastinal node-negative lung adenocarcinoma. Eur J Cardiothorac Surg. 2016;49(1):e9–e15. https://doi.org/10.1093/ejcts/ezv316.
19. Yoshizawa A, Motoi N, Riely GJ, Sima CS, Gerald WL, Kris MG, Park BJ, Rusch VW, Travis WD. Impact of proposed IASLC/ATS/ERS classification of lung adenocarcinoma: prognostic subgroups and implications for further revision of staging based on analysis of 514 stage I cases. Mod Pathol. 2011;24(5):653–64. https://doi.org/10.1038/modpathol.2010.232.

20. Yotsukura M, Yasuda H, Shigenobu T, Kaseda K, Masai K, Hayashi Y, Hishida T, Ohtsuka T, Naoki K, Soejima K, Betsuyaku T, Asamura H. Clinical and pathological characteristics of EGFR mutation in operable early-stage lung adenocarcinoma. Lung Cancer. 2017;109:45–51. https://doi.org/10.1016/j.lungcan.2017.04.014.
21. Zhang J, Wu J, Tan Q, Zhu L, Gao W. Why do pathological stage IA lung adenocarcinomas vary from prognosis?: a clinicopathologic study of 176 patients with pathological stage IA lung adenocarcinoma based on the IASLC/ATS/ERS classification. J Thorac Oncol. 2013;8(9):1196–202. https://doi.org/10.1097/JTO.0b013e31829f09a7.
22. Zhao ZR, To KF, Mok TS, Ng CS. Is there significance in identification of non-predominant micropapillary or solid components in early-stage lung adenocarcinoma? Interact Cardiovasc Thorac Surg. 2017;24(1):121–5. https://doi.org/10.1093/icvts/ivw283.
23. Zhao ZR, Xi SY, Li W, Situ DR, Chen KM, Yang H, XD S, Lin YB, Long H. Prognostic impact of pattern-based grading system by the new IASLC/ATS/ERS classification in Asian patients with stage I lung adenocarcinoma. Lung Cancer. 2015;90(3):604–9. https://doi.org/10.1016/j.lungcan.2015.10.026.
24. Zugazagoitia J, Enguita AB, Nunez JA, Iglesias L, Ponce S. The new IASLC/ATS/ERS lung adenocarcinoma classification from a clinical perspective: current concepts and future prospects. J Thorac Dis. 2014;6(Suppl 5):S526–36. https://doi.org/10.3978/j.issn.2072-1439.2014.01.27.

Chapter 2
Practical Reviews on the Anatomy of the Chest

Guozhen Zhang and Xiangpeng Zheng

2.1 Normal Anatomy of the Lung

2.1.1 Pulmonary Alveolus

The intrapulmonary bronchi divide and subdivide throughout the entire organ, constituting the bronchial trees. Each of the smallest subdivisions distally connects a pulmonary lobule (i.e., secondary pulmonary lobule), known as lobular bronchiole with a diameter of less than 1.0 mm. After entering the lobule, the lobular bronchiole continuously divides into respiratory bronchioles, about 0.5 mm in diameter, and finally reaches the terminals of the bronchial trees, composed of alveolar ducts and bulging sacs, and pulmonary alveoli.

Several alveoli converge into a single chamber, the alveolar sac. Each alveolus is surrounded by a blood capillary network, where gaseous exchanges take place, oxygen diffusing from the alveolar lumen into the capillary and carbon dioxide diffusing in the opposite direction crossing the alveolar walls. The pulmonary alveolus is a hollow cavity found in the lung parenchyma, as the terminal of 24-grade bronchial trees and the place of the external respiration. In adults, there are about 300–400 million alveoli. Their average diameter is 0.2 μm, with a total surface area of nearly 100 m^2, which is a few times larger than human skin surface area.

The alveoli arise from the walls of the sacs as diverticula. The alveoli alveolar epithelium comprises two major cell types and related supporting structures.

G. Zhang (✉)
Department of Radiology, Fudan University Huadong Hospital, Shanghai, China
e-mail: cjr.zhangguozhen@vip.163.com

X. Zheng
Department of Radiation Oncology, Fudan University Huadong Hospital, Shanghai, China

X. Zheng et al. (eds.), *Early-stage Lung Cancer*,
https://doi.org/10.1007/978-981-10-7596-4_2

2.1.1.1 Type I Alveolar Cells

The majority of alveolar surface is lined by these cells, which are usually extremely thin (about 0.1 μm), tightly attached to the basement membrane, and lack proliferative capability. The type I cell is a complex branched cell with multiple cytoplasmic plates that are substantially attenuated and relatively devoid of organelles; these plates represent the gas exchange surface in the alveolus. Under electron microscopy, there is a basement membrane below the alveolar epithelium and outside the alveolar capillary endothelium. The air exchange between alveoli and capillaries occurs crossing through at least four layers of structures, i.e., the alveolar epithelium, the epithelial basement membrane, vascular endothelial basement membrane, and endothelial cells. Hence, type I alveolar cells are mainly involved in gas exchange. In interstitial pneumonia, edema and inflammatory cell infiltration may occur in alveolar septa and affect pulmonary ventilation.

2.1.1.2 Type II Alveolar Cells

Type II alveolar cells are cubical or round and protruding into the alveolar cavity, with round nuclei and foamy cytoplasm, located among type I alveolar cells. These cells act as the "caretaker" of the alveolar compartment. They respond to damage of the vulnerable type I cells by dividing and acting as progenitor cells for both type I and type II cells. Alveolar type II cells form 63% of the epithelial lining cells but cover only 3% of the surface area. They have many features in common with highly metabolically active cells: abundant mitochondria, endoplasmic reticulum, polyribosomes, and Golgi apparatus. However, the most characteristic features are the microvilli around the apex and the rich osmiophilic lamellated inclusion bodies in the cytoplasm. These lamellar bodies are the site of storage of surfactant, the protein-lipid mixture that lines the alveolar compartment [1]. Type II cells synthesize, store, and release pulmonary surfactant into the alveolar cavities, where it acts to optimize conditions for gas exchange. The surfactant reduces surface tension at the gas-liquid interface and allows surface tension to vary directly with the radius of the alveolus, to maintain the consecutive gaseous exchange by inspiratory and expiratory movements. Deficiency or degeneration of surfactant caused pulmonary atelectasis. To identify cancer cells, deriving from the type I or II alveolar cells has no clinical significance.

2.1.1.3 Clara Cells

In distal airways, Clara cells are present. These cells are nonciliated without mucus secretion. In human lungs, Clara cells comprise 15–20% of distal airway epithelial cells. Under light microscopy, cells are columnar and dome-like with shallow stained cytoplasm and the apical part protruding into the lumen. The electron microscope shows that there exist numerous secretory granules with low-electron density in the cytoplasm at the top of cells. Clara cells have active proliferation, differentiation, and secretion function, which are involved in the repair process of bronchial epithelial damage. Clara cell secretory protein (CCSP) is the most important secretory product of Clara cells. It has many biological activities, including anti-inflammation, anti-fibrosis, and antitumor invasion which are closely related to various lung diseases. In addition, the CCSP also plays an important physiological role in organ protection, airway epithelial renewal, damage repair, biotransformation of exogenous chemicals, and distal airway fluid balance regulation.

2.1.1.4 Alveolar Macrophage

The alveolar macrophages are derived from blood monocytes and transformed to dust cells after engulfing dust particles. And heart failure cells are the alveolar macrophages containing hemosiderin, the decomposition products of hemoglobin, in patients with heart failure or chronic pulmonary edema.

2.1.1.5 Alveolar Sac, Duct, and Pore

The alveolar sac is a capsule composed of many pulmonary alveoli, connecting with the alveolar ducts, and each branch of alveolar ducts has two to three alveolar sacs. The pulmonary alveoli are communicated with each other by alveolar pores (also known as the pores of Kohn), and the pulmonary alveoli connect with the terminal bronchioles by the canals of Lambert (Fig. 2.1). Typically, one to six alveolar pores are seen in the alveolar wall. With the pulmonary alveoli expanding, these pores could be fully opened as the communication channels for air exchange in adjacent pulmonary alveoli. Moreover, collateral ventilation could be established through the alveolar pores to compensate limited gas exchange when a bronchus or its subdivisions are partly or completely blocked.

2.1.1.6 Alveolar Septa

The thin layer of connective tissues between the adjacent alveoli is known as alveolar septum, which contains abundant capillary networks, elastic fibers, reticular fibers, and collagenous fibers. The reticular fibers, elastic fibers, and a few collagenous fibers compose the framework of alveolar capillaries, and due to the presence of elastic fibers, the alveoli maintain good elasticity. In cases of chronic bronchitis or bronchial asthma, excessive expansion destructs the elastic fibers, and the involved pulmonary alveoli lose the elasticity, resulting in emphysema and impaired pulmonary function. Additionally, alveolar septa contain rich lymphatic vessels and nerve fibers. As the capillary permeability increases from various reasons, such as chemical toxins, plasma components will seep into the connective tissues, resulting in pulmonary interstitial edema.

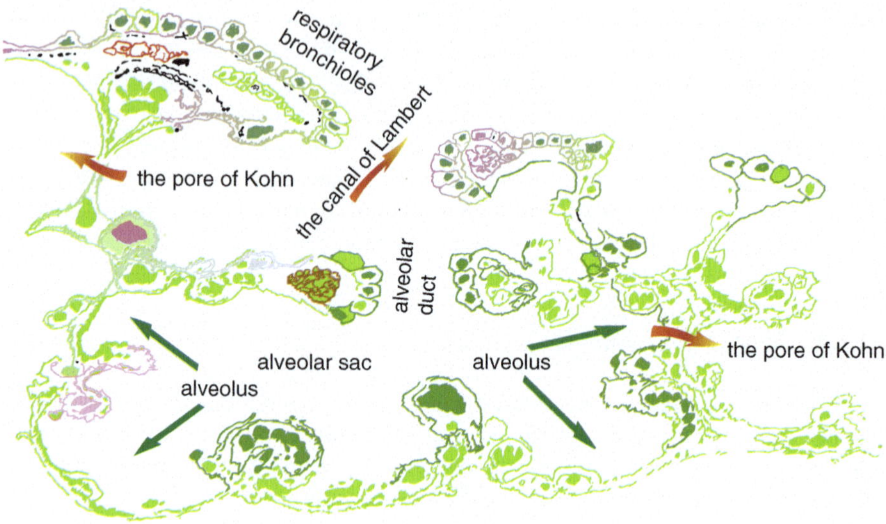

Fig. 2.1 The pores of Kohn and the canals of Lambert

2.1.2 *Pulmonary Vessels*

The lungs have two functionally distinct vascular systems: pulmonary system and bronchial system. The former is the functional vascular system of the lung, while the latter from the systemic circulation provides nutrients to pulmonary structures.

Pulmonary arteries, originating from the base of pulmonary conus of the right ventricle, divide into branches which accompany the bronchial trees and end in a dense capillary network in the walls of the alveoli. The small pulmonary veins originate from the capillary network in alveolar walls and converge more and more widely in the process of concentric reflux, ultimately forming superior and inferior pulmonary veins into the left atrium. The branches of the pulmonary artery accompany closely the homonymous bronchi at a particular distribution pattern, i.e., in the front and outside of the bronchi. Unlike the pulmonary arteries, the pulmonary veins have fewer branches and weaker relationship with the bronchi. The distribution of its branches is not consistent with that of bronchi, but common in the back and inside of the homonymous bronchus. In the pulmonary segments, the distribution of segmental arteries is consistent with that of segmental bronchi, but the segmental veins can be divided into the inner-segment branch and the intersegment branch. The former is smaller and located within the pulmonary segments, collecting part of returning venous blood of corresponding lung segments. The latter is thicker and accepting the venous return from two adjacent lung segments, thus distributed between the adjacent lung segments and not accompanied by bronchi and arteries. It is clinically relevant and significant to recognize and distinguish pulmonary veins

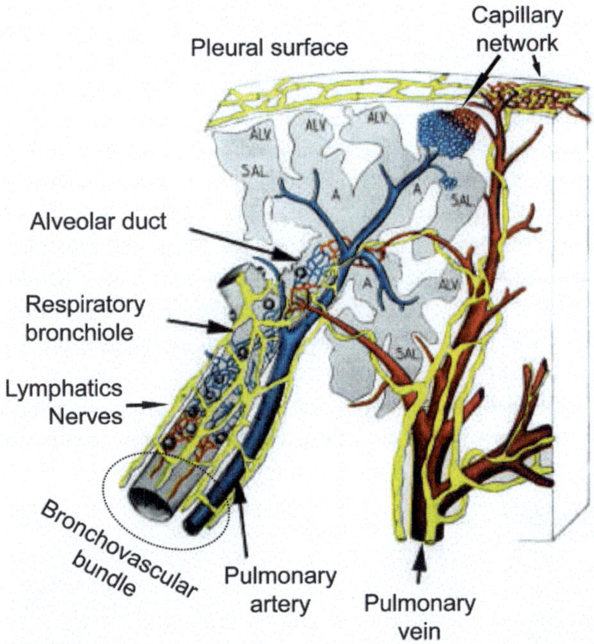

Fig. 2.2 The intersegmental and intrasegmental blood vessels in a primary pulmonary lobule. According to Miller, the primary pulmonary lobule is composed of alveolar ducts, atria (A), alveolar sacs (SAL), and alveoli (A) distal to the respiratory bronchiole, along with their associated blood vessels, nerves, and connective tissues (From Miller WS. The lung. Springfield, IL: Charles C Thomas; 1947:75)

and arteries since intersegmental veins can be used to acknowledge individual segments in imaging diagnosis and segmentectomy (Fig. 2.2).

Bronchial arteries are the nutrient vessels of the lung, supplying blood to the bronchus, lung parenchyma, pleura, and bronchial and intrapulmonary lymph nodes. Physiological anastomosis commonly exists between the terminal branches of pulmonary arteries and bronchial arteries to link the systemic circulation with the pulmonary circulation with co-distribution in the alveolar walls. It has been proved that the ligation of bronchial arteries below the lobe level would not cause the severe damage to distal bronchi and lung tissues.

Bronchial arteries vary in number and origin, usually only one in the right and two in the left, occasionally four to five on each side. They may be alone or in conjunction with intercostal artery arise from the descending aorta. Less frequently, they may come from the subclavian artery, the innominate artery, the internal thoracic artery, or even the intercostal artery. The left bronchial artery is about 1.1–1.5 mm in diameter, starting from the descending aorta at the level of fifth to sixth thoracic vertebra, while the right bronchial artery usually has a rectangular opening to the right wall of the descending aorta with a diameter of about 2 mm.

The bronchial arteries normally receive only about 1% of the total cardiac output and help maintain airway and lung function. They provide systemic blood supply to the trachea, bronchi, bronchial branches, esophagus, and visceral pleura. They also supply blood to the vasa vasorum of the thoracic aorta and pulmonary arteries as well as to the nerves, pulmonary veins, and lymph nodes in the thorax [2]. Besides, communications between bronchial arteries and pulmonary artery, intercostal artery, and Adamkiewicz artery are frequently observed (Fig. 2.3). Bronchial arteries create arterial plexus (i.e., the bronchial arterial plexus) in the bronchial wall adventitia. Some send out branches penetrating through the muscular layer into the submucosa and form a thin capillary plexus to supply nutrition for bronchial mucosa, the wall of pulmonary arteries, veins, and the visceral pleural membrane. About two-thirds of blood flows in the bronchial arteries are drained into bronchial veins, and the remaining one-third are collected into the azygos vein in the right and the hemizygos vein in the left and then to the superior vena cava.

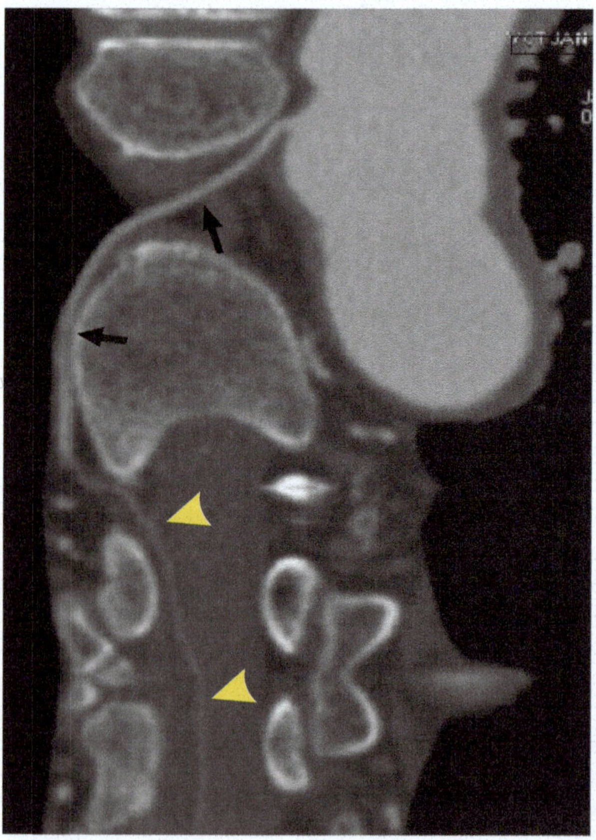

Fig. 2.3 The right bronchial artery (arrow) arises from the descending aorta and gives the Adamkiewicz artery (arrowhead)

The systemic circulation of the lungs mainly arises from the bronchial artery and bronchial vein and to a small extent from intercostal and inferior phrenic arteries. Although the bronchial circulation accounts for only a small proportion of the total blood flow in healthy people, it plays a vital role in maintaining the airway and lung function. Especially in many pathological conditions, bronchial circulation is more malleable in plasticity and plays a more important role. For example, in the development of lung cancer, bronchial circulation is considered as the major momentum. The hemodynamics of the blood supply system may change abnormally in the pathological state. CT perfusion imaging (CTPI) may be used to assess the hemodynamic changes in pulmonary microcirculation by analyzing the perfusion variations.

For a long time, there have been controversies on the relative proportion of the blood supply from pulmonary and bronchial circulatory systems in certain lung diseases. Early in the 1960s, autopsy-based reports revealed that lung cancers received blood supplies from both circulatory systems, confirmed in numerous subsequent studies. However, some researchers firmly believed that bronchial arterial system was the sole vascular supporting system for lung cancers. Hence, it is important to revisit and reemphasize the origin and amount of blood supply related to lung diseases for understanding the occurrence, development, and diagnosis, as well as decision making of treatment and the prognosis.

The bronchial arterial system is considered as the principal vascular system in the development and progression of lung cancers. In contrast, pulmonary arteries contribute a relatively small portion of blood supply of lung cancers, which is more evident in peripheral lung cancers, especially those located in the subpleural area. Occasionally, lung cancers may receive blood supply from bilateral bronchial arteries or other systemic arteries. The blood supply of lesions at the upper lobe tends to be from branches of the subclavian artery, and those lesions at lower lobes are usually supplied by the proper esophageal artery or phrenic artery. For centrally located lesions, blood supply may be from branches of systemic circulation in the mediastinum. Since both bronchial artery and pulmonary artery can participate in the blood supply to lung cancers, transbronchial arterial infusion chemotherapy alone may not be adequate for effective control of lung cancer in some cases.

In addition, intercommunication between two circulatory systems can be found in tuberculosis, similar to lung cancers. The underlying mechanism is the tuberculosis-induced damages to vascular bed. Due to the higher pressure in pulmonary artery system than that in the bronchial artery system, a bronchial-pulmonary arterial fistula would generate and account for the hemoptysis commonly seen in patients with tuberculosis and lung cancers. Imaging assessment of blood supply can also be used to evaluate the disease activity, a reliable approach for pretreatment prediction and posttreatment outcome evaluation.

On CT scan, the common manifestation of bronchial and pulmonary vessels is dependent on their size and path. Air-containing bronchi present as hollow tubular or circular structures, while blood vessels appear as high-density solid tubular or nodular opacities. Regarding density or morphological features, pulmonary arteries and veins usually have no difference. According to their positional relationship with the corresponding bronchus mentioned above, it is possible to distinguish arteries from veins. Additionally, tracking the interested vascular structure in consecutive slices could be helpful to identify its origin or branches. Figure 2.4 shows the diagrammatic relative position of bronchioles, pulmonary and bronchial vessels, and alveoli in a pulmonary lobule.

2.1.3 Secondary Pulmonary Lobule

The secondary pulmonary lobule is a fundamental unit of lung structure with irregularly polyhedral shape and varying size from 1 to 2.5 cm in diameter in most locations. Each of the lobes has about 50–80 pulmonary lobules. Each lobule is composed of a central bronchovascular bundle and dozens of peripheral pulmonary acinus and marginated by connective tissue and the interlobular septa.

On thin-section CT, several of lobular components are usually visible, including the interlobular septa and septal structures, the centrilobular region and centrilobular structures, and the lobular parenchyma. Interlobular septa vary in amount and thickness, thickest and richest in peripheral lungs, such as the apical aspect of the upper lobes and the anterior and diaphragmatic surfaces of the lower lobes, and along the mediastinal pleural surfaces. In the subpleural area, septa could be up to 0.1 mm in thickness. Lobules are supplied by arteries and bronchioles measuring approximately 1 mm in diameter, while intralobular terminal bronchioles and arteries measure about 0.7 mm in diameter and acinar bronchioles and arteries range from 0.3 to 0.5 mm in diameter. On thin-section CT scans, a linear, branching, or dot-like opacity seen in the center of a lobule or within 1 cm of the pleural surface represents the intralobular artery branch or its divisions. The visibility of bronchioles in healthy subjects depends on the wall thickness of the bronchiole, rather than its diameter. For a 1-mm bronchiole supplying a secondary lobule, the wall thickness measures approximately 0.15 mm [3]. The central lobular structure, known as the bronchovascular bundle, is constituted by bronchioles (or terminal bronchioles), small arterioles, and some supportive connective tissues. The structure of pulmonary lobule and alveolus is shown in Figs. 2.4 and 2.5.

The recognition of lung abnormalities relative to the structures of the secondary lobule is fundamental to the interpretation of thin-section CT scans. How to distinguish vessels from pulmonary micronodules on CT imaging? The following principles may be helpful: (1) The cross section of a vessel is frequently escorted by a bronchus in similar size, generating a diamond-on-ring appearance. (2) In comparison with adjacent known vessels, a pulmonary nodule may have different features such as size or density from the vessels. (3) To observe the suspected nodule in consecutive images, a vessel would be visualized in mutiple consecutive images with gradual size change, while a small nodule may be only seen in several images with the largest dimension measured in some middle

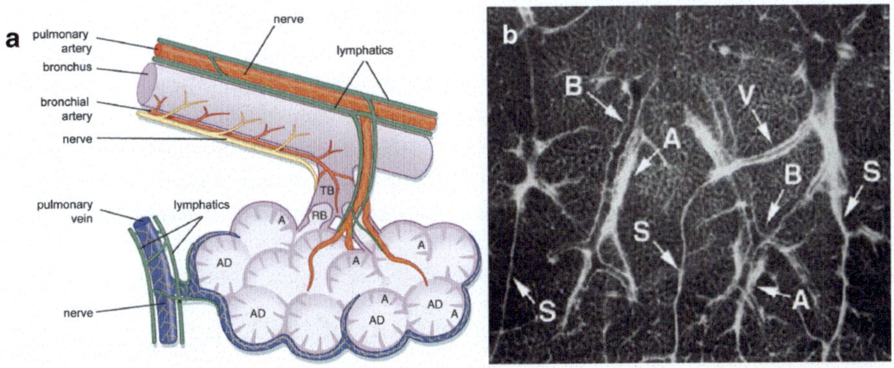

Fig. 2.4 The relative position of bronchioles, vessels, and alveoli in a pulmonary lobule (**a**) Diagrammatic illustration. *A* alveolus, *AD* alveolar duct, *RB* respiratory bronchioles, *TB* terminal bronchiole (From *Koeppen & Stanton: Berne AND Levy Physiclogy, 6th Edition*. Reprinted with permission) (**b**) Radiograph of 1-mm lung slice taken from peripheral lower lobe. Two well-defined secondary pulmonary lobules are visible. Lobules are marginated by thin interlobular septa (S)-containing pulmonary vein (V) branches. Bronchioles (B) and pulmonary arteries (A) are centrilobular (From *Itoh H*, et al. *Diffuse lung disease: pathologic basis for the high-resolution computed tomography findings. J Thorac maging 1993;8:176–188*. Reprinted with permission)

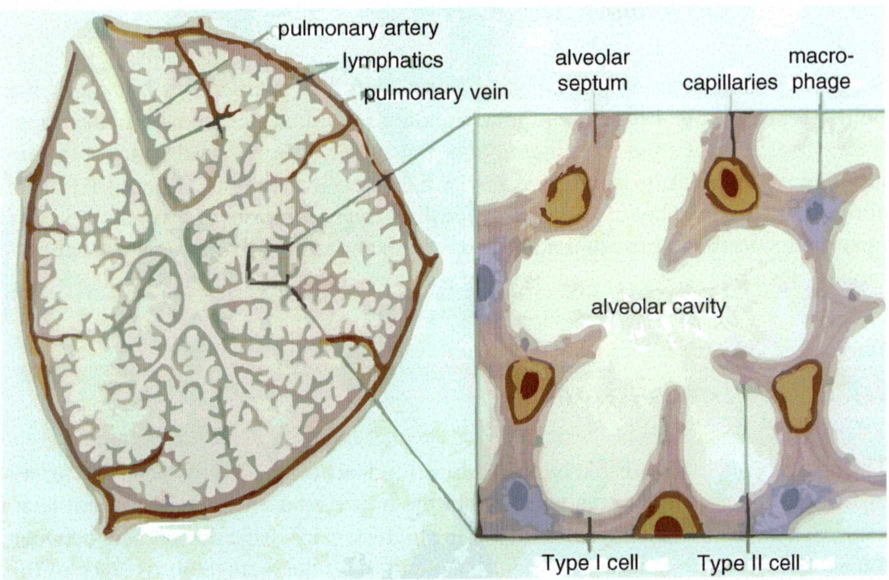

Fig. 2.5 Diagram of the secondary pulmonary lobule and alveolus a secondary pulmonary lobule is composed of dozens of acini which comprise numerous alveoli. Alveolar septa are located between adjacent alveoli, containing abundant capillaries, reticular fibers, and elastic fibers (around the alveolus)

images. (4) The images of vessels are subject to patient's position on CT table, prone or supine or lateral, due to the gravity effect. However, pulmonary nodules are less likely subject to scanning position. (5) Image post-processing is helpful. In the multiplanar reformation images, a vessel could appear a tubular structure when reformation plane is parallel to its path and a dot-like opacity when perpendicular. However, for a pulmonary nodule, the refomation plane may have limited impacts on its appearance, and the largest dimension is typically found in the median images among reformatted images.

2.2 Cross-Sectional Imaging Anatomy of the Lung

On CT imaging, recognition of pulmonary segments is based on segmental bronchi located in the center of the segments. Lobules and segments can be identified in consecutive slices through the upper, middle, and lower lobes of the lung. Figure 2.6 shows seven representative cross sections on CT imaging from the apex of the lung to the diaphragm. Figure 2.7 lists major structures within each section, including bronchi, segments, and mediastinal contents.

2.2.1 The Level above Aortic Arch

Several circular or comma-shaped opacities can be visualized in bilateral lung fields, representing bronchovascular bundles in apical segments of the upper lobes (Fig. 2.7a). Cupula of pleurae over the apex pulmonis, both extending into the root of the neck together, are also called cervical pleura. It could be 2 cm above the medial clavicle, probably with a manifestation of irregular patchy opacity due to thickening and adhesion, which should be distinguished from pulmonary lesions.

2.2.2 The Level of Aortic Arch

The apical bronchus is visible by the mediastinum accompanied by the apical artery inside and the apical vein outside. Within the upper lobe, the apical segment is an area bounded by the medial extremity of the high-density stripe demarcated between the anterior segment and the posterior segment, the intersegmental tributary of the apical segmental vein at the margin of the mediastinum, and the cross section of the posterior segmental vein (Fig. 2.7b). The major fissure in the left lung is located at a higher level than that in the right lung, so the upper segment (the posterior segment) of the left lower lobe is seen at this level. At this and following levels, serous pericardium reflexes along the roots of large vessels forming serous spaces. Those with larger sizes are named sinus, such as transverse sinus and oblique sinus, while

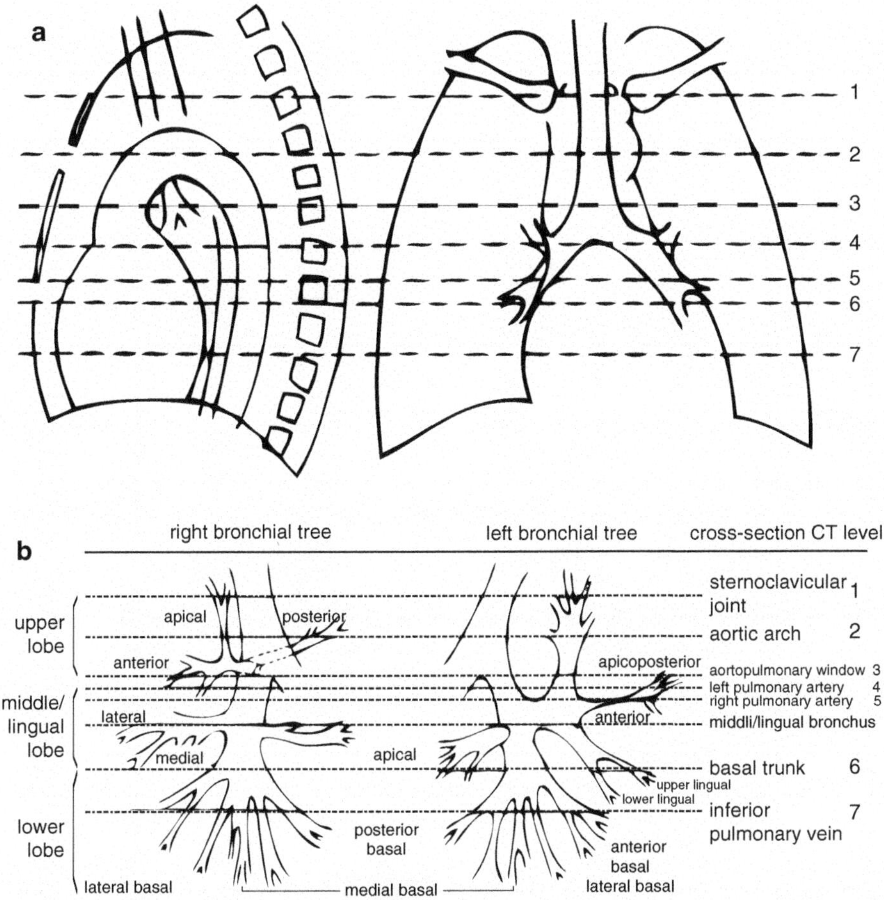

Fig. 2.6 Diagrams of seven representative transverse cross sections of the lung. (**a**) The projection of distribution map of cross sections in the lung. (**b**) Major bronchial structures corresponding to each section

the smaller spaces are named recess, such as superior recess by heart and superior aortic recess (Fig. 2.7c). These recesses or sinuses could expand with appearance mimicking lymph nodes if excessive fluid accumulates in physiological or pathological conditions.

2.2.3 The Level of Left Pulmonary Artery

In this level, the right upper lobe bronchial trunk and the long axis of its anterior and posterior segmental bronchus can be visible in right lung field. The apical vein appears circular, located between anterior and posterior segmental bronchi; the

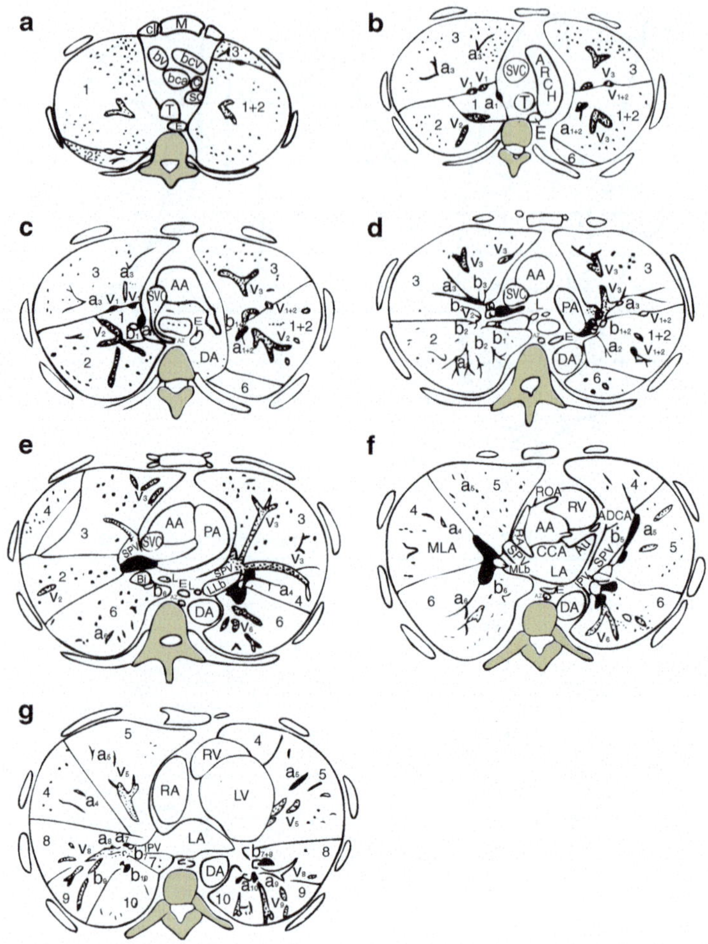

Fig. 2.7 Major anatomical structures on sketched CT images from seven representative cross-sectional levels (**a**) Sternoclavicular joint level. (**b**) Aortic arch level. (**c**) Aortic window. When fluid accumulation occurs in the superior recess by the heart and transverse sinus, the recess may appear a circular (axial views) or elongated (coronal and sagittal views) low-density opacity, which should not be misdiagnosed as enlarged lymph nodes. (**d**) The left pulmonary artery window level. (**e**) The right pulmonary artery window level. (**f**) The level above the basal trunk. (**g**) Inferior pulmonary vein level. (*These drawings were elaborately produced by the late professor Zongwen Shen from the former Shanghai Medical University, with reference to cross-sectional anatomy and CT scans of corpses*) *Abbreviations: A* artery, *AA* ascending aorta, *ADCA* anterior descending coronary arteries, *ARCH* aorta arch, *Au* auricular appendix, *Az* azygos vein, *B* bronchi, *b* segmental bronchus, *bca* brachiocephalic artery, *bv* brachiocephalic vein, *Bi* bronchus intermedius, *CA* cephalic artery, *RCA* right coronary artery, *Cl* clavicle, *DA* descending aorta, *E* esophagus, *IAR* inferior aortic recess, *ILA* inferior lobar artery, *ILB* inferior lobar bronchus, *IPV* inferior pulmonary vein, *IV* innominate vein, *IVC* inferior vena cava, *L* lymph, *LA* left atrium, *LCA* left coronary artery, *LLb* lingular lobe bronchus, *LPAR* left pulmonary artery recess, *LPVR* left pulmonary vein recess, *LSPV* left superior pulmonary vein, *LV* left ventricle, *M* sternum, *MLA* middle lobar artery, *MLb* middle lobar bronchus, *OS* oblique sinus, *PA* pulmonary artery, *PCR* postcaval recess, *RA* right atrium, *RCA* right coronary artery, *RIPV* right inferior pulmonary vein *RPA* right pulmonary artery, *RPAR* right pulmonary artery recess, *RSPV* right superior pulmonary vein, *RV* right ventricle, *RVOT* right ventricular outflow tract *SA* subclavian artery, *SAR* superior aortic recess, *SPV* superior pulmonary vein, *SVC* superior vena cava, *T* trachea, *TD* thoracic duct, *Th* thymus, *TS* transverse sinus, *V* vein

posterior vein can be used to distinguish anterior and posterior segments in the right upper lobe.

A hypovascular zone in the left lung, representing the interlobar fissure, extends from the interlobar artery posterolaterally. Within the left upper lobe, an imaginary line dividing the anterior segment from the apical-posterior segment is drawn slightly anterior to the apical-posterior segmental bronchus. In the anterior segment, the anterior segmental bronchus runs anteriorly and horizontally (Fig. 2.7d). Located anteriorly to the anterior bronchus is the inferior branch of the anterior segmental artery. Close to the mediastinum, intrasegmental vein courses posteriorly to drain into the superior pulmonary vein. In the apical-posterior segment, there is a transverse apical-posterior segmental artery without escort by bronchus.

The boundary between mediastinum and lungs is evident in the right with a remarkable longitudinal linear opacity with lipid density, but not visible in the left. Hence, an imaginary line from the proximal of the first branch of the left pulmonary artery and the starting point of the left upper lobe bronchus is considered as the boundary line. The superior aortic recess can be seen in this section.

2.2.4 The Level by Right Pulmonary Artery Trunk

This section passes through the upper level of the intermediate bronchus. In the right lung, a hypovascular zone extending laterally between the interlobar artery and intermediate bronchus represents the right interlobar fissure, the horizontal fissure (transverse fissure, accessory interlobular fissure). An imaginary line is drawn from the upper division of the superior pulmonary vein dividing into the lateral and anterior areas. The lateral area is named as the lateral segment of the middle lobe, and the posterior triangular portion of the anterior area is an avascular plane of the para-interlobar fissure, and its anterior portion is the anterior segment of the upper lobe.

In the left lung, lingual lobe bronchus and vessels are visible. At this section, the major structures in the right lung include the anterior segment of the upper lobes, lateral segment of the middle lobe, and the upper segment of the lower lobe, while in the left the anterior segment and superior lingual segment of upper lobe and upper segment of the lower lobe (Fig. 2.7e).

In cases with pleural metastases, the horizontal fissure may be involved with imaging features of miliary distribution of bead-like nodular lesions, which should be distinguished from intrapulmonary metastases (Fig. 2.8a). Occasionally, prominent right hilar soft tissue collections are seen in or near the right hilum, superior to the right interlobar pulmonary artery and medial to the right superior pulmonary vein as illustrated in the anatomical section (Fig. 2.8b, c). These abnormalities are considered due to normal accumulations of hilar lymph nodes, fatty tissue, and connective tissues, measuring from 3 to 15 mm with more than one-half exceeding 10 mm. If there exists difficulty in differentiation with pulmonary diseases, such as pulmonary artery embolism or lymphadenopathy, contrast-enhancement thin-slice CT scan could be helpful. Additionally, encapsulated localized effusions in fissures are easily mistaken as pulmonary lesions, which could be differentiated with the assistance of image post-processing and contrast-enhancement scanning (Fig. 2.9).

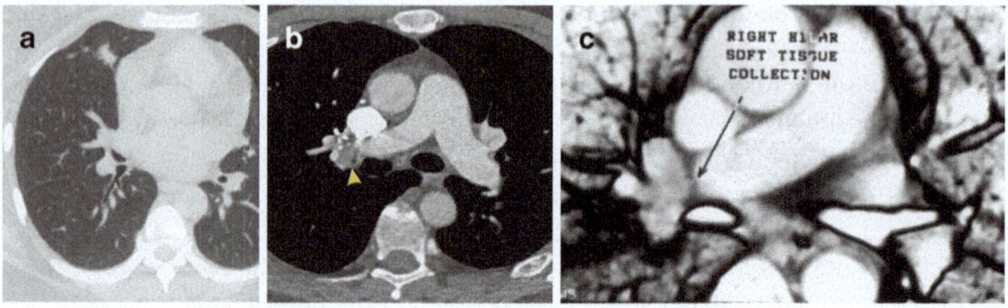

Fig. 2.8 Miliary metastases on the interlobar fissure and the right hilar soft tissue collections. (**a**) Miliary metastases on the right interlobar fissure. (**b**) Right hilar soft tissue collections (arrowhead). (**c**) Right hilar soft tissue collections and the low-density boundary line between the right lung and mediastinum (arrow)

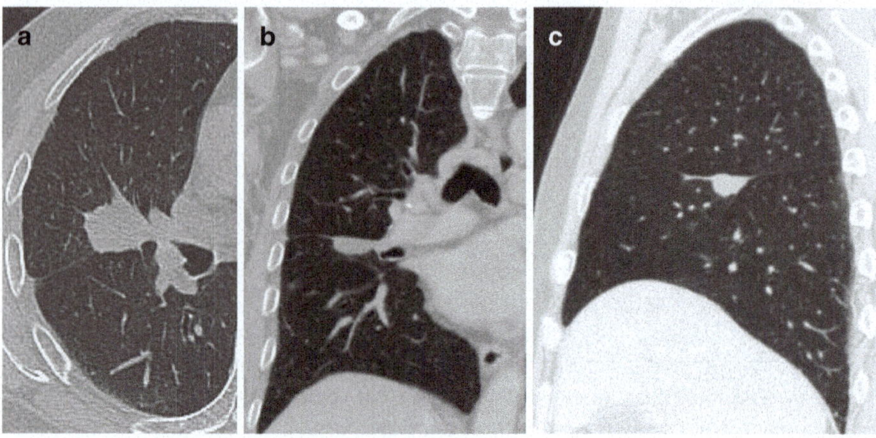

Fig. 2.9 Encapsulated effusions in fissures. The effusions are easily misdiagnosed as intrapulmonary lesion in axial images. (**a**) In coronal (**b**) and sagittal (**c**) views, the effusions are clearly visualized between interlobular fissures

In this section, transverse sinus (TS), the superior aortic recess (SAR), and bilateral pulmonary artery recesses are observed (Fig. 2.10).

2.2.5 The Level of Interlobular Artery

This is a section passing through the basal trunk (Fig. 2.7). The bilateral hypovascular zones extending laterally from the lateral border of the lower lobe arteries represent the interlobar fissures. Within the middle lobe, an imaginary line drawn anterolaterally between the lateral and medial segmental bronchi arteries and veins demarcates the lateral segment and the medial segment. Within the left upper lobe,

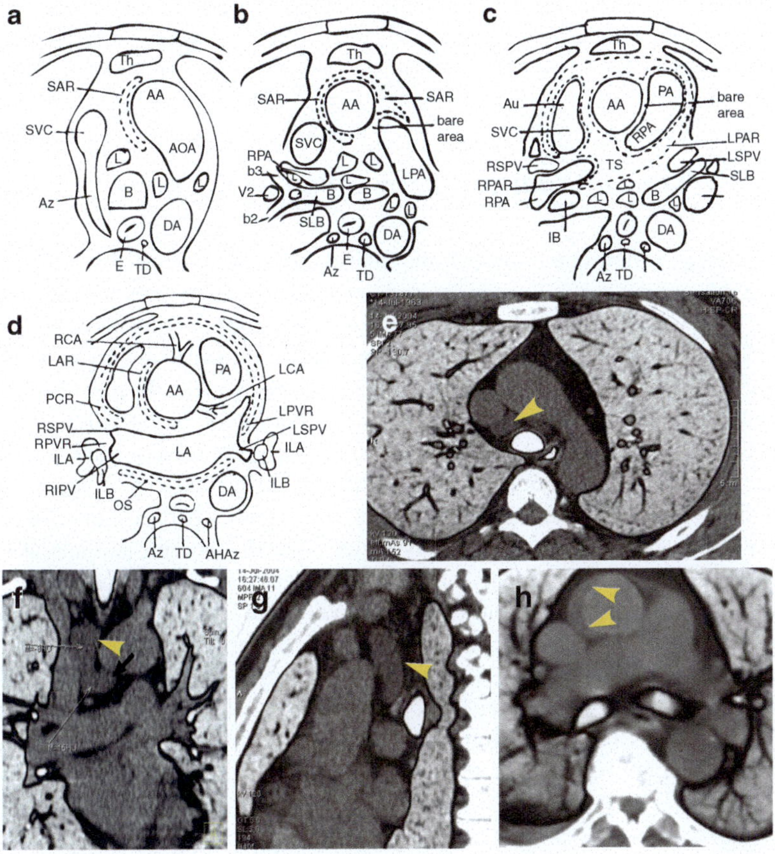

Fig. 2.10 Pericardial recesses and sinuses (**a–d**) The locations of pericardial recesses and sinuses in cross-sectional anatomy (dotted line) (**a**, aortic arch level; **b**, left pulmonary artery level; **c**, right pulmonary artery level; **d**, aortic root level) (**e–h**) Fluid accumulation is seen in the superior aortic recess (SAR), and pericardial recesses and sinuses (arrowhead) are variably dilated filled with components with liquid density of 8 HU. (**e**) Axial CT image at the level of aortic arch; (**f**) and (**g**) are coronal and sagittal views, respectively. (**h**) CT at the level of right pulmonary artery shows a recess wrapping around the ascending aorta *Abbreviations: AA* ascending aorta, *DA* descending aorta, *L* lymph node, *LPR* left lung recess, *MPA* main pulmonary artery, *OS* oblique sinus, *RPA* right pulmonary artery, *SAR* superior aortic recess, *SVC* superior vena cava, *TS* transverse sinus

an intersegmental tributary of the superior segmental vein courses posteromedially between the long stripe-shaped superior segmental bronchus and the round section of the inferior segmental bronchus. Finally, it drains into the lingular vein. It is a landmark that demarcates the superior segment and the inferior segment of the lingular lobe. The portion located anteromedially to the lingular lobe is still the anterior segment of the upper lobe.

In addition, at this level, the inferior aortic recess (IAR) and the oblique sinus (OS) can be visible. Left pulmonary artery recess (LPAR) is located between the left atrial appendage and left superior pulmonary vein (LSPV). Right pulmonary artery recess is between right superior pulmonary vein (RSPV) and right inferior pulmonary vein (Fig. 2.10).

2.2.6 The Level of Bilateral Inferior Pulmonary Veins

This image is a section going through the inferior pulmonary veins (Fig. 2.7g). The bilateral hypovascular zones, located anterior to the inferior pulmonary vein at the margin of the mediastinum and extending laterally, represent the interlobar fissures. Within the right lower lobe, the medial basal segmental artery is situated laterally to the homonymous bronchus. The medial basal segment is located medially to medial basal artery and bronchus and adjacently to the proximal portion of the inferior pulmonary vein. After giving off the lateral basal segmental bronchus, the basal trunk continues inferiorly to the posterior basal segmental bronchus. The higher-level tributary of the anterior division of the inferior pulmonary vein which passes between anterior artery anteriorly and lateral bronchus posteriorly divides into the anterior and lateral basal segments. The higher-level tributary of the intermediate division separates the lateral basal segment from the posterior basal segment. Within the left lower lobe, the division of the segments is similar in appearance to that found on the right lower lobe.

The anterior parietal layer of the pericardium is visible about 2 mm in thickness. On the contrary, the visceral layer is too thin to be visualized in the physiological state. The thickness of pericardium adjacent to the right ventricle may be up to 7 mm and should not be considered as the pericardial thickening.

2.3 Updates on Regional Lymph Node Classification for Lung Cancer

It is important to accurately group the regional lymph nodes associated with lung cancer for staging, treatment, and prognosis of the disease. Local and regional lymph nodes of lung cancer include pulmonary, hilar, mediastinal, supraclavicular, and infraclavicular lymph node zones. Up to 2009, there existed two grouping systems for the regional lymph nodes in lung cancer, that is, AJCC/Naruke system endorsed by the Japan Lung Cancer Society and the American Joint Committee on Cancer (AJCC) and MD-ATS system supported by American Thoracic Society (ATS).

The AJCC/Naruke system was initially proposed in 1978. In this system, lymph nodes are divided into superior and inferior mediastinal and intrapulmonary zones. Furthermore, the superior mediastinal zone includes (1) the most superior mediastinal, (2) upper paratracheal, (3) prevascular and retrotracheal, (4) lower paratracheal, (5) aortic window, and (6) para-aortic (ascending aorta, aortic arch, and phrenic). The inferior mediastinal zone includes (7) subcarinal, (8) paraesophageal, and (9) pulmonary ligament (including the bilateral pulmonary vein). Intrapulmonary lymph node zone includes (10) hilar, (11) interlobar, (12) lobar, (13) segmental, and (14) intrapulmonary. In order to define intrathoracic lymph nodes more precisely from the anatomical perspective, ATS system was established based on the AJCC/Naruke system in 1983. Thirteen years later, the AJCC and Union for International Cancer Control (UICC) proposed MD-ATS system with the intention to integrate both ATS and AJCC/Naruke systems. However, this classification system was only accepted in North America. The rest of the world, including Europe, Japan, and China, continued using the AJCC/Naruke system. Multiple differences in the descriptors for mediastinal lymph nodes existed between the systems of AJCC and ATS, for example, level 1 lymph nodes in the AJCC system corresponding to levels 1 + 2 in the ATS system, and levels 2, 3, 4R, and 4 L in the AJCC system corresponded to levels 4R and 4 L in the ATS system. Perhaps the most significant discrepancy was that level 7 subcarinal lymph nodes in the ATS system were equivalent to levels 7 + 10 in the AJCC system. As a result, lung cancers with positive level 10 lymph nodes were staged N1 by ATS system but N2 by AJCC system.

To solve these discrepancies and facilitate worldwide communication, the International Association for the Study of Lung Cancer (IASLC) International Staging Committee were commissioned by AJCC and UICC to develop a revised lymph node classification system for the forthcoming UICC/AJCC 7th Edition for lung cancer TNM staging in 1998. After years of endeavors and dedications from numerous international experts, the IASLC lymph node classification was published in 2007 [4]. According to the IASLC system, the regional lymph nodes are divided into 7 zones and 14 stations, including supraclavicular zone (station 1); superior mediastinal zone (stations 2R, 2L, 3a, 3p, 4R, 4L); aortopulmonary AP zone (stations 5, 6); inferior mediastinal zone, including subcarinal zone (station 7) and the lower zone (station 8, 9); hilar/interlobar zone (stations 10, 11); and peripheral zone (stations 12, 13, 14). The detailed information regarding individual lymph node station is described in Table 2.1 and Fig. 2.11.

Compared with the previous classification systems of MD-ATS and AJCC/Naruke, IASLC map clarified preexisting confusions and redefined the scope and boundaries of each lymph node station to minimize the uncertainty and randomness in the clinical application of the system. The major revisions or updates include the following. (1) The supraclavicular and sternal notch lymph nodes, which were not previously identified as a lymph node station, are now clearly described as level 1 to facilitate differentiation from intrathoracic nodes. The sternal notch serves as the border between the levels 1 and 2. (2) The discrepancies between levels 2 and 4 have been resolved with more precise definitions. The left lateral wall of the trachea is set as the boundary between the right- and left-sided levels 2 and 4. The extent of level 5 is reduced, with its lower border adjusted to the upper rim of the left main pulmonary artery. At the same time, the upper limit of level 10L expands to the upper rim of the left main pulmonary artery, belonging to N2. (3) Considering that lymphatic system in the superior mediastinum predominantly collects the right paratracheal area with extension beyond the midline of the trachea, the boundary between the

Table 2.1 Regional nodal stations of lung cancer in IASLC classification system

Zone	Nodal stations and anatomic boundaries
Supraclavicular zone	#1 low cervical, supraclavicular and sterna notch lymph nodes
	Upper border: lower margin of cricoid cartilage
	Lower border: clavicles bilaterally and in the midline, the upper border of the manubrium
	1R and 1L, respectively, represent the right and left side of the lymph node
	The midline of the trachea serves as the border between 1R and 1L
Superior mediastinal	#2 Upper paratracheal lymph nodes
	2R—Upper border: apex of right lung and, in the midline, the upper border of the manubrium
	Lower border: intersection of caudal margin of innominate vein with the trachea
	2L—Upper border: apex of left lung and, in the midline, the upper border of the manubrium
	Lower border: superior border of the of aortic arch
	The left lateral border of the trachea (not the midline of the trachea) serves as the border between 2R and 2L
	#3 Prevascular and retrotracheal lymph nodes
	3a: Prevascular lymph node
	Right side
	Upper border: apex of lung
	Lower border: level of tracheal carina
	Anterior border: posterior aspect of sternum
	Posterior border: anterior border of superior vena cava
	Left side
	Upper border: apex of lung
	Lower border: level of tracheal carina
	Anterior border: posterior aspect of sternum
	Posterior border: left common carotid artery
	3p: Retrotracheal lymph node
	Upper border: apex of lung
	Lower border: level of tracheal carina
	#4 Lower paratracheal lymph nodes
	4R: Right paratracheal lymph nodes and pretracheal lymph nodes extending to the left lateral border of trachea
	Upper border: intersection of caudal margin of innominate vein with the trachea
	Lower border: lower edge of venae azygos
	4L: Nodes to the left of the left lateral border of the trachea, medial to the ligamentum arteriosum
	Upper border: upper margin of aortic arch
	Lower bound: upper rim of left main pulmonary artery

Table 2.1 (continued)

Zone	Nodal stations and anatomic boundaries
Aortopulmonary AP zone	#5 Subaortic(aortopulmonary window)lymph nodes
	Upper border: lower margin of aortic arch
	Lower border: upper rim of left main pulmonary artery
	Left border: ligamentum arteriosum
	#6 Paraaortic lymph nodes
	Anterior and left lateral to the ascending aorta and aortic arch
	Upper border: a line tangential to the upper border of the aortic arch
	Lower border: the lower border of the aortic arch
Inferior mediastinal zone	#7 Subcarinal lymph nodes
	Upper border: the tracheal carina
	Lower border: the upper border of the lower lobe bronchus on the left; the lower border of the bronchus intermedius on the right
	#8: Subcarinal paraesophageal lymph nodes
	The lymph nodes located below the subcarinal lymph nodes and along the esophagus
	Upper border: the upper border of the lower lobe bronchus on the left; the lower border of the bronchus intermedius on the right
	Upper border: the diaphragm
	#9 Pulmonary ligament lymph nodes
	Lymph nodes within the pulmonary ligament
	Upper border: the inferior pulmonary veins
	Lower: the diaphragm
Hilar and interlobar zone	#10 Hilar lymph nodes
	Lymph nodes immediately adjacent to the mainstem bronchus and hilar vessels (including the proximal segment of the pulmonary veins and the main pulmonary artery)
	Upper border: the lower rim of the azygos vein on the right; upper rim of the pulmonary artery on the left
	Lower border: lobar bronchial opening bilateral
	#11 Interlobar lymph nodes
	Between the origin of the lobar bronchi
	11s: between the upper lobe bronchus and bronchus intermedius on the right
	11i: between the middle and lower lobe bronchi on the right
Peripheral zone	#12 Lobar nodes
	Adjacent to the lobar bronchus
	#13 Segmental lymph nodes
	Adjacent to the segmental bronchus
	#14 Subsegmental lymph nodes
	Adjacent to the subsegmental bronchus

(From *Rusch VW*, et al. *(2009) The IASLC lung cancer staging project: a proposal for a new international lymph node map in the forthcoming seventh edition of the TNM classification for lung cancer. Journal of thoracic oncology: official publication of the International Association for the Study of Lung Cancer 4 (5):568-577*. Reprinted with permission)

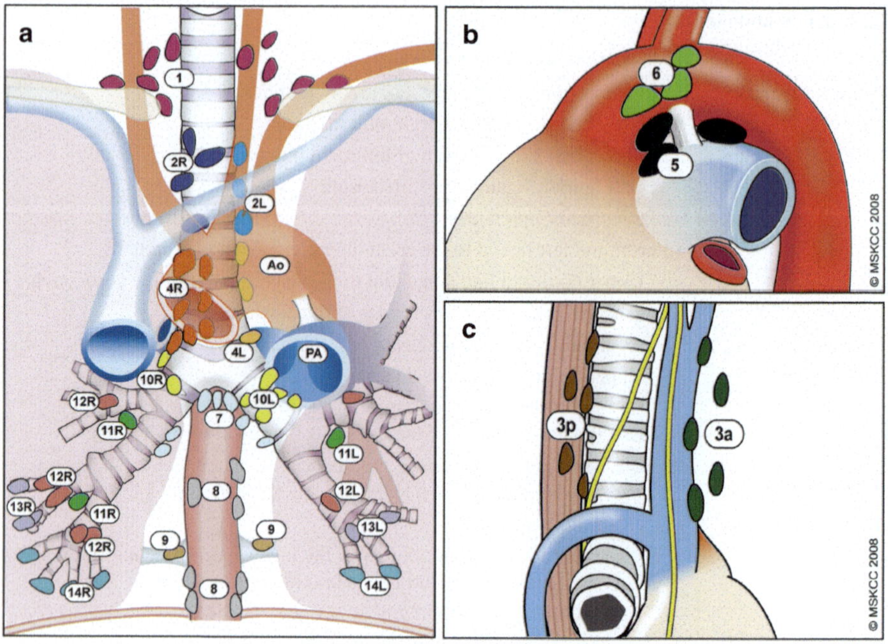

Fig. 2.11 Illustrations of the International Association for the Study of Lung Cancer (IASLC) lymph node map. (**a**) Distribution of lymph nodes by stations, except stations 3, 5, and 6. (**b**) The position of stations 5 and 6 lymph nodes. (**c**) The position of stations 3a and 3p lymph nodes. (From *AJCC/UICC 7th Edition TNM Stage*. Reprinted with permission)

right- and left-sided levels 2 and 4 has been moved leftward to the left lateral wall of the trachea. The midline lymph nodes of a left lung cancer should be designated N3 by current system instead of N2. In contrast, for a right lung cancer, the midline lymph nodes should be classified as N2 by current system instead of N3. (4) The arbitrary designation of the anterior tracheal lymph nodes in the previous AJCC system has been eliminated because these nodes are not reliably distinguishable from levels 2 and 4 and are generally removed en bloc with level 4 during a mediastinal component of systematic nodal dissection from the right. The designation of prevascular and retrotracheal nodes as 3a and 3p has been retained and clarified [5]. (5) The entire subcarinal group of lymph nodes, previously designated as level 7 in the ATS map but levels 7 and 10 in the AJCC map, are now defined as level 7, with clarified anatomic borders. (6) As an anatomical landmark with more imaging and surgical recognition, the lower margin of the azygos vein on the right and the upper rim of the pulmonary artery replaced the pleural fold and became the border between the levels 4 and 10. (7) Similarly, more precise definitions have been made for the designation of level 10 and 11. As a result, levels 10R and 10L are now classified as N2 instead of N1. (8) Certain lymph node stations with similar outcome data are grouped into a zone. The zone concept is valuable for oncologists and radiologists when dealing with large nodal masses that involve multiple nodal stations [5].

Despite that IASLC system has improved the recognition of the scope of involved lymph nodes, uncertainties are not completely eliminated, and some gray areas still remain. In fact, some definitions or pitfalls in current classification system limit the clinical performance, for example, in the context of radiation therapy, as stated below [6]. (1) The relative location variation in lung apex and clavicle probably causes difficulties in determination of levels 1, 2, or 3, resulting in an uncertainty of an N2 or N3 disease; (2) The boundaries between levels 10R and 4R, and 10L and 4L, are ambiguous, likely leading to mistakenly staging N1 or N2 stages, especially when lymph nodes are located in the front of the tracheal bifurcation; (3) The arterial ligament, serving as the boundary of lymph nodes between levels 4L and 5, is not easily visualized on CT images; (4) The extent of level 7 is expanded in both anterior and posterior directions, which requires more practice in accurate recognition; (5) Level 10 extends further medially toward the carina. The implication of this change is that N1 regions extend further than previously. CT-based separation of levels 10 and 11 can be challenging.

References

1. Ward HE, Nicholas TE. Alveolar type I and type II cells. Aust NZ J Med. 1984;14(5 Suppl 3):731–4.
2. Walker CM, Rosado-de-Christenson ML, Martinez-Jimenez S, Kunin JR, Wible BC. Bronchial arteries: anatomy, function, hypertrophy, and anomalies. Radiographics. 2015;35(1):32–49. https://doi.org/10.1148/rg.351140089.
3. Webb WR. Thin-section CT of the secondary pulmonary lobule: anatomy and the image—the 2004 Fleischner lecture. Radiology. 2006;239(2):322–38. https://doi.org/10.1148/radiol.2392041968.
4. Zielinski M, Rami-Porta R. Proposals for changes in the Mountain and Dresler mediastinal and pulmonary lymph node map. J Thorac Oncol. 2007;2(1):3–6. https://doi.org/10.1097/JTO.0b013e31802bff98.
5. Rusch VW, Asamura H, Watanabe H, Giroux DJ, Rami-Porta R, Goldstraw P. The IASLC lung cancer staging project: a proposal for a new international lymph node map in the forthcoming seventh edition of the TNM classification for lung cancer. J Thorac Oncol. 2009;4(5):568–77. https://doi.org/10.1097/JTO.0b013e3181a0d82e.
6. Pitson G, Lynch R, Claude L, Sarrut D. A critique of the international association for the study of lung cancer lymph node map: a radiation oncology perspective. J Thorac Oncol. 2012;7(3):478–80. https://doi.org/10.1097/JTO.0b013e318249a9c6.

Suggested Readings

1. American Joint Committee on Cancer AJCC cancer staging manual. 7th ed. New York: Springer.
2. American Thoracic Society Medical section of the American Lung Association. Clinical staging of primary lung cancer. Am Rev Respir Dis. 1983;127(5):659–64. https://doi.org/10.1164/arrd.1983.127.5.659.
3. Ashida C, Zerhouni EA, Fishman EK. CT demonstration of prominent right hilar soft tissue collections. J Comput Assist Tomogr. 1987;11(1):57–9.

4. Goldstraw P, Crowley J, Chansky K, Giroux DJ, Groome PA, Rami-Porta R, Postmus PE, Rusch V, Sobin L. The IASLC Lung Cancer Staging Project: proposals for the revision of the TNM stage groupings in the forthcoming (seventh) edition of the TNM Classification of malignant tumours. J Thorac Oncol. 2007;2(8):706–14. https://doi.org/10.1097/JTO.0b013e31812f3c1a.
5. Itoh H, Murata K, Konishi J, Nishimura K, Kitaichi M, Izumi T. Diffuse lung disease: pathologic basis for the high-resolution computed tomography findings. J Thorac Imaging. 1993;8(3):176–88.
6. Mountain CF, Dresler CM. Regional lymph node classification for lung cancer staging. Chest. 1997;111(6):1718–23.
7. Naruke T, Suemasu K, Ishikawa S. Lymph node mapping and curability at various levels of metastasis in resected lung cancer. J Thorac Cardiovasc Surg. 1978;76(6):832–9.
8. Shen ZW, Zhang GZ, Cao Y. Division of lobes and segments of lung on CT scan and topographical relation of segmental bronchi and related vessels. Chin Med J. 1988;101(10):723–30.

Chapter 3
Lung Cancer Screening

Xiangpeng Zheng and Guozhen Zhang

3.1 Lung Cancer Screening: Chest Radiography Versus Computed Tomography

3.1.1 Chest Radiography

Lung cancer remains the highest incidence and the leading cause of cancer death in China. Lack of typical symptoms in patients with early-stage lung cancers and subsequent misdiagnosis account for the high mortality to some extent. This situation can be partly solved with lung cancer screening. Both chest radiography and LDCT can be used for this purpose. As the basic imaging examination of respiratory disease, chest radiography utilizes X-rays to capture imaging of diseases and normal anatomy at a single film, well known as plain film. With higher resolution than fluoroscopy, plain film can display fine lesions with records for consultation and follow-up comparison. For comprehensive evaluation of the location and morphological features of lesions, posteroanterior and lateral films are generally required. However, for assessment of miliary, micronodular, reticular, or honeycomb-like lesions with bilateral diffuse distribution, a posteroanterior film may suffice for diagnostic purpose. Incorrect radiography position, improper filming parameters, or filming at expiratory phase could cause information loss and subsequent misdiagnosis.

The development of computer technology and storage capacities has revolutionized radiography with digitalization. Computed radiography (CR) is the early

X. Zheng (✉)
Department of Radiation Oncology, Fudan University Huadong Hospital, Shanghai, China
e-mail: zhengxp@fudan.edu.cn

G. Zhang
Department of Radiology, Fudan University Huadong Hospital, Shanghai, China

X. Zheng et al. (eds.), *Early-stage Lung Cancer*,
https://doi.org/10.1007/978-981-10-7596-4_3

digital imaging system, using a photostimulable phosphor image receptor plate to store the energy of transmitted X-ray as a latent imaging, which can be transformed into digital signals with laser scanning and displayed on monitors. CR systems have been widely used in hospitals due to their compatibility with existing radiography equipment and accelerate the digitalization in conventional radiography. CR imaging has some advantages, including post-processing, superior density resolution, and high tolerance, which allow better visualization of vessels, bronchi, mediastinal structures, mammal tissues, and lesions subject to be missed in the conventional radiography with less radiation dose. High tolerance facilitates application of CR systems in a certain environment with unstable electric power supply, such as bedside radiography in the units of emergency or intensive care, by adaptive mechanism for maintaining consistent density response. More recently, full-field digital amorphous silicon flat-panel X-ray detector radiography systems based on cesium iodide and amorphous silicon have become commercially available, referred to as direct radiography (DR). Compared to CR systems, DR imaging systems do not require laser scanning for image display, so DR is also referred to as DDR (direct digital radiography). Additionally, DR system has a superior spatial resolution up to 2560 × 3072, fully sufficing to diagnostic requirements of the vast majority of clinical diseases. Other advantages of this technology include high detection efficiency and rapid image display. These systems have excellent image quality and allow a significant reduction in effective dose compared with either conventional film-screen or storage phosphor-based CR systems. Practically, CR is eventually replaced by DR. However, both systems have cons, especially in temporal resolution. Low response rate (several seconds) limits the visualization of those organs with involuntary motions or evaluation of those organs with voluntary motions. Image compression for archiving and decompression for reading may compromise image quality and influence the analysis of subtle changes in the lungs.

Retrospective analysis revealed that approximately 90% of misdiagnosis of small lung cancers might have abnormal imaging manifestations in chest radiography. The underlying reasons for the misdiagnosis could be particular locations (such as behind the heart, in the apical or hilar zone, or close to the ribs or diaphragm), the inexperience of reading skill, or disturbance by coexisting abnormalities. Researches have shown that artificial intelligence-based computer-aided detection and diagnosis (CAD) system could be applied to process digitalized chest radiography images and mark suspected opacities for radiologists' discretion and diagnosis, which may improve detection accuracy of small pulmonary nodules and reduce the incidence of misdiagnosis as well as time in the interpretation of images.

To perform the pulmonary nodule detection, a CAD system commonly has four step-by-step operations: segmentation of the lungs, detection of the candidate nodules, characteristic analysis, and elimination of false positives. After decades of development and evolution, current commercial CAD systems have achieved great advances in sensitivity and accuracy of detection of pulmonary nodules. For example, the IQQA™-Chest developed by EDDA Technology inte-

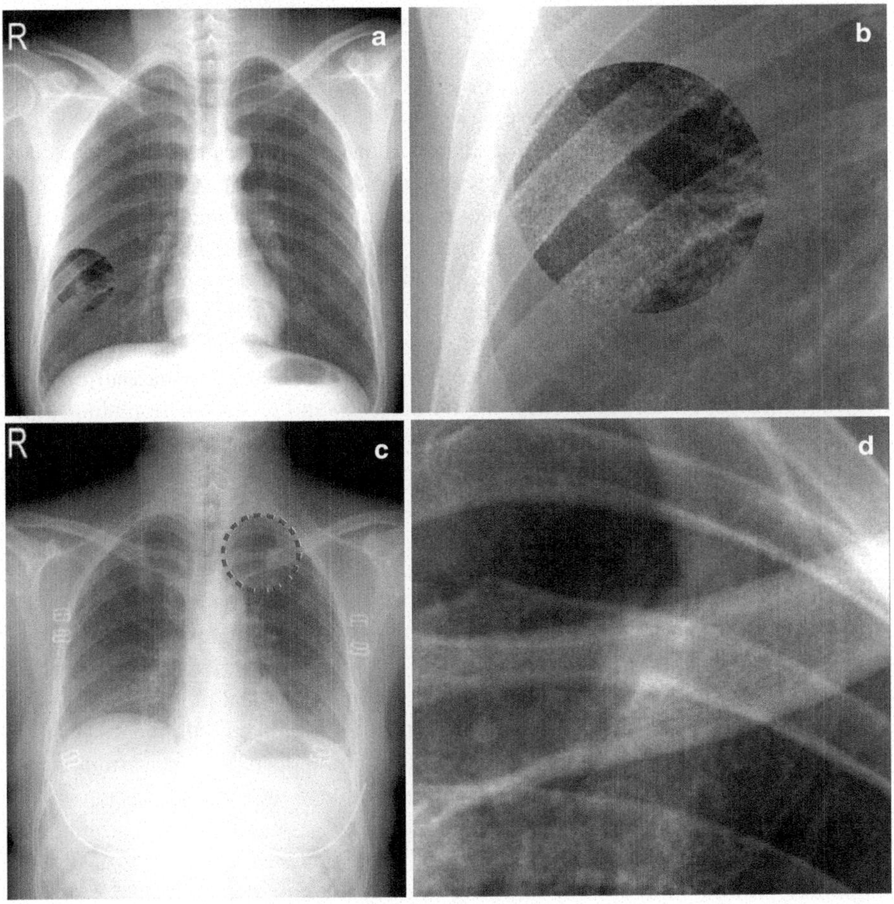

Fig. 3.1 Application of CAD in chest imaging (the intelligent/interactive IQQA™-Chest). (**a**, **b**) A chest DR image (**a**) was processed with enhanced display mode, and a small nodule (arrowhead in **b**) readily omitted on the unprocessed image was observed. (**c**, **d**) In another case, an adenocarcinoma-proven nodular lesion (arrowhead in **d**) was clearly shown on the DR image (**c**) processed with enhanced display mode (Courtesy of Drs. Jianzhong Qian and Xiaolan Zeng, EDDA Technology, Inc.)

grates enhanced display techniques, auto-segmentation, and other advanced imaging analysis functions to interpret chest images and even generate structured preliminary reports for radiologists (Fig. 3.1).

According to the results reported by Abe et al. [1] on large-scale observer tests at the 1996–2001 RSNA scientific assemblies, the CAD application significantly improved the diagnostic accuracy of radiologists, reduced omission rate, and interpretation time. Shiraishi and colleagues developed a computerized scheme for detection of lung nodules in chest radiographs, achieving sensitivity of 70.5% and 4.9 false positives per image in PA views only, 60.7% sensitivity and 1.7 false positives per image in lateral views only, and 86.9% sensitivity and 6.6 false positives in combination of PA and lateral views [2]. They concluded that the CAD scheme by the use of lateral-view images had the potential to improve the overall performance for detection of lung nodules on chest radiographs when combined with a conventional CAD scheme for standard PA views.

Chest tomosynthesis once was considered as an evolutionary technique with the potential of substantial improvement over chest radiography for evaluation of subtle lung diseases by providing reconstructed sectional images and overcoming the interferences from overlapping structures. Prior to the advent of chest CT scans, chest tomosynthesis was used frequently to evaluate suspected pulmonary nodules. However, due to operational complexity, positioning difficulty, and poor image quality, this technique was quickly abandoned with the clinical adaption of computed tomography. In the past decade, tomosynthesis revived with the contributions from advances in computer science, digital detector, and reconstruction algorithm. And digital tomosynthesis (DT) has been developed with simplified operation and improved image quality, which echoes the increasing concern about radiation dose from CT [3]. DT uses a set of projection images acquired as the X-ray tube moves along a presetting path to reconstruct multiple sectional images, which improves the visibility of anatomy compared with radiographic imaging. A recent study evaluated DT and conventional chest radiography for the detection and management of pulmonary nodules. The results showed that DT outperformed conventional radiography in all nodule size categories, case-level sensitivity, and case management decision-making assistance owing to a reduction in anatomical noise or composite artifact, better depth localization, and contrast resolution. In comparison to CT, DT has advantages in aspects of low cost and less radiation dose. DT has various clinical applications, including as a case-solving technique in the diagnosis of equivocal or suspected pulmonary lesions on chest radiography, as a tool for the intrapulmonary metastasis surveillance for patients with malignancies, and as a tool for the follow-up of pulmonary nodules and lung cancer screening detection.

3.1.2 Computed Tomography (CT)

3.1.2.1 Conventional CT

CT has a higher density resolution than conventional radiography (0.2% versus 5%). In chest radiography, overlapping structures are projected in a two-dimensional film or screen which apparently causes difficulty in detecting small lesions, either intrapulmonary or extrapulmonary. However, the cross-sectional imaging acquisition and sophisticated post-processing techniques in CT provide comprehensive information of normal anatomies and abnormalities with little interference from adjacent structures. Therefore, CT has been the indispensable and the most valuable imaging modality for evaluation of thoracic diseases. With administration of contrast media, CT imaging could provide additional information related to vasculatures for assessment and differential diagnosis of suspected pulmonary nodular diseases. The essence of thoracic CT imaging can be summarized as "scanning with thin-slice thickness, applying contrast media, quantitative measurement, and image post-processing." It has been suggested that LDCT should replace conventional radiography as the imaging tool for lung cancer screening. The vast majority of early-stage adenocarcinoma less than 10 mm in diameter with a ground-glass feature (AIS or MIA, probably) may have negative signs in conventional radiography and PET imaging. In addition, amounting evidence has shown that the detection rate of small lung cancer within nonsmoking, over 40-year-old females, especially those in menopause, rises quickly. Whether the NCCN guidelines on lung cancer screening should be revised to include this vulnerable population merits further investigation and discussion.

As the major precedent in lung cancer screening using CT, the Early Lung Cancer Action Project (ELCAP) initiated the first large-scale study of the early diagnosis of lung cancer in 31,567 cigarette smokers with the use of annual screening in 1993, involving more than 38 institutions for 7 countries [4]. After a long-term follow-up, a total of 484 lung cancers were screened out, and 86% were clinical stage I disease. Of the 375 participants who underwent resection (producing the estimated overall cure rate of 80%), 347 had pathological stage I cancer, and their estimated 10-year survival rate was 94%. The operative mortality rate is as low as 0.5%. This study provides solid evidence that CT screening can dramatically improve the early detection rate of small lung cancer by up to 80% for clinical stage I. Inspired by I-ELCAP, multiple international lung cancer screening trials have been conducted, including National Lung Screening Trial, which will be discussed in the following section.

3.1.2.2 CT Angiography (CTA)

As one of the important CT applications, CTA requires bolus injection of contrast agent from peripheral veins and fast acquisition of thin-slice imaging with full coverage of regions of interest. Multiplanar reformation and other post-processing techniques are employed to facilitate better visualization of vasculatures and/or lesions. CTA is safe, noninvasive, and readily used for assessment of veins, arteries, and parenchyma with dependent on acquisition time. In comparison to Doppler ultrasound and magnetic resonance angiography (MRA), CTA possesses several advantages including excellent quality of reformatted imaging; multidimensional displays; less subject to motion artifacts from respiration, swallowing, or peristalses; and differential diagnosis of vascular plaques. Angiogenesis plays critical roles in tumor development. Thus, accurate recognition of vascular changes is essential for tumor assessment.

3.1.2.3 Clinical Applications of Image Post-processing

Primary axial CT images are reconstructed using raw scanning data. Based on axial images, multiplanar images could be reformatted and displayed in two-dimensional or three-dimensional view, including MPR, CPR, SSD, VR, MIP,

Table 3.1 Comparison of commonly used image post-processing techniques

Technique	Indications	Advantages	Limitations
Multiplanar reformation (MPR)	Whole-body imaging	No learning curve required. Should be part of the routine image review for almost every type of examination. It is often used in daily CT as supplements to regular cross-sectional images	Not a 3D imaging technique
Maximum intensity projection (MIP)	Blood vessels	Versatile, simple, and quick technique to demonstrate vessels. Combining with the MIP slab to show more or less anatomical structures	Dense structures in the same images, such as bones, may obscure the vessels dense vessel calcification renders MIP images almost useless
Curved planar reformations (CPR)	Tortuous and calcified vessels, pancreas, bile ducts, ureters, spine, mandible, and many others	Single best way to show a luminal narrowing in calcified or tortuous vessels or stent patency	Can be time-consuming and cumbersome to generate images if automated software not available
Surface shaded display (SSD)	Musculoskeletal (MSK) imaging	An excellent 3D technique to demonstrate anatomy and pathology of osseous structures	Inside part of the structures cannot be viewed, and greatly affected by the threshold, easy to create a false image
Volume rendering (VD)	Any examination that would benefit from 3D imaging	Most versatile and useful 3D imaging technique. Can benefit a wide range of vascular and nonvascular cases, particularly when combined with effective segmentation techniques	Vessel calcification is a significant limitation effective use improves significantly with experience
CT virtual endoscopy (CTVE)	Colon, airways, blood vessels, and other hollow organs	Allows the user to look inside a blood vessel or hollow organ at the surface of that structure	Use limited to certain types of examinations. Can be time-consuming to be used effectively

and CTVE. Table 3.1 summarizes the advantages and disadvantages of these image post-processing techniques and clinical applications. Again, the distinction between reconstruction and reformation is the usage of raw imaging data or reconstructed images. To be emphasized, for those small pulmonary lesions less than 10 mm, proper combination of post-processing techniques in addition to axial imaging is essential for recognition and characterization of subtle features.

3.1.2.4 Spectral CT

Energy spectral imaging represents a significant advance in CT acquisition and reconstruction techniques. The same object is simultaneously scanned by two energy levels of X-rays. In GE-manufactured CT, a technique called fast kV switching between 80 and 140 kVp is utilized, while in Siemens-manufactured CT, the imaging acquisition is implemented with dual sources of 80 and 120 kVp. Datasets acquired could be used to reconstructed images corresponding to each integral energy level from 40 keV through 120 or 140 keV, hence monochromatic spectral imaging. Unlike the conventional single kVp images, in monochromatic imaging, images corresponding to any specified photon energy (keV) can be reconstructed based on CT scan data. At a given keV, the characteristics of the object are revealed as if it was imaged with a monochromatic beam at the same keV. The merits of monochromatic imaging include less radiation dose, improved contrast-to-noise ratio, accurate quantification of the images, and images free of beam hardening-related artifacts. Monochromatic imaging allows examination of tissues that attenuate multiple energy level X-rays (hence, deriving of a HU curve), which will help differentiate tissues that have identical attenuation (CT HU numbers) with standard CT imaging. This approach had been proven with dual-energy CT imaging. However, monochromatic imaging expands this application by providing more energy level choices, which appears to render this approach more practical in comparison with previously reported results for dual-energy CT [5].

In thoracic imaging, spectral CT has shown promising results, especially in the differentiation of pulmonary nodules. A retrospective study with small samples revealed that there existed statistically significant differences in iodine concentration, spectral curve slope, and CT attenuation value at 40 keV between pneumonia and malignant tumors and between squamous carcinoma and adenocarcinoma. However, these results should be validated in well-designed, large-sample, double-blind randomized prospective clinical trials.

3.1.2.5 CT Perfusion Imaging

Perfusion is the transport of blood to a unit volume of tissue per unit of time and usually refers to the blood transport at the capillary level. CT perfusion is based on the increase and subsequent decrease of contrast agent concentrations in tissues as a function of time [6]. Perfusion imaging has controversial values in differential assessment of small lung cancer, especially those presenting as ground-glass opacities. Pontana et al. investigated the feasibility of lung perfusion with dual-energy multidetector row CT in recognizing ground-glass opacities of vascular origin instead of bronchioloalveolar origin [7]. Another study from Lv et al. showed that in combination with morphological features of ground-glass nodules, perfusion-weighted CT imaging could provide additional information (such as blood flow, blood volume, mean transit time, and permeability surface related to nodules) for better differentiation between malignant and benign lesions [8]. However, perfusion imaging has inherent limitations. Among them, the high radiation exposure is one of the most serious issues with this technique. In the context of early detection and screening programs, exposure to high radiation is not acceptable. In addition, the lack of standards on CT perfusion data acquisition and reporting has been another challenge for a more widespread use of CT perfusion imaging, which affects the reproducibility of any reported results related to perfusion studies. The last but not the least, since tumors are spatially and temporally heterogeneous, functional assessment derived from a single tumor level (or time) may not reflect perfusion in the tumor as a whole. Overall, as a promising technique, CT perfusion has roles in early diagnosis of lung cancers and assessment of therapeutic efficacies, but several issues such as radiation dose, reproducibility, protocol standardization, and motion correction need to be solved.

3.1.3 Image Post-processing for Assessment of Small-Sized Pulmonary Nodules

Advances in CT imaging techniques not only improve the detection rate of pulmonary nodules but also push the minimal size of detected nodules to new levels. Currently, with the submillimeter-thickness images, 1–2 mm nodules can be visualized, and more nodules of larger than 3 or 4 mm are reported. Radiologically, traditional experiences in the analysis of pulmonary nodules, such as lobulation and spiculation, may not be applicable in the evaluation of these subcentimeter nodules. For accurate analysis of these small-sized nodules, sophisticated imaging techniques and protocols are required, from data acquisition to reconstruction to image post-processing. And image post-processing may be more frequently utilized in the analysis of subcentimeter nodules than larger nodules. Since most of subcentimeter lung cancers are in a preinvasive or minimally invasive stage, pulmonary parenchyma or alveolar structures are preserved to some extent. To detect those subtle changes from very early-stage lung cancers, radiologists should be extremely cautious and experienced in image post-processing.

Multidetector 16-slice and above CT scaners with isotropic acquisition and reconstruction have dramatically improved image quality of multiplanar reformations, which obviously benefit comprehensive assessment of nodules from any direction if necessary or even use a curved reformation to better track the relationship between nodules and tubular structures such as bronchus or blood vessel. To obtain better quality of reformatted images, a dataset of images reconstructed with thin-slice thickness ($\leq$1 mm preferred) should be stored in workstations or PACS system immediately following the acquisition of raw data. Otherwise, once the raw data has been deleted from the CT workstation, it is impossible to conduct reconstruction. As a routine protocol in our radiology department, 1 mm slice thickness images are reconstructed with overlap over 50% immediately after imaging acquisition and sent to PACS for archiving.

Analysis of the relationship between subcentimeter nodules and blood vessels is much more valuable than larger nodules. As addressed above, subcentimeter nodules may represent the very early-stage lung cancer, and their development demands recruitment of new blood vessels from pre-existing vessels in surrounding tissues (known as sprouting angiogenesis). The presence or detection of sprouting vessels is a reliable imaging feature characteristic of a potential lung cancer. Three-dimensional images would be helpful to recognize angiogenesis, especially in cases that the paths of new vessels are perpendicular to the scanning plane. Among multiplanar reformations, curved planar reformation (CPR) probably is the best method for evaluation of vessels and their relationship with suspected nodules. Technically, CPR is a way to display tubular structures for diagnostic purposes by generating longitudinal cross sections in order to show their lumen, wall, and surrounding tissue in a curved plane. The CPR operation requires training and knowledge of pulmonary vessels (Fig. 3.2). The post-processing workstations and protocols may vary among commercial providers. If the relationship between nodules and vessels cannot be determined in CPR images, which may occur occasionally, a combination of other views such as MIP may be helpful to get a better result.

For those nodules with solid components, three-dimensional display with the assistance of volume rendering could be useful to better understand the shape, margin, and volume of nodules and the nodule-lung interface. And the nodular volume could be used in the follow-up evaluation by calculation of volume doubling time. And tumor volume has been reported as a much more sensitive and accurate parameter for assessment of tumor growth than dimensional measurement. In addition, three-dimensional rendering of bronchial and vascular images facilitates accurate localization of lesions and recognition of bronchial or vascular variants or abnormalities for planning surgical procedures.

3.2 Low-Dose CT in Lung Cancer Screening

Radioactivity is present throughout the universe. Besides common resources such as cosmic radiation, terrestrial radiation sources (e.g., uranium, thorium, and radium in the soil and building materials), radon, and medical radiation examination, many consumer products have trace concentration of radioactivity. For example, anything rich in potassium, such as bananas and salt substitutes, has certain concentrations of ^{40}K, and it is estimated that the radiation exposure from consuming a banana (150 g) is approximately 0.0001 mSv, 1% of the average daily exposure to radiation. Hence, the banana equivalent dose (BED) is used to indicate certain radiation exposure for educational purpose. This external and ingested radiation collectively contributes to each of our personal doses throughout life. Table 3.2 lists radiation doses received in certain daily living activities or radiation accidents.

Radiation exposure has long been proven to be carcinogenesis, and there exists a stochastic effect between radiation dose and cancer risk which may vary with individuals receiving the same amount of dose. As the primary target of ionizing radia-

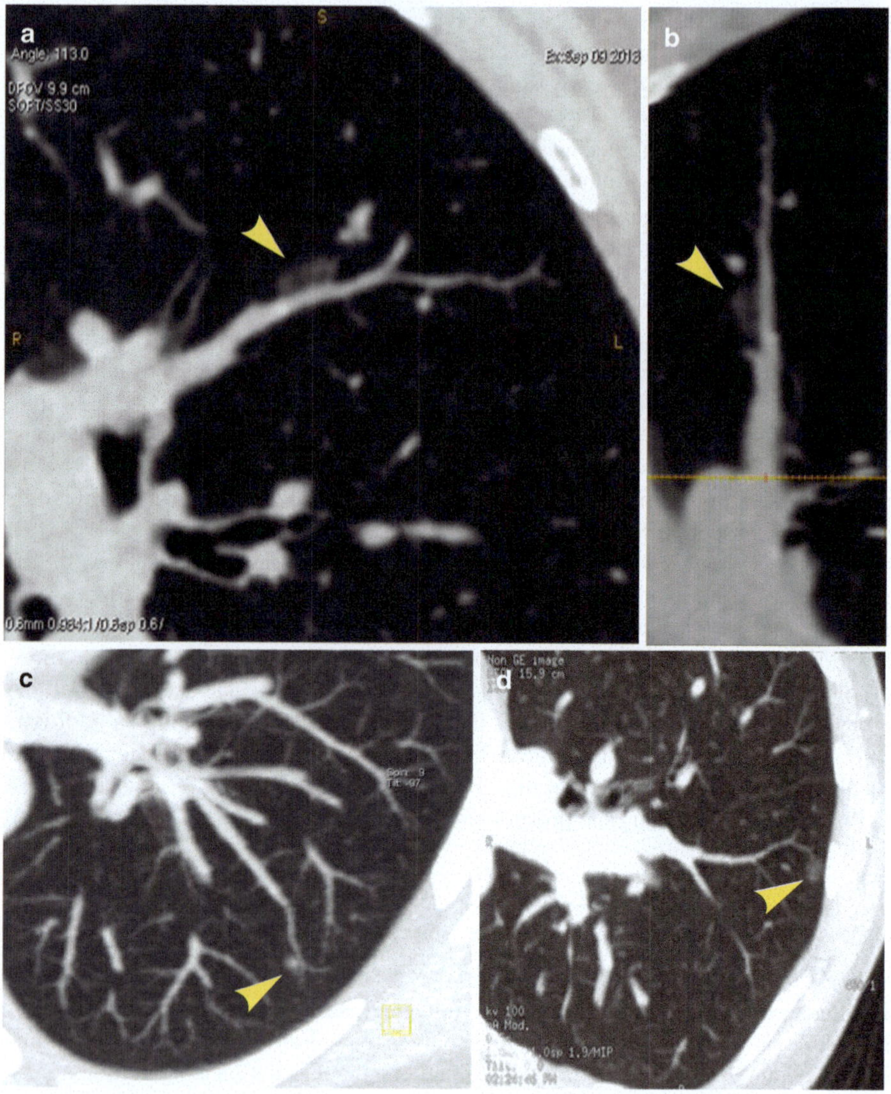

Fig. 3.2 Image post-processing for small pulmonary nodules. (**a**, **b**) A small part-solid ground-glass nodule (arrowhead) abuts a vessel in the left upper lobe (**a** Stretched CPR view of the vessel, **b** straightened CPR view of the vessel). (**c**, **d**) A small subpleural ground-glass nodule (arrowhead) is seen in the left lower lobe (**c** MIP image, **d** stretched CPR view of the adjacent vessel)

tion, nuclear DNA could be induced to produce single-strand breaks or double-strand breaks, which if not properly and promptly repaired would cause cell death or mutation leading to cancer in the future (10–20 years later). Worldwide, the annual radiation dose from natural sources by an adult is in the range of 2.0–4.0 mSv, and in China, it is approximately 2.3 mSv.

Table 3.2 Radiation exposures in daily living or accidents

Radiation source	Dose (mSv)
Eating one banana (150 g)	0.0001
Watching TV 2 h per day for a year	0.001
Living within 5 miles of a nuclear power plant for a year	0.001~0.02
1-hour airplane flight	0.01
A PA chest X-ray	0.02
Yearly limit on radiation exposure to a single person	1
Normal yearly background dose (about 85% is from natural sources, and the rest is from medical scans)	~4
Radiation worker 1-year dose limit	50
Severe radiation poisoning, in some cases fatal	2000~4000
Death (fatal radiation)	>4000

Source: https://en.wikipedia.org/wiki/Banana_equivalent_dose

Modern medicine has increasing reliance on diagnostic imaging, every aspect from disease diagnosis to treatment evaluation. More than a half of diagnostic imaging examinations are performed using ionizing radiation-based modalities, such as radiography, CT, and nuclear medicine. As a consequence, patients receive increasing medical radiation exposure. In the early 1980s, the yearly per capita radiation dose was 3.6 mSv averaged over the US population. Medical radiation contributed only 0.54 mSv to this annual dose, with the remainder coming from radon, soil, construction materials, and cosmic rays. In 2006, medical radiation contributed 3 mSv to the annual dose, raising the per capita dose to 6.2 mSv averaged over the US population [9]. Advances in multidetector CT and post-processing have led to increased utilization of CT cross-sectional imaging to approximately 88 million scans in 2010, an over 20-fold increase since 1980. This increase has resulted in an ~600% increase in US per capita exposure to ionizing radiation from medical procedures from 1980 to 2006, with CT imaging contributing to nearly 50% of this increase.

3.2.1 Historical Views of Low-Dose CT

According to statistical data released by World Health Organization, the incidence and mortality of lung cancer in 2012 worldwide reached new high levels, approximately 1.8 million and 1.6 million, respectively. In coming decades, lung cancer will remain as the top malignancy in most countries and as the priority of cancer research. In comparison to chest radiography, CT has dramatically improved the management of lung cancer, from detection to staging to therapeutic assessment. Furthermore, CT-based lung cancer screening has been proven to be effective in early detection (subsequent intervention) of lung cancer in asymptomatic patients with or without cancer-related risks. In this context, advances in CT manufacturing technologies and scanning techniques to decrease radiation dose to patients are critically necessary. Hence, low-dose CT (LDCT) has been gaining more attention and clinical acceptance.

Actually, CT scanning with low-dose setting in clinics is not a novel or even recent idea. The first published article on low-dose CT scanning can be dated back to 1981. Rüegsegger et al. [10] developed a special purpose low-dose CT system to quantify trabecular bone in patients suffering immobilization or postmenopausal osteoporosis for assessment of therapeutic response. Due to the limited tissue resolution, most of earliest LDCT studies in the 1980s were in the field of orthopedics, such as evaluation of osteoporosis, bone development in pediatric patients, and pelvimetry.

The first report on LDCT for lungs was published in 1990. In this study, Naidich et al. [11] assessed two sets of images obtained at routine scanning settings (120 kVp, 140 mAs) and low-dose settings (120 kVp, 10 mAs) regarding the clarity of lung anatomy, the presence of artifacts, and the extent of graininess. Their results showed that high-quality, diagnostic images of the lung could be obtained with a very low radiation dose and the visualization of parenchymal structures was not affected, thanks to inherent excellent contrast in the lungs. As the conclusion, low-dose CT was indicated as a screening procedure, in particular for populations at high risk for developing lung cancer, and for use in the pediatric population. This would be the first time that LDCT was suggested for lung cancer screening. Ever since, LDCT has been gradually utilized in assessment of lung diseases and even expanded into extrathoracic sites. One of the frequent concerns with LDCT is the imaging sensitivity, i.e., whether CT images with lower dose would omit small lesions and compromise the diagnostic accuracy. Many investigators have conducted researches on the impact of low-dose settings (e.g., 40 mAs, 80 mAs) on lung CT image quality and diagnostic consistency in comparison to routine scans. Zwirewich et al. evaluated the efficacy of high-resolution LDCT in the assessment of lung parenchyma [12]. There was no significant difference in performance between LDCT and conventional scans on visualization of vessels, bronchi, and anatomy of secondary pulmonary lobules, and on characterization of the extent and distribution of reticulation, honeycomb cysts, and thickened interlobular septa. LDCT might have low performance in the evaluation of subtle pulmonary changes, such as ground-glass opacity (failure rate, 20%) and emphysema (failure rate, 11%), which, however, was not statistically different from conventional scans. Both scans were judged equally diagnostic in 97% of cases. Lee et al. compared the accuracy of thin-section LDCT to thin-section conventional CT in the diagnosis of chronic infiltrative lung disease (CILD) and found a high confidence level in the diagnosis of 61% versus 63% and accuracy of 90% versus 96% without statistical significance [13].

In early years, image noise and artifacts were severe in LDCT images, which in some cases could affect final image interpretation. With the advances in computer technology and CT hardware in the past decades, numerous improvements have been achieved in LDCT at every aspect, such as image quality, acquisition time, radiation dose, and noise inhibition. Most of mainstream CT machines have integrated LDCT scanning mode and adaptive statistical iterative reconstruction for individualized CT scanning and radiation dose optimization/minimization. Recently, concepts such as "green CT" or "ultralow-dose CT" have been proposed or advertised in magazines or brochures by some CT manufacturers, which reflects the technological advancement, meanwhile inevitably causing conceptual confusion due to inconsistent terminology.

3.2.2 The Definition of Low-Dose CT

Despite that the term of LDCT has been used for more than three decades, there lacks a consistent and scientific definition for LDCT. According to "the NCCN Guidelines: Lung Cancer Screening," the radiation dose from LDCT is 10–30% of the dose from conventional CT scans. Specifically, LDCT scanning protocol should include at least the following parameters: in a small patient with BMI $\leq$ 30, acquisition with 100–20 kVp and $\leq$40 mAs and total radiation exposure $\leq$3 mSv and in a large patient with BMI > 30, acquisition with 120 kVp and $\leq$60 mAs and total radiation exposure $\leq$5 mSv (Fig. 3.3). Other prerequisites include CT scanner detectors ($\geq$16), scan acquisition time ($\leq$10 s), slice width ($\leq$1.5 mm), slice interval ($\leq$slice width), and maximum inspiration. Recently, ultralow-dose CT (ULDCT) scanning has been proposed. ULDCT uses a radiation dose level equivalent to chest X-ray with iterative reconstruction technique but preserves nodular detectability on chest CT images. The radiation dose with ULDCT could be as low as 0.2 mSv, one tenth of the dose from LDCT.

3.2.3 The Benefits of LDCT Screening for Lung Cancer

Lung cancer screening using helical LDCT scans has many benefits especially for individuals at an increased risk for lung cancer, including decreased lung cancer mortality, improvement of the quality of life or lifestyles, and collateral gains from detection of extrapulmonary diseases that require treatment.

As the most influential clinical trial on lung cancer screening using LDCT, the National Lung Screening Trial (NLST) recruited 53,454 patients with high-risk factors of lung cancer to compare the efficacy of LDCT in comparison to chest radiography [14]. The rate of positive screening tests was 24.2% with low-dose CT and 6.9% with radiography. The incidence of and deaths from lung cancer in the LDCT group were 645 and 247 per 100,000 person-years and 572 and 309 in the radiography group, which was converted to a relative reduction of 20% in mortality from lung cancer with LDCT. According to a recent study, assuming the screening regimens adopted in the NLST are fully implemented in the United States, effective lung cancer screening may prevent more than 12,000 premature lung cancer deaths per year.

In addition to NLST, two European randomized trials, the Dutch-Belgian NELSON trial and UK Lung Screen (UKLS), are designed to assess LDCT screening for lung cancer. The UKLS pilot trial demonstrated that it is possible to detect lung cancer at an early stage and deliver potentially curative treatment in over 80%

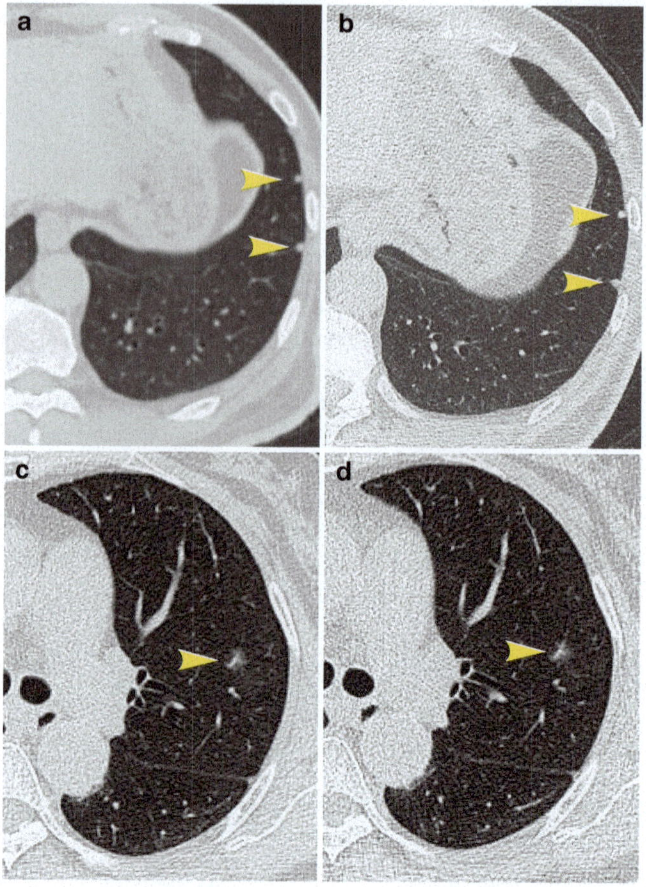

Fig. 3.3 Comparative study of radiation dose and image quality of routine CT (imaging parameter, 100 kVp, 80 mAs, 5 mm slice thickness) and LDCT (imaging parameter, 100 kVp, 40 mAs, 5-mm slice thickness). (**a**, **b**) A small nodular lesion (arrowhead) was seen in a 64-year-old male patient. (**a**), routine CT (DLP 161 mGy cm = 2.2 mSv); (**b**), LDCT (DLP 25 mGy cm = 0.35 mSv). (**c**, **d**) A 69-year-old female patient received right upper lobectomy for lung cancer in 2012. On 1-year follow-up CT, a ground-glass opacity (arrowhead) was found in the left upper lobe. Five months later, another follow-up CT was performed. (**a**), routine CT (DLP 105 mGy cm = 1.47 mSv); (**b**), LDCT (DLP 35 mGy cm = 0.49 mSv)

of cases [15]. Results of the Nelson and UKLS trials confirm the NLST findings of the superiority of LDCT screening over radiotherapy in separate cohorts. With LDCT screening, the detection rate of stage IA lung cancer increases from 35.1% to 93%. In combination with the results from the nonrandomized single-armed I-ELCAP study, LDCT is undoubtedly the most effective screening tool for early detection of lung cancer with adequate sensitivity and accuracy and acceptable radiation dose.

Besides the direct benefit of reducing lung cancer mortality, the adoption of LDCT screening would increase the awareness of lung cancer and risks related to lung cancer in public. The detection rate of any pulmonary nodule is as high as 80% in persons receiving LDCT scans. Most of these nodules are benign possibly related to the medical history of tuberculosis, pneumonitis, asymptomatic inflammation, or other benign processes. Some patients may seek medical counseling, which could be an opportunity for education of lung cancer and lifestyle improvement, in particular smoking cessation for smokers. According to a study conducted by Townsend et al. on the impacts of CT screening on smoking cessation, smokers with abnormal CT findings were more likely to be abstinent from smoking. Hence, low-dose chest CT screenings could be an effective persuasive weapon for smoking cessation and represent teachable opportunities to enhance motivation for smoking abstinence [16].

3.2.4 The Potential Harms of LDCT Screening for Lung Cancer

Certainly, lung cancer screening may do harms to individuals. These harms or controversies are related to several aspects: the safety of multiple LDCT scanning and the secondary cancer risk from radiation exposure, overdiagnosis, unnecessary testing or procedures due to false-positive results, underdiagnosis due to false-negative results, economic burden to the individual and society, and psychological stress.

Croswell et al. conducted a randomized trial to estimate rates of cumulative false-positive results in LDCT screening and unnecessary diagnostic procedures. Risks for false-positive results on LDCT lung cancer screening tests are substantial, 21% after one screening and 33% after two screenings, leading to a total of 7% of participants with false-positive results receiving invasive procedures. In addition, false-positive results increase the probability of further overuse of imaging examinations, such as conventional chest CT with or without contrast media and PET/CT, which imposes more radiation exposure as well as economic burdens to patients.

Some collateral benefits from lung cancer screening may not be just beneficial. Patients with asymptomatic pneumonitis may receive antibiotics for prophylaxis. Some patients with coronary artery calcifications may be recommended for further cardiac CT imaging to exclude potential soft plaques. These collateral findings plus incidentally detectable benign or indeterminate pulmonary nodules could cause psychological stress in some patients.

3.2.5 The Strategies for Optimization of LDCT Screening for Lung Cancer

Lung cancer screening using LDCT has potential benefits and harms. So the question is how to implement LDCT screening properly. Apparently, those abovementioned factors related to benefits and harms should be taken into consideration and balanced to generate an individualized screening strategy.

1. Is LDCT lung cancer screening really needed?
   The answer to this question is straightforward. The NLST trial showed that 40% of cancers detected in LDCT screening arm were stage IA, in comparison with 21% in radiography group. Apparently, lung cancer screening using LDCT improves early detection and subsequent therapeutic outcomes and prognosis.
2. Are there better approaches than LDCT for lung cancer screening?
   A useful and efficient screening tool should be affordable and easy to administer, widely available to the population for which it is intended, of adequate sensitivity and specificity, and highly reproducible. Many approaches have been investigated as screening tools for lung cancer, including conventional radiography, sputum cytology, biomarkers from blood and exhaled breath, and autofluorescence bronchoscopy. Except for LDCT, most of these modalities have been proven to be low-throughput for screening purpose or are not yet commercially available in clinic setting. Currently, the position of LDCT as the screening approach for lung cancer is solid and unreplaceable.
3. How to solve problems related to false-positive and false-negative results and overdiagnosis?
   In comparison to the high sensitivity of LDCT scans, specificity is relatively low. Specificity requires not only the performance of imaging acquisition but also more experiences and skills of radiologists on differential diagnosis of suspected lesions. In the NCCN guidelines on lung cancer screening, false-positive and false-negative phenomena in LDCT screening have been discussed in detail. In brief, false-positive rate of noncalcified nodules larger than 4 mm on LDCT screening of high-risk populations is in 10–43% range. The false-negative rate currently is unavailable. Detection errors could be due to subtle lesions, lesions overlapping with normal pulmonary structures, or disturbance from evident pre-existing lung diseases, such as tuberculosis, emphysema, or postoperative changes (Fig. 3.4). More training on CT interpretation and interactive discussion on suspicious cases, in combination with the use of computer-assisted diagnosis system if possible, may help to decrease false-positive and false-negative results.

   Overdiagnosis refers to histologically confirmed lung cancers identified through screening that would not affect the patient's lifetime if left untreated. Overdiagnosis and related overtreatment have been extensively discussed in prostate cancer, the top malignancy in men in western countries, leading to the strategy of active surveillance for low-risk patients and reserving treatment for only those patients whose tumors show evidence of progression. Earlier studies suggested that chest radiograph screening might have an overdiagnosis rate of roughly 25%. The overdiagnosis rate for LDCT screening cannot yet be estimated and cannot be completely eliminated. It is believed to be most probably in the 2–10% range. The number of overdiagnosed cancers can be further reduced to less than 5% with careful exclusion of indolent lesions based on CT imaging features and growth rate. Again, improvements in interpretation skills of CT imaging are favorable to reduce overdiagnosis.

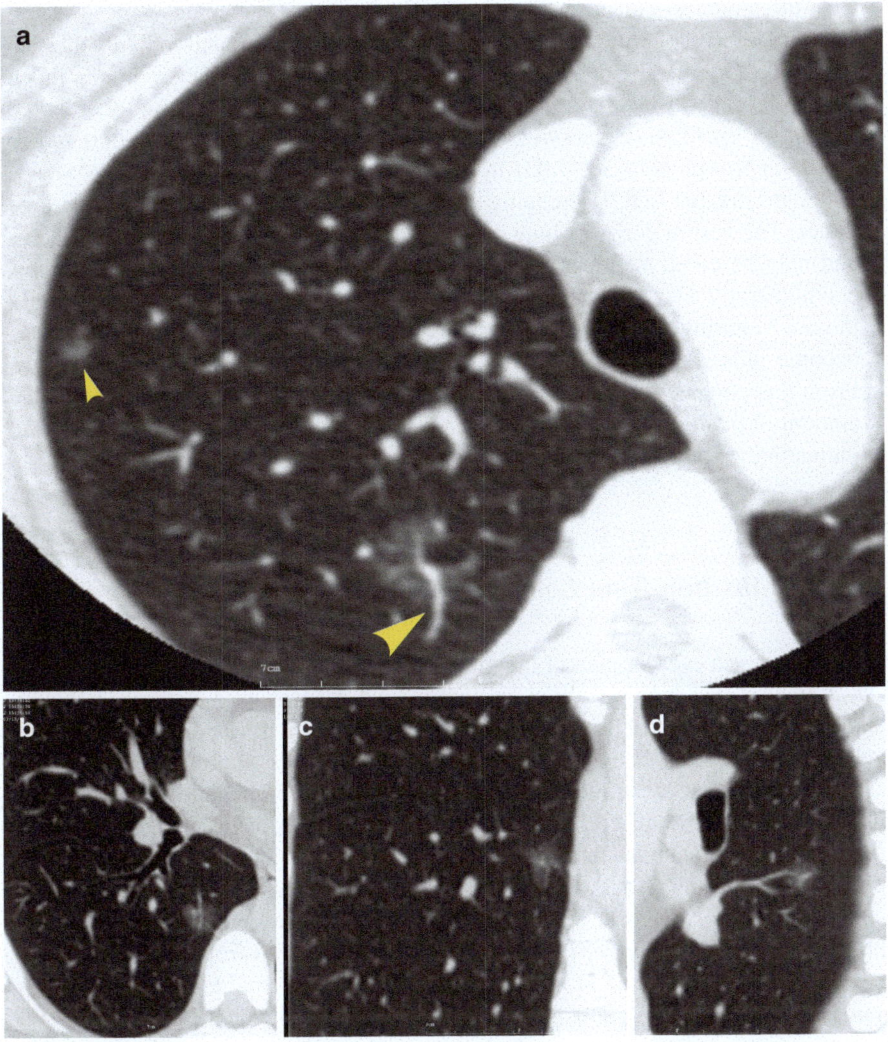

Fig. 3.4 AIS detected in LDCT lung cancer screening. (**a**) Two nodular lesions were found in the left upper lobe. The pure GGN in the subpleural region was measured 3 mm in diameter without microvascular migration, indicative of AAH; the semisolid GGN (arrowhead) close to thoracic vertebrae was 10 mm in diameter with evident microvascular (connect) connection, indicative of AIS, proven by surgical pathology. (**b–d**) A 6 mm mGGN was seen in the paravertebral region of the superior segment of the right lower lobe. Contrast-enhancement CT showed microvascular migration into the lesion in the axial view (**b**) and the characteristic CTA-TA sign in MPR images (**c**, **d**), indicative of AIS. The lesion was resected via VATS and pathologically proved to be AIS

4. Cost-effectiveness considerations in LDCT lung cancer screening.
   The increased economic burden on both healthcare system and individuals is an inevitable topic in the debate of lung cancer screening. However, this is much more relevant in western countries than in China. Taking China and the United States, for example, the service fee for an LDCT chest scan and report is 200 RMB (approximately 30 USD) in China and 527 USD in the United States, which means that LDCT screening in China costs only 1/17 of that in the United States. The vast majority of lung cancers detected in screening are in early stage and may be cured with surgery alone, and no adjuvant therapy (radiotherapy, chemotherapy, even targeted therapy) is required. In many countries, especially those developing countries, the expense in the treatment of advanced cancers has become unbearable burdens, economically, emotionally, and psychologically. From this perspective, LDCT screening at a small cost will save a considerable amount of healthcare resources, preserve the quality of life of the sufferers, and maintain the stability of suffered families.

3.2.6 Transition from Low Dose to Right Dose

With advances in every aspect of imaging acquisition and processing, the quality of LDCT images has achieved dramatic improvements. However, compared to conventional CT, LDCT still has some limitations, especially in visualization of spatial and temporal nuances. In assessment of pulmonary nodules, the sensitivity of LDCT is size-related: 67%, 89%, and 100% for those <3 mm, 4–5 mm, and >6 mm, respectively. This sensitivity discrepancy should be taken into consideration when LDCT images are interpreted and analyzed.

Theoretically, any dose level of radiation exposure has a risk of secondary malignancy, hence the stochastic effect (Fig. 3.5). As discussed previously, in the past three decades, the yearly per capita radiation dose received from medical purpose increases by 500%, from 0.54 mSv to 3 mSv. Healthcare providers have put a great endeavor to study the relationship between exposure of medical radiation and secondary cancers, and no clear conclusion has been reached. No prospective epidemiologic study with nonirradiated control subjects has quantitatively demonstrated adverse effects of radiation at doses less than about 100 mSv. However, social media widely and fanatically report that any articles suggesting radiation, as used in medicine, is harmful and can cause cancer, which to some extent misleads the public and even physicians other than radiologists to avoid CT examinations even if strongly indicated, and may do real harms to patients. The risks of radiation exposure in medical imaging should not be either neglected or exaggerated. Technological advances have created LDCT scanning techniques and will continue pushing the radiation dose to a new low level.

Low-dose scanning or LDCT has been one of the most misused radiological terms. In the editorial of Radiology, Bankier and Kressel analyzed the usage of LDCT in scientific articles, "Any definition of low dose is substantially limited by

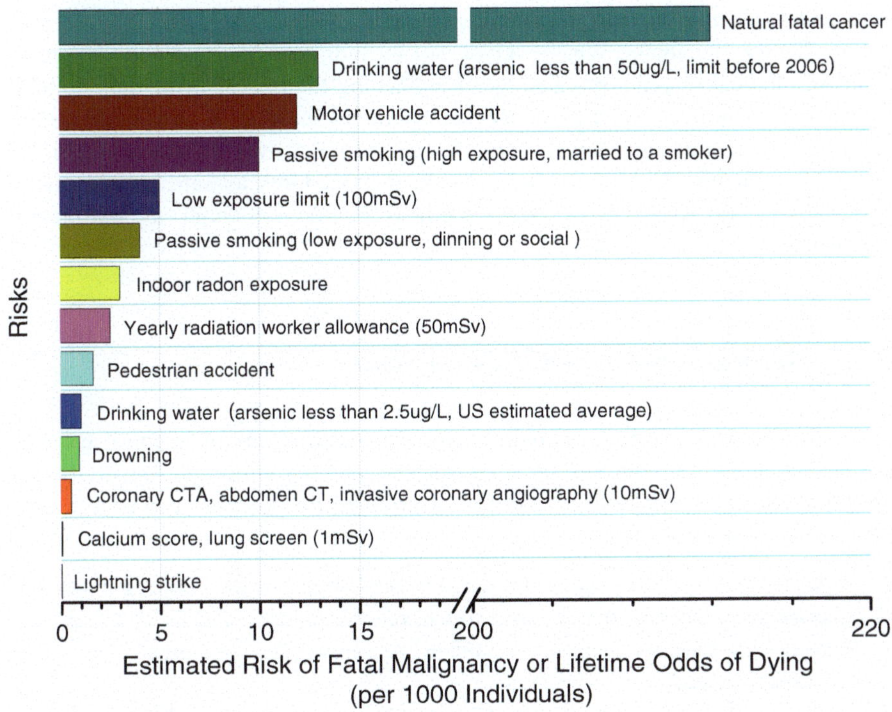

Fig. 3.5 Estimated risks of fatal malignancy or death resulting from radiation exposure and the lifetime odds of dying as a result of selected activities of everyday life (From *Gerber TC, et al. Circulation, 2009, 119:1056–65*. Reprinted with permission)

its relativistic foundation" [17]. According to them, the descriptive term of low dose should be abandoned and substituted with reporting comparable, accurate, and measurable dose-related parameters, including volume CT dose index (CTDIvol), dose length product (DLP), the size-specific dose estimate (SSDE), and effective diameter. The authors believed that rather than vague qualifiers, these parameters would warrant the clinical applicability and reproducibility of radiological studies, especially those related to dose comparison.

For many decades, all radiation exposures in medical practices are governed by the ALARA (as low as reasonably achievable) principle for radiation protection by minimizing all exposure and applying limits for controlling occupational and general public exposures. This principle implies that no unnecessary exposure should be allowed, no exposure at all should be permitted without considering the benefits, and equipment and facilities should be designed so that exposure of personnel and the public is kept to a minimum and not up to a standard. However, the ultimate problem is determining what is "reasonable." There is also the question: How much expense is justified to reduce the exposure of personnel by a given amount? The practice of extremely reducing radiation dose at the cost of diagnostic accuracy is not acceptable and against ethics, because that could put the patient at the risk of receiving more radiation instead due to repeated scanning. Therefore, the low radiation dose is not the sole goal in the usage of medical radiation. Initiatives, such as Image Gently and Image Wisely, advocated by radiological organizations aim to improve medical imaging practice by strengthening the rule of using only enough radiation to acquire needed diagnostic information, in other words, applying the right dose to capture the right images. Besides ALARA, two additional principles are recommended, ASARA (to keep medical procedures as safe as reasonably achievable) and AHARA (to keep medical benefits as high as reasonably achievable).

3.2.7 Indications for LDCT Chest Scan

Retrospective and prospective studies have showed that low-dose spiral CT is a cost-effective and reliable tool for lung cancer screening with high sensitivity and specificity at an acceptable radiation dose. Currently, the consensus on LDCT indications has been generated, including:

1. High-risk populations (age in the range of 55–74 years old, smoking history of 30 pack-year, current smoker, etc.) should receive annual LDCT chest scan.
2. Nonsmoking females over 45 years old are recommended for annual LDCT lung cancer screening.
3. Patients with indeterminate solitary or multiple nodules could be followed up using LDCT. If suspicious of aggression, the lesion(s) should be reexamined using conventional CT with or without administration of contrast medium.
4. Follow-up and therapeutic assessment in patients with malignancies, either intrapulmonary or extrapulmonary.
5. CT-guided percutaneous biopsy of intrapulmonary lesions.
6. Infant and children patients if CT scanning is required.
7. Other extrathoracic anatomies with excellent inherent contrast, such as sinuses and bones, may be examined using LDCT scanning mode.

3.3 Lung Cancer Screening: Guidelines and Beyond

A malignancy can be better prognostic if given treatment in an earlier stage. Cancer screening intends to advance cancer detection to an earlier stage to initiate effective (definitive mostly) treatments timely and improve overall treatment outcomes ultimately. Several malignancies can be effectively screened using currently available imaging techniques and/or blood tests, including cervical cancer, colon cancer, breast cancer, and lung cancer. Worldwide, large-scale randomized lung screening studies have been conducted, and results confirmed the effectiveness of lung cancer screening. In 2011, the results of lung cancer screening in the Prostate, Lung, Colorectal, and Ovarian (PLCO) Cancer Screening Trial were reported with conclusion that annual chest radiographic screening for 3–4 years did not show any effect on the cumulative lung cancer mortality during a 13-year follow-up period, which was once considered a hit on lung cancer screening [18]. Specifically, what the PLCO trial proved is the minimal effectiveness of chest radiography in lung cancer screening instead of lung cancer screening itself. In the same year, the milestone National Lung Screening Trial (NLST) showed that a 20.0% decrease in mortality from lung cancer was observed in the low-dose CT group as compared with the radiography group, strongly supporting the effectiveness of lung cancer screening in reducing mortality and the value of low-dose CT as the screening tool. Since then, low-dose CT scan has been gradually accepted as the standard procedure for lung cancer screening with replacement of chest radiography. In the United States, the Centers for Medicare and Medicaid Services (CMS) issued a National Coverage Determination in early 2015 supporting annual lung cancer screening with LDCT for asymptomatic individuals aged 55–77 years who have a tobacco smoking history of at least 30 pack-years and who are either currently smoking or had quit less than 15 years earlier. In China, low-dose CT lung cancer screening has been included in the coverage of the national health system since 2010, much earlier than the United States.

With the worldwide adoption of LDCT for lung cancer screening, considering the much higher radiation exposure than chest radiography and the risk of radiation-induced secondary malignancy, many guidelines from authoritative organizations have been published. Among them, the National Comprehensive Cancer Network (NCCN) [19] is the first and updates the guideline regularly (annually or semiannually). The latest guideline is version 2.2018 with many updates from the previous version. The NCCN guideline has received supports and endorsement from multiple professional societies and governmental agencies, including the International Association for the Study of Lung Cancer (IASLC), US Preventive Services Task Force (USPSTF), American Cancer Society (ACS), and American College of Chest Physicians (ACCP).

3.3.1 Lung Cancer Risk Assessment

There are many risk factors related to lung cancer such as smoking history (previous or current), secondhand smoke exposure, radon gas exposure, occupation-related exposure, history of cancer, family history of cancer, chronic pulmonary disease (such as COPD, lung fibrosis, etc.), hormone replacement therapy, etc.

Tobacco smoking has long been considered as a major modifiable risk factor related to the development of lung cancer. And it is estimated that tobacco smoking may be accountable for 85% of all lung cancer-related deaths. Tobacco smoking is also associated with other cancers, such as bladder cancer, esophageal carcinoma, and pancreatic carcinoma. Each year, in the United States, about half a million of deaths in adults are smoking-related, while worldwide deaths from smoking tobacco-related diseases are predicted to be over 10 million by 2020. The first report on causal relationship between smoking and lung cancer could be dated back to 80 years ago. Despite the unceasing controversy, the link between the risk of developing lung cancer and the smoking habitat has been gradually established. Smoking cessation and tobacco control have remained the top priority of lung cancer control and prevention.

Among more than 7000 chemical compounds identified in tobacco smoke, more than 50 are known carcinogens. Besides, 93 chemicals found in tobacco products have been listed as harmful and potentially harmful constituents by the Food and Drug Administration. The risk rate for lung cancer in smokers is reported to be approximately 20-fold higher than in nonsmokers. Moreover, the risk cannot be immediately decreased by smoking cessation. The former smokers still hold a higher risk for lung cancer than never-smokers, and reportedly it may take 10–15 years for former smokers to have the similar risk to never-smokers.

Pack-year history of smoking (defined as packs of cigarettes smoked per day × years of smoking) is the common parameter used for measuring the smoking severity and stratification of smokers for analysis of the relationship between smoking and smoke-related lung cancer risk. In the NCCN guidelines and NLST clinical trial, individuals (aged 55–74 years) with a 30 or more pack-year history of smoking tobacco or less than 15 years smoking cessation are enrolled into the highest-risk group for lung cancer. Currently, reliable data are unavailable to support the relationship between secondhand smoke or passive smoke and lung cancer. Thus, secondhand smoke is not considered to confer a high risk for exposed individuals. As a result, these populations shall not be regarded as proper candidates for lung cancer screening in the NCCN guidelines.

Besides tobacco smoking, occupational history may have a certain link with the development of lung cancer. Some industrial chemical agents have been identified as carcinogens in the lungs, including arsenic, asbestos, nickel, beryllium, silica, etc. For population who have potential occupational exposure to these chemicals, the estimated mean risk rate for the development of lung cancer is 1.59 in comparison to those who have not. Among them, smokers have a much higher risk of lung cancer than nonsmokers.

History of malignancy has been reported a risk factor for lung cancer, probably also for any other cancers, partly due to intrinsic genetic susceptibility and toxicity from previous treatment, such as chemotherapy and/or radiation therapy. Lung cancer has been reported as a second primary tumor in patients with previous malignancies, such as lymphomas, head and neck cancers, lung cancers, and esophageal cancers. For example, those small lung cancer survivors could have a 3.5-fold increase in the risk for developing a new primary lung cancer, while chest radiation and administration of alkylating agents increase the relative risk by 12 and 8.4, respectively [20]. Family history of malignancy is another risk that should be taken into consideration. Despite being less significant than individual history of malignancy, clinical data suggested that those having first-degree relatives suffering from lung cancer faced an increased risk for lung cancer, a reported RR of 1.8. The lung cancer risk is increased in patients with pulmonary diseases (such as COPD and diffuse pulmonary fibrosis). The reason is related to the etiology of these chronic diseases, the same as previously mentioned smoke, occupational exposure history, etc.

Based on the available data, and NLST clinical trial data, the NCCN Panel stratifies population into three risk groups, high, moderate, or low risk for lung cancer

Table 3.3 Risk assessment of lung cancer according to the NCCN

Risk status	Risk factors
High risk	• Age 55–74 years, ≥30 pack-year history of smoking, and smoking cessation <15 years • Age ≥ 50 years and ≥20 pack-year history of smoking and coexisting additional risk factors that increase the predicted risk of lung cancer to ≥1.3%
Moderate risk	Age ≥ 50 years and ≥20 pack-year history of smoking or secondhand smoke exposure. No additional risk factors
Low risk	Age < 50 years and/or <20 pack-year history of smoking

(Table 3.3). And individuals with the high risk for lung cancer are strongly recommended for LDCT screening, while individuals at moderate- or low-risk groups may not gain benefits from screening in balance with the potential risks from radiation examination and collateral effects.

3.3.2 Age Impact on Lung Cancer Screening

The median age of lung cancer patients at diagnosis is 70 years. Approximately half of lung cancers are diagnosed in patients aged 55–74 years while less than one third in older patients aged 75–84 years. Therefore, it is uncertain by what age the lung cancer screening should stop. The NCCN guidelines acknowledge that individuals with high-risk factors who are older than 74 years are also eligible for LDCT screening. Recent recommendations from USPSTF recommend LDCT for individuals aged 55–80 years with high-risk factors. Thus, annual LDCT seems reasonable for those individuals with high-risk factors older than 74 years but having good performance status eligible for definitive treatment with curative intent, e.g., surgery, chemoradiation, or stereotactic body radiation therapy (SBRT). In other words, annual LDCT should not be canceled until individuals are no longer eligible for definitive treatment. The appropriate screening interval or frequency is not determined. Semiannual, annual, or biannual screening may be appropriate in certain population having nodules with different biological behaviors. Typically, a relative frequent screening procedure is recommended initially to calculate the volume doubling time as a measurement of biological behavior.

3.3.3 The Principles in Radiological Assessment of Pulmonary Nodules Detected in LDCT Screening

Depending on the internal characteristics of detected nodules, they can be classified into three types, i.e., solid nodule, part-solid nodule, and nonsolid nodule. Part-solid nodule is also named part-solid ground-glass nodule (pGGN) or mixed GGN (mGGN) or semisolid GGN (ssGGN). Likewise, the nonsolid nodule is also named pure GGN (pGGN). The probability of malignancy corresponding to three groups is 59%, 48%, and 11%, separately. Clinically, some of pGGN may be diminished spontaneously without any treatment during the follow-up, but the probability of malignancy for a persistent pGGN will be as high as up to 75% reported. Pathologically, the malignant pGGN frequently represents preinvasive diseases, AAH or AIS, occasionally MIA. The 10-year survival rate of preinvasive diseases with surgical resection is reported to be approximately 100%. Those mGGN and solid nodules, if malignant, usually are in more advanced stage than pGGN, likely MIA or invasive carcinoma. The 5-year survival rate is above 90% if standard surgical resection is performed. Hence, early detection and proper treatment improve the overall survival, which is believed the ultimate approach to cure lung cancer.

For an incidentally detected nodule, initial radiological assessment should be differential diagnosis between benign or malignant. What should be kept in mind is that the majority of initially detected pulmonary nodules are benign, probably resulting from previous pneumonia, or just idiopathic. Despite the excellent prognosis of surgical treatment in early-stage lung cancer, surgery should not be given to any nodules without definitive diagnosis or high probability of malignancy to avoid overtreatment or unnecessary thoracotomy. Some radiological features may be helpful in differentiating a suspected pulmonary nodule.

The volume doubling time (VDT) is an essential characteristic in differentiation of benign and malignant nodules by measuring growth rate. Benign lesions tend to grow very fast or slow with primary lung cancers in between. A prespecified analysis based on the NELSON trial conducted by Horeweg et al. showed that for nodules with a diameter of 5–10 mm or volume of 100–300 mm^2, VDT could be a reliable differential parameter. Those nodules with VDT more than 600 days are at neglectable risk of malignancy. In contrast, those with VDT less than 600 days should be closely monitored or further evaluated with other advanced imaging modalities or biopsy due to significantly increasing risk of lung cancer [21]. Specifically, the probabilities of malignancy in nodules with VDT $\geq$ 600 days, 400–600 days, or $\leq$400 days are 0.8% (0.4–1.7%), 4.0% (1.8–8.3%), and 9.9% (6.9–14.1%), respectively. Apparently, larger nodules have increasing risks with reported probability of 16.9% for nodules $\geq$300 mm^3 in volume and 15.2% for nodules $\geq$10 mm in diameter, warranting immediate diagnostic workups. Regarding size, lung cancer probability was 0.4% (0.2–0.7%) in participants with a nodule smaller than 5 mm and not significantly different from participants without nodules. However, the probability increased to 1.3% (1.0–1.8%) if nodules had a diameter of 5–10 mm and 15.2% (12.7–18.1%) if nodules were bigger than 10 mm. Since most of pGGNs and mGGNs grow slowly, follow-ups are routinely required for VDT evaluation. Depending on the calculated VDT, a better follow-up strategy including interval and contrast use could be established for each nodule or individualized follow-up.

3.3.4 Guidelines: More Is Less or Less Is More?

With the increasing incidence and awareness of incidentally detected pulmonary nodules, dozens of guidelines or consensuses on the management have been published in professional journals from international organizations to national organizations to even local societies. Most of them are from multidisciplinary experts with varying compositions for particular emphasis on certain perspectives. Representative and extensively used guidelines are the NCCN guideline, the ACCP guideline [22], and the Fleischner Society guideline [23].

This is the best of times, and this is the worst of times. We have so many guidelines and options available for reference, whereas so many controversies and even conflicts between guidelines confuse us. Therefore, more guidelines do not necessarily mean more efficacy or higher effectiveness in the implementation of guideline. On the contrary, more guidelines may cause less effectiveness and low compliance in clinical practice due to confusing information from different guidelines. Mets et al. conducted a survey study to assess the awareness and conformance to the Fleischner Society recommendations for the management of subsolid pulmonary nodules (SSN) in daily clinical practice. The good news was that the recommendations had been widely disseminated. And the bad news was that heterogeneous implementation was subject to the clinical experience, practice pattern, patient throughput, and individual preference [24]. Undoubtedly, the inter-guideline heterogeneity is much larger, which certainly compromises the concordance in clinical practice. Therefore, a united and generalized guideline with less confusing information would significantly improve the compliance and benefit the implementation of lung cancer screening and management of detected pulmonary nodules.

There exists no agreement on from which age should the screening be initiated as well as the time of duration in current guidelines. Most guidelines are based on the risk stratification model, and those with high risk are the screening candidates. Hence, the majority of candidates are over 50 or 55 years old. However, those risk models for lung cancer have inherent flaws since the data those models rely on do not reflect the current situation, i.e., more subcentimeter early-stage lung cancers are found in the younger population, especially never-smoking women, with a pathological predominance of adenocarcinoma instead of smoking-related squamous cell carcinoma. Smoking remains the major issue in relatively elderly population, whereas other factors play more roles in younger patients, such as genetic mutation, hormonal variation, and even emotional or environmental factors.

In our practice, the youngest lung cancer patient is a 15-year-old girl. And patients in 20s or 30s are not rare. Therefore, in our opinion, the starting age for the initial screening should be as early as possible. The year of a man or woman into a career may be an optimal time. The real value of this initial screening is stored as a baseline chest CT imaging. As far as the next screening or the screening interval, it should be dependent on the findings in the initial imaging. If negative and without other risk factors, every 5 years may be an optional interval. Otherwise the interval should be individualized based on the probability of malignancy of the findings plus other risk factors.

Regarding the duration, in the latest update of NCCN guideline, it has been revised to "Annual LDCT until patient is no longer a candidate for definitive treatment" from the previous "Annual LDCT for 2 years or consider annual LDCT until the patient is no longer a candidate for definitive treatment." However, in the Fleischner Society guideline, the recommended duration for suspected GGNs is 5 years annually or biannually. Considering the extremely indolent biological behavior in some preinvasive lesions and numerous reports that progression occurs in nodules followed up for more than 5 years, the 5-year duration may be not adequate, and, in our opinion and in our practice, the NCCN guideline is preferred.

Most guidelines are based on western population, mainly reflecting the epidemiology of lung cancer in western countries, especially industrialized developed countries. Apparently certain variation in the epidemiology and etiology exists between western countries and other countries. In Asia, despite that ACCP guidelines are widely followed, practitioners should be beware of some caveats and avoid applying indiscriminately. One of the major issues related to the development of lung cancer in Asia is the air pollution indoors and outdoors. The high incidence of adenocarcinoma in female nonsmokers is another epidemiological feature of lung cancer in Asia, implying that nonsmoking women should not be excluded from screening population without any discretion. Furthermore, considering the high prevalence of granulomatous disease and other infectious diseases in Asian population, pulmonary nodules should be carefully evaluated on the basis of extensive differential diagnosis. Hence, the majority of lung cancer risk probability algorithms developed using non-Asian data may not be applicable to Asian population. A longer surveillance period starting from a younger population than that recommended by the ACCP seems more practical and meaningful in Asia (the Asia guideline) [25]. Therefore, the implementation of lung cancer screening and management should be optimized with patient individualization and nation-based/region-based population individualization on the basis of a generalized guideline.

Other issues related to lung cancer screening and management are briefly addressed as the following:

1. All the screening and follow-up CT should be used of low-dose technique, such as scanning voltage should be 100–120 kVp, current 40–60 mAs, or lower condition. However, if the evaluation of mediastinum or lymph nodes is required, conventional scan condition should be applied, and if necessary, the contrast agent should also be used.
2. The newly detected nodule is typically defined as a lesion with average diameter $\geq$ 3 mm, average diameter = (nodule max diameter + distance of vertical radial line)/2. The standard for nodule enlargement is defined as follows: for <15 mm nodule or multiple nodules or subsolid nodule, average diameter of any nodule or solid area increases $\geq$2 mmd, while for $\geq$15 mm nodule, the average diameter increases by 15%.

3. For all GGN/GGO or subsolid lesion, the evaluation should be based on thin (slice thickness < 1.5 mm) CT radiological image in order to exclude any existence of the solid part. If the lesion has a solid part, it should be managed by the principle of subsolid nodule.
4. Regarding the value of PET/CT in lung cancer screening, due to the indolent biological and metabolic features, most of preinvasive and part of minimally invasive diseases are negative in FDG-PET scanning, especially those subcentimeter lesions. Hence, false-negative results are frequent in stage IA diseases. Those containing significant solid component may be the proper candidates for FDG-PET examination.
5. Administration of a broad-spectrum antibiotic with anaerobic coverage was once recommended when multiple nodules are present and occult infection or inflammation is a possibility but has been deleted in the latest update of NCCN guideline. In contrast, the empirical antibiotic treatment is suggested in the Asia guideline. In our practice, patients with newly detected nodules in follow-up chest CT, either single or multiple, are prescribed with antibiotics for a 2-week course.

Lung cancer screening and the management of detected pulmonary nodules require organized stepwise, comprehensive strategies, which are well summarized by Fintelmann et al. [26] into a ten-pillar model with components of eligibility, education, examination ordering, image acquisition, image review, communication, referral network, quality improvement, reimbursement, and research frontiers.

References

1. Abe H, MacMahon H, Engelmann R, Li Q, Shiraishi J, Katsuragawa S, Aoyama M, Ishida T, Ashizawa K, Metz CE, Doi K. Computer-aided diagnosis in chest radiography: results of large-scale observer tests at the 1996-2001 RSNA scientific assemblies. Radiographics. 2003;23(1):255–65. https://doi.org/10.1148/rg.231025129.
2. Shiraishi J, Li F, Doi K. Computer-aided diagnosis for improved detection of lung nodules by use of posterior-anterior and lateral chest radiographs. Acad Radiol. 2007;14(1):28–37. https://doi.org/10.1016/j.acra.2006.09.057.
3. Bertolaccini L, Viti A, Terzi A. Digital tomosynthesis in lung cancer: state of the art. Ann Transl Med. 2015;3(10):139. https://doi.org/10.3978/j.issn.2305-5839.2015.06.03.
4. Henschke CI, Yankelevitz DF, Libby DM, Pasmantier MW, Smith JP, Miettinen OS. Survival of patients with stage I lung cancer detected on CT screening. N Engl J Med. 2006;355(17):1763–71. https://doi.org/10.1056/NEJMoa060476.
5. Zheng X, Ren Y, Phillips WT, Li M, Song M, Hua Y, Zhang G. Assessment of hepatic fatty infiltration using spectral computed tomography imaging: a pilot study. J Comput Assist Tomogr. 2013;37(2):134–41. https://doi.org/10.1097/RCT.0b013e31827ddad3.
6. Kim SH, Kamaya A, Willmann JK. CT perfusion of the liver: principles and applications in oncology. Radiology. 2014;272(2):322–44. https://doi.org/10.1148/radiol.14130091.
7. Pontana F, Remy-Jardin M, Duhamel A, Faivre JB, Wallaert B, Remy J. Lung perfusion with dual-energy multi-detector row CT: can it help recognize ground glass opacities of vascular origin? Acad Radiol. 2010;17(5):587–94. https://doi.org/10.1016/j.acra.2009.12.013.

8. Lv Y, Jin Y, Xu D, Yan Q, Liu G, Zhang H, Yuan D, Bao J. Assessment of 64-slice spiral computed tomography with perfusion weighted imaging in the early diagnosis of ground-glass opacity lung cancer. J BUON. 2016;21(4):954–7.
9. Hendee WR, O'Connor MK. Radiation risks of medical imaging: separating fact from fantasy. Radiology. 2012;264(2):312–21. https://doi.org/10.1148/radiol.12112678.
10. Ruegsegger P, Anliker M, Dambacher M. Quantification of trabecular bone with low dose computed tomography. J Comput Assist Tomogr. 1981;5(3):384–90.
11. Naidich DP, Marshall CH, Gribbin C, Arams RS, McCauley DI. Low-dose CT of the lungs: preliminary observations. Radiology. 1990;175(3):729–31. https://doi.org/10.1148/radiology.175.3.2343122.
12. Zwirewich CV, Mayo JR, Muller NL. Low-dose high-resolution CT of lung parenchyma. Radiology. 1991;180(2):413–7. https://doi.org/10.1148/radiology.180.2.2068303.
13. Lee KS, Primack SL, Staples CA, Mayo JR, Aldrich JE, Muller NL. Chronic infiltrative lung disease: comparison of diagnostic accuracies of radiography and low- and conventional-dose thin-section CT. Radiology. 1994;191(3):669–73. https://doi.org/10.1148/radiology.191.3.8184044.
14. Aberle DR, Adams AM, Berg CD, Black WC, Clapp JD, Fagerstrom RM, Gareen IF, Gatsonis C, Marcus PM, Sicks JD. Reduced lung-cancer mortality with low-dose computed tomographic screening. N Engl J Med. 2011;365(5):395–409. https://doi.org/10.1056/NEJMoa1102873.
15. Field JK, Duffy SW, Baldwin DR, Brain KE, Devaraj A, Eisen T, Green BA, Holemans JA, Kavanagh T, Kerr KM, Ledson M, Lifford KJ, McRonald FE, Nair A, Page RD, Parmar MK, Rintoul RC, Screaton N, Wald NJ, Weller D, Whynes DK, Williamson PR, Yadegarfar G, Hansell DM. The UK lung cancer screening trial: a pilot randomised controlled trial of low-dose computed tomography screening for the early detection of lung cancer. Health Technol Assess. 2016;20(40):1–146. https://doi.org/10.3310/hta20400.
16. Townsend CO, Clark MM, Jett JR, Patten CA, Schroeder DR, Nirelli LM, Swensen SJ, Hurt RD. Relation between smoking cessation and receiving results from three annual spiral chest computed tomography scans for lung carcinoma screening. Cancer. 2005;103(10):2154–62. https://doi.org/10.1002/cncr.21045.
17. Bankier AA, Kressel HY. Through the looking glass revisited: the need for more meaning and less drama in the reporting of dose and dose reduction in CT. Radiology. 2012;265(1):4–8. https://doi.org/10.1148/radiol.12121145.
18. Oken MM, Hocking WG, Kvale PA, Andriole GL, Buys SS, Church TR, Crawford ED, Fouad MN, Isaacs C, Reding DJ, Weissfeld JL, Yokochi LA, O'Brien B, Ragard LR, Rathmell JM, Riley TL, Wright P, Caparaso N, Hu P, Izmirlian G, Pinsky PF, Prorok PC, Kramer BS, Miller AB, Gohagan JK, Berg CD. Screening by chest radiograph and lung cancer mortality: the prostate, lung, colorectal, and ovarian (PLCO) randomized trial. JAMA. 2011;306(17):1865–73. https://doi.org/10.1001/jama.2011.1591.
19. National Comprehensive Cancer Network Lung Cancer Screening (Version 2.2018). https://www.nccn.org/store/login/login.aspx?ReturnURL=https://www.nccn.org/professionals/physician_gls/pdf/lung_screening.pdf. Accessed 20 Aug 2017.
20. Wood DE, Eapen GA, Ettinger DS, Hou L, Jackman D, Kazerooni E, Klippenstein D, Lackner RP, Leard L, Leung AN, Massion PP, Meyers BF, Munden RF, Otterson GA, Peairs K, Pipavath S, Pratt-Pozo C, Reddy C, Reid ME, Rotter AJ, Schabath MB, Sequist LV, Tong BC, Travis WD, Unger M, Yang SC. Lung cancer screening. J Natl Compr Cancer Netw. 2012;10(2):240–65.
21. Horeweg N, van Rosmalen J, Heuvelmans MA, van der Aalst CM, Vliegenthart R, Scholten ET, ten Haaf K, Nackaerts K, Lammers JW, Weenink C, Groen HJ, van Ooijen P, de Jong PA, de Bock GH, Mali W, de Koning HJ, Oudkerk M. Lung cancer probability in patients with CT-detected pulmonary nodules: a prespecified analysis of data from the NELSON trial of low-dose CT screening. Lancet Oncol. 2014;15(12):1332–41. https://doi.org/10.1016/s1470-2045(14)70389-4.

22. Gould MK, Fletcher J, Iannettoni MD, Lynch WR, Midthun DE, Naidich DP, Ost DE. Evaluation of patients with pulmonary nodules: when is it lung cancer?: ACCP evidence-based clinical practice guidelines (2nd edition). Chest. 2007;132(3 Suppl):108s–30s. https://doi.org/10.1378/chest.07-1353.
23. MacMahon H, Naidich DP, Goo JM, Lee KS, Leung ANC, Mayo JR, Mehta AC, Ohno Y, Powell CA, Prokop M, Rubin GD, Schaefer-Prokop CM, Travis WD, Van Schil PE, Bankier AA. Guidelines for management of incidental pulmonary nodules detected on CT images: from the Fleischner society 2017. Radiology. 2017;284(1):228–43. https://doi.org/10.1148/radiol.2017161659.
24. Mets OM, de Jong PA, Chung K, Lammers JJ, van Ginneken B, Schaefer-Prokop CM. Fleischner recommendations for the management of subsolid pulmonary nodules: high awareness but limited conformance—a survey study. Eur Radiol. 2016;26(11):3840–9. https://doi.org/10.1007/s00330-016-4249-y.
25. Bai C, Choi CM, Chu CM, Anantham D, Chung-Man Ho J, Khan AZ, Lee JM, Li SY, Saenghirunvattana S, Yim A. Evaluation of pulmonary nodules: clinical practice consensus guidelines for Asia. Chest. 2016;150(4):877–93. https://doi.org/10.1016/j.chest.2016.02.650.
26. Fintelmann FJ, Bernheim A, Digumarthy SR, Lennes IT, Kalra MK, Gilman MD, Sharma A, Flores EJ, Muse VV, Shepard JA. The 10 pillars of lung cancer screening: rationale and logistics of a lung cancer screening program. Radiographics. 2015;35(7):1893–908. https://doi.org/10.1148/rg.2015150079.

Suggested Readings

1. Gerber TC, Carr JJ, Arai AE, Dixon RL, Ferrari VA, Gomes AS, Heller GV, McCollough CH, McNitt-Gray MF, Mettler FA, Mieres JH, Morin RL, Yester MV. Ionizing radiation in cardiac imaging: a science advisory from the American Heart Association Committee on Cardiac Imaging of the Council on Clinical Cardiology and Committee on Cardiovascular Imaging and Intervention of the Council on Cardiovascular Radiology and Intervention. Circulation. 2009;119(7):1056–65. https://doi.org/10.1161/circulationaha.108.191650.
2. Andy Adam AKD, Gillard J, Schaefer-Prokop C, Grainger RG. Grainger & Allison's diagnostic radiology. 6th ed. New York: Churchill Livingstone; 2014.
3. Balkman JD, Mehandru S, DuPont E, Novak RD, Gilkeson RC. Dual energy subtraction digital radiography improves performance of a next generation computer-aided detection program. J Thorac Imaging. 2010;25(1):41–7. https://doi.org/10.1097/RTI.0b013e3181aa34ed.
4. Bankier AA, MacMahon H, Goo JM, Rubin GD, Schaefer-Prokop CM, Naidich DP. Recommendations for measuring pulmonary nodules at CT: a statement from the Fleischner society. Radiology. 2017;285(2):584–600. https://doi.org/10.1148/radiol.2017162894.
5. Bray F, Jemal A, Grey N, Ferlay J, Forman D. Global cancer transitions according to the Human Development Index (2008-2030): a population-based study. Lancet Oncol. 2012;13(8):790–801. https://doi.org/10.1016/s1470-2045(12)70211-5.
6. Croswell JM, Baker SG, Marcus PM, Clapp JD, Kramer BS. Cumulative incidence of false-positive test results in lung cancer screening: a randomized trial. Ann Intern Med. 2010;152(8):505–512, w176-580. https://doi.org/10.7326/0003-4819-152-8-201004200-00007.
7. Damilakis JE, Tsouderos JG. Optimal CT settings for head imaging in the paediatric patient. An analysis of absorbed dose. Eur J Radiol. 1989;9(1):48–50.
8. Dobbins JT 3rd, McAdams HP, Sabol JM, Chakraborty DP, Kazerooni EA, Reddy GP, Vikgren J, Bath M. Multi-institutional evaluation of digital tomosynthesis, dual-energy radiography, and conventional chest radiography for the detection and management of pulmonary nodules. Radiology. 2017;282(1):236–50. https://doi.org/10.1148/radiol.2016150497.

9. Firmino M, Angelo G, Morais H, Dantas MR, Valentim R. Computer-aided detection (CADe) and diagnosis (CADx) system for lung cancer with likelihood of malignancy. Biomed Eng Online. 2016;15:2. https://doi.org/10.1186/s12938-015-0120-7.
10. Galea A, Durran A, Adlan T, Gay D, Riordan R, Dubbins P, Williams MP. Practical applications of digital tomosynthesis of the chest. Clin Radiol. 2014;69(4):424–30. https://doi.org/10.1016/j.crad.2013.10.019.
11. Gilkeson RC, Sachs PB. Dual energy subtraction digital radiography: technical considerations, clinical applications, and imaging pitfalls. J Thorac Imaging. 2006;21(4):303–13. https://doi.org/10.1097/01.rti.0000213646.34417.be.
12. Hasan N, Kumar R, Kavuru MS. Lung cancer screening beyond low-dose computed tomography: the role of novel biomarkers. Lung. 2014;192(5):639–48. https://doi.org/10.1007/s00408-014-9636-z.
13. Hoffman RM, Sanchez R. Lung cancer screening. Med Clin North Am. 2017;101(4):769–85. https://doi.org/10.1016/j.mcna.2017.03.008.
14. International Agency for Research on Cancer GLOBOCAN2012 (IARC), Section of Cancer Information. http://globocan.iarc.fr/Pages/fact_sheets_cancer.aspx.
15. Jha P, Ramasundarahettige C, Landsman V, Rostron B, Thun M, Anderson RN, McAfee T, Peto R. 21st-century hazards of smoking and benefits of cessation in the United States. N Engl J Med. 2013;368(4):341–50. https://doi.org/10.1056/NEJMsa1211128.
16. Linet MS, Slovis TL, Miller DL, Kleinerman R, Lee C, Rajaraman P, Berrington de Gonzalez A. Cancer risks associated with external radiation from diagnostic imaging procedures. CA Cancer J Clin. 2012;62(2):75–100. https://doi.org/10.3322/caac.21132.
17. Loeb S, Bjurlin MA, Nicholson J, Tammela TL, Penson DF, Carter HB, Carroll P, Etzioni R. Overdiagnosis and overtreatment of prostate cancer. Eur Urol. 2014;65(6):1046–55. https://doi.org/10.1016/j.eururo.2013.12.062.
18. Ma J, Ward EM, Smith R, Jemal A. Annual number of lung cancer deaths potentially avertable by screening in the United States. Cancer. 2013;119(7):1381–5. https://doi.org/10.1002/cncr.27813.
19. Mortani Barbosa EJ Jr. Lung cancer screening overdiagnosis: reports of overdiagnosis in screening for lung cancer are grossly exaggerated. Acad Radiol. 2015;22(8):976–82. https://doi.org/10.1016/j.acra.2014.10.011.
20. Nagatani Y, Takahashi M, Murata K, Ikeda M, Yamashiro T, Miyara T, Koyama H, Koyama M, Sato Y, Moriya H, Noma S, Tomiyama N, Ohno Y, Murayama S. Lung nodule detection performance in five observers on computed tomography (CT) with adaptive iterative dose reduction using three-dimensional processing (AIDR 3D) in a Japanese multicenter study: comparison between ultra-low-dose CT and low-dose CT by receiver-operating characteristic analysis. Eur J Radiol. 2015;84(7):1401–12. https://doi.org/10.1016/j.ejrad.2015.03.012.
21. Schauer DA, Linton OW. NCRP report no. 160, ionizing radiation exposure of the population of the United States, medical exposure—are we doing less with more, and is there a role for health physicists? Health Phys. 2009;97(1):1–5. https://doi.org/10.1097/01.HP.0000356672.44380.b7.
22. Smith RA, Andrews KS, Brooks D, Fedewa SA, Manassaram-Baptiste D, Saslow D, Brawley OW, Wender RC. Cancer screening in the United States, 2017: a review of current American Cancer Society guidelines and current issues in cancer screening. CA Cancer J Clin. 2017;67(2):100–21. https://doi.org/10.3322/caac.21392.
23. Sudarski S, Hagelstein C, Weis M, Schoenberg SO, Apfaltrer P. Dual-energy snap-shot perfusion CT in suspect pulmonary nodules and masses and for lung cancer staging. Eur J Radiol. 2015;84(12):2393–400. https://doi.org/10.1016/j.ejrad.2015.09.024.
24. Suramo I, Torniainen P, Jouppila P, Kirkinen P, Lahde S. A low-dose CT-pelvimetry. Br J Radiol. 1984;57(673):35–7. https://doi.org/10.1259/0007-1285-57-673-35.
25. Tammemagi MC, Church TR, Hocking WG, Silvestri GA, Kvale PA, Riley TL, Commins J, Berg CD. Evaluation of the lung cancer risks at which to screen ever- and never-smokers: screening rules applied to the PLCO and NLST cohorts. PLoS Med. 2014;11(12):e1001764. https://doi.org/10.1371/journal.pmed.1001764.

26. Travis LB, Gospodarowicz M, Curtis RE, Clarke EA, Andersson M, Glimelius B, Joensuu T, Lynch CF, van Leeuwen FE, Holowaty E, Storm H, Glimelius I, Pukkala E, Stovall M, Fraumeni JF Jr, Boice JD Jr, Gilbert E. Lung cancer following chemotherapy and radiotherapy for Hodgkin's disease. J Natl Cancer Inst. 2002;94(3):182–92.
27. van Iersel CA, de Koning HJ, Draisma G, Mali WP, Scholten ET, Nackaerts K, Prokop M, Habbema JD, Oudkerk M, van Klaveren RJ. Risk-based selection from the general population in a screening trial: selection criteria, recruitment and power for the Dutch-Belgian randomised lung cancer multi-slice CT screening trial (NELSON). Int J Cancer. 2007;120(4):868–74. https://doi.org/10.1002/ijc.22134.
28. Vock P, Szucs-Farkas Z. Dual energy subtraction: principles and clinical applications. Eur J Radiol. 2009;72(2):231–7. https://doi.org/10.1016/j.ejrad.2009.03.046.
29. Wang G, Zhang C, Li M, Deng K, Li W. Preliminary application of high-definition computed tomographic gemstone spectral imaging in lung cancer. J Comput Assist Tomogr. 2014;38(1):77–81. https://doi.org/10.1097/RCT.0b013e3182a21633.

Chapter 4
PET/CT for the Assessment of Pulmonary Nodules

Yihui Guan

4.1 An Overview of PET/CT Imaging

Using hybrid co-registration of both functional and structural information, PET/CT can provide valuable information in lesion characterization, quantification, localization, metabolic and biologic status, and staging (Table 4.1). Oncologic evaluation remains as one of the major clinical indications of PET/CT examination. In most cases of malignancy, tumor cells are characterized by distinctly increased glucose metabolism. ^{18}F-FDG, the most commonly used radiopharmaceutical, is an analogue of glucose and detained in the tumor cell after hexokinase phosphorylation to FDG-6-phosphate which is unable to participate in downstream metabolism. PET/

Table 4.1 Comparison and complementary interpretation between PET and CT

PET	CT	Complementary interpretation
Molecular information	Structural and anatomical imaging	Molecular imaging
High sensitivity and specificity	High spatial and tissue resolution, precise localization	Increased diagnostic reliability due to comprehensive assessment
Abnormal	Abnormal	Reliable positive diagnosis
Normal	Normal	Reliable negative diagnosis
Abnormal	Normal	Physiological uptake/false positivity/early-stage malignancy
Normal	Abnormal	Avoid missing or misdiagnosing benign or some malignant lesions with false negativity in PET imaging

Y. Guan
Department of Nuclear Medicine, Fudan University Huashan Hospital, Shanghai, China
e-mail: guanyihui@hotmail.com

X. Zheng et al. (eds.), *Early-stage Lung Cancer*,
https://doi.org/10.1007/978-981-10-7596-4_4

CT can detect ^{18}F-FDG uptake and therefore provide valuable information on tumor metabolism as well as precise localization of primary and metastases if present for disease evaluation and outcome assessment.

4.1.1 PET/CT Imaging Protocol

For PET/CT examination, patients are required to fast for at least 6 h before receiving an intravenous injection of 370–555 MBq (10–15 mCi) ^{18}F-FDG. The injection site should be on the limb contralateral to the known lesion. During the injection of FDG and the subsequent uptake phase, patients should remain seated or recumbent and silent to minimize FDG uptake in muscles. The scan begins 1 h after the injection. Firstly, low-dose CT images are acquired from the head to the mid-femur using scanning parameters as planned. The regular acquisition time for PET scan is 2 min/bed. For those patients less than 60 kg and those who may be of poor compliance during the imaging course, the acquisition time can be shortened to 1–1.5 min/bed. On the other hand, the acquisition time should be prolonged to 3–4 min/bed for those overweight patients or the patients with a small lesion. An additional delay scan (2–3 h postinjection versus 1-hour postinjection for the regular scan) may be performed if necessary. After scanning, the PET images are attenuation corrected, reconstructed, and fused with CT images. Since the diagnosis of small pulmonary nodules rely much on accurate morphological features, an additional diagnostic CT scan would be needed in most cases. We recommend to acquire diagnostic CT images after PET/CT evaluation as a routine procedure in patients with small-sized pulmonary lesions.

4.1.2 Analysis of PET/CT Imaging

1. *Visual inspection*: Qualitative visual inspection of the presence of "hot" tumor is the most basic analytical method in the clinic. Abnormal hypermetabolic lesions throughout the body should be spotted and distinguished from physiological uptake and inflammatory lesions (false positive). A delay scan would be performed in some occasions if necessary. Generally, the glucose uptake of a thoracic lesion is compared with that of the mediastinal blood pool and categorized into four grades as the following: grade I, no glucose uptake; grade II, mild glucose uptake, lower than that of the mediastinal blood pool; grade III, moderate glucose uptake, similar to that of the mediastinal blood pool; and grade IV, significant glucose uptake, higher than that of the mediastinal blood pool.
2. *Semiquantitative analysis*: The standardized uptake value (SUV) is the most frequently used semiquantitative analysis approach for measurement of FDG uptake. Since the absolute quantity of regional FDG uptake depends on glucose metabolic rate as well as the injected dose and the body weight, the semiquantitative results should be corrected with the latter two variables. In most commercial PET/CT workstations and softwares, SUV can be calculated automatically by drawing a

region of interest (ROI) on PET images, using the following equation: SUV = tissue FDG concentration defined by ROI/(injected FDG dose/body weight). Both the maximum and mean SUV within the ROI (SUVmax and SUVmean) can be obtained. As one of the most common diagnostic metrics, however, SUVmean is more susceptible to ROI delineation than the SUVmax. Thus, to ensure reproducibility, SUVmax should be reported with SUVmean, especially for those lesions with heterogeneous uptake. Other SUV-affecting factors include the interval between injection and acquisition, reconstruction parameters as well as the precision of body weight and injected dose. A standardized procedure is favorable to minimize the uncertainties. The blood glucose level during the injection is another important factor. Since glucose can competitively inhibit the injected ^{18}F-FDG, an increased blood glucose level would inhibit FDG uptake in lesions, resulting in lowered SUV values. It is also noteworthy that the distribution of FDG in adipose tissues is relatively limited. Therefore the application of body weight to standardize the distribution volume may result in overestimation of SUV for those who are overweighted or obese. Hence, some investigators have proposed the application of lean body weight and body surface area instead of body weight for standardization. In conclusion, all factors mentioned above need to be considered for achieving as accurate SUV values as possible. In the past, SUVmean of 2.5 was recommended as a cutoff value for differentiating active (malignant) lesions from inactive (benign) lesions. However, it has been acknowledged that there exist significant limitations in characterizing pulmonary nodules using SUV alone. Instead, comprehensive evaluation including the location, size, morphology, quantity, and radioactive homogeneity of pulmonary nodules as well as clinical information and results from other examinations is the approach for accurate assessment of pulmonary nodules.

3. *T/B or L/B*: T/B or L/B is the ratio between the radioactivity of the target (T) or lesion (L) and that of the background (B). They can be served as surrogate semi-quantification indices when SUV is unavailable or inaccurate. However, their application is limited in the clinical practice due to the susceptibility to various factors.
4. *Comprehensive analysis of PET/CT*: PET/CT has the advantages of both PET and CT. Functional information acquired by PET and morphological information obtained from CT provide more comprehensive characterization and localization information for lesions than PET or CT alone. It is noteworthy that various CT imaging post-processing techniques such as multiple planar reformation and virtual endoscopy may offer additional diagnostic information.

4.2 Current Status and Advancements of PET/CT Assessment of Pulmonary Micronodules

4.2.1 Solitary Pulmonary Nodule (SPN)

It is estimated that the discovery rate of the pulmonary nodular lesions in conventional chest X-ray is only 0.2%, while the rate is about 40–60% in high-resolution CT. Most of the lesions are benign. For the remaining malignancies, high differential accuracy is required in need of early detection and treatment to reduce tumor mortality rate. A "solitary pulmonary nodule (SPN)" is a term to describe a well-circumscribed solitary round solid opaque lesion measuring ≤30 mm in diameter on a conventional chest X-ray. In a high-resolution CT study for lung cancer screening, the baseline detection rate of small nodular lesions is 8–51%. The nodules are usually multiple, 96% of the noncalcified nodules are ≤10 mm, and 72% of them are ≤5 mm. The nodular lesions measuring ≤10 mm in diameter are concluded as small pulmonary nodules due to the difficulty in determining their nature.

Small pulmonary nodules can be classified into three groups, solid nodules, pure ground-glass nodules (pGGs), and semisolid GGNs (sGGNs). Most solid nodules are solitary with well-circumscribed or ill-circumscribed margin in the pulmonary parenchyma measuring ≤10 mm on CT images. Pure GGNs are hazy nodular findings on high-resolution CT with increased attenuation and preservation of bronchial and vascular structures. The density of pGGNs is typically homogeneous. Such ground-glass nodules generally progress slowly and may remain stable for years. Those persistent pGGNs have an increasing probability of carcinoma in situ or atypical adenomatous hyperplasia. sGGNs contain a variable amount of solid component. If unchanged with antibiotic treatment or slowly growing in multiple follow-up CT scans, the potential of malignancy increases, especially minimally invasive adenocarcinoma.

4.2.2 The Analysis Methods of Small Pulmonary Nodule on ^{18}F-FDG PET/CT Imaging

Integrated PET/CT allows morphological and functional imaging to be carried out in a single imaging procedure which has been gradually applied in the assessment of pulmonary nodules. The study from Yi et al. showed that the sensitivity, specificity, and accuracy of contrast-enhanced CT and PET/CT is 81%, 93%, and 85% and 96%, 88%, and 93%, respectively. The combination of PET and CT has been proven more accurate for lesion location and characterization than the results obtained from PET separately. With more information on the morphology of the pulmonary lesions, it is possible to differentiate benign lesions with morphological alterations but without FDG uptake from malignancies which are FDG-negative. At the same time, the quantitative features of PET/CT have increasing impacts in oncology trials and clinical practice. The PET/CT is more sensitive and more accurate than PET alone in the diagnosis of lung cancer (Fig. 4.1).

Recent reviews showed that the diagnostic sensitivity of lung cancer using ^{18}F-FDG PET/CT ranges from 72 to 94%. The limitation of the most researches is the application of a single SUV cutoff value. In addition, the application of a single SUVmax cutoff value in SPN diagnosis and differentiation is even more limited. Since the nodule is small, the partial volume effect (PVE) may lead to miscalculation of the SUVmax. Besides, the phenomenon, which less regional radioactivity resulting from fewer activated tumor cell aggregation, is more obvi-

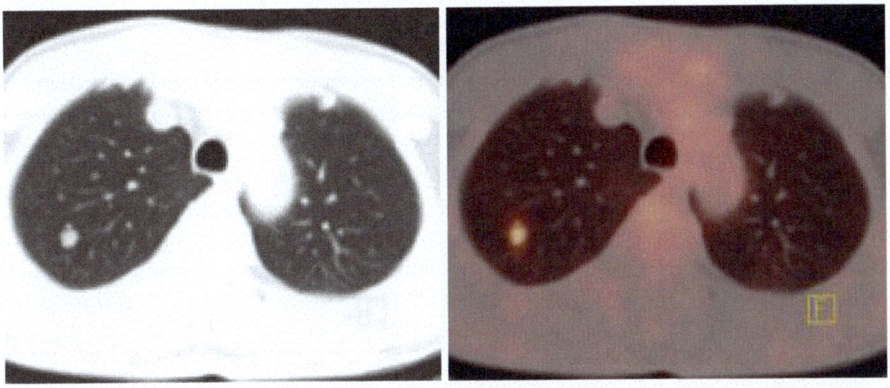

Fig. 4.1 Male, 53 years old. Chest CT showed a nodule (6 mm × 7 mm) in the right upper lobe. The nodule had fine spiculation and lobulation, indicative of malignancy. PET scan showed increased FDG metabolism with early SUVmax = 3.7 and delayed SUVmax = 4.1, supporting the suspicion of malignancy. The surgical pathologic results confirmed an adenocarcinoma

ous in the pure ground-glass nodules. A GGN <5 mm usually lacks metabolic activity and appears negative uptake of FDG. A prospective research studied 344 US veterans with pulmonary nodules with a purpose to overcome limitations by reporting likelihood ratios (LRs) in five different categories, definitely benign (dB), probably benign (pB), indeterminate (Int), probably malignant (pM), and definitely malignant (dM). In comparison to low LRs in the first four categories (0.03–3.2), the dM category had significantly high LR value, 9.9 (range from 5.4 to 18.3), three times as high as that in pM category. This result indicated that the degree of fluorodeoxyglucose (FDG) uptake was strongly associated with malignancy [1]. In this study, according to the FDG uptake in the nodules relative to the mediastinal blood pool, if the uptake of any point within nodules greater than in blood pool (a SUV of 2.5), probably malignant was considered, while if the uptake of all points within nodules much greater than in blood pool (a SUV of 2.5), definitely malignant was considered. To improve diagnostic accuracy, dual time point measurements of FDG uptake have been investigated and proved to be of use. However, Barger and Nandalur conducted a systematic review to assess the value of dual time point measurements and concluded otherwise: the dual time point measurement performed no better than single time point measurement. The pooled sensitivity and specificity of single time point and dual time point FDG-PET for characterizing pulmonary nodules are 96.8% and 77.8%, and 85% and 77%. In this study, data from 10 studies involving a total of 890 nodules from 816 patients were analyzed [2]. As an additional finding, the value of dual time point imaging was even more limited in most of the FDG-negative pulmonary nodules.

Pathologically, a small-sized malignant pulmonary nodule could be atypical adenomatous hyperplasia (AAH), adenocarcinoma in situ (AIS), minimally invasive adenocarcinoma (MIA), and lepidic-predominant adenocarcinoma (LPA). Slow-growing and hypometabolic squamous cell carcinoma is rarely seen. It is usually mildly metabolic active. In most cases, typical imaging features of lung cancer on CT would be adequate for the establishment of malignancy. Those lesions in the bottom of the lungs adjacent to the diaphragm can easily be affected by motion artifacts, resulting in a hypometabolic appearance on PET. Lesions ≤5 mm could also be hypometabolic due to partial volume effect. Hence in these cases, CT could be of more values in diagnosis. In clinical practice, respiratory motion artifacts could be minimized by advancing scanning techniques and reconstruction methods. For example, the 4D respiratory-gated scanning and PSF reconstruction techniques can improve the detection rate of small and micronodules, thus improving the diagnostic accuracy of PET/CT. More attention should be paid to small malignant lesions with low or no FDG uptake on PET because of partial volume effect (Fig. 4.2).

In conclusion, the diagnostic values of single cutoff SUV and dual time point imaging in small pulmonary nodules are limited. It is necessary to include as many as possible information, such as FDG uptake, clinical risk index and CT morphological information, and/or adopting T/B and L/B, to evaluate any suspicious lesions comprehensively.

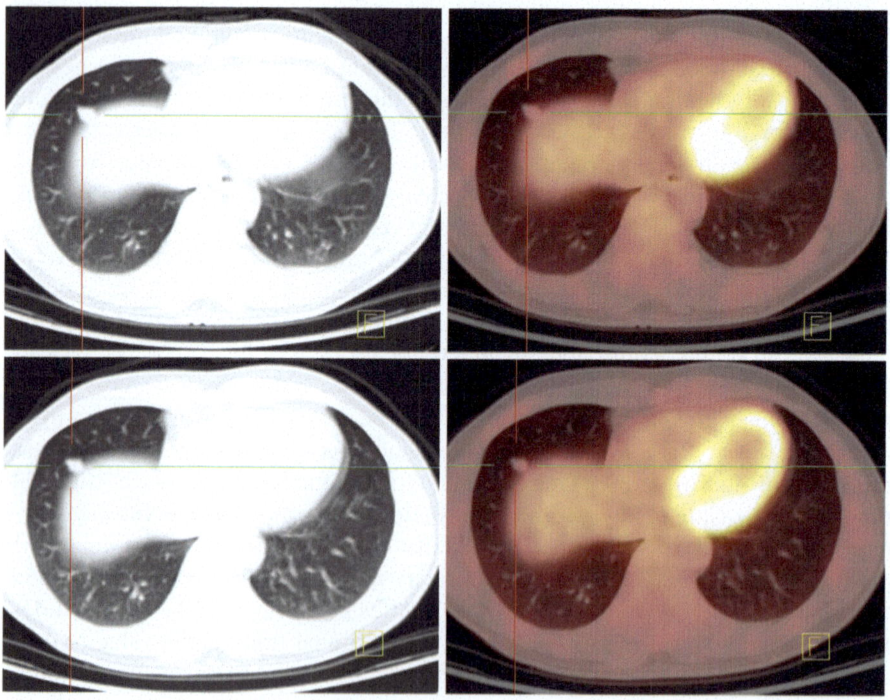

Fig. 4.2 Male, 68 years old. A small nodule was incidentally detected in the right lower lobe adjacent to the diaphragm. No abnormal FDG uptake was seen on PET. Three years later, the follow-up CT showed no change in size and morphology. Mild FDG uptake was seen on PET with SUVmax = 0.9. Surgical pathologic examinations confirmed poorly differentiated adenocarcinoma

4.2.3 ^{18}F-FDG PET/CT Imaging in Small Pulmonary Nodules

4.2.3.1 Risk Stratification of Small Pulmonary Nodules

In 2005, the American Fleischner Society guidelines advocated to perform potential malignant risk evaluation of indeterminate small pulmonary nodules and quantify risk factors among clinical characteristics using probabilistic prediction models. Four independent risk factors were generated, including smoking history, age, the size of the nodule, and the duration of smoking cessation with risk ratios of 7.9, 2.2, 1.1, and 1.6, respectively. The malignancy probability of small pulmonary nodules can be roughly divided into three categories: low risk (≤5%), moderate risk (5–65%), and high risk (>65%). Low-risk clinical factors include young age, minimal history of smoking, the absence of cancer history, regular margin and small size, location in the upper lobe, etc. Clinical factors related to the high risk include elderly, history of heavy smoking, the presence of cancer history, irregular margin and spiculation, and/or location in the upper lobe. As for the nodules with a moderate risk, they may have some of clinical features listed above.

4.2.3.2 ^{18}F-FDG PET/CT in Small Pulmonary Nodules

CT Imaging Findings

Small pulmonary nodules, especially those measuring ≤8 mm, are usually PET-negative (no FDG uptake). Diagnostic CT is needed in these cases to acquire more morphological information to increase the diagnostic accuracy (Fig. 4.3).

The following are common imaging characteristics seen in benign lesions:

(a) Dense and uniform calcification. In a lung cancer screening study, calcification is present in 14% of small nodules whose CT value is > 164 HU with a similar density close to the rib. Typical calcification in benign lesions is stratiform, central type, or popcorn-like. The first two signs are usually seen in inflammatory granuloma, while the last one is a typical sign of hamartoma. Calcification is also present in 15% of malignant nodules with irregular or punctate appearance.
(b) Internal lipid density is another characteristic in benign lesions, specifically in hamartoma.
(c) Polymorphism. The morphology is a nonspecific imaging feature. However, a study showed that 24% of the small polygonal nodules are benign, especially those adjacent to the pleura. The plane adjacent to the pleura is linear, while other planes are sunken because of contraction of the lesion. The study also showed that the ratio of the maximum transverse/orthodox diameter was even more meaningful in differentiating benign lesions from malignancy. The ratio larger than 1.78 (tubular and flattened) was suggestive of benignity. Malignant nodules tend to infiltrate in all directions. The sensitivity and specificity of poly-

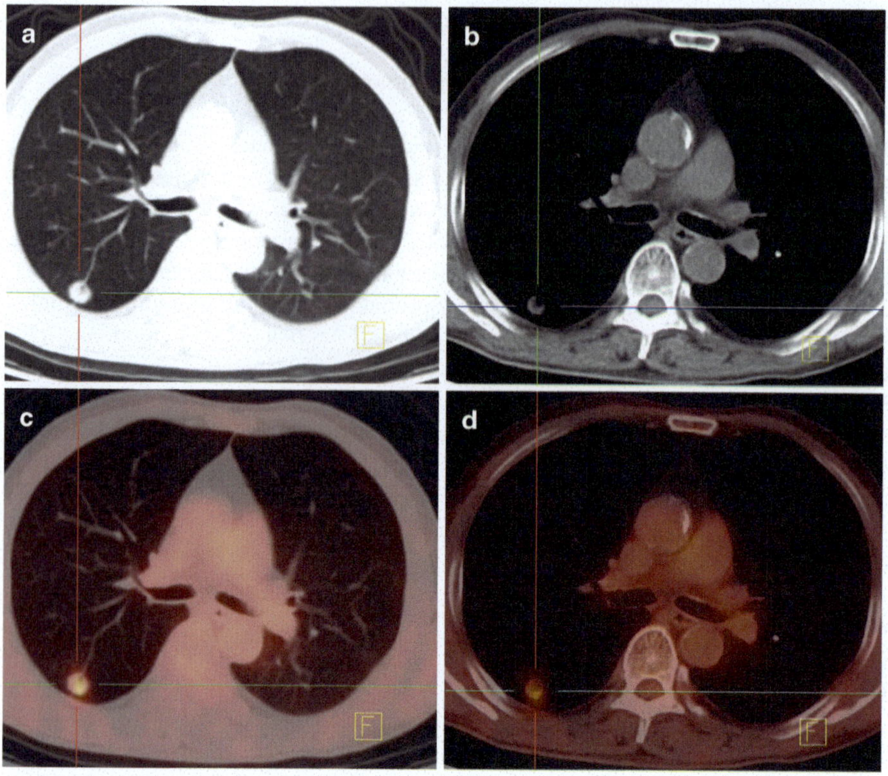

Fig. 4.3 Male, 50 years old. A cough and expectoration for more than 1 month. Thoracic CT revealed a solid nodule in the right upper lobe with bubble lucencies, lobulation, and spiculation signs (**a**, **b**). PET scan showed abnormally elevated FDG uptake. Initial SUVmax = 3.5, delayed SUVmax = 4.3 (**c**, **d**). Surgical pathologic examinations confirmed adenocarcinoma

morphism (tubular or flattened) in diagnosing subpleural, solid lesions benign is 61% and 100%, respectively. Additionally, the nodal or cluster-like distribution of two or more separate lesions measuring ≤10 mm is indicative of infection.

These imaging characteristics of malignancy lesions are listed as follows:

(a) Lobulation and spiculation. Lobulation and spiculation are common seen in malignant tumors, especially larger tumors. It is reported that lobulation is present in 33–100% of malignant tumors, while spiculation is seen in less than 50% of malignant nodules.
(b) Density. A nodule with ground-glass density has an increasing risk of being malignant in comparison to those without. It has been reported that 19% of the uncalcified lesions are nonsolid. Most of them are pure or partial ground-glass and 34% are malignant. Pure ground-glass lesions are usually small and homogeneous in density, in which spiculation is rarer than that in solid lesions. With the nodular volume and density increasing, the disease may have invasiveness increasingly. Compared to the pure ground-glass nodules and solid nodules, the mixed ground-

glass nodules are more polymorphic with central bubble-like lucencies. Focal fibrosis is commonly seen in cigarette smokers due to interstitial pneumonia associated with respiratory bronchiolitis and desquamative interstitial pneumonia. Some of these lesions may be absorbed within 3 months spontaneously.

(c) Air bronchogram sign, bubble-like lucency sign, and cavitation. In a radiologic-pathologic correlation study, 80% of the malignant lesions had at least one of these three signs (Fig. 4.4).

PET Imaging

Considering the performance, the radiation burden and expense, and the use of FDG-PET scanning in small pulmonary nodules, particularly those with ground-glass components, should be cautioned and meet the cost-effectiveness requirement. For those nodules with discordant findings between CT scan and clinical evaluations, PET scan could be a good supplemental examination to clarify the discordance. Lung cancers at their very early developmental stage may be biologically indolent and at low metabolic activity, implying that malignancy should not be excluded solely by negative PET scan results. In such circumstance, comprehensive assessment of clinical history, CT findings, PET results, and nodular dynamic changes in multiple follow-up images if available is of importance. Studies have revealed an inverse correlation between the FDG uptake and treatment outcomes. Those patients with hypometabolic tumors may have a favorable prognosis than those with the same tumors but at an active metabolic status. Hence, in patients with solid nodules and negative (hypometabolic) PET scan results, surveillance is required for at least 2 years to exclude potential malignancy. Needle biopsy is commonly required in tumors with a high probability of malignancy but negative PET scan results.

Integrated PET/CT scanners combine CT and FDG-PET imaging capability in a single unit and facilitate precise localization of lesions with abnormal FDG uptake or assessment of the metabolic status of lesions found in anatomic CT images. Although characterization and cancer staging are considered as two common indications for PET scanning, PET is more frequently used as a qualitative diagnosing tool.

According to the updated ACCP guidelines, PET is recommended for evaluation of extrathoracic metastasis in patients with surgically curable pulmonary nodules and otherwise normal chest CT. Biopsy of PET-vivid lesions, including mediastinal lymph nodes, is necessary for accurate preoperative staging. Two randomized clinical trials showed that PET scan could decrease the rate of nonradical surgery. Fischer et al. found that 52% of patients with pulmonary nodules received futile thoracotomies using conventional imaging modalities for preoperative assessment, while the number decreased to 35% in the group including PET/CT in preoperative assessment [3]. Futile thoracotomy was defined as benign lung lesion, exploratory thoracotomy, pathologic N2 disease, stage IIIb or IV disease, inoperable T3 or T4 disease, or recurrence or death within 1 year of surgery. This result was subsequently confirmed by numerous studies, including Van Tinteren et al. In their study, 41% patients had a futile thoracotomy in the arm of conventional workup (CWU), compared with 21% in

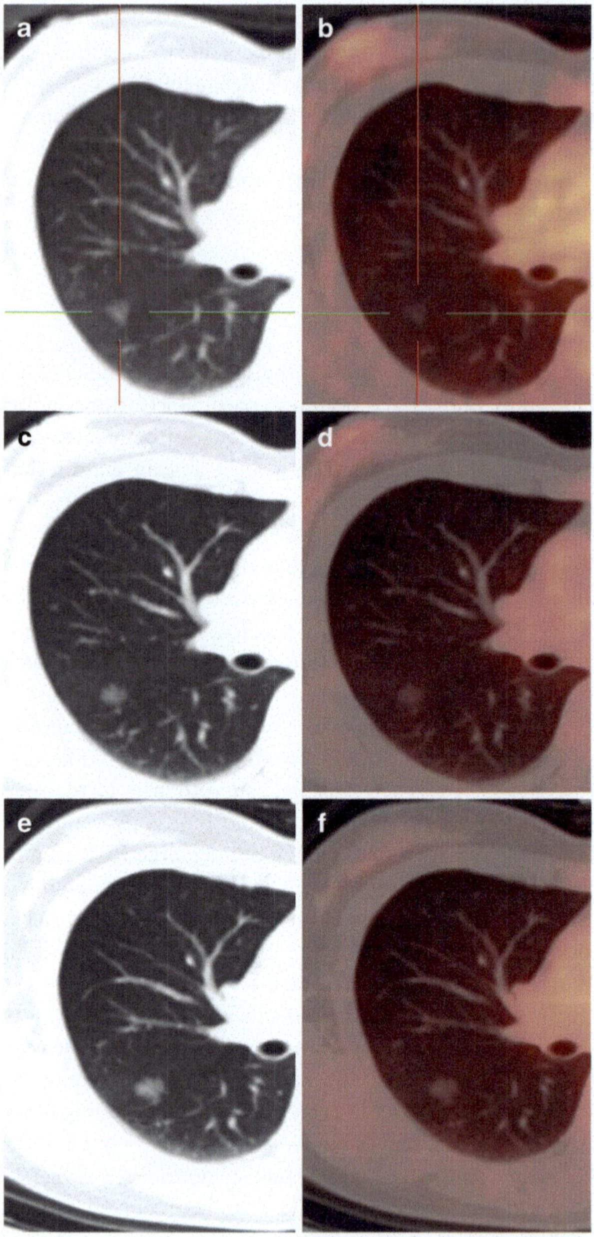

Fig. 4.4 Female, 56 years old. A GGN was incidentally detected in the right lower lobe without abnormal FDG uptake. After that, the lesion was routinely followed up. Comparative analysis of three consecutive follow-up CT scans (**a**, **b**; **c**, **d**; **e**, **f**) revealed a slow growth pattern with mildly elevated FDG uptake (higher than the pulmonary background) with SUVmax = 0.6. Surgical pathologic examinations confirmed adenocarcinoma in situ

the arm of CWU + PET, implying that addition of PET to conventional workup prevented unnecessary surgery in one out of five patients with suspected non-small cell lung cancer [4]. Three other randomized trials showed that PET imaging could detect distant metastasis and lymph node involvement which eventually derived about 14–17% of the cases to receive the nonsurgical treatment. Large-scaled studies based on the US National Cancer Data Base and Surveillance Epidemiology concluded that PET scan is beneficial for preoperative staging of pulmonary nodules.

According to ACCP clinical guidelines, recommendations are provided regarding the necessity of PET/CT examination in the assessment of small pulmonary nodules measuring ≤10 mm with high pretest probability of lung cancer. PET/CT is recommended for the individuals with a solid indeterminate nodule measuring 8–10 mm in diameter and low to moderate pretest probability of malignancy (5–65%). PET/CT is not recommended for individuals with a solid indeterminate nodule measuring 8–10 mm and a high pretest probability of malignancy (>65%); nonetheless, PET/CT may be indicated for pretreatment staging purpose among those patients with nodules strongly suspected of malignancy. Surveillance with serial CT scans (2 years at least, and 3 years for the pure GGO) is recommended for individuals with a solid indeterminate nodule measuring 8–10 mm when clinical probability of malignancy is low (30–40%) and the lesion is not hypermetabolic on PET. Surgical diagnosis is recommended for individuals with a solid indeterminate nodule measuring 8–10 mm when the nodule is intensely hypermetabolic by PET. PET/CT is recommended for individuals with a part-solid nodule measuring >8 mm following chest CT at 3 months and individuals with a part-solid nodule measuring >15 mm directly, but not for individuals with a part-solid lesion in which the solid component measures ≤8 mm for characterization. In conclusion, PET/CT is recommended for individuals with a solid or part-solid nodule and moderate probability of malignancy and for pretreatment staging.

False-Positive and False-Negative Results

As discussed previously, lung cancers at their very early developmental stage, such as lepidic-predominant adenocarcinomas (AIS or MIA), mucinous adenocarcinomas, and carcinoid tumors, may be biologically indolent and at low metabolic activity, resulting in false-negative PET findings. In the meanwhile, false-positive PET results in pulmonary nodules may reflect the complexity of underlying pathogenesis. Besides lung cancers, many benign processes could produce focal pulmonary nodule(s), such as chronic pneumonia, pulmonary pseudotumor, mycoses, tuberculoma, and sarcoidosis (Fig. 4.5). Paradoxically, false-positive PET results should be considered as an alert to clinicians to be aware of the presence of an active infectious or inflammatory condition that might require specific treatment. In addition, FDG-PET images can be used for precise tissue biopsy. With the functional information, PET imaging can distinguish metabolically active portions of lesions from necrotic areas. A biopsy on the active portions should be most likely to yield a definitive pathologic result, avoiding repeated biopsy and expenditure. Solid nodules with

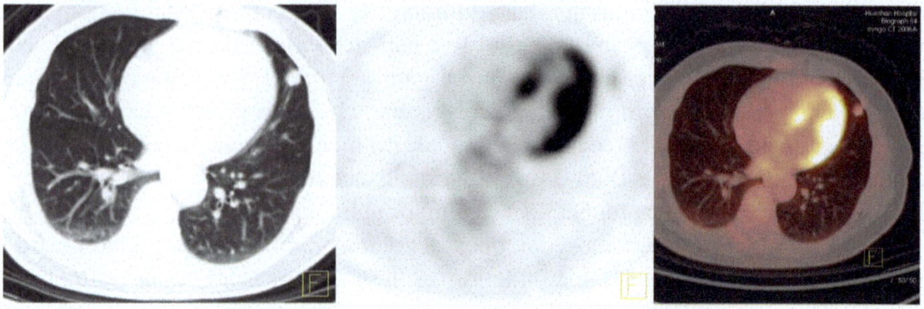

Fig. 4.5 Male, 68 years old. A cough and expectoration without bloody phlegm for more than 1 month. Chest CT revealed an 8 mm × 9 mm solid nodule in the lingular lobe of the left lung with elevated FDG uptake. Initial SUVmax = 2.85, delayed SUVmax = 3.91. Malignancy was highly suspected. Surgical pathologic examinations confirmed inflammatory granuloma

homogeneous attenuation are more likely to be malignant if signs of lobulation, coarse spiculation, or pleural retraction are present. Due to the high false-negative rates in the biopsy and PET scan in small lesion ≤8 mm, thoracotomy may be required for both diagnostic and curative purposes in cases with increasing suspicion of malignancy. Clinically, the management of asymptomatic small pulmonary nodules depends mainly on image findings. When malignancy is highly suspected, PET scan, CT-guided percutaneous lung biopsy, or VATS can be conducted.

4.3 Conclusion

In the oncological situation, PET/CT examination has numerous valuable roles, such as differential diagnosis, staging/restaging, and treatment outcome monitoring. As lung cancer screening techniques advance, the detection rate of small-sized especially subcentimeter pulmonary nodules is increasing. Characterization and clinical management of these small pulmonary nodules are challenging. Although limited, ^{18}F-FDG PET/CT has its unique values in the assessment of small pulmonary nodules. Clinical trials or well-designed retrospective studies need to be conducted to further optimize the application of PET imaging and interpretation of imaging findings in the diagnosis and management of early-stage lung cancer.

References

1. Fletcher JW, Kymes SM, Gould M, Alazraki N, Coleman RE, Lowe VJ, Marn C, Segall G, Thet LA, Lee K. A comparison of the diagnostic accuracy of 18F-FDG PET and CT in the characterization of solitary pulmonary nodules. J Nucl Med. 2008;49(2):179–85. https://doi.org/10.2967/jnumed.107.044990.
2. Barger RL Jr, Nandalur KR. Diagnostic performance of dual-time 18F-FDG PET in the diagnosis of pulmonary nodules: a meta-analysis. Acad Radiol. 2012;19(2):153–8. https://doi.org/10.1016/j.acra.2011.10.009.

3. Fischer B, Lassen U, Mortensen J, Larsen S, Loft A, Bertelsen A, Ravn J, Clementsen P, Hogholm A, Larsen K, Rasmussen T, Keiding S, Dirksen A, Gerke O, Skov B, Steffensen I, Hansen H, Vilmann P, Jacobsen G, Backer V, Maltbaek N, Pedersen J, Madsen H, Nielsen H, Hojgaard L. Preoperative staging of lung cancer with combined PET-CT. N Engl J Med. 2009;361(1):32–9. https://doi.org/10.1056/NEJMoa0900043.
4. van Tinteren H, Hoekstra OS, Smit EF, van den Bergh JH, Schreurs AJ, Stallaert RA, van Velthoven PC, Comans EF, Diepenhorst FW, Verboom P, van Mourik JC, Postmus PE, Boers M, Teule GJ. Effectiveness of positron emission tomography in the preoperative assessment of patients with suspected non-small-cell lung cancer: the PLUS multicentre randomised trial. Lancet. 2002;359(9315):1388–93.

Suggested Readings

1. Balogova S, Huchet V, Kerrou K, Nataf V, Gutman F, Antoine M, Ruppert AM, Prignon A, Lavolee A, Montravers F, Mayaud C, Cadranel J, Talbot JN. Detection of bronchioloalveolar cancer by means of PET/CT and 18F-fluorocholine, and comparison with 18F-fluorodeoxyglucose. Nucl Med Commun. 2010;31(5):389–97. https://doi.org/10.1097/MNM.0b013e3283369654.
2. Buchbender C, Herbrik M, Treffert J, Forsting M, Bockisch A, Antoch G, Heusner TA. Virtual 18F-FDG PET/CT bronchoscopy for lymph node staging in non-small-cell lung cancer patients: present and future applications. Expert Rev Med Devices. 2012;9(3):241–7. https://doi.org/10.1586/erd.12.9.
3. Cha MJ, Lee KS, Kim HS, Lee SW, Jeong CJ, Kim EY, Lee HY. Improvement in imaging diagnosis technique and modalities for solitary pulmonary nodules: from ground-glass opacity nodules to part-solid and solid nodules. Expert Rev Respir Med. 2016;10(3):261–78. https://doi.org/10.1586/17476348.2016.1141053.
4. Chao F, Zhang H. PET/CT in the staging of the non-small-cell lung cancer. J Biomed Biotechnol. 2012;2012:783739. https://doi.org/10.1155/2012/783739.
5. Chiu CF, Lin YY, Hsu WH, Chen CY, Yeh JJ, Kao CH. Shorter-time dual-phase FDG PET/CT in characterizing solid or ground-glass nodules based on surgical results. Clin Imaging. 2012;36(5):509–14. https://doi.org/10.1016/j.clinimag.2011.11.032.
6. Chun EJ, Lee HJ, Kang WJ, Kim KG, Goo JM, Park CM, Lee CH. Differentiation between malignancy and inflammation in pulmonary ground-glass nodules: the feasibility of integrated (18)F-FDG PET/CT. Lung Cancer. 2009;65(2):180–6. https://doi.org/10.1016/j.lungcan.2008.11.015.
7. Divisi D, Barone M, Zaccagna G, Crisci R. Fluorine-18 fluorodeoxyglucose positron emission tomography in the management of solitary pulmonary nodule: a review. Ann Med. 2017;49:626–35. https://doi.org/10.1080/07853890.2017.1339906.
8. Gomez-Caro A, Boada M, Cabanas M, Sanchez M, Arguis P, Lomena F, Ramirez J, Molins L. False-negative rate after positron emission tomography/computer tomography scan for mediastinal staging in cI stage non-small-cell lung cancer. Eur J Cardiothorac Surg. 2012;42(1):93–100; discussion 100. https://doi.org/10.1093/ejcts/ezr272.
9. Gould MK, Ananth L, Barnett PG. A clinical model to estimate the pretest probability of lung cancer in patients with solitary pulmonary nodules. Chest. 2007;131(2):383–8. https://doi.org/10.1378/chest.06-1261.
10. Gould MK, Donington J, Lynch WR, Mazzone PJ, Midthun DE, Naidich DP, Wiener RS. Evaluation of individuals with pulmonary nodules: when is it lung cancer? Diagnosis and management of lung cancer, 3rd ed: American College of Chest Physicians evidence-based clinical practice guidelines. Chest. 2013;143(5 Suppl):e93S–e120S. https://doi.org/10.1378/chest.12-2351.
11. Hattori A, Matsunaga T, Takamochi K, Oh S, Suzuki K. Clinical significance of positron emission tomography in subcentimeter non-small cell lung cancer. Ann Thorac Surg. 2017;103(5):1614–20. https://doi.org/10.1016/j.athoracsur.2016.09.059.

12. Hattori A, Suzuki K, Matsunaga T, Fukui M, Tsushima Y, Takamochi K, Oh S. Tumour standardized uptake value on positron emission tomography is a novel predictor of adenocarcinoma in situ for c-stage IA lung cancer patients with a part-solid nodule on thin-section computed tomography scan. Interact Cardiovasc Thorac Surg. 2014;18(3):329–34. https://doi.org/10.1093/icvts/ivt500.
13. Kernstine KH, Grannis FW Jr, Rotter AJ. Is there a role for PET in the evaluation of subcentimeter pulmonary nodules? Semin Thorac Cardiovasc Surg. 2005;17(2):110–4. https://doi.org/10.1053/j.semtcvs.2005.04.004.
14. Kozower BD, Meyers BF, Reed CE, Jones DR, Decker PA, Putnam JB Jr. Does positron emission tomography prevent nontherapeutic pulmonary resections for clinical stage IA lung cancer? Ann Thorac Surg. 2008;85(4):1166–1169; discussion 1169-1170. https://doi.org/10.1016/j.athoracsur.2008.01.018.
15. Lasnon C, Hicks RJ, Beauregard JM, Milner A, Paciencia M, Guizard AV, Bardet S, Gervais R, Lemoel G, Zalcman G, Aide N. Impact of point spread function reconstruction on thoracic lymph node staging with 18F-FDG PET/CT in non-small cell lung cancer. Clin Nucl Med. 2012;37(10):971–6. https://doi.org/10.1097/RLU.0b013e318251e3d1.
16. Minamimoto R, Senda M, Jinnouchi S, Terauchi T, Yoshida T, Uno K, Iinuma T, Murano T, Nakashima R, Inoue T. Detection of lung cancer by FDG-PET cancer screening program: a nationwide Japanese survey. Anticancer Res. 2014;34(1):183–9.
17. Murakami S, Saito H, Sakuma Y, Kondo T, Oshita F, Ito H, Tsuboi M, Hasegawa C, Yokose T, Kameda Y, Nakayama H, Yamada K. Prognostic value of preoperative FDG-PET in stage IA lung adenocarcinoma. Eur J Radiol. 2012;81(8):1891–5. https://doi.org/10.1016/j.ejrad.2011.04.007.
18. Naidich DP, Bankier AA, MacMahon H, Schaefer-Prokop CM, Pistolesi M, Goo JM, Macchiarini P, Crapo JD, Herold CJ, Austin JH, Travis WD. Recommendations for the management of subsolid pulmonary nodules detected at CT: a statement from the Fleischner society. Radiology. 2013;266(1):304–17. https://doi.org/10.1148/radiol.12120628.
19. Nair VS, Barnett PG, Ananth L, Gould MK. PET scan 18F-fluorodeoxyglucose uptake and prognosis in patients with resected clinical stage IA non-small cell lung cancer. Chest. 2010;137(5):1150–6. https://doi.org/10.1378/chest.09-2356.
20. Nitadori J, Bograd AJ, Morales EA, Rizk NP, Dunphy MP, Sima CS, Rusch VW, Adusumilli PS. Preoperative consolidation-to-tumor ratio and SUVmax stratify the risk of recurrence in patients undergoing limited resection for lung adenocarcinoma </=2 cm. Ann Surg Oncol. 2013;20(13):4282–8. https://doi.org/10.1245/s10434-013-3212-2.
21. Ost D, Fein AM, Feinsilver SH. Clinical practice. The solitary pulmonary nodule. N Engl J Med. 2003;348(25):2535–42. https://doi.org/10.1056/NEJMcp012290.
22. Park HK, Jeon K, Koh WJ, Suh GY, Kim H, Kwon OJ, Chung MP, Lee KS, Shim YM, Han J, Um SW. Occult nodal metastasis in patients with non-small cell lung cancer at clinical stage IA by PET/CT. Respirology. 2010;15(8):1179–84. https://doi.org/10.1111/j.1440-1843.2010.01793.x.
23. Park SY, Cho A, WS Y, Lee CY, Lee JG, Kim DJ, Chung KY. Prognostic value of total lesion glycolysis by 18F-FDG PET/CT in surgically resected stage IA non-small cell lung cancer. J Nucl Med. 2015;56(1):45–9. https://doi.org/10.2967/jnumed.114.147561.
24. Qiu ZX, Cheng Y, Liu D, Wang WY, Wu X, WL W, Li WM. Clinical, pathological, and radiological characteristics of solitary ground-glass opacity lung nodules on high-resolution computed tomography. Ther Clin Risk Manag. 2016;12:1445–53. https://doi.org/10.2147/tcrm.s110363.
25. Saisho S, Yasuda K, Maeda A, Yukawa T, Okita R, Hirami Y, Shimizu K, Nakata M. Role of 2-[18F]fluoro-2-deoxyglucose positron emission tomography in preoperative management of solid-type small-sized lung cancer. Ann Nucl Med. 2013;27(6):515–22. https://doi.org/10.1007/s12149-013-0715-7.
26. Sayyouh M, Vummidi DR, Kazerooni EA. Evaluation and management of pulmonary nodules: state-of-the-art and future perspectives. Expert Opin Med Diagn. 2013;7(6):629–44. https://doi.org/10.1517/17530059.2013.858117.
27. Shibata H, Nomori H, Uno K, Iyama K, Tomiyoshi K, Nakashima R, Sakaguchi K, Goya T, Takanami I, Koizumi K, Suzuki T, Kaji M, Horio H. 11C-acetate for positron emission tomography imaging of clinical stage IA lung adenocarcinoma: comparison with 18F-fluorodeoxyglucose for imaging and evaluation of tumor aggressiveness. Ann Nucl Med. 2009;23(7):609–16. https://doi.org/10.1007/s12149-009-0278-9.

28. Shiono S, Abiko M, Okazaki T, Chiba M, Yabuki H, Sato T. Positron emission tomography for predicting recurrence in stage I lung adenocarcinoma: standardized uptake value corrected by mean liver standardized uptake value. Eur J Cardiothorac Surg. 2011;40(5):1165–9. https://doi.org/10.1016/j.ejcts.2011.02.041.
29. Shiono S, Abiko M, Sato T. Limited resection for clinical stage IA non-small-cell lung cancers based on a standardized-uptake value index. Eur J Cardiothorac Surg. 2013;43(1):e7–e12. https://doi.org/10.1093/ejcts/ezs573.
30. Shiono S, Yanagawa N, Abiko M, Sato T. Detection of non-aggressive stage IA lung cancer using chest computed tomography and positron emission tomography/computed tomography. Interact Cardiovasc Thorac Surg. 2014;19(4):637–43. https://doi.org/10.1093/icvts/ivu188.
31. Sun JS, Park KJ, Sheen SS, Yoon JK, Yoon SN, Lee KB, Hwang SC. Clinical usefulness of the fluorodeoxyglucose (FDG)-PET maximal standardized uptake value (SUV) in combination with CT features for the differentiation of adenocarcinoma with a bronchioloalveolar carcinoma from other subtypes of non-small cell lung cancers. Lung Cancer. 2009;66(2):205–10. https://doi.org/10.1016/j.lungcan.2009.01.009.
32. Swensen SJ, Silverstein MD, Ilstrup DM, Schleck CD, Edell ES. The probability of malignancy in solitary pulmonary nodules. Application to small radiologically indeterminate nodules. Arch Intern Med. 1997;157(8):849–55.
33. Takenaka T, Yano T, Morodomi Y, Ito K, Miura N, Kawano D, Shoji F, Baba S, Abe K, Honda H, Maehara Y. Prediction of true-negative lymph node metastasis in clinical IA non-small cell lung cancer by measuring standardized uptake values on positron emission tomography. Surg Today. 2012;42(10):934–9. https://doi.org/10.1007/s00595-012-0277-7.
34. Tsutani Y, Miyata Y, Nakayama H, Okumura S, Adachi S, Yoshimura M, Okada M. Solid tumor size on high-resolution computed tomography and maximum standardized uptake on positron emission tomography for new clinical T descriptors with T1 lung adenocarcinoma. Ann Oncol. 2013;24(9):2376–81. https://doi.org/10.1093/annonc/mdt230.
35. Uehara H, Tsutani Y, Okumura S, Nakayama H, Adachi S, Yoshimura M, Miyata Y, Okada M. Prognostic role of positron emission tomography and high-resolution computed tomography in clinical stage IA lung adenocarcinoma. Ann Thorac Surg. 2013;96(6):1958–65. https://doi.org/10.1016/j.athoracsur.2013.06.086.
36. Waki A, Fujibayashi Y, Yokoyama A. Recent advances in the analyses of the characteristics of tumors on FDG uptake. Nucl Med Biol. 1998;25(7):589–92.
37. Wang YC, Tseng HL, Lin YH, Kao CH, Huang WC, Huang TC. Improvement of internal tumor volumes of non-small cell lung cancer patients for radiation treatment planning using interpolated average CT in PET/CT. PLoS One. 2013;8(5):e64665. https://doi.org/10.1371/journal.pone.0064665.
38. Yi CA, Lee KS, Kim BT, Choi JY, Kwon OJ, Kim H, Shim YM, Chung MJ. Tissue characterization of solitary pulmonary nodule: comparative study between helical dynamic CT and integrated PET/CT. J Nucl Med. 2006;47(3):443–50.
39. Yonemori K, Tateishi U, Uno H, Yonemori Y, Tsuta K, Takeuchi M, Matsuno Y, Fujiwara Y, Asamura H, Kusumoto M. Development and validation of diagnostic prediction model for solitary pulmonary nodules. Respirology. 2007;12(6):856–62. https://doi.org/10.1111/j.1440-1843.2007.01158.x.
40. Yoshioka M, Ichiguchi O. Selection of sublobar resection for c-stage IA non-small cell lung cancer based on a combination of structural imaging by CT and functional imaging by FDG PET. Ann Thorac Cardiovasc Surg. 2009;15(2):82–8.
41. Zhang WD, Guan YB, Li CX, Huang XB, Zhang FJ. Pulmonary mucosa-associated lymphoid tissue lymphoma: computed tomography and (1)(8)F fluorodeoxyglucose-positron emission tomography/computed tomography imaging findings and follow-up. J Comput Assist Tomogr. 2011;35(5):608–13. https://doi.org/10.1097/RCT.0b013e318227a661.
42. Zhou J, Li Y, Zhang Y, Liu G, Tan H, Hu Y, Xiao J, Shi H. Solitary ground-glass opacity nodules of stage IA pulmonary adenocarcinoma: combination of 18F-FDG PET/CT and high-resolution computed tomography features to predict invasive adenocarcinoma. Oncotarget. 2017;8(14):23312–21. https://doi.org/10.18632/oncotarget.15577.

Chapter 5
Tumor Dormancy and Angiogenesis-Dependent Progression

Xiangpeng Zheng, Ming Li, and Guozhen Zhang

5.1 Tumor Dormancy, Progression and Angiogenesis

The formation and development of a tumor is a complex, multistep process involving genetic mutations in single cells, immune imbalances in microenvironments, and the effects of tumor promoters. Taking lung adenocarcinoma as an example, the hypothesis of multistep tumorigenesis, in which some, if not all, lung adenocarcinomas arise from preneoplastic AAH lesions, progress to AIS and MIA, and eventually develop into invasive adenocarcinomas, was proposed over two decades ago. It has increasingly been accepted given expanding evidence from numerous pathological and molecular investigations [1].

According to the IASLC/ATS/ERS classification of lung adenocarcinoma, both AAH and AIS are classified as preinvasive lesions. The progression from preinvasive diseases to invasive diseases (such as MIA and IAC) can be a slow process lasting several years or even decades [2]. During this period, tumor cells remain in a state of growth inertia or dormancy. Once the tumor escapes the dormant state because of the interactions of various intrinsic or extrinsic factors, its development gains momentum, with continuous proliferation characterized by accelerated progression, shortening of the volume doubling time, and the presentation of certain clinical symptoms. Biologically, a variety of molecular events are involved in malignant progression, and epigenetic transition of tumor cells and angiogenesis is with the dominating significance by exerting determinant influences on tumor development and the clinical presentation. Investigations into the interaction between tumor progression and angiogenesis have shown that tumors without

X. Zheng (✉)
Department of Radiation Oncology, Fudan University Huadong Hospital, Shanghai, China
e-mail: zhengxp@fudan.edu.cn

M. Li • G. Zhang
Department of Radiology, Fudan University Huadong Hospital, Shanghai, China

X. Zheng et al. (eds.), *Early-stage Lung Cancer*,
https://doi.org/10.1007/978-981-10-7596-4_5

angiogenesis tend to hibernate due to a limited nutritional supply, whereas those with active angiogenesis resulting from predominant proangiogenic effects gain the ability to sustain clonal expansion, stromal invasion, and eventually distant metastasis, which indirectly explains the clinical observation of persistent ground-glass opacities on chest CT scans.

5.1.1 Tumor Dormancy

Tumor dormancy refers to a "steady state" in which fully transformed tumor cells are viable but temporarily lose their capacity for linear growth, progression, and expansion into a clinically detectable lesion. This is a common phenomenon in biology and is one of the hallmarks of cancer biological behavior. The state of dormancy could apply to the early stages of primary cancer; to the remnants of surgically resected or medically controlled primary tumors, which could serve as "seeds" for disease recurrence; and to "dormant" micrometastases, which could, after a latency period, be "reactivated" and evolve into clinical disease [3].

Various hypotheses have been proposed to explain tumor dormancy with corresponding clinical and experimental evidence. Based on the underlying mechanisms, tumor dormancy can be categorized into two types: cellular dormancy and angiogenic dormancy. In cellular dormancy, either solitary or a small group of cells remain quiescent (a state known as "reversible cell cycle arrest"), driven by cell-related intrinsic or extrinsic factors from microenvironments, and primarily characterized by a constant cell amount and tumor volume resulting from a dynamic balance between cell proliferation and apoptosis, as well as reduced cellular mobility. Experimental research has revealed that initial tumor cell microfoci in mouse lungs consist of 1–30 cells, most (if not all) of which are in the G0 or early G1 phase of the cell cycle. A more advanced phase of lung micrometastases comprises avascular deposits that form cuffs around pre-existing vessels, thin layers on the pleural surface, or spheroid colonies of about 10^3–10^5 cells, depending on the tumor type. Avascular micrometastases remain in a steady state with a high proliferation index, a high apoptotic index, and no necrosis [4]. In contrast, angiogenic dormancy results from an inadequate capacity for vessel recruitment in early-stage tumors or micrometastases. It is well established that tumor growth beyond the size of 1–2 mm or the volume of 2 mm^3 is angiogenesis-dependent; without vessel proliferation, the metabolic activity and proliferation ability of tumor cells will be compromised due to an insufficient nutritional supply.

A nonangiogenic and dormant tumor is characterized by seven features [5, 6]:

1. Self -limitation in tumor growth *in vivo* to a diameter up to approximately 1 mm.
2. Inability to induce angiogenic activity characterized by the lack or relative absence of intra-tumor microvessels or by active repulsion of existing blood vessels in the local microenvironment.

3. Production of similar or greater amounts of antiangiogenic (i.e., thrombospondin-1) than proangiogenic (i.e., VEGF, bFGF) factors.
4. Dynamic equilibrium between active tumor cell proliferation and apoptosis *in vivo* and metabolic activity during the dormancy period.
5. Possibility of cloning from a human angiogenic tumor, because human tumors are heterogeneous and contain a mixture of nonangiogenic and angiogenic tumor cells.
6. Inability to spontaneously metastasize from the microscopic dormant state.
7. No harm being caused to the host until they switch to the angiogenic phenotype.

As described above, no neovascularization is observed in the dormant tumor. A break in the dormancy state is related to the activation of an angiogenic switch and subsequent angiogenesis. With the improvement in blood circulation and a sufficient supply of oxygen and nutrition, tumor cells have an increased metabolic and proliferation activity, driving disease progression toward more advanced stages.

5.1.2 Tumor Angiogenesis

The sustainable development of a tumor relies on adequate vasculature and a sufficient blood supply. In 1974, Folkman postulated that the growth of tumors *in vivo* occurs in two distinct phases, namely, avascular and vascular phases [7]. The initial avascular phase is characterized by the slow development of the tumor cell population with a proliferation index of 12% and an apoptosis index varying between 4 and 7.5%. Consequently, the tumor has a significant volume doubling time, even after several years. Due to the lack of an efficient blood supply, nutrients and waste products are transported by diffusion. The subsequent vascular phase is characterized by neovascularization and the formation of a tumor blood circulation system. With a sustainable nutrient supply and an improved microenvironment, the balance between proliferation and apoptosis is disrupted, the cell proliferation is predominating, and tumors are growing faster with an increased risk of distant metastasis via the lymphatic or vascular routes.

Early in 1973, Gimbrone et al. conducted a classic experiment on the assessment of neovascularization using a model of an intraocular tumor [8]. Tumor cells were implanted in the iris and anterior chamber of rabbit eyes. The cells in the iris induced novel microvascular trees toward the tumor cell foci which consequently grew rapidly, whereas those in the anterior chamber showed no signs of growth and a lack of neovascularization. These observations indicated that neovascularization is essential for tumor growth and appears to be directly mediated by a humoral factor from viable tumor cells or through intermediary interaction with host tissues.

As previously discussed, without a sufficient and sustainable nutrient supply, tumor cells can enter a state of long-term dormancy, and the tumor size is beyond the limit of clinical detection using the imaging modalities that are currently available. Besides organic nutrients, oxygen is essential for tumor growth and should be transported to tumor area via blood circulation. Likewise, oxygen has a limited diffusion distance in the microenvironment, as the distance from the vessels increases, the oxygen tension decreases. The effective oxygen diffusion distance varies with tissues, in a range of 70 to about 150 μm, and tumor cells over 200 μm away physically remain in a hypoxic status. Thomlinson et al. investigated oxygen diffusion by using bronchial carcinoma and showed that with a radius of less than about 160 μm, no necrosis was evident in small tumor cords, whereas a tumor cord with a radius exceeding 200 μm was always with a necrotic center. As the diameter of the necrotic area increased, the thickness of the sheath of viable tumor cells remained essentially constant at 100–180 μm [9]. Without a continuous oxygen supply from vascular penetration, tumor size remains relatively constant. Therefore, to overcome the restriction of nutrients on growth, tumors should recruit and develop their own vascular system, a process called angiogenesis, that is closely related to the mechanism of angiogenic switch.

5.1.2.1 Angiogenic Switch

The underlying mechanism and timing of dormant tumor cells emerging from quiescence are not yet fully understood. Mounting evidence shows that distinct microvascular development is involved in the regulation of this process. Mature blood vessels produce signals that sustain tumor cell quiescence, whereas sprouting microvasculature provides stimuli that reactivate dormant tumor cells [10]. The hallmark of the transition from the avascular to the vascular phase is angiogenesis, microvasculature sprouting from pre-existing vessels. The onset of angiogenesis relies primarily on the activation of the angiogenic switch, a concept describing a permanent change in the angiogenic capacity of the tumor with the potential to convey tumorigenic properties to tumor cells [11]. As a discrete event, the angiogenic switch can be triggered by various signals, including genetic mutations, metabolic stress (e.g., hypoxia, low pH conditions, low sugar concentration, etc.), mechanical stress (e.g., from cell proliferation), and the immune/inflammatory response (infiltration of immune cells and/or inflammatory cells due to local tissue damage, etc.). These signals alone or in combination exert impacts on the production of angiogenesis-related proangiogenic or antiangiogenic factors to regulate endothelial proliferation, stabilize neovasculature structures, and promote their maturation. Table 5.1 lists major angiogenesis activators and inhibitors as well as their functional mechanisms of action.

The initiation and maintenance of angiogenesis is a process that is subject to the relative concentrations of activators and inhibitors produced by tumor cells and/or stromal cells in the microenvironment. If angiogenesis activators prevail, bone marrow-derived endothelial precursor cells and/or angiogenesis-related inflammatory cells can migrate toward the tumors and facilitate the activation of the angiogenic

Table 5.1 Angiogenesis activators and inhibitors [12]

Activators	Function	Inhibitors	Function
VEGF family members	Stimulate angio-/vasculogenesis, permeability, leukocyte adhesion	VEGFR-1; soluble VEGFR-1; soluble NRP-1	Sink for VEGF, VEGF-B, PlGF
VEGFR, NRP-1	Integrate angiogenic and survival signals	Ang2	Antagonist of Ang1
Ang1, Tie2	Stabilize vessels, inhibit permeability	TSP-1, TSP-2	Inhibit endothelial migration, growth, adhesion, and survival
PDGF-BB and receptors	Recruit smooth muscle cells	Angiostatin and related plasminogen kringles	Suppress tumor angiogenesis
TGF-β1, endoglin, TGF-β receptors	Stimulate extracellular matrix production	Endostatin (collagen XVIII fragment)	Inhibit endothelial survival and migration
FGF, HGF, MCP-1	Stimulate angio-/arteriogenesis	Vasostatin; calreticulin	Inhibit endothelial growth
Integrins $\alpha_v\beta_3$, $\alpha_v\beta_5$, $\alpha_5\beta_1$	Receptors for matrix macromolecules and proteinases	Platelet factor-4	Inhibits binding of bFGF and VEGF
VE-cadherin; PECAM (CD31)	Endothelial junctional molecules	TIMPs; MMP inhibitors; PEX	Suppress pathological angiogenesis
Ephrins	Regulate arterial/venous specification	Meth-1; Meth-2	Inhibitors containing MMP, TSP and disintegrin domains
Plasminogen activators, MMPs	Remodel matrix, release and activate growth factors	IFN-α, -β, -γ; IP-10, IL-4, IL-12, IL-18	Inhibit endothelial migration; downregulate bFGF
PAI-1	Stabilize nascent vessels	Prothrombin kringle-2; antithrombin III fragment	Suppress endothelial growth
NOS; COX-2	Stimulate angiogenesis and vasodilation	Prolactin (Mr, 16 K)	Inhibits bFGF/VEGF
AC133	Regulate angioblast differentiation	VEGI	Modulate cell growth
Chemokines	Pleiotropic role in angiogenesis	Fragment of SPARC	Inhibit endothelial binding and activity of VEGF
Id1/Id3	Determine endothelial plasticity	Osteopontin fragment	Interfere with integrin signaling
		Maspin	Protease inhibitor
		Canstatin, proliferin-related protein, restin	Mechanisms unknown

switch and subsequent transition from the avascular to vascular phase. Besides the activation of the angiogenic switch, a sustained production of angiogenic factors is equally important for tumor progression, which is reflected by the "spike hypothesis" [13]. Per this hypothesis, there exist an induction threshold and a maintenance threshold of angiogenic factors for neoangiogenesis. The induction threshold may be physically represented by the number of angiogenic factors required to turn quiescent endothelial cells into proliferating cells and is conceivably higher than the levels required to keep them proliferating, which is referred to as the maintenance threshold. In most cancers, the induction threshold is overcome by the sustained production of angiogenic factors by the tumor cells themselves, and the progressive tumor growth occurs. Alternatively, cancer cells may lack sufficient angiogenic potential, and a short-term exogenous "spike" of angiogenic factors within the tumor microenvironment could suffice to initiate the process of angiogenesis and tumor growth [11].

In addition, as one of the many discrete steps in the tumor progression, angiogenesis itself is a complex, multistep process that follows tissue-specific regulations. In those tissues that are deficient in vasculature such as the epidermis, the activation of neoangiogenesis mainly relies on the overproduction of proangiogenic factors. In contrast, in those tissues with ample blood supply such as the pancreas, the inhibition or decreased production of anti-proangiogenic factors may play a dominant role in the initiation of neoangiogenesis.

5.1.2.2 Process of Angiogenesis

New vessel formation in tumors can occur in several ways, including sprouting, intussusception, incorporation of bone marrow-derived endothelial precursors, vasculogenic mimicry, and by the co-opting of pre-existing vessels by tumor cells. Among these methods, bone marrow-derived endothelial precursor cells are involved in the *de novo* formation of new vessels, which, in combination with sprouting, is the major angiogenic approach. Generally, angiogenesis refers to the sprouting approach; the host vascular network is expanding by the budding of endothelial sprouts or the formation of bridges. Angiogenesis can be divided into four steps: (1) activation of endothelial cells lining small pre-existing vessels, (2) degradation of the extracellular matrix, (3) migration and proliferation of endothelial cells in the alignment of a hollow tube, and (4) interconnection of hollow tubes.

As listed in Table 5.1, sprouting angiogenesis is regulated by numerous molecules. Initially, pre-existing host vessels dilate in response to VEGF with increasing permeability. Simultaneously, Ang2 and proteinases mediate dissolution of the existing basement membrane and interstitial matrix. Endothelial precursors are mobilized and recruited into the tumor matrix under the stimulation of VEGF, bFGF, IGF-1, and granulocyte-macrophage colony-stimulating factor (GM-CSF). Numerous molecules, including VEGF, Ang1, and bFGF, stimulate endothelial proliferation, migration, and assembly, and the migration of endothelial cells is regulated by cell-matrix receptors such as $\alpha v\beta 3$ and $\alpha v\beta 5$. Structurally, nascent vessels are unstable, and microvasculature formation and regression coexist. Using a spheroid model of ovarian carcinoma in nude mice, Gilead et al. showed that the cycles of vascular development and regression preceded the exit of the implanted spheroids from dormancy, and the neovasculature underwent maturation by formation of a new basement membrane and investment of new vessels through the recruitment of pericytes and smooth muscle cells before the initiation of tumor growth [14]. During the maturation process, PDGF-BB recruits smooth muscle cells, whereas signaling by TGF-1 and Ang1/Tie2 stabilizes the interaction between endothelial and smooth muscle cells. Proteinase inhibitors (e.g., PAI-1) prevent degradation of the provisional extracellular matrix around nascent vessels. Only when a stable, sustained, and efficient circulatory system is established within tumors and between tumors and the host vascular network do hibernating tumors awake from the dormant state and progressive development occurs.

After series of complicated molecular and biological events, tumors establish their own circulatory system derived from the pre-existing host vascular network. The stability and maintenance of neovasculatures largely depend on the concentrations of angiogenic factors (primary VEGF and Ang1) and the fate of endothelial cells. In an adult, quiescent endothelial cells can survive for several years (Fig. 5.1).

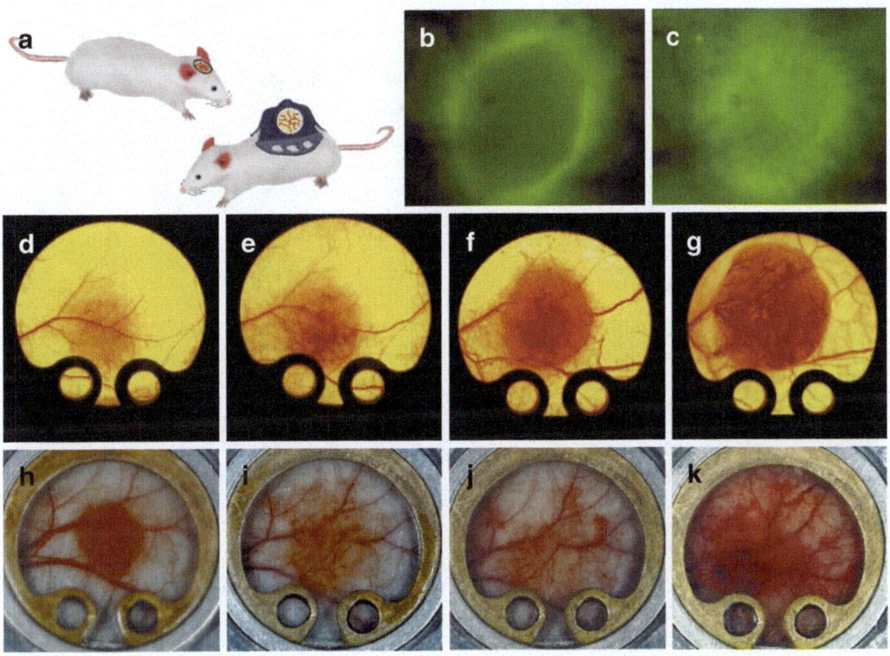

Fig. 5.1 Intravital microscopic observation of angiogenesis. (**a**) The tumor xenograft animal model. (**b**, **c**) VEGF promoter activity, as monitored by GFP intensity, on days 7 and 14 in murine mammary carcinoma growing in the dorsal window. (**d–g**) Angiogenesis and tumor growth in a 5-, 10-, 15-, and 20-day-old human colon adenocarcinoma in the dorsal window. (**h–k**) Angiogenesis during tumor regression and relapse following hormone ablation therapy of a hormone (androgen/testosterone)-dependent murine mammary carcinoma (From: *Jain RK* et al. *Endothelial cell death, angiogenesis, and microvascular function after castration in an androgen-dependent tumor: role of vascular endothelial growth factor. Proc Natl Acad Sci USA. 1998;95:10820–5.* Reprinted with permission)

5.1.2.3 Structural and Functional Features of Tumor Vessels

Unlike physiological angiogenesis in normal tissues or organs, tumor angiogenesis is a process that lacks proper control or regulation. Consequently, newly formed tumor vessels are structurally and functionally abnormal [12].

1. Chaotic architecture and blood flow. Due to an imbalance in angiogenic activators and inhibitors, neovessels in tumors are highly disorganized. Morphologically, tumor vessels are tortuous and dilated, have uneven diameters, and display excessive branching and shunts. These structural abnormalities disturb blood circulation, leading to chaotic and reduced or even reversed blood flow in some areas within tumors, eventually resulting in a hypoxic and acidic microenvironment (Fig. 5.2). Furthermore, hypoxia may select for the clonal expansion of

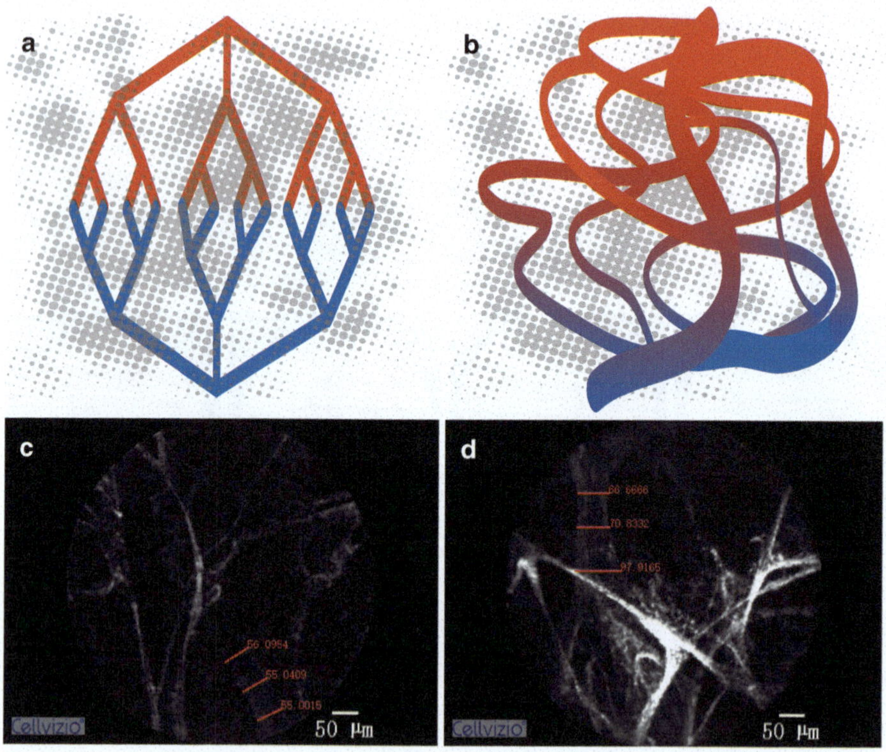

Fig. 5.2 Structural comparison between normal and tumor microvasculature. (**a**) Schematic illustration of microvasculature in physiological condition or benign diseases. Microvessels distribute homogeneously and display regular branching. (**b**) Schematic illustration of microvasculature in malignant tumors. Tumor blood vessels are typically dilated and tortuous, with abnormal branching patterns, dead ends, and no organization into arterioles, capillaries, and venules. (**c, d**) Intravital assessment of microvessels of inflammatory lesion (**c**) and lung adenocarcinoma (**d**) with transbronchial confocal endoscopy. (**c**) Normal capillaries are observed with a homogeneous diameter of approximately 55 μm. (**d**) In contrast, microvessels in adenocarcinoma appear rigid and irregularly dilated, with diameters ranging from 56 to 97 μm

cells that have lost their apoptotic response to hypoxia, which may promote tumor malignancy, invasiveness, and resistance to therapies [15]. Vascular normalization is a strategy involving the administration of certain antiangiogenic agents to prune nascent vessels and consequently improve blood circulation.
2. High vascular permeability. Microscopically, nascent vessels are distinct from normal vessels. Numerous abnormal openings including endothelial fenestrae, vesicles, and transcellular holes (about 0.6 μm) can be observed on vascular walls (Fig. 5.3). In addition, inter-endothelial junctions or pores have a diameter up to 1.5 μm [16]. In some regions, the basement membrane is discontinuous or absent due to a proliferative mismatch between endothelial and smooth muscle cells. These defects render neovessels highly leaky, allowing excessive plasma contents into the extravascular space and tumor microenvironment, as well as facilitating the hematogenous dissemination of tumor cells. Consequently, there is an increase in the interstitial pressure, which further inhibits the extravasation and diffusion of nutrients and therapeutic agents within tumors. Antiangiogenic therapy has the potential to overcome an unfavorable microenvironment and improve therapeutic outcome.
3. Nonuniform surface markers. Tumors stimulate angiogenesis to secure a blood supply for the growing tumor. The activated endothelial cells and pericytes in this neovasculature express cellular adhesion molecules or other surface markers that are not present or are barely detectable with extremely low levels in normal mature vessels. Moreover, the endothelial cells of tumor lymphatics also express tumor-specific markers. These distinct molecules or surface markers are known as vascular zip codes, signatures of tumor neovasculatures. In addition to tumor cells, stromal cells within tumors up-express or down-express certain molecules contributing to the complexity of tumor microenvironment. The chaotic blood circulation and the heterogeneous expression of adhesion molecules in combination may account for reduced interaction between leukocytes and endothelial cells and the selectively adhesion of activated lymphocytes to tumor vessels.

Besides nutrients and an oxygen supply through blood perfusion, tumor neovessels have paracrine functions. Endothelial cells lined neovessels secrete various growth factors and cytokines in a paracrine pattern which stimulates and maintains the proliferation of endothelial cells via a positive feedback loop that includes tumor cells. Consequently, tumor progression and invasiveness are accelerated.

5.2 Imaging Assessment of Microvasculature in Pulmonary Ground-Glass Nodules

5.2.1 Imaging Modalities for Microvasculature

Tumor blood vessels not only provide blood to the tumor, but also reflect the change in biological tumor behavior, from the inertia of a dormant state, progressing to a malignant and invasive state. Therefore, early identifying tumor angiogenesis

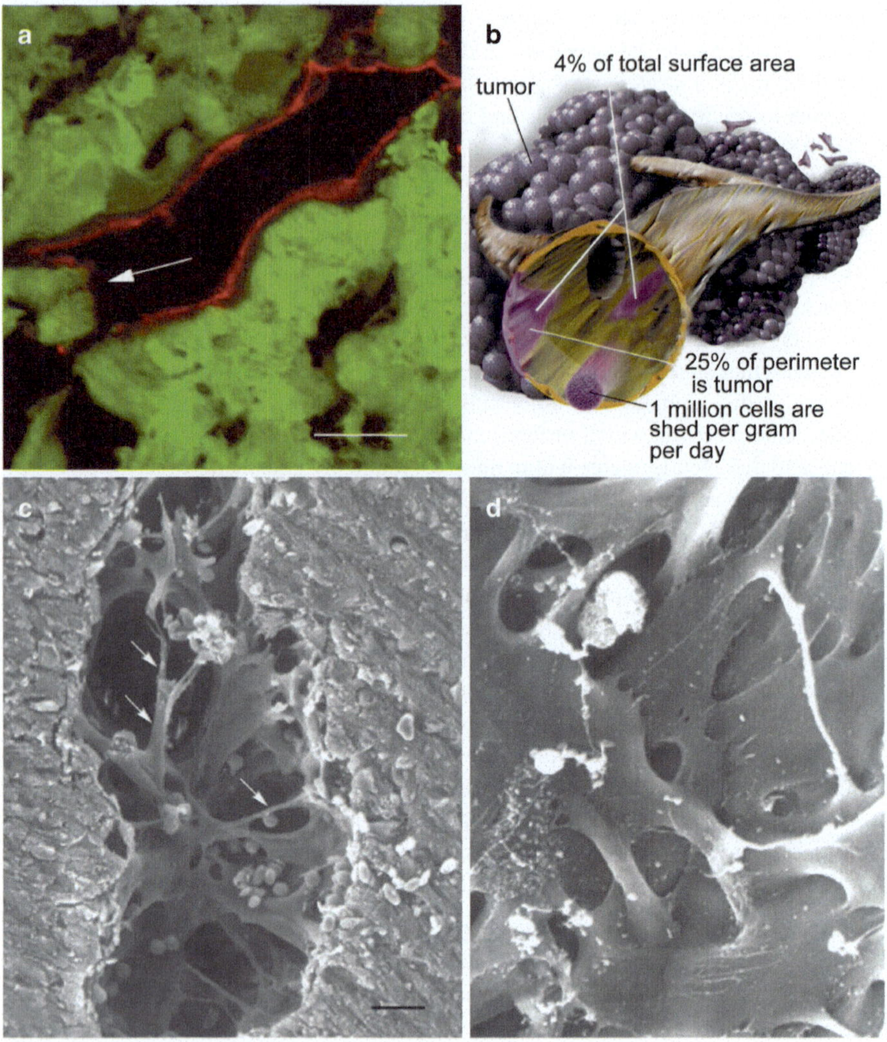

Fig. 5.3 Chaotic and mosaic vessels in tumors. (**a**) Cancer cell in the lining of a tumor vessel, referred to as a mosaic vessel. Cellular components of the vascular wall in a human colon carcinoma xenograft: cancer cells [green fluorescence, green fluorescent protein (GFP)] and endothelial cells (red fluorescence, CD31/CD105 antibody detected with cyanine 5 and lectin fluorescence to mark perfused vessels). The width of the endothelial gap exposing cancer cells to the vessel lumen is about 20 μm. (**b**) Quantification of mosaic vessels. In colon carcinoma, about 15% of tumor vessels are mosaic in nature, and cancer cells occupy about 4% of the total vascular surface area. If each of these cells intravasates in 2 days, the tumor will shed about 10^6 cells per day, per gram of tumor. (**c, d**) Scanning electron microscopy of the luminal surface of a blood vessel in a murine mammary tumor showing various abnormalities. Bar length represents 15 μm. (**c**) Abnormal endothelial cells partition the lumen (arrowheads). (**d**) Multiple intercellular openings (arrows) on the order of 1–5 μm (From *Carmeliet P, Jain RK. Angiogenesis in cancer and other diseases. Nature. 2000;407(6801):249–57*. Reprinted with permission)

phenomena is important for determining the dynamic development of the tumor, as well as to allow for the timely completion of interventions. Clinicians now have available a variety of imaging technologies, including CT, MRI, etc., that can help to evaluate new blood vessels to a degree. These methods have both advantages and disadvantages. Table 5.2 briefly compares the application of different image techniques in the assessment of tumor microvasculature.

Table 5.2 Contrast application of different image techniques in assessing tumor microvasculature

Image technology	Contrast agent	Sensitivity	Size of voxel	Advantages	Limitations
MRI	Gd-DTPA, USPIO	+++	1.5 mm (dynamic state); 0.4–0.8 mm (static state)	Low toxicity of contrast medium; functional diversity; multiple sequence parameter imaging; sensitivity to vascular size; no radiation risk	Easily affected by movement; limited in scanning layer; device dependencies
	Hb, Hydrogen	+			
MD CT	Iodine—containing contrast agent	+	0.5–0.8 mm	The quality of the vascular image is directly related to the concentration of contrast agent in the vasculature	Low sensitivity of contrast; toxicity; risk of ionizing radiation
PET	$H_2{}^{15}O$, ^{11}C-CO, $C^{15}O$	+++++	3–4 mm	Quality of image is directly related to the concentration of contrast; whole-body imaging	Short half-life
SPECT	^{99m}Tc-RBC	++++	5–6 mm	Imaging quality correlates with the amount of radioisotope accumulated in lesions; whole-body imaging	
Ultrasound	Microbubble	++++	0.5 mm	Microbubble is limited to the vascular lumen; ultrasound has high sensitivity for detecting the microbubble	Limited penetration of ultrasound; affected by the cavity viscera; operator dependent
Near-infrared spectroscopy	Hb, HbO_2	+	1–2 cm	Portable; low cost	Limited penetration depth; lack of equipment standards

MDCT, the imaging method noted in Table 5.2, enables good resolution of small blood vessels; although its sensitivity is poor, the rapid speed scanning makes the breathing movements and viscera peristalsis having only a little effect on the CT image. CT imaging has an advantage compared to other techniques, particularly for air-filled lungs, because the presence of air allows for good contrast resolution. Therefore, MDCT is the preferred method for the examination of small nodules and lung cancer.

Presently, in the examination of sub-centimeter lung nodules, the effectiveness of a contrast-enhanced scanning is controversial. Some clinicians believe that the enhanced scanning has no practical significance. However, contrast administration is indispensable for observing blood vessel formation. The importance of the contrast enhancement in the sub-centimeter nodules rests on two points:

First, most nodules form blood vessels when their diameter is greater than 2 mm. The introduction of contrast medium obviously helps to identify those blood vessels, particularly when the lesion is a ground-glass nodule (GGN). CT enhancement scanning can show that tiny blood vessels move into the nodules, interconnecting there and forming what is known as the "CT angiogram of tumor angiogenesis" sign or CTA-TA sign. This sign is important for identifying progression of the tumor from the inertia of a dormant state to an invasive state. Atypical adenomatous hyperplasia lesions (AAH) in the lung are usually isolated, without the formation of new blood vessels; during follow-up, if new blood vessels have formed, this may suggest that the lesion has exited the AAH stage. For AIS and IAC, the tumor microvascular CT sign is more significant.

Second, most sub-centimeter nodules are classified as pGGNs and mixed GGNs, and determining the content of solid components or any changes is very important for assessing the progress of the nodules. Usually, any changes in the solid content are evaluated subjectively by directly observing the unenhanced CT image; at other times, the CT value is measured. Both these methods have limitations and can easily lead to underestimation of the lesion. This is because the wall of the tumor capillaries is incomplete at the early formation stage, and the plasma composition can easily access the stroma of the lesion. On the unenhanced CT image, stroma cannot be distinguished from interstitial hyperplasia. Some studies have confirmed that before and after enhancement, the change in the CT value of GGNs has a clear linear relationship with the increase of the solid component; if the CT value increases 100 HU on the enhanced CT image, the solid components of the lesion increase by about 10%. Enhanced CT examination, therefore, helps to more accurately and quantitatively determine the change in the solid component of the lesion.

5.2.2 *Radiologic-Pathologic Correlation Between GGNs and Pulmonary Vessels*

Blood vessels play a major role in determining the nature of pulmonary nodules in the bronchus. In 1993, Gaeta and others published a classic article about the relationships between nodules and the tumor-bronchus. They divided the relationships between the tumor-bronchus and nodules into five types: (a) bronchus cutoff by the tumor, (b) bronchus contained within the tumor, (c) bronchus compressed by the tumor, (d) thickening and smooth narrowing of the bronchus leading to the tumor, and (e) thickening and irregular narrowing of the bronchus leading to the tumor. The paper analyzed the relationship between pulmonary nodules and blood vessels. With the broad acceptance of low-dose multidetector spiral CT in lung cancer screening, the number of GGNs detected has increased dramatically. It has been reported that the proportion of malignancy in GGNs is higher than in solid pulmonary nodules (SPNS), and most are atypical adenomatous hyperplasia (AAH), adenocarcinoma in situ (AIS), and minimally invasive adenocarcinoma (MIA). Benign lesions, such as focal fibrosis, inflammation, or alveolar hemorrhage, may also be discovered, so an accurate differential diagnosis is very important.

Retrospective analysis has demonstrated that some common imaging features of malignant nodules, such as lobulation, pleural indentation, spiculation, and the "vascular convergence sign," are seldom seen in very early-stage malignant GGNs, such as small GGNs and pGGNs. If these imaging features continue to be used to determine which tumors are benign or malignant, this may easily lead to misdiagnosis and missed diagnoses, as the progression of biological characteristics of early tumor depends on angiogenesis. A careful analysis and summary of CT image features of the new blood vessels in the lesions can help determine the nature of the lesion more accurately.

In 1993, the MDCT was under development, and the thinnest slice thickness of reconstructed CT images was 2 mm. After 20 years of development, the reconstructed slice thickness could be as low as 0.625 mm. With improved imaging resolution and the application of CTA, MDCT could demonstrate the relationship between GGNs and bronchial blood vessels more clearly. The bronchial and pulmonary arteries are at the level of the corresponding bronchi in anatomical structure, and the bronchial branch can, therefore, be seen, as can also the arteries and their physical relationship with the nodules (Fig. 5.4).

To analyze tumor microvascular status using CT, contrast-enhanced scanning needs to be undertaken, with image reconstruction using slice thickness not more than 1 mm. The thin reconstruction image is sent to a post-processing workstation for subsequent post-processing, including MPR, MIP, and VR. To clearly demonstrate the relationships between nodule and vessels, a single dimensional imaging may not be adequate. Blood vessel analysis (from the lesion to the hilum) is performed with regard to vascular morphology and vascular relationships with GGN lesions. Under normal conditions, the diameter of the pulmonary vessels gradually decreases from the hilum toward the periphery. If the diameter of the vascular segment within the lesions is larger than the proximal segment (before entering the lesions) or if the lesion vessels are apparently wider than other vessels at the same branch level, the vessels are considered as abnormal widening. The vessels are considered to be distorted or rigid if they deviate from the expected normal course. Multiple supplying vessels with different sources of origin, converging toward a lesion, are most likely indicative of increased blood circulation. To further clarify the affiliations of supplying vessels, vascular courses are traced slice-wise back-

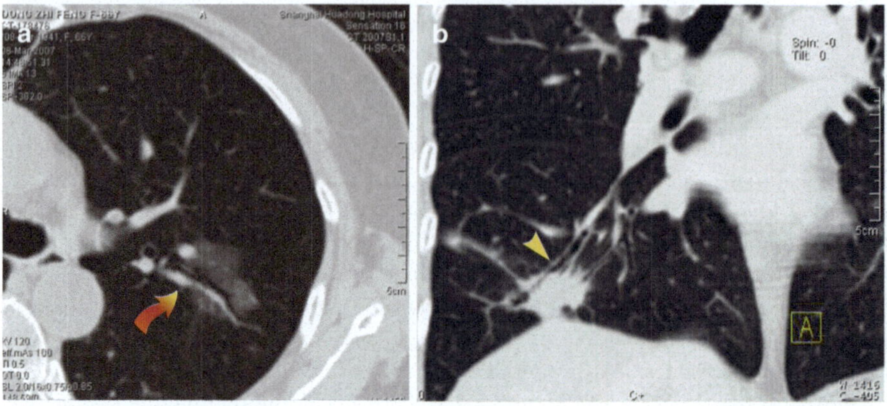

Fig. 5.4 The parallel distribution of pulmonary and bronchial arteries. (**a**) Pulmonary artery in GGN images appears rigid and narrow (arrow). (**b**) Bronchial artery within the nodules appears rigid and narrow (arrowhead)

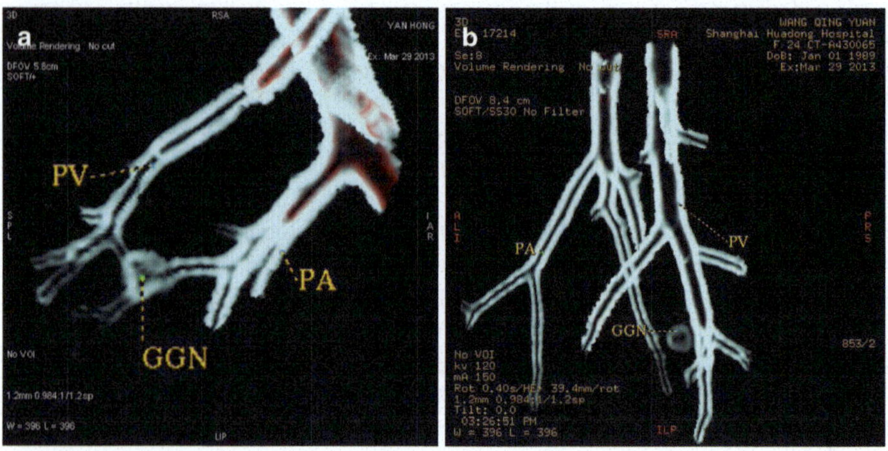

Fig. 5.5 The relationship between the nodules and pulmonary arteriovenous system. (**a**) At the edge of the GGN, there is a fine arteriovenous system entering the nodule. (**b**) The edge of the GGN has no fine arteriovenous system entering the nodule. *GGN* ground-glass nodule, *PA* pulmonary artery, *PV* pulmonary vein

ward to major vessels in the hilum, and the original tumor vascular vessel, pulmonary artery, pulmonary vein, or bronchial artery is identified to determine the lesion's original blood supply system (Fig. 5.5).

Based on the relationships between the bronchi and pulmonary nodules devised by Gaeta, the relationships between the nodules and vessels can be divided into four types (Figs. 5.6 and 5.7).

Type I, passing by. Lesion is isolated and vessels pass by the GGNs without detectable supplying branches to the lesions.

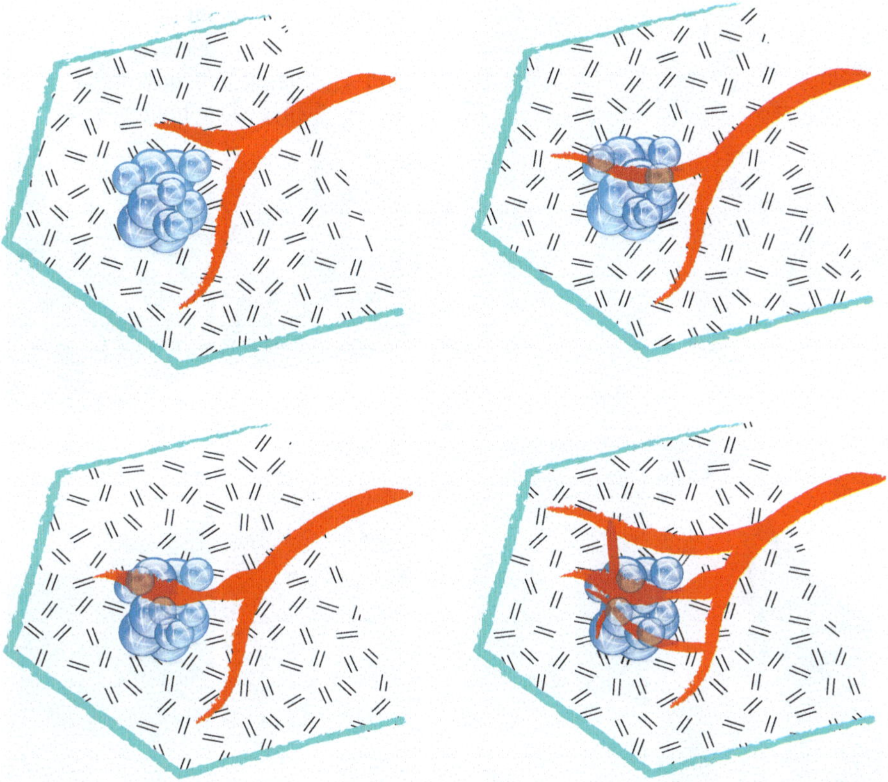

Fig. 5.6 Pattern diagrams of the relationships between the lesion and vessels. I, (pass by) Lesion is isolated; the vessels pass by the GGNs without detectable supplying branches to the lesions. II, (pass through) Vessels pass through the lesions without obvious morphological changes in the traveling path or size. III, (distorted/dilated) Vessels within the lesions are tortuous or rigid without an increase in number. IV, (complicated) More complicated vasculature other than that described in the types above within the GGNs; e.g., coexistence of irregular vascular dilation and vascular convergence from multiple supplying vessels

Type II, passing through. Vessels pass through the lesions without any obvious morphological changes in the traveling path or size.

Type III, distorted or dilated. Vessels within the lesions are tortuous or rigid without an increase in number.

Type IV, complicated or mixed. More complicated vasculatures other than the aforementioned types within the GGNs are observed, such as coexistence of irregular vascular dilation and vascular convergence from multiple supplying vessels.

The relationships between GGNs and large blood vessels can be divided into three categories: A, vessel is derived from the pulmonary artery or bronchial artery; B, vessel enters the pulmonary vein; and C, vessel is derived from the pulmonary artery or bronchial artery and entering the pulmonary vein.

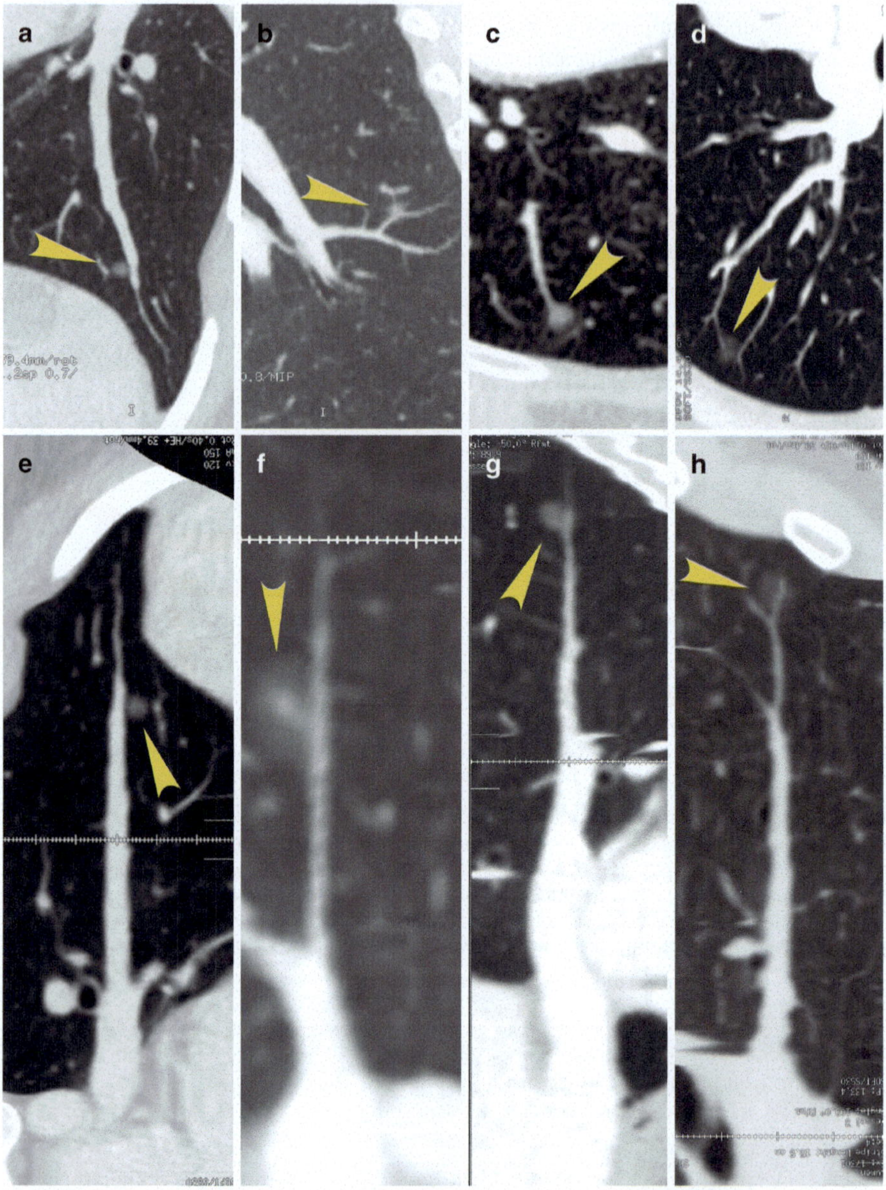

Fig. 5.7 Pattern diagrams of the relationships between the GGNs (arrowhead) and vessels. I (**a**, **b**) Lesion is isolated; vessels pass by the GGNs without detectable supplying branches to the lesions. II (**c**, **d**) Vessels pass through the lesions without any obvious morphological changes in the traveling path or size. III (**e**, **f**) Only one blood vessel passes through the lesion, and the vessels within the lesions are tortuous or rigid without any increase in number. IV (**g**, **h**) Two or more vessels pass through the lesion and form branches within the lesion; branches are connected; coexistence of irregular vascular dilation and vascular convergence from multiple supplying vessels

Table 5.3 Incidence of GGN-vessel relationship types in three GGN groups

GGN groups	The relationship between a GGN and vessels			
	Type I	Type II	Type III	Type IV
Benign group	0[a] (0.0%)[b]	9 (90.0%)	0 (0.0%)	1 (10.0%)
Preinvasive group	6 (25.0%)	16 (66.67%)	2 (8.3%)	0 (0.0%)
Invasive adenocarcinoma group	3 (4.0%)	33 (44.6%)	19 (25.7%)	19 (25.7%)

[a]Case(s) corresponding to specific type and group
[b]Proportion of a particular type in the corresponding group

Table 5.4 Subgroup analysis: the incidence of GGN-vessel relationship type in MIA and IAC

Subgroup	The relationship between a GGN and vessels			
	Type I	Type II	Type III	Type IV
MIA	3[a] (7.7%)[b]	19 (48.7%)	5 (12.8%)	12 (30.8%)
IAC	0 (0.0%)	14 (40.0%)	14 (40.0%)	7 (20.0%)

[a]Case(s) corresponding to specific type and group
[b]Proportion of a particular type in the corresponding group

Based on all these characteristics, we studied 108 GGNs (98 malignant cases and 10 benign), and all underwent resection using video-assisted thoracoscopy or thoracotomy surgery [17]. These cases were comprised of all the specimen that can be seen after surgery, with slices measuring within 15 mm. Representative hematoxylin-eosin-stained sections were reviewed. For the cases of equivocal pathological classification noted under light microscopy, immunohistochemical analysis was performed for clarification. The diagnosis of malignant lesions was made based on the new pulmonary adenocarcinoma classification, 2011 edition; 7 AAHs, 17 AISs, 39 MIAs, and 35 IACs were discovered. The results of the analysis are shown in Table 5.3.

Many studies have demonstrated that relationships between SPNs and vessels [particularly the vascular convergence sign (VCS)] are valuable for estimation of the malignancy potential of SPNs. VCS is thought to occur because of significant reactive fibrous connective tissue proliferation pulling the nearby blood vessels into the nodules. Fibrosis in the damaged lung and tumor proliferation cause destruction that leads to the collapse of the bracket structure, shrinkage, and pulling of the nearby vessels. Therefore, VCS can also be seen in benign lesions. In addition, the tumor microvascular CT sign can only be shown clearly after image post-processing, but CVS does not need to perform any image post-processing; a simple unenhanced examination can demonstrate it. In this study, the GGN-vessel relationships were categorized into four types. The statistical analysis indicated that when the relationship was type III or IV (particularly type IV), there was a very high likelihood of the GGNs being malignant invasive adenocarcinoma, with MIA more likely than IAC. In contrast, most of the benign and preinvasive cases were seen in type I or type II GGN-vessel relationships (Tables 5.3 and 5.4).

In terms of histopathology, AIS often originates in bronchial mucous epithelium or alveolar epithelium, and the bronchioles may appear rigid, narrowed, pulled to the side, or truncated. The pulmonary artery travels along the bronchiole, and when the image shows a truncated or rigidly retracted bronchiole, the pulmonary artery often also has similar morphological changes. Early on, the bronchioles can appear as narrow, rigid, or stretched, etc.; severe damage is manifested as truncation. The pulmonary vein does not travel along with the bronchiole. It lies at a certain distance from the bronchus and has a variety of forms, and the edge can be rigid, stretchy, narrow, or truncated.

Some studies have indicated that disease progression from AAH or MIA to IAC is a complicated, polygene-involved dynamic process. MIA or IAC may gradually develop from AAH and AIS. Interstitial fiber hyperplasia within the lesion is the primary contributing factor to type III and IV vascular morphological changes. This presumption encompasses the findings of Noguchi regarding the mechanism of VSC formation, leading to the conclusion that the course of adjacent vessels is dependent on the location of the lesions, particularly when the disease infiltrates the bronchovascular bundle and interlobular septa. As a result, involved vessels might appear distorted, rigid, or concentrated toward the lesion. Thus, it is reasonable to postulate that the vascular convergence sign commonly seen in SPNs will ultimately be observed in GGNs along with their progression. Specifically, the type IV GGN-vessel relationship resembles VCS to some degree. The invasive adenocarcinoma group is comprised of two subgroups, MIA and IAC. Subgroup analysis showed that MIA and IAC had different patterns of the GGN-vessel relationship. Type III vascular morphological changes were observed more often in the IAC than MIA subgroup, indicating that with increasing malignancy, fiber hyperplasia stimulated by malignant tissues may become more severe, and subsequently, the impact on the vasculature may become more aggravated. Furthermore, tumor metabolism is faster than in normal tissues; therefore, the blood supply demanded by the tumors is much higher than in normal tissues. These mechanisms indirectly lead to vessel proliferation and irregular luminal dilation. Some studies have shown that endogenous and/or extrinsic tumor angiogenesis and neovascularization could be the driving factors of vascular abnormalities observed in malignant early-stage lung cancers.

This study showed that the type II GGN-vessel relationship was common among benign and malignant GGN groups. In our opinion, any space-occupying lesion in the lung can form a spatial relationship with its adjacent structures. Therefore, even if the lesion and its associated vessel have no internal contact, the lesion can be seen as the vessel travels through the GGN because it is located in the normal line of the vascular path. If the blood vessel only travels through the GGNs without distortion, rigidity, enlargement, or aggregation, it will be of no value for diagnosis of the lesion. Hyperplasia of fiber composition, which occurs in the process of inflammation, can also affect the local small blood vessels, but the vessels did not demonstrate a distorted performance in the benign lesion group in our study. This may be because we choose the GGNs in which the ground-glass opacity comprised more than 50% of the area of the lesion on CT, so the focal fibrous hyperplasia was not significant, producing no effect on the local small blood vessels. With inflammation, granulation tissue, new blood capillary hyperplasia, and local blood flow all increase. This can also lead to the vessels appearing enlarged, but in this study, ten benign lesions were not associated with dilated vessels, and this may be due to the

GGNs that were selected. The GGO comprised more than 50% of the area of the lesion on CT, so the lesions were not in the acute phase, inflammation was not obvious, and blood flow did not increase.

SPN-vessel relationships can not only facilitate the estimation of the malignant potential of nodules, but some studies have also shown that the affiliation of tumor-supplying vessels, pulmonary arteries, and veins can also be used as an indication of differentiation. If pulmonary veins are involved with SPNs, lung cancer should be suspected. This is because with the increase in tumor growth and its frequent invasion adjacent to the lung and sub-lung segments, the pulmonary vein is located in the surrounding parts of the lung lobules, and it is therefore more susceptible to becoming involved and may provide a blood supply to the tumors. Other studies have shown that most vasculature in the VCS is not comprised of vessels that supply blood to tumors or tumor blood vessels. In the present study, there were no significant differences between vessel categories among the three GGN groups ($p > 0.05$); therefore, the vessel categories were unrelated to the three GGN groups ($p = 0.217$), and these categories had no diagnostic value for the differential diagnosis of the lesion.

Through the study of the CTA-TA sign, it is evident that vascular categories (pulmonary artery or pulmonary vein) have no differential value in the evaluation of pulmonary nodules, when the relationship between the lesions and vessels appear to be type III and type IV. Moreover, when vessels within the lesions are tortuous or rigid without any increase in the number or more complicated vasculature other than that previously described within the GGNs, the coexistence of irregular vasculature dilation and vascular convergence from multiple supplying vessels was shown to highly indicate malignant lesions.

References

1. Chapman AD, Kerr KM. The association between atypical adenomatous hyperplasia and primary lung cancer. Br J Cancer. 2000;83(5):632–6. https://doi.org/10.1054/bjoc.2000.1317.
2. de Bruin EC, McGranahan N, Mitter R, Salm M, Wedge DC, Yates L, Jamal-Hanjani M, Shafi S, Murugaesu N, Rowan AJ, Gronroos E, Muhammad MA, Horswell S, Gerlinger M, Varela I, Jones D, Marshall J, Voet T, Van Loo P, Rassl DM, Rintoul RC, Janes SM, Lee SM, Forster M, Ahmad T, Lawrence D, Falzon M, Capitanio A, Harkins TT, Lee CC, Tom W, Teefe E, Chen SC, Begum S, Rabinowitz A, Phillimore B, Spencer-Dene B, Stamp G, Szallasi Z, Matthews N, Stewart A, Campbell P, Swanton C. Spatial and temporal diversity in genomic instability processes defines lung cancer evolution. Science. 2014;346(6206):251–6. https://doi.org/10.1126/science.1253462.
3. Akslen LA, Naumov GN. Tumor dormancy—from basic mechanisms to clinical practice. APMIS. 2008;116(7–8):545–7. https://doi.org/10.1111/j.1600-0463.2008.01209.x.
4. Demicheli R. Tumour dormancy: findings and hypotheses from clinical research on breast cancer. Semin Cancer Biol. 2001;11(4):297–306. https://doi.org/10.1006/scbi.2001.0385.
5. Naumov GN, Folkman J, Straume O, Akslen LA. Tumor-vascular interactions and tumor dormancy. APMIS. 2008;116(7–8):569–85. https://doi.org/10.1111/j.1600-0463.2008.01213.x.
6. Naumov GN, Akslen LA, Folkman J. Role of angiogenesis in human tumor dormancy: animal models of the angiogenic switch. Cell Cycle. 2006;5(16):1779–87. https://doi.org/10.4161/cc.5.16.3018.

7. Folkman J. Proceedings: Tumor angiogenesis factor. Cancer Res. 1974;34(8):2109–13.
8. Gimbrone MA Jr, Leapman SB, Cotran RS, Folkman J. Tumor angiogenesis: iris neovascularization at a distance from experimental intraocular tumors. J Natl Cancer Inst. 1973;50(1):219–28.
9. Thomlinson RH, Gray LH. The histological structure of some human lung cancers and the possible implications for radiotherapy. Br J Cancer. 1955;9(4):539–49.
10. Weis SM, Cheresh DA. A wake-up call for hibernating tumour cells. Nat Cell Biol. 2013;15(7):721–3. https://doi.org/10.1038/ncb2794.
11. Moserle L, Amadori A, Indraccolo S. The angiogenic switch: implications in the regulation of tumor dormancy. Curr Mol Med. 2009;9(8):935–41.
12. Carmeliet P, Jain RK. Angiogenesis in cancer and other diseases. Nature. 2000;407(6801):249–57. https://doi.org/10.1038/35025220.
13. Indraccolo S, Favaro E, Amadori A. Dormant tumors awaken by a short-term angiogenic burst: the spike hypothesis. Cell Cycle. 2006;5(16):1751–5. https://doi.org/10.4161/cc.5.16.2985.
14. Gilead A, Neeman M. Dynamic remodeling of the vascular bed precedes tumor growth: MLS ovarian carcinoma spheroids implanted in nude mice. Neoplasia. 1999;1(3):226–30.
15. Giaccia AJ. Hypoxic stress proteins: survival of the fittest. Semin Radiat Oncol. 1996;6(1):46–58. https://doi.org/10.1053/srao0060046.
16. Jain RK, Tong RT, Munn LL. Effect of vascular normalization by antiangiogenic therapy on interstitial hypertension, peritumor edema, and lymphatic metastasis: insights from a mathematical model. Cancer Res. 2007;67(6):2729–35. https://doi.org/10.1158/0008-5472.can-06-4102.
17. Gao F, Li M, Ge X, Zheng X, Ren Q, Chen Y, Lv F, Hua Y. Multi-detector spiral CT study of the relationships between pulmonary ground-glass nodules and blood vessels. Eur Radiol. 2013;23(12):3271–7. https://doi.org/10.1007/s00330-013-2954-3.

Suggested Readings

1. Aguirre-Ghiso JA. Models, mechanisms and clinical evidence for cancer dormancy. Nat Rev Cancer. 2007;7(11):834–46. https://doi.org/10.1038/nrc2256.
2. Aoki T, Tomoda Y, Watanabe H, Nakata H, Kasai T, Hashimoto H, Kodate M, Osaki T, Yasumoto K. Peripheral lung adenocarcinoma: correlation of thin-section CT findings with histologic prognostic factors and survival. Radiology. 2001;220(3):803–9. https://doi.org/10.1148/radiol.2203001701.
3. Fridman WH, Dieu-Nosjean MC, Pages F, Cremer I, Damotte D, Sautes-Fridman C, Galon J. The immune microenvironment of human tumors: general significance and clinical impact. Cancer Microenviron. 2013;6(2):117–22. https://doi.org/10.1007/s12307-012-0124-9.
4. Henschke CI, Yankelevitz DF, Mirtcheva R, McGuinness G, McCauley D, Miettinen OS. CT screening for lung cancer: frequency and significance of part-solid and nonsolid nodules. AJR Am J Roentgenol. 2002;178(5):1053–7. https://doi.org/10.2214/ajr.178.5.1781053.
5. Jain RK. Normalization of tumor vasculature: an emerging concept in antiangiogenic therapy. Science. 2005;307(5706):58–62. https://doi.org/10.1126/science.1104819.
6. Kakinuma R, Ohmatsu H, Kaneko M, Eguchi K, Naruke T, Nagai K, Nishiwaki Y, Suzuki A, Moriyama N. Detection failures in spiral CT screening for lung cancer: analysis of CT findings. Radiology. 1999;212(1):61–6. https://doi.org/10.1148/radiology.212.1.r99jn1461.
7. Kim HY, Shim YM, Lee KS, Han J, Yi CA, Kim YK. Persistent pulmonary nodular ground-glass opacity at thin-section CT: histopathologic comparisons. Radiology. 2007;245(1):267–75. https://doi.org/10.1148/radiol.2451061682.
8. Knighton D, Ausprunk D, Tapper D, Folkman J. Avascular and vascular phases of tumour growth in the chick embryo. Br J Cancer. 1977;35(3):347–56.

9. Lee HJ, Goo JM, Lee CH, Yoo CG, Kim YT, Im JG. Nodular ground-glass opacities on thin-section CT: size change during follow-up and pathological results. Korean J Radiol. 2007;8(1):22–31. https://doi.org/10.3348/kjr.2007.8.1.22.
10. Mori K, Saitou Y, Tominaga K, Yokoi K, Miyazawa N, Okuyama A, Sasagawa M. Small nodular lesions in the lung periphery: new approach to diagnosis with CT. Radiology. 1990;177(3):843–9. https://doi.org/10.1148/radiology.177.3.2243999.
11. Noguchi M, Morikawa A, Kawasaki M, Matsuno Y, Yamada T, Hirohashi S, Kondo H, Shimosato Y. Small adenocarcinoma of the lung. Histologic characteristics and prognosis. Cancer. 1995;75(12):2844–52.
12. Soda H, Nakamura Y, Nakatomi K, Tomonaga N, Yamaguchi H, Nakano H, Nagashima S, Anami M, Hayashi T, Tsukamoto K, Kohno S. Stepwise progression from ground-glass opacity towards invasive adenocarcinoma: long-term follow-up of radiological findings. Lung Cancer. 2008;60(2):298–301. https://doi.org/10.1016/j.lungcan.2007.09.001.
13. Travis WD, Brambilla E, Noguchi M, Nicholson AG, Geisinger KR, Yatabe Y, Beer DG, Powell CA, Riely GJ, Van Schil PE, Garg K, Austin JH, Asamura H, Rusch VW, Hirsch FR, Scagliotti G, Mitsudomi T, Huber RM, Ishikawa Y, Jett J, Sanchez-Cespedes M, Sculier JP, Takahashi T, Tsuboi M, Vansteenkiste J, Wistuba I, Yang PC, Aberle D, Brambilla C, Flieder D, Franklin W, Gazdar A, Gould M, Hasleton P, Henderson D, Johnson B, Johnson D, Kerr K, Kuriyama K, Lee JS, Miller VA, Petersen I, Roggli V, Rosell R, Saijo N, Thunnissen E, Tsao M, Yankelewitz D. International Association for the Study of Lung Cancer/American Thoracic Society/European Respiratory Society International Multidisciplinary Classification of Lung Adenocarcinoma. J Thorac Oncol. 2011;6(2):244–85. https://doi.org/10.1097/JTO.0b013e318206a221.
14. Udagawa T, Fernandez A, Achilles EG, Folkman J, D'Amato RJ. Persistence of microscopic human cancers in mice: alterations in the angiogenic balance accompanies loss of tumor dormancy. FASEB J. 2002;16(11):1361–70. https://doi.org/10.1096/fj.01-0813com.
15. Uhr JW, Marches R. Dormancy in a model of murine B cell lymphoma. Semin Cancer Biol. 2001;11(4):277–83. https://doi.org/10.1006/scbi.2001.0383.
16. Yang Z, Sone S, Takashima S, Li F, Honda T, Yamanda T. Small peripheral carcinomas of the lung: thin-section CT and pathologic correlation. Eur Radiol. 1999;9(9):1819–25.
17. Zhang L, Yankelevitz DF, Carter D, Henschke CI, Yip R, Reeves AP. Internal growth of nonsolid lung nodules: radiologic-pathologic correlation. Radiology. 2012;263(1):279–86. https://doi.org/10.1148/radiol.11101372.
18. Zwirewich CV, Vedal S, Miller RR, Muller NL. Solitary pulmonary nodule: high-resolution CT and radiologic-pathologic correlation. Radiology. 1991;179(2):469–76. https://doi.org/10.1148/radiology.179.2.2014294.

Part II
Imaging Assessment of Pulmonary Nodules

Chapter 6
Pure Ground-Glass Nodules

Guozhen Zhang and Xiangpeng Zheng

6.1 Nomenclature and Management Guidelines of Incidentally Detected Pulmonary Nodules

6.1.1 Nomenclature of Incidentally Detected Pulmonary Nodules

Founded in 1969 in memory of the renowned radiologist, Felix Fleischner, the Fleischner Society is dedicated to the diagnosis and treatment of diseases of the chest through extensive international collaboration between researchers and clinicians. The Society is well known for its regular publications on thoracic diseases. In 1971, leaders of the Society acknowledged the need to compile a standardized nomenclature of thoracic radiology for facilitating communication among radiologists. With contributions from numerous members, the Nomenclature Committee, with the authorization of the Society, proposed special reports in May 1983 and published the first version of the *Glossary of Terms for Thoracic Radiology* in 1984, a collection of major radiologic terms and their definitions, as well as explanations used in chest radiography [1]. In 1996, because of the increasing clinical application of computed tomography, the committee edited a *Glossary of Terms for CT of the Lung* to standardize the use of CT terms in thoracic imaging [2]. The classic publication, *Glossary of Terms for Thoracic Imaging*, was announced in 2008 as an extended and integrated version of previous publications, with special emphasis on clarifying ambiguous terms and focusing on the description of techniques and features in thoracic imaging [3]. In addition, a glossary of terms related to HRCT was

G. Zhang (✉)
Department of Radiology, Fudan University Huadong Hospital, Shanghai, China
e-mail: cjr.zhangguozhen@vip.163.com

X. Zheng
Department of Radiation Oncology, Fudan University Huadong Hospital, Shanghai, China

X. Zheng et al. (eds.), *Early-stage Lung Cancer*,
https://doi.org/10.1007/978-981-10-7596-4_6

included in Webb's *Edited HRCT of the Lung* in 1991. This book was revised in 1993 and the fifth edition was published in 2015.

According to the 2008 version of the *Glossary of Terms for Thoracic Imaging* from the Fleischner Society and the classifications of pulmonary nodules proposed by the International Early Lung Cancer Action Program (I-ELCAP), there is consensus on the nomenclature of incidentally detected pulmonary nodules. Ground-glass opacity (GGO) represents a nonspecific CT finding and appears as a hazy area with increasing attenuation and intact bronchial and vascular markings. If the abnormal area is localized, the term "focal GGO (fGGO)" applies. The etiology of GGO varies and includes the partial filling of airspace due to the mild accumulation of fluid and cellular debris, partial collapse of alveoli due to poor ventilation, increased capillary blood, or interstitial thickening. In contrast to obscured vasculature and bronchial structures in pulmonary consolidation, these structures appear to be discernible within GGO lesions. Based on the solid component, GGO can be divided into pure GGO (pGGO) and mixed GGO (mGGO). In the former, no solid component exists in the lesion, whereas in the latter, some amount of solid component can be found. Furthermore, GGNs represent a specific type of GGO with rounded or oval morphology and well- or poorly defined margin. Again, GGNs can be divided into pure GGNs without a solid component and partly solid GGNs with soft-tissue attenuation components. The latter is synonymous with semisolid GGN or mixed GGN.

According to the glossary for thoracic imaging from the Fleischner Society, a nodule on a lung CT is defined as a rounded or irregular opacity, well- or poorly margined, and up to 3 cm in diameter, whereas a micronodule is a discrete, small, round, and focal opacity less than 3 mm in diameter. When multiple micronodules are found diffusely distributed throughout the lungs, this is known as a miliary pattern. Apparently, nodular lesions range from 3 mm to 3 cm and include T1a and T1b diseases. In the era of low-dose CT screening of lung cancer, this definition is somewhat lacking practicality as increasing numbers of smaller nodules (subcentimeter nodules, in particular) are detected. For further analysis of nodular lesions and better guidance of treatment, a revision of the nodular classification system is required. Throughout this book, we use nodule, small nodule, micronodule, and miliary nodule to describe opacities with the aforementioned morphological features and a diameter of >20 mm to approximately ≤30 mm, >10 mm to approximately ≤20 mm, >4 mm to approximately ≤10 mm, and ≤4 mm (Table 6.1).

Table 6.1 Pulmonary nodule classification, based on diameters in CT imaging

Classification	Fleischner society	Revised classification used in this book
Miliary nodule	≤3 mm, multiple, diffuse distribution	≤4 mm, solitary or multiple
Micronodule	≤3 mm	>4 mm – ≤10 mm
Small nodule	/	>10 mm – ≤20 mm
Nodule	>3 mm – ≤30 mm	>20 mm – ≤30 mm

6.1.2 Summary of Recommendations from the Fleischner Society for the Management of Subsolid Pulmonary Nodules Detected on CT

In 2011, an international interdisciplinary group of experts in oncology, thoracic surgery, radiology, pathology, and molecular biology from IASLC, ATS, and ERS reached consensus on the diagnostic pathologic classification of pulmonary adenocarcinoma, which represented and reflected numerous advances in multifaceted research and bore significance in guiding multidisciplinary treatment and predicting prognosis. With the incidence of pathologically proven, nonsolid peripheral carcinoma soaring, the need to standardize glossaries related to pulmonary nonsolid nodules and management strategy is urgent. In 2005, the Fleischner Society published a statement on the management of incidentally radiologically detected pulmonary nodules. Eight years later in 2013, an update was announced with emphasis on nonsolid pulmonary nodules. Based on the most recent progress, the updated guideline proposed six major recommendations for solitary and multiple nonsolid nodules (three for each type). Each guideline item was supplemented with specific explanations and a rationale for the points covered (further details in Chap. 3: Lung Cancer Screening). Considering the high heterogeneity in the genomics and proteomics of adenocarcinoma, the complexity of the microenvironment and controversy over the optimal management strategy, the Fleischner guideline is far from complete and will require ongoing revisions in the future.

As low-dose CT is increasingly used in lung cancer screening, the amount of small pulmonary hazy opacities that are undetectable in traditional chest plain films has increased. Studies have shown that the probability of malignancy in ground-glass lesions can be higher than in solid lesions, suggesting that attention should be placed in CT imaging on those lesions with a ground-glass presentation. A pure ground-glass opacity (pGGO) presents as a hazy opacity with CT values of −450 to −650 HU and frequent visualization of fine vasculature and variable air bubbles or air bronchograms within the opacity in the lung window setting but cannot be seen in the mediastinal window setting. Pathologically, pGGN is a nonspecific imaging entity, possibly due to reduced air filling in the alveoli, increasing quantity of cells, pulmonary epithelial proliferation, septal thickening, or partial obliteration of a terminal bronchus. Statistical data have shown that approximately 43% of subcentimeter adenocarcinomas are solitary pGGNs without a clear solid component within the hazy nodular lesions. After proper surgical removal, the 7-year overall survival is 100%. In contrast, about 30% of adenocarcinomas are solitary pGGNs with variable amounts of solid component (called mixed nodules or mixed ground-glass nodules (mGGN)). These diseases have a relatively poor prognosis—approximately 60% 7-year overall survival. Another 27% of subcentimeter adenocarcinomas present as multiple pulmonary lesions, and these have the worst prognosis. An incidentally detected GGN could represent a persistent GGN if the nodule does not respond to empirical antibiotic treatment or continues growing during follow-up. In comparison with other GGNs, persistent GGNs carry a higher risk of being malignant and should be thoroughly evaluated by a multidisciplinary team. As the CT microangiogram is visualized, there should be a high suspicion for adenocarcinoma in situ (AIS). The "CT microangiogram" sign or CTA-TA sign is defined as an abnormal microvessel (neo-vessel) sprouting from the adjacent pulmonary vessel (vein or artery), migrating toward and infiltrating into the nodule, and intercommunicating with other neo-vessels within the nodule (neo-vessel mobilization and intercommunication). Hence, the imaging diagnosis of pulmonary AIS can be simplified to "persistent GGN plus CT microangiogram." According to the 7th version of the TNM staging of pulmonary adenocarcinoma, AIS is classified as stage 0, whereas in the 8th version, AIS is listed as a stage IA disease. As preinvasive disease, AIS represents the earliest step in the development sequence of lung cancer and is deemed the foundation of pathological diagnosis of microinvasive adenocarcinoma, as well as the key issue for further improving the clinical treatment outcome of lung cancer with the "triple early" strategy, i.e., early detection, early diagnosis, and early treatment. Thus, it is vital for thoracic oncologists, pathologists, and radiologists for the accurate radiologic and pathologic diagnosis of AIS.

In plain chest radiography, pulmonary AIS is commonly neglected due to its small size or misdiagnosed as inflammation or infiltrative tuberculosis due to its ill-defined margins and lack of solid components. Ground-glass opacities can be seen in many parenchymal and interstitial entities, including hypersensitive alveolitis, interstitial pneumonitis, pulmonary alveolar proteinosis, lipoid pneumonia, sarcoidosis, idiopathic interstitial fibrosis, and bronchiolitis obliterans organizing pneumonia, so the differential diagnosis should be considered fully for every GGN case.

6.1.3 The 2011 Version of the Pathological Classification of Pulmonary Adenocarcinoma

According to the international interdisciplinary classification published in 2011, pulmonary adenocarcinoma can be divided into four categories: adenocarcinoma in situ (AIS), minimally invasive adenocarcinoma (MIA), invasive adenocarcinoma (IAC), and variants of invasive adenocarcinoma (VIA). Further descriptions regarding each category can be found in Chap. 1.

In the revised classification, the terms "bronchioloalveolar carcinoma (BAC)" and "mixed adenocarcinoma" are abandoned and replaced with AIS and MIA. Most of the previously diagnosed adenocarcinomas with bronchioloalveolar components should be reclassified into the MIA category following the current system. Accordingly, the imaging evaluation and descriptions should be updated to reflect the revised system. Considering that radiological imaging plays an increasing role in the detection and diagnosis of early-stage small cell lung cancer, the committee placed particular emphasis on the proper utilization and integration of imaging, while lung cancers are diagnosed and classified. Table 6.2 briefly lists the revised

Table 6.2 Radiologic-pathologic correlation in Noguchi system and IASLC/ATS/ERS system

Noguchi system (1995)	IASLC/ATS/ERS system (2011)	CT imaging features
	AAH	GGN (avascular stage)
Type A: Localized bronchioloalveolar carcinoma (LBAC)	AIS	GGN (hypovascular stage)
Type B: LBAC with foci of collapsed alveolar structure	AIS	GGN (external angiogenesis stage)
Type C: LBAC with foci of active fibroblastic proliferation	MIA	GGN/PSN (internal angiogenesis stage)
	IAC	PSN/SN, Solid component +++
Type D: Poorly differentiated adenocarcinoma	VIA	PSN/SN, Solid component ++++
Type E: Tubular adenocarcinoma		
Type F: Papillary adenocarcinoma with compressive and destructive growth		

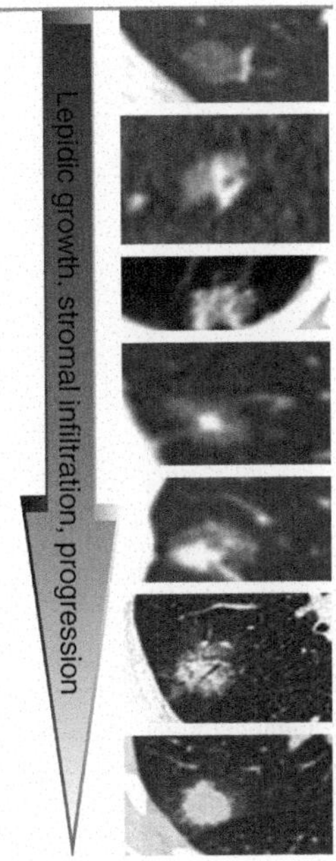

AAH atypical adenomatous hyperplasia, *AIS* adenocarcinoma in situ, *GGN* ground-glass nodule, *IAC* invasive adenocarcinoma, *MIA* minimally invasive adenocarcinoma, *LBAC* localized bronchioloalveolar carcinoma, *PSN* partially solid nodule, *SN* solid nodule, *VIA* variants of invasive adenocarcinoma

classification system in comparison with the Noguchi system, as well as the corresponding characteristic CT imaging features.

Regarding any suspicious nodule detected on CT imaging, either pGGN, subsolid, or solid, radiologists should attempt to provide a thorough assessment from the following five items: localization, quantitation, qualification, morphological characterization, and staging if malignancy is suspected. As the earliest phase of preinvasive disease, AAH manifests as a pGGN with a diameter $\leq$ 5 mm, whereas AIS is commonly larger than 5 mm with cubic, columnar, goblet, or hobnail-like neoplastic cells growing along the pre-existing alveolar structures in a lepidic pattern but lacking stromal, vascular, or pleural invasion. In contrast with avascular AAH, small vascular branches from adjacent pre-existing vessels proliferate and grow into AIS lesions (Fig. 6.1).

Radiologically, minimally invasive adenocarcinoma commonly manifests as a ground-glass nodule with a limited number of solid components, and less than 5 mm in diameter. On thin-sliced CT imaging, particularly with contrast media

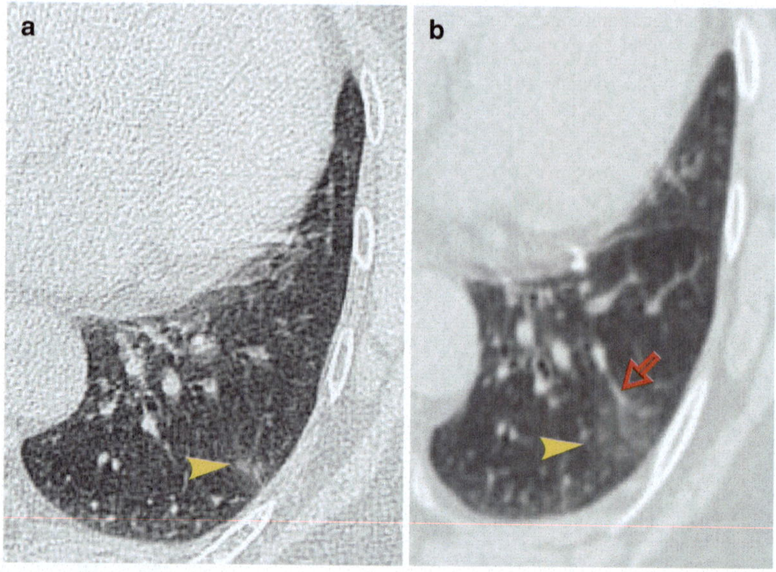

Fig. 6.1 After 8 years of consecutive follow-up, an AAH lesion gradually evolved into an AIS lesion in a 65-year-old female patient. A pure ground-glass nodule with an ill-defined margin was occasionally detected in the lateroposterior segment of the left lower lobe. With antibiotic administration, no clear response was seen. AAH was clinically suspected, and annual low-dose CT follow-up was suggested. At the eighth annual CT scanning, the lesion had grown and neo-vessels eventually migrated into the lesion, radiologically indicating AIS, which was proven by pathological examination after surgical removal with video-assisted thoracoscopic surgery (VATS)

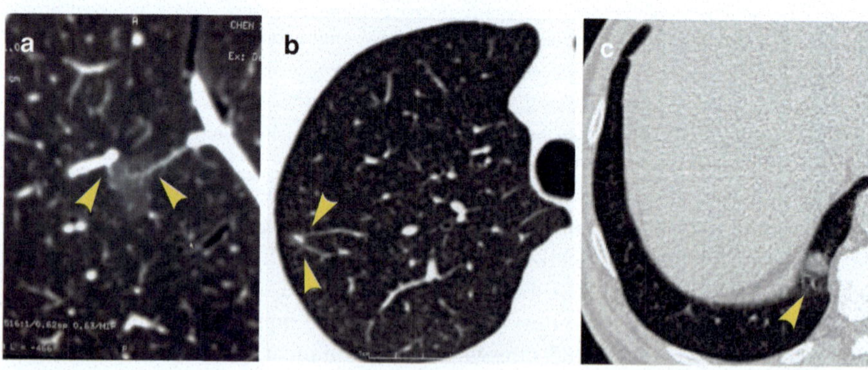

Fig. 6.2 Neo-vessels migrate into MIA. (**a**) Neo-vessels (arrowhead) originating from two pre-existing intrapulmonary vessels (branches of the pulmonary artery) migrate into the lesion and subdivide into interconnecting microvessels. (**b**) Same radiologic findings as in (**a**). Clear solid component is seen in the center of this lesion. (**c**) Lesions located at the paravertebral costodiaphragmatic recess are subject to respiratory movement. For better characterization of the vascular relationship, views of multiplanar reformation (MPR) may be necessary for extracting additional information, as in this patient

enhancement, nutrient neo-vessels move into and interconnect in the lesion, establishing intratumoral vasculature (Figs. 6.2 and 6.3). Most invasive adenocarcinomas present as solid nodules, a few as semisolid nodules, and rare ones as pure ground-glass nodules. Characteristic deep lobulation and short spiculation are usually seen

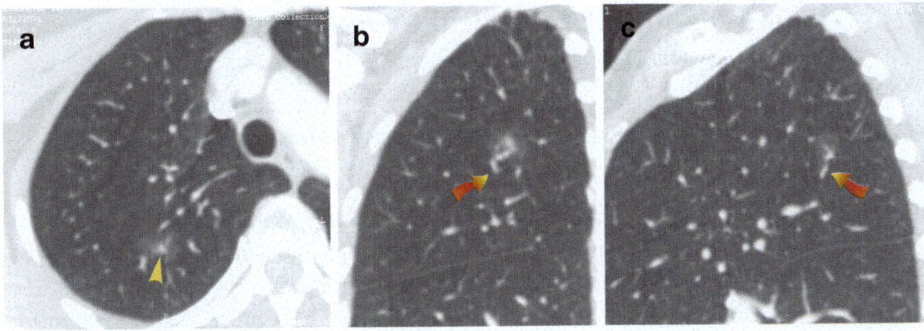

Fig. 6.3 CT microangiogram in MIA. Image from a 52-year-old female patient. On the magnified axial CT image (**a**), a 12-mm diameter semisolid nodule (arrowhead) is seen with an approximately 2 mm dense invasive component. On the coronal (**b**) and sagittal (**c**) views, a neo-vessel (arrow) is clearly visualized migrating into the lesion. Within the lesion, microvascular interconnection and enhancement are observed

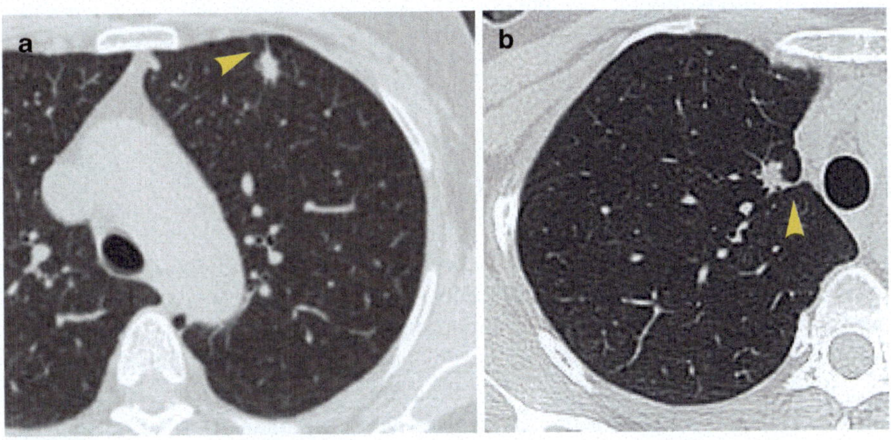

Fig. 6.4 CT findings in IAC. On axial images, two solid nodules are detected: a 15-mm diameter nodule in the posterior segment of the left upper lobe (**a**) and a 10-mm diameter nodule in the apical segment of the right upper lobe (**b**). Both nodules demonstrate typical signs such as deep lobulation, spiculation, and pleural indentation (arrowhead), strongly suggestive of invasive adenocarcinoma, which was proven by surgical pathological examination

(Fig. 6.4). CT imaging can provide a panoramic view of the pulmonary nodule, visual differentiation, as well as quantitative analysis of the intratumoral solid component and ground-glass component, which compensate to some extent for the limits (due to undersampling) in pathological evaluations. With the capability of visualizing the tumor and its adjacent structures, and discerning the density variation of various components, CT has been used to guide pathologists to conduct biopsies accurately or to sample surgical specimens. By way of analogy, radiologic imaging discovers the forest, while pathologic imaging reveals the leaves and tree trunks. Overall, accurate imaging evaluation and pathologic diagnosis of a given pulmonary nodule require comprehensive analysis from interdisciplinary and multidimensional perspectives.

6.2 CT Findings and Pathological Correlation of Pure Ground-Glass Nodules

6.2.1 CT Scanning and Reconstruction Techniques

Pure ground-glass nodules have a slightly higher density than pulmonary parenchyma. The density discrepancy between the nodule and surrounding structures can become even smaller when the breath-holding maneuver is performed poorly during imaging acquisition, leading to a misdiagnosis. Therefore, a strict scanning protocol including breathing control and optimal scanning parameter settings should be implemented to assure imaging quality and reproducibility. For example, the tube current should be within the range of 100–300 mA. pGGNs can be detected using low-dose CT scanning. For the 5–9 mm pGGNs, re-scanning with standard non-LDCT parameters is mandatory for further characterizing lesions, if contrast media allows visualization. Imaging reconstruction should use a small slice thickness (≤1.0 mm) without a slice interval. Thicker slice imaging can lead to a nodule being missed or misclassification of a solid nodule as pGGN due to a partial volume effect.

6.2.2 Pure Ground-Glass Nodule (pGGN)

pGGNs have significant relevance in the clinical setting. In lung cancer screening with conventional chest radiography, 70% of missing lesions manifest as pure ground-glass opacities in CT imaging. Additionally, miliary lesions less than 4 mm in diameter are predisposed to be neglected or omitted, even in CT imaging. To avoid such incidences, radiologists should read consecutive thin-sliced (1 mm or less) axial images as well as multiplanar reformation images. Even though thin-sliced CT has adequate capability for visualizing pGGNs, distinguishing between benign and malignant disease remains challenging. However, invasive procedures (e.g., biopsy) are not required in most of cases at the initial time of detection. Considering the small size and inert growth behavior, patients should be advised that lesions are at the benign stage but should also be routinely followed up with low-dose CT for at least 3 years or more. Most benign nodules shrink or even vanish during follow-up, and only a small proportion remains the same size. In contrast, if consecutive follow-up imaging series demonstrate that nodular lesions gradually grow with an increasing solid component that is contrast-enhanced and with proliferating vasculature (called "the quadruplet pattern"), there should be high suspicion for malignant disease (Fig. 6.5).

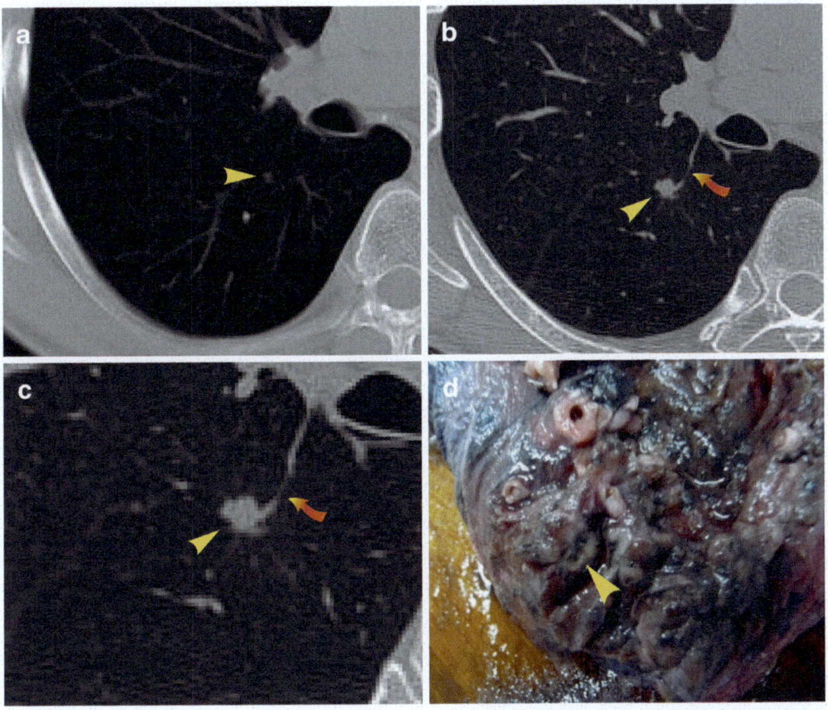

Fig. 6.5 A miliary nodule evolved into adenocarcinoma over the 3.5-year follow-up. (**a**) A miliary nodule (arrowhead) was detected in the superior segment of the right lower lobe and was classified as indeterminate; regular follow-up was advised. (**b**) Forty-two years later, a follow-up CT revealed the quadruplet pattern: larger size, higher density, greater vasculature, and contrast-enhanced, indicating that the lesion had evolved into invasive adenocarcinoma (arrowhead). (**c**) Magnified view of the lesion (arrowhead) in panel B showed the vasculature (arrow) and lobulation. (**d**) In the surgical specimen, a 10-mm IAC was seen (arrowhead)

6.2.3 Atypical Adenomatous Hyperplasia (AAH)

The incidence of AAH in general population and the population over 60 years of age is reportedly 2.8% and 6.6%, respectively. In patients with a history of pulmonary adenocarcinoma, AAH is far more frequently detected than in other populations, with a reported prevalence of 10–23.2%. In the 2011 version of the pathologic classification of lung adenocarcinoma, AAH was categorized as preinvasive disease. On thin-sliced CT imaging, AAH manifests as a round or oval pGGN without a solid component, marginal spiculation, or pleural indentation. A CT microangiogram sign should not be seen. Microscopically, there exists extensive focal hyperplasia of pulmonary terminal tissues and replacement of normal pulmonary epithelium by atypical cubical or cylindrical epithelium, growing sparsely along the alveoli or respiratory terminal bronchi in a lepidic pattern (Fig. 6.6).

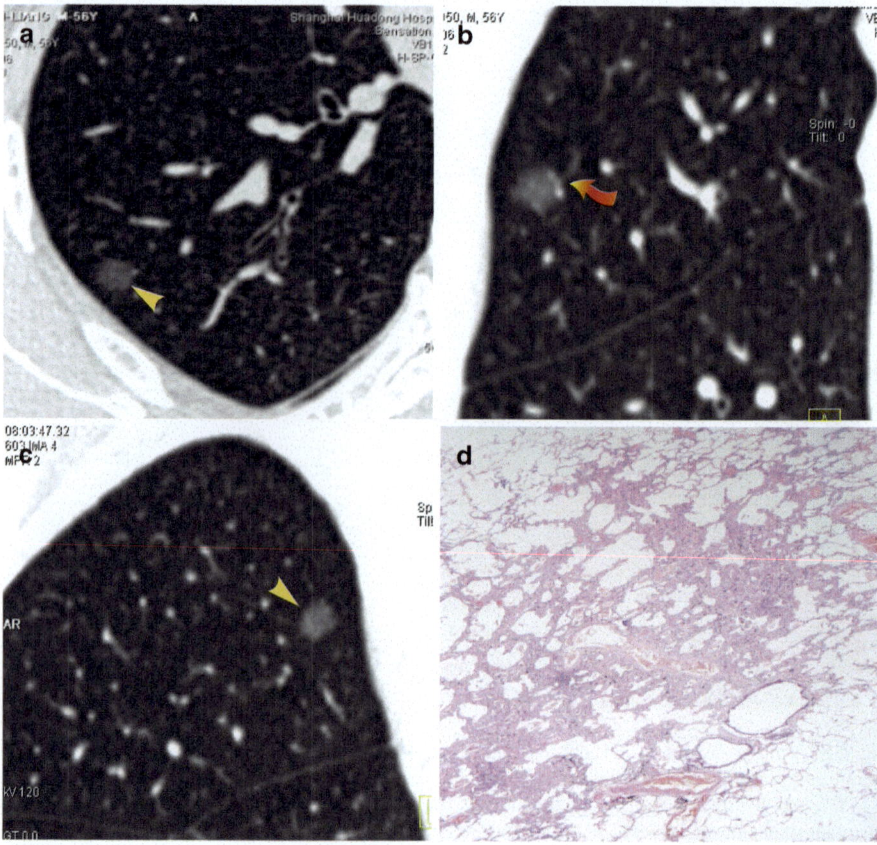

Fig. 6.6 CT findings and pathological features of pulmonary AAH. (**a**) A 5 mm pGGN (arrowhead) seen in the posterior segment of the right upper lobe. (**b**) The nodule gradually enlarged over the 3-year follow-up. No spiculation was observed, but a small amount of neovasculature (arrow) was evident along the margin in the coronal reformation view. (**c**) In the sagittal view, the neovasculature was not seen within the nodule (arrowhead), a typical characteristic for differentiation from AIS. (**d**) AAH was proven by surgical pathology

Initially, AAH was found incidentally in the surgical specimens of lung cancer. Since then, more AAH lesions have been recognized in low-dose CT screening for lung cancer in high-risk populations. Considering that there exists a certain similarity in the morphological and molecular features between AAH and early-stage lung cancer, AAH has been classified as a precancerous lesion or well-differentiated adenocarcinoma. Due to their small size and low density, these lesions tend to be neglected or missed in conventional radiography. Kawakami et al. published a retrospective analysis on 17,919 individuals screened for lung cancer by CT scanning [4]. Among them, ten AAH nodules were detected in nine asymptomatic subjects. Histopathologically, AAH appears as a focal, round nodular lesion with well-marginated borders and atypical cuboidal to low columnar pneumocytes. These cells proliferate sparsely along

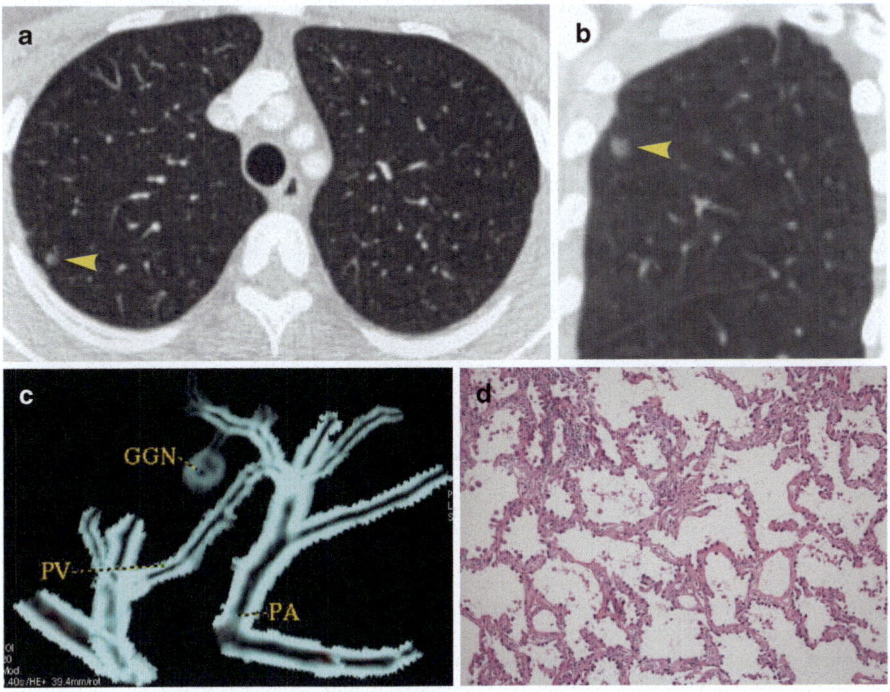

Fig. 6.7 CT findings and pathological features of AAH. (**a**) A 4.3 mm pGGN was seen in the apicoposterior segment of the right upper lobe (arrowhead). (**b**) In the coronal view, the lesion appeared to be solitary without obvious supplying vessels (arrowhead). (**c**) No direct relationship was seen between the nodular lesion and adjacent pulmonary vessels observed with three-dimensional volume rendering (VR). (**d**) Surgical pathology showed intact alveolar structures and abnormal proliferating pneumocytes, characteristic of AAH (HE stain, ×100). Abbreviations: *PV* pulmonary vein, *PA* pulmonary artery, *GGN* ground-glass nodule

slightly thickened alveolar septa or respiratory bronchioles with dense nuclei, obscure nucleoli, and few mitotic figures. Within AAH lesions, residual airspace can frequently be seen (Fig. 6.7). According to a report by Nakata et al. on 305 cases of pulmonary nodules, 7% were GGNs and 22.7% of the GGN lesions were pathologically proved to be AIS. Therefore, it is necessary to conduct routine low-dose CT for GGN follow-up. A persistent GGN that does not disappear or shrink in size during follow-up imaging carries a high probability of becoming AAH or AIS.

Current research supports the hypothesis that AAH lesions originate from the proliferation of cancer stem cells which develop from bronchioalveolar stem cells (BACSs) [5]. AAH can be incidentally seen in resected lung specimens and detected in low-dose CT screening for lung cancer in high-risk populations. Due to certain similarities in morphological and biological features of early-stage lung adenocarcinoma, AAH has been deemed the precursor lesion for adenocarcinoma. AAH lesions could be stable in size and density for a long follow-up period of up to 8–10 years. In cases of multiple AAHs, follow-up CT scanning may indicate that some lesions

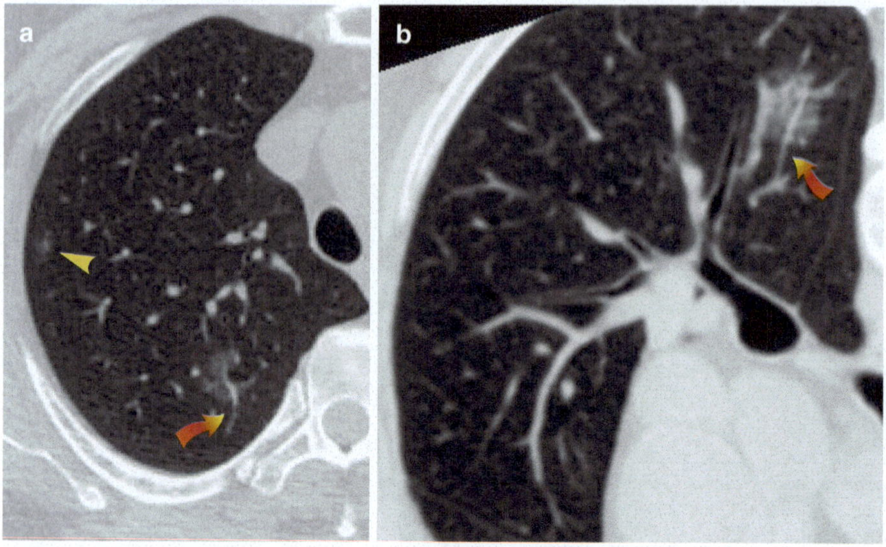

Fig. 6.8 Coexisting of AAH (arrowhead) and AIS (arrow) with supplying vessels. (**a**) Two GGNs were detected in the right upper lobe with measurements of 5 mm (arrowhead) and 12 mm diameter. A supplying vessel was seen with the larger nodule (arrow). (**b**) In oblique reformation, more details of the 12 mm lesion are displayed, including multiple supplying vessels (arrow) and proliferating intratumoral microvasculature, as well as solid components. Surgical pathology confirmed AAH for the smaller nodule and AIS for the larger nodule

progress to AIS and/or even MIA, a phenomenon known as synchronous multiple primary lung cancer (SMPLC) or metachronous multiple primary lung cancer (mMPLC), depending on the interval of occurrence of multiple malignant lesions (Fig. 6.8). Further details regarding SMPLC and MMPLC can be found in Chap. 10.

6.3 CT Findings, Pathological Correlation, and Differential Diagnosis of Adenocarcinoma in Situ

The development and progression of AIS are a multistep process involving multiple genes. A regional pulmonary stem cell population located at the bronchioalveolar duct junction has been identified as bronchioalveolar stem cells (BASCs) with the capability of self-renewal and multipotency in clonal assays. BASCs play a critical role in distal lung homeostasis by maintaining bronchiolar Clara cells and alveolar cells with resistance to bronchiolar and alveolar damage. Under the excitation of environmental factors and/or induction of internal cytokines or genetic mutations (e.g., K-ras mutation), BASCs can be transformed into malignant cells, giving rise to adenocarcinoma. The continuum between the precursor lesions AAH and AIS to MIA has been proven to be a stepwise evolution modulated by molecular alterations through the activation of oncogene mutation and inactivation of tumor suppressor genes by epigenetic changes or loss of heterozygosity [6]. There exists no absolute boundary between each step temporally or spatially. Thus all pathological findings can be found coexisting in a single lesion with a predominant type. Hence, in AIS disease, diverse radiological features can be found but pGGO predominates.

Due to low-dose CT lung cancer screening, the proportion of AIS in lung cancer continuously increased from approximately 5% in the 1980s up to 30% currently. More than half of the AIS patients living today are women and 62% are nonsmokers. Most patients have no cancer-related clinical symptoms, and the lesions are incidentally detected at chest CT scanning. Compared with other types of lung adenocarcinoma, the prognosis of AIS is excellent, with a 7-year overall survival of up to 100%. However, misdiagnosis of AIS is frequently observed in routine medical practice due to lack of experience, resulting in inaccurate management and unsatisfactory outcomes. Studies have failed to reveal specific clinical symptoms or hematological biomarkers that relate to AIS, and currently, imaging examination remains the first-line tool for AIS evaluation. Therefore, thoracic radiologists assume more responsibility for AIS diagnosis and differentiation than do other specialists.

Radiologically, AIS greatly resembles AAH. On thin-sliced CT imaging, most AIS lesions manifest as well-marginated focal GGO no more than 3 cm in diameter. Typical imaging features of AIS that differ from AAH include microvessels of less than 2 mm in diameter migrating into the lesion and bifurcating into smaller branches, i.e., the characteristic CTA-TA sign (Figs. 6.9 and 6.10).

In terms of the size and density, AAH is usually less than 5 mm diameter and of low density (around −600 HU) and can be stable for several years. Compared to AIS, AAH is poorly defined and lacks the CTA-TA sign in contrast-enhanced imaging. Most AIS lesions are above 5 mm in diameter, ranging from 5 mm to 30 mm. Of note, small AIS

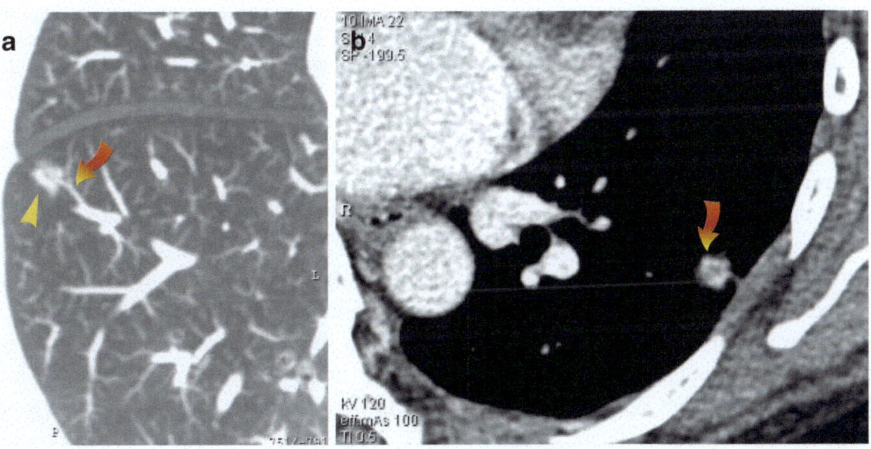

Fig. 6.9 CTA-TA sign. (**a**) Axial MIP demonstrates migration of supplying microvessels (arrow) into the nodular lesion (arrowhead). (**b**) Contrast-enhanced image shows enhanced microvessels (arrow) in the periphery of the lesion

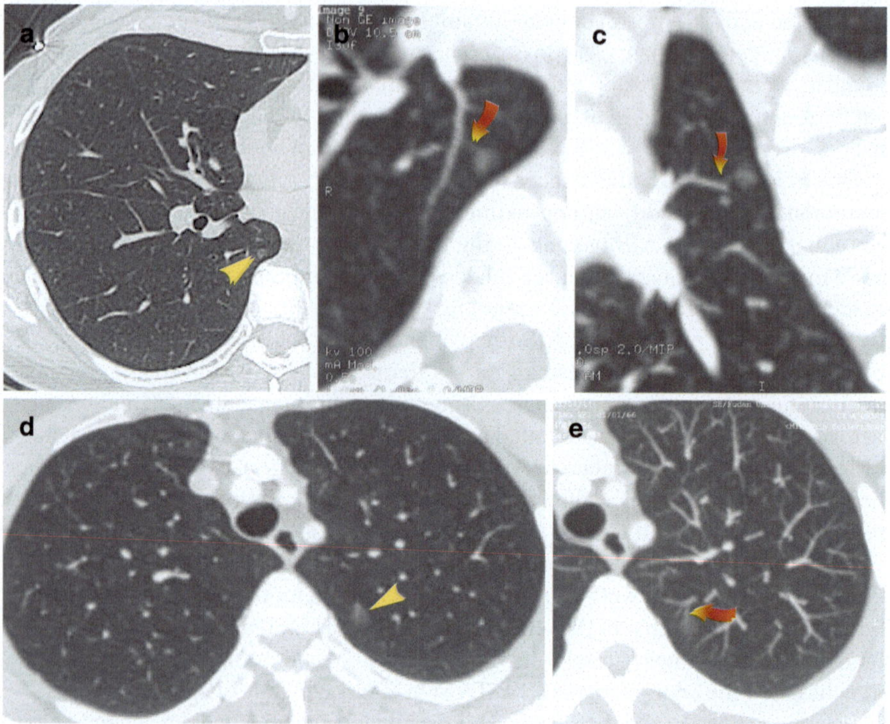

Fig. 6.10 AIS. (**a–c**) The patient was a 45-year-old female. A GGN of 4.5 mm diameter was seen in the medial segment of the right lower lobe. (**d**, **e**) The patient was a 50-year-old female. A GGN of 7 mm diameter was seen in the apical segment of the left upper lobe. In both cases, axial imaging was not adequate for evaluation of microvessels inside and surrounding the lesions (arrowhead). Image post-processing, including CPR (**b**, **c**) and MIP (**e**) provided additional information about the lesions and microvessels from multiple directions and views, i.e., small vessels migrating into the lesions and dot-like or linear enhanced microvessels seen inside the lesions, which are the key features differentiating AIS from AAH. Both patients underwent VATS, which confirmed the diagnosis of AIS

lesions of less than 5 mm diameter are not rare. In this case, evaluation of the existence of a relationship between microvessels and the lesions bears importance for the differential diagnosis (Fig. 6.11). AIS is slightly denser than AAH. Using the absolute CT number to determine the progression from AAH to AIS, a 100 HU increment of the lesion in consecutive follow-up CT scans has been shown to be clinically relevant and can be used as the second differential point, in addition to the CTA-TA sign.

As previously described in AIS, neoplastic cells grow along pre-existing alveolar structures (lepidic growth) without displaying stromal, vascular, or pleural invasion (hence, noninvasive adenocarcinoma). Papillary or micropapillary patterns and intra-alveolar tumor cells are absent. Most AIS cases are nonmucinous, comprising type II pneumocytes and/or Clara cells, whereas in mucinous AIS, tall columnar

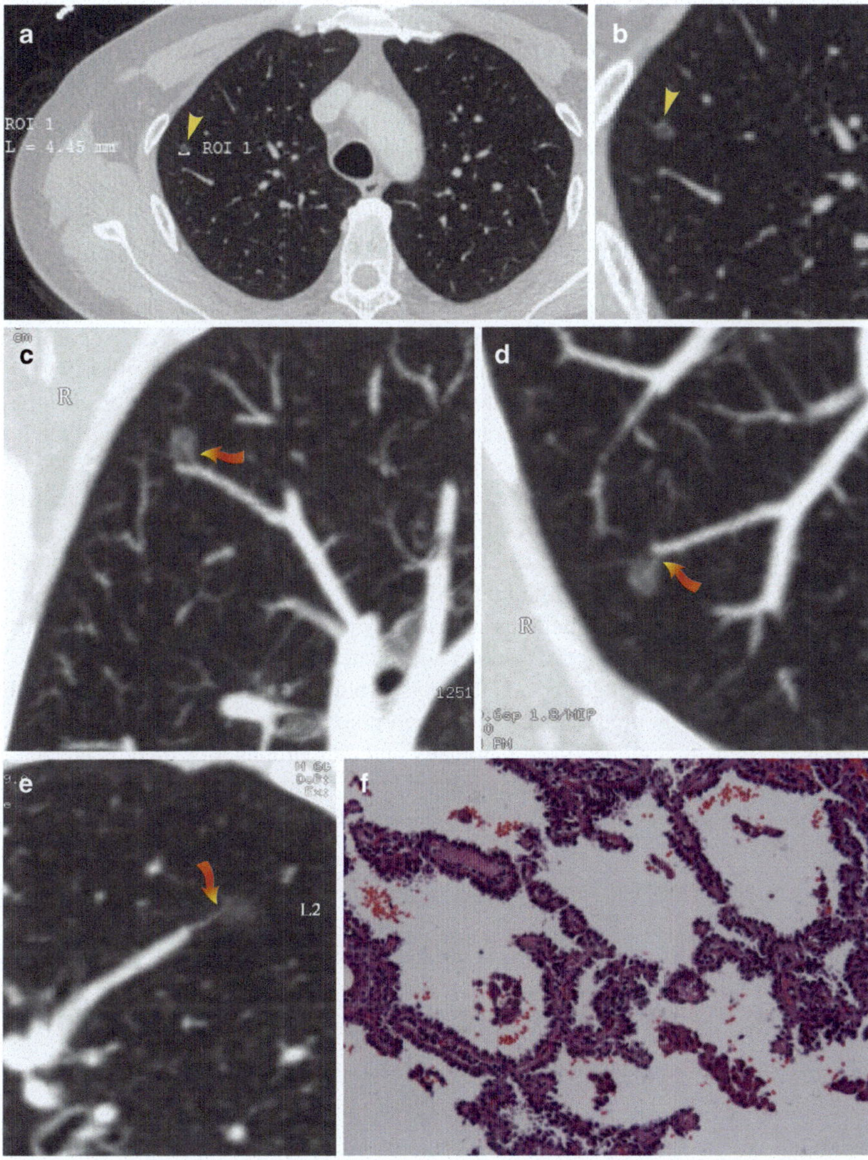

Fig. 6.11 Imaging differentiation of AIS and AAH. The patient is a 59-year-old male. The axial image showed a GGN (arrowhead in **a**, **b**) of 4.4 mm in diameter, and microvessels associated with the lesions could be evaluated. The image post-processing (MIP in **c**, **d**; CPR in **e**) revealed a small vessel of less than 2 mm (arrow) diameter, growing into the lesion and giving rise to smaller branches, i.e., the CTA-TA sign, not seen in AAH lesions. (**f**) Surgical pathology confirmed the diagnosis of AIS, 4.4 mm in diameter, intact alveolar structure, and lepidic growth of nonmucinous tumor cells (HE, × 200)

cells with basal nuclei and abundant cytoplasmic mucin or goblet cells can be observed. Residual airspace can be seen in AIS but alveolar structures remain intact (Fig. 6.12). In contrast, AAH is a localized, small proliferation of mild to moderately atypical type II pneumocytes and/or Clara cells lining the alveolar walls and sometimes the respiratory bronchioles. Atypical cells appear rounded, cuboidal, low columnar, or "peg"-shaped, with round to oval nuclei and intercellular gaps frequently seen, which signifies the third differential point between AIS and AAH. Due to the continuum of morphologic changes between AAH and AIS, both diseases can coexist in the same or separate lobe. In the 2011 international multidisciplinary classification of lung adenocarcinoma publication, AIS was officially recognized as a second preinvasive lesion for lung adenocarcinoma, in addition to AAH. According to the TNM staging system, AIS is classified as stage 0 (TisN0M0) with a 5-year overall survival of 95 to 100%. However, the 5-year overall survival for all lung cancers is only 16% globally and even lower in China, which is mainly ascribed to a high percentage of advanced diseases at detection. Therefore, the key to early detection, early diagnosis, early intervention, and better outcome of lung cancer is the accurate imaging evaluation of AIS [7].

In the revised IASLC/ATS/ERS classification of lung adenocarcinoma, mucin-producing adenocarcinoma of the lung (MPA) has no longer been classified as an independent entity but as a mucinous subcategory in related types such as mucinous AIS and mucinous MIA, etc. Mucinous adenocarcinoma possesses unique pathological features, represented by mucin pools containing islands of small atypical cells characterized by moderate-sized, pleomorphic nuclei with an open chromatin pattern and indistinct nucleoli [8]. Clinically and radiographically, there is no clear distinction between the mucinous and other types of adenocarcinomas. However, mucinous adenocarcinoma has a poor prognosis, primarily due to its prevalence in

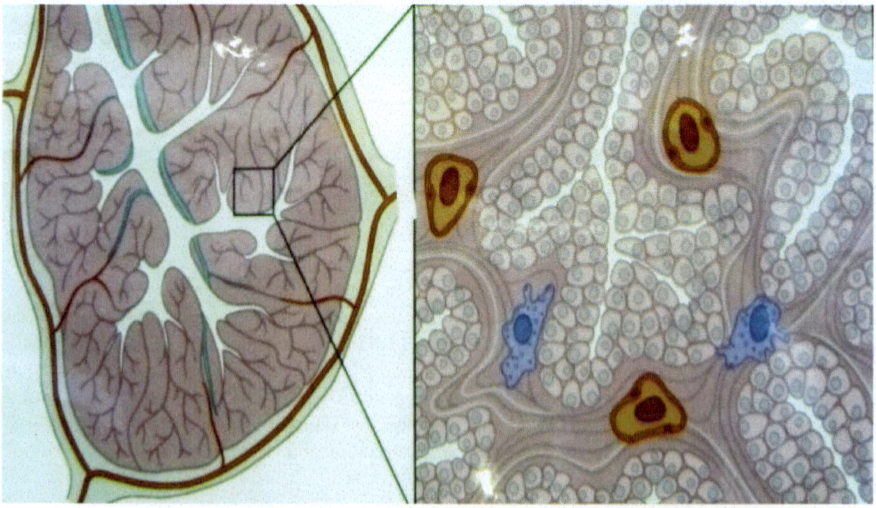

Fig. 6.12 The development of AIS. (**a**) Tumor cells proliferating along pre-existing alveolar wall without stromal invasion. (**b**) Enlarged view of the alveolar surface

the elderly population and a lack of specific symptoms leading to a definitive diagnosis at the advanced stage and the impossibility of surgical treatment. On CT imaging, MPA can manifest with various features, including GGN, focal consolidation, multicystic lesions, cavitation, bubble-like lucency, air bronchograms, and widening of lobular septa. In three-fourths of cases, the central zone of the lesion appears as low density due to the existence of a mucin pool, generating the typical "central bubble" CT sign (Fig. 6.13). The definitive diagnosis of MPA requires pathological examination, and surgical resection is the standard treatment.

Transformation of normal cells into abnormal ones is a biological event at the molecular level with certain changes in various genes or proteins. At the preinvasive stage of AAH, transformed cells undergo slow clonal proliferation and apoptosis, which renders the lesion stable, inert, dormant, and even reversible to normal conditions. This stage can last a long time (up to dozens of years). Most AAH lesions do

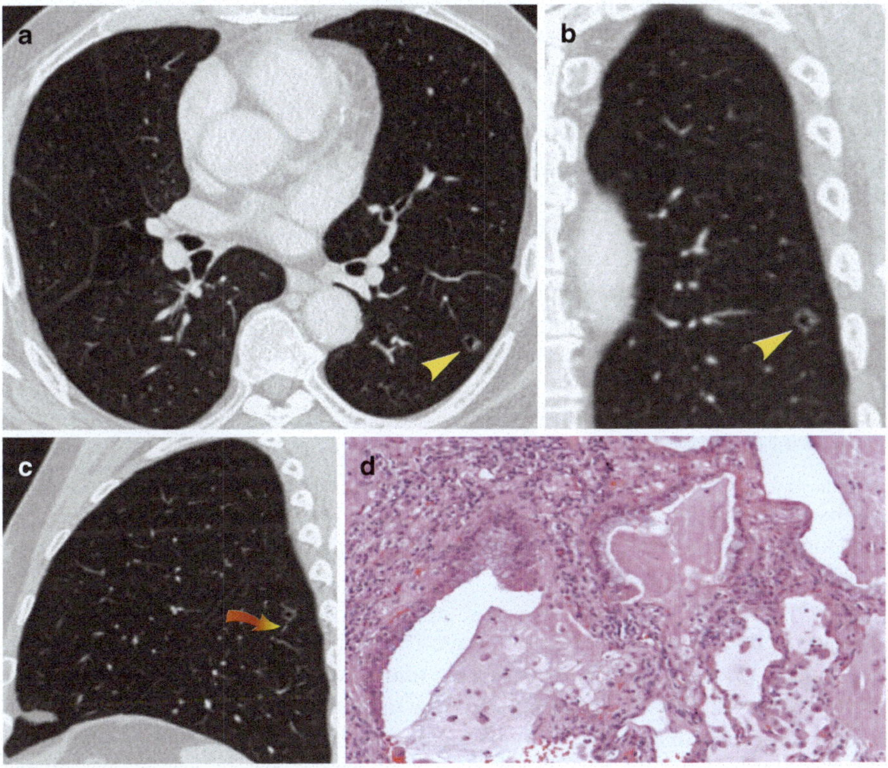

Fig. 6.13 Mucinous AIS. (**a**) The patient was a 74-year-old male. A 9 mm lesion with a "central bubble" sign in the left lower lobe (arrowhead). (**b**) After a 10-year follow-up, the lesion remained stable in shape, size, density, and location without specific malignant features on nonenhancement CT imaging (arrowhead). (**c**) With administration of contrast media and image post-processing, a small vessel was observed migrating into the lesion, a sign indicating malignancy (arrow). (**d**) Surgical pathology confirmed mucinous AIS (10 × 6 mm) with interstitial pneumonitis (HE stain, × 100 magnification)

not have a direct supplying blood circulation (avascular phase) under the balance of proangiogenic factors and antiangiogenic factors and absorb nutrition diffusing within the extracellular matrix from adjacent vessels, which further limits the tumor growth potential. If the angiogenic balance is broken with the proangiogenic factors dominating, neovascularization will occur with the replacement of the avascular phase by the vascular phase, indicating that the lesion is continuing to develop toward the next stage, AIS. Hence, vascular proliferation or neovascularization is one of the macroscopic markers of disease progression with the potential of detection using modern imaging modalities, particularly CT.

Earlier studies revealed that neovascularization influenced wound healing with prognostic value [9]. In the 1990s, Weidner et al. proposed a definition of microvessel density (MVD) and a measurement methodology, finding that there was a significant correlation between the incidence of metastases and MVD in histologic sections of breast and prostate cancer [10, 11]. Thereafter, related research on various solid tumors showed that higher MVD measurement implied a higher tumor growth rate and predicted increasing metastatic risks and poor overall survival. MVD can be used as an independent prognostic factor for the assessment of malignant solid tumors. In lung cancer, a negative correlation has been observed between MVD and postoperative survival time. To a certain extent, average MVD reflects the tumor biological behavior and microenvironmental condition and may have influences on proliferation, progression, invasion, and metastasis of tumor cells.

Angiogenic stimuli produced by the tumor cells, such as VEGF, induce endothelial cells of the adjacent vessels to migrate into the perivascular space. Proliferating endothelial cells adhere to each other and create a blood vessel sprout, accompanied by basement membrane formation and pericyte attachment [12]. The sprout grows continuously and penetrates the tumor to provide nutrition (external vasculogenesis). Within the tumor, the sprout fuses with other sprouts and the pre-existing vasculature to build new circulatory systems for sustainable tumor development (internal vasculogenesis). In addition, the tumor cells can receive nutrition and metastasize via pre-existing interstitial lymphatics. As described above, angiogenesis itself is a complex, multistep process that follows stage- and tissue-specific regulations from the avascular phase to external vasculogenesis and to internal vasculogenesis (Fig. 6.14).

Based on microvascular characterization and distribution, the pulmonary adenocarcinoma nodule can be divided into three zones: (1) outer zone, or the peripheral area, comprised of an actively proliferating tumor cell population and highly dense microvessels. The amount and structure of the microvessels correlate with the metastatic risks; (2) median zone, or transitional area, located between the outer zone and central zone; and the (3) central zone, where pulmonary structures lose their intactness and remodel with neovascularization and matrix reproduction. On contrast-enhanced CT images of AIS/MIA disease, intratumoral microvessels can be better visualized with the characteristic CTA-TA sign (Fig. 6.15). The differentiation between AIS and MIA relies on the size of the migrating vessels surrounding

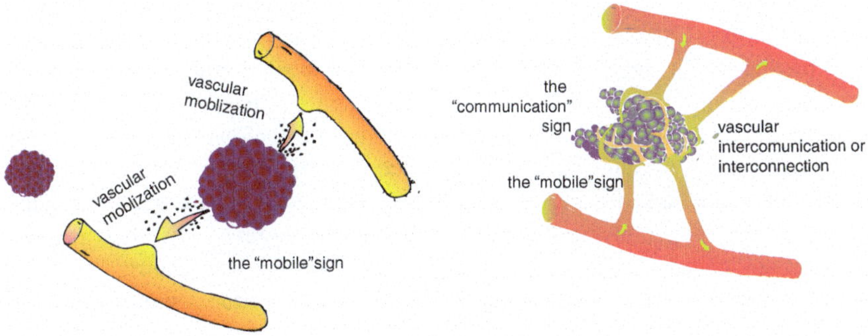

Fig. 6.14 The “neo-vessel mobilization and intercommunication” phenomenon. (**a**) Avascular phase. In this stage, the tumor size is too small to require a direct blood supply. (**b**) Neo-vessel mobilization (external vascular phase). Stimulated by proangiogenic factors, new vascular buds (neo-vessels) sprouting from pre-existing vessels adjacent to the tumor are mobilized to grow toward the tumor. (**c**) Neo-vessel intercommunication (internal vascular phase). Neo-vessels grow into the tumor and intercommunicate with each other to establish the intratumoral capillary network (namely, “vascular interconnection”), through which the tumor can metastasize distantly

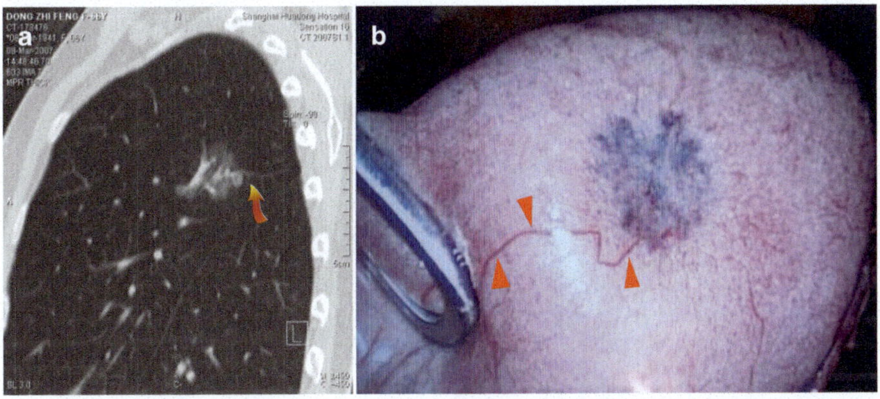

Fig. 6.15 Correlation between the CTA-TA sign and surgical findings. (**a**) Microvessels (arrow) migrate into the tumor and become components of intratumoral microvascular networks which can be significantly enhanced on imaging with contrast media. (**b**) On the direct surgical view from VATS, a tortuous vessel (arrowhead) is connected to the tumor

the lesion and the number of interconnecting vessels within the lesion: larger migrating vessels (≥2 mm in diameter) and more interconnecting vessels are seen in MIA than in AIS.

Two decades ago, it was impossible to assess in vivo MVD in a pulmonary nodule using noninvasive procedures. Then, most studies on MVD were based on surgical specimens using immunohistochemical methodologies, such as VIII-Ag, avidin-biotin-peroxidase complex, anti-CD34 monoclonal antibody, and the labeled streptavidin-biotin (LSAB) method. With advancement in imaging technology and contrast media, MVD can be readily measured in vivo using noninvasive contrast CT scanning for the differential diagnosis, treatment evaluation, and prognostic assessment. For accurate assessment of MVD and the correlation between microvessels and pulmonary nodules, image post-processing (including MIP, CPR, and MPR) should be applied (if necessary) for better visualization of the anatomic relationship (Fig. 6.16). Notably, traditionally well-known imaging signs, such as deep lobulation, spiculation, pleural indentation, and air bronchograms, are less commonly seen in preinvasive diseases or MIA but more frequently in invasive or advanced diseases.

Clarifying the relationships between the bronchus, pulmonary vessels, and nodules facilitates the differential diagnosis of nodules. Anatomically, both bronchial arteries and pulmonary arteries accompany the corresponding bronchus and further subdivide into capillaries, distributing around and supporting the alveolar and bronchial walls, as well as the visceral pleura. The enhancement of lung cancer is not proportional to the size of the external vessels. However, the average and peak enhancement of the tumor correlates with the internal neovasculature (size range,

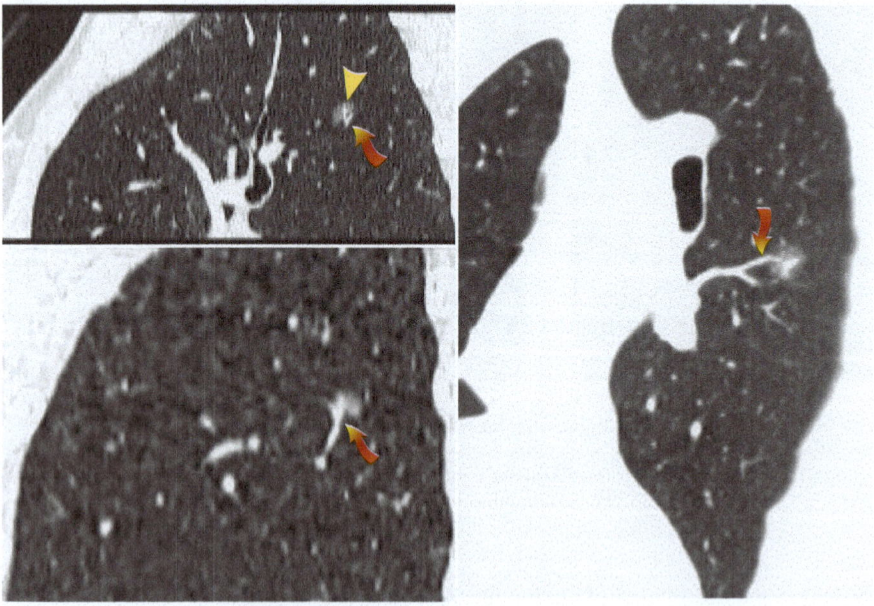

Fig. 6.16 CTA-TA sign and image post-processing. (**a**) A supplying microvessel (arrow) migrates into the nodule (arrowhead) on the sagittal view. (**b**) The correlation between the microvessel (arrow) and the nodule is better seen on the coronal view. (**c**) The oblique reformation reveals the microvessel originating from the pulmonary artery (arrow)

0.02–0.10 mm) and lower enhancement (≤20 HU), indicating a lower density of neovasculature and a better prognosis, and vice versa. The involvement of the pulmonary veins has been reported as being valuable in the imaging diagnosis of lung cancer [13]. Once pulmonary veins are encroached by a mass, lung cancer should be strongly suspected. In addition, part of the tumor blood circulation can originate from the pulmonary venous system.

As the characteristic imaging feature in distinguishing peripheral small/subcentimeter lung cancer from other benign pulmonary nodules, the CTA-TA sign is distinct from the well-known vascular convergence sign (VCS). As a CT imaging sign, VCS describes the relationship between SPNs and vessels, i.e., one or multiple vessels dragged toward and passing through lesions or being truncated at the edge of lesions [14]. Involved vessels appear tortuous, rigid, or irregularly dilated and link to pulmonary arteries or pulmonary veins. VCS was reported in 93% of carcinomas and 12.5% of nonneoplastic lesions. In addition to dilated vessels, VCS may consist of collapsed bronchioles, reactive connective tissues, and embolized lymphatics. Pathologically, VCS reflects the involvement of preexisting vessels with resistance to the returning venous circulation due to tumor compression and tumor emboli at the venous section adjacent to the mass, instead of neoangiogenic amateur structures observed in the CTA-TA sign functioning as the supplying circulation. Specifically, VCS is a late sign of the mass occupation effect of lung cancer resulting from squeezing and compressing adjacent vascular and nonvascular structures, while the CTA-TA sign represents the very early neoangiogenic stage of lung cancer development. Hence, the involved vessels in VCS are more dilated, irregular, and larger than those in the CTA-TA sign.

Besides lung cancer, ground-glass opacity can be seen in other pulmonary parenchymal and interstitial diseases because of the infiltration of inflammatory cells within alveolar cavities and/or walls. The distribution or location of GGOs may vary with diseases: centrilobular in allergic alveolitis and interstitial pneumonitis, panlobular in alveolar proteinosis, lipoid pneumonia, sarcoidosis, and *Pneumocystis jirovecii* pneumonia, or marginal in idiopathic pulmonary fibrosis and bronchiolitis obliterans with organizing pneumonia.

If an incidental GGN in an otherwise healthy patient does not respond to experimental antibiotics or grows and represents the typical CTA-TA sign in a follow-up CT, there should be a high suspicion for AIS. This can be summarized in the following formulation for the imaging diagnosis of AIS:

$$\text{AIS} = \text{persistent GGNs} + \text{CTA} - \text{TA}\,\textit{sign}$$

Despite the fact that the CTA-TA sign has a high specificity in differentiating peripheral subcentimeter lung adenocarcinoma from benign lesions, this formulation should be applied with caution, with additional consideration of the previous medical history, physical examination, and other imaging findings to avoid possible misdiagnosis or overdiagnosis (Figs. 6.17 and 6.18).

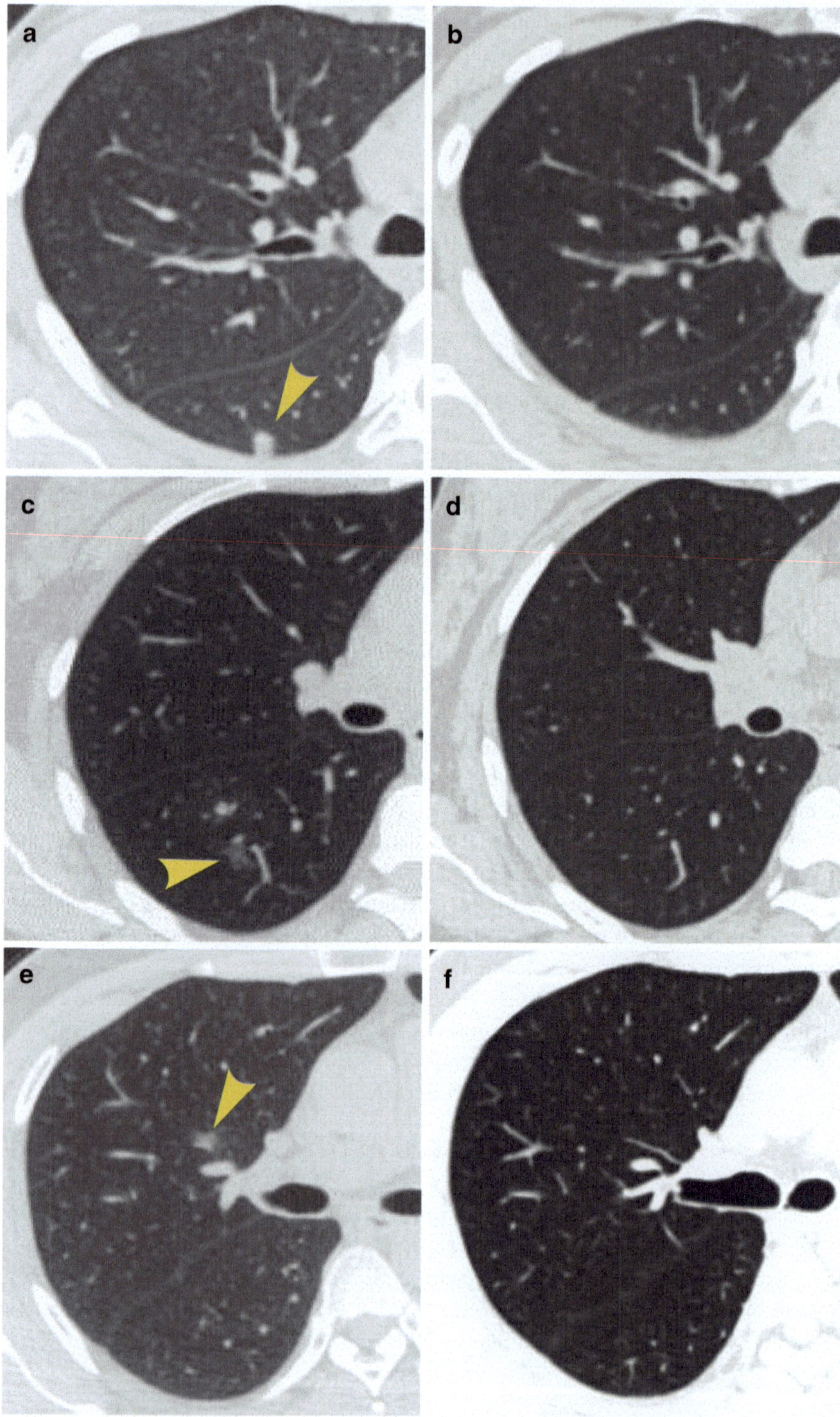
a
b
c
d
e
f

Fig. 6.17 Anti-inflammation in the diagnostic differentiation of nodules. (**a**, **b**) A benign solid micronodule of 8 mm diameter (**a**, arrowhead) was incidentally detected in the superior segment of the right lower lobe during an annual lung cancer screen in a 45-year-old female patient. After antibiotic treatment, the nodule had disappeared by the 3-month follow-up CT (**b**). (**c**, **d**) A benign semisolid GGN of 6 mm diameter (**c**, arrowhead) was found in the superior segment of the right lower lobe in a 48-year-old female patient; it had completely regressed after antibiotic administration by the 2-month follow-up visit (**d**). (**e**, **f**) A benign semisolid GGN of 7 mm (**e**, arrowhead) diameter was in the anterior segment of the right upper lobe in an otherwise healthy 31-year-old male patient; it disappeared after antibiotic administration by the 2-month follow-up visit (**f**)

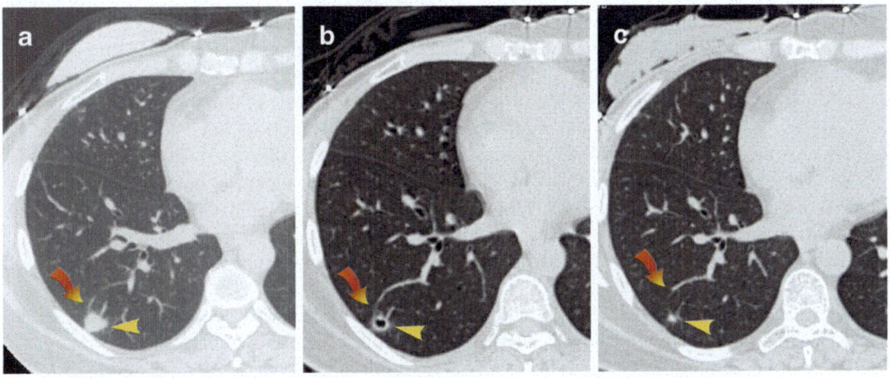

Fig. 6.18 Benign solitary nodule. (**a**) The patient is a 40-year-old female with a history of Stage I breast cancer, status post-surgery. At the 1-year follow-up CT imaging, a solid nodule with a diameter of 11 mm (arrowhead) was detected in the posterior segment of the right lower lobe with several supplying microvessels (arrow), and this was suggestive of metastatic disease. The patient declined any invasive procedures to make a definitive diagnosis, and oral anti-inflammation medicine was prescribed. (**b**) After 2 months of anti-inflammatory treatment, the solid component dramatically decreased, with central cavitation (arrowhead) and regression of the supplying microvessels (arrow). (**c**) Five months later, the nodule continued shrinking with a residual lesion of 3 mm diameter (arrowhead), and the supplying microvessels had completely disappeared (arrow)

References

1. Tuddenham WJ. Glossary of terms for thoracic radiology: recommendations of the Nomenclature Committee of the Fleischner Society. AJR Am J Roentgenol. 1984;143(3):509–17. https://doi.org/10.2214/ajr.143.3.509.
2. Austin JH, Muller NL, Friedman PJ, Hansell DM, Naidich DP, Remy-Jardin M, Webb WR, Zerhouni EA. Glossary of terms for CT of the lungs: recommendations of the Nomenclature Committee of the Fleischner Society. Radiology. 1996;200(2):327–31. https://doi.org/10.1148/radiology.200.2.8685321.
3. Hansell DM, Bankier AA, MacMahon H, McLoud TC, Muller NL, Remy J. Fleischner Society: glossary of terms for thoracic imaging. Radiology. 2008;246(3):697–722. https://doi.org/10.1148/radiol.2462070712.

4. Kawakami S, Sone S, Takashima S, Li F, Yang ZG, Maruyama Y, Honda T, Hasegawa M, Wang JC. Atypical adenomatous hyperplasia of the lung: correlation between high-resolution CT findings and histopathologic features. Eur Radiol. 2001;11(5):811–4. https://doi.org/10.1007/s003300000790.
5. Kim CF, Jackson EL, Woolfenden AE, Lawrence S, Babar I, Vogel S, Crowley D, Bronson RT, Jacks T. Identification of bronchioalveolar stem cells in normal lung and lung cancer. Cell. 2005;121(6):823–35. https://doi.org/10.1016/j.cell.2005.03.032.
6. Kim H, Park CM, Koh JM, Lee SM, Goo JM. Pulmonary subsolid nodules: what radiologists need to know about the imaging features and management strategy. Diagn Interv Radiol. 2014;20(1):47–57. https://doi.org/10.5152/dir.2013.13223.
7. Travis WD, Brambilla E, Noguchi M, Nicholson AG, Geisinger KR, Yatabe Y, Beer DG, Powell CA, Riely GJ, Van Schil PE, Garg K, Austin JH, Asamura H, Rusch VW, Hirsch FR, Scagliotti G, Mitsudomi T, Huber RM, Ishikawa Y, Jett J, Sanchez-Cespedes M, Sculier JP, Takahashi T, Tsuboi M, Vansteenkiste J, Wistuba I, Yang PC, Aberle D, Brambilla C, Flieder D, Franklin W, Gazdar A, Gould M, Hasleton P, Henderson D, Johnson B, Johnson D, Kerr K, Kuriyama K, Lee JS, Miller VA, Petersen I, Roggli V, Rosell R, Saijo N, Thunnissen E, Tsao M, Yankelewitz D. International association for the study of lung cancer/american thoracic society/european respiratory society international multidisciplinary classification of lung adenocarcinoma. J Thorac Oncol. 2011;6(2):244–85. https://doi.org/10.1097/JTO.0b013e318206a221.
8. Brownlee NA, Mott RT, Mahar A, Roggli VL. Mucinous (colloid) adenocarcinoma of the lung. Arch Pathol Lab Med. 2005;129(1):121–2. https://doi.org/10.1043/1543-2165(2005)129<121:mcaotl>2.0.co;2.
9. Leibovich SJ, Wiseman DM. Macrophages, wound repair and angiogenesis. Prog Clin Biol Res. 1988;266:131–45.
10. Weidner N, Carroll PR, Flax J, Blumenfeld W, Folkman J. Tumor angiogenesis correlates with metastasis in invasive prostate carcinoma. Am J Pathol. 1993;143(2):401–9.
11. Weidner N, Semple JP, Welch WR, Folkman J. Tumor angiogenesis and metastasis—correlation in invasive breast carcinoma. N Engl J Med. 1991;324(1):1–8. https://doi.org/10.1056/nejm199101033240101.
12. Bergers G, Benjamin LE. Tumorigenesis and the angiogenic switch. Nat Rev Cancer. 2003;3(6):401–10. https://doi.org/10.1038/nrc1093.
13. Mori K, Saitou Y, Tominaga K, Yokoi K, Miyazawa N, Okuyama A, Sasagawa M. Small nodular lesions in the lung periphery: new approach to diagnosis with CT. Radiology. 1990;177(3):843–9. https://doi.org/10.1148/radiology.177.3.2243999.
14. Yang X, Yan H, Liu H, Xie Y, Hu M, Soimakallio S. Vascular manifestations of small solitary pulmonary masses. Angiographic-pathologic correlations and clinical significance. Investig Radiol. 1996;31(5):275–9.

Suggested Readings

1. Aberle DR, Berg CD, Black WC, Church TR, Fagerstrom RM, Galen B, Gareen IF, Gatsonis C, Goldin J, Gohagan JK, Hillman B, Jaffe C, Kramer BS, Lynch D, Marcus PM, Schnall M, Sullivan DC, Sullivan D, Zylak CJ. The National Lung Screening Trial: overview and study design. Radiology. 2011;258(1):243–53. https://doi.org/10.1148/radiol.10091808.
2. Akashita S, Tachibana Y, Sakamaki K, Sogawa K, Inoue T. Detection of pure ground-glass nodules in the lung by low-dose multi-detector computed tomography, with use of an iterative reconstruction method: a comparison with conventional image reconstruction by the filtered back-projection method. Jpn J Radiol. 2015;33(3):113–21. https://doi.org/10.1007/s11604-014-0384-z.

3. Ashida C, Zerhouni EA, Fishman EK. CT demonstration of prominent right hilar soft tissue collections. J Comput Assist Tomogr. 1987;11(1):57–9.
4. Bach PB, Mirkin JN, Oliver TK, Azzoli CG, Berry DA, Brawley OW, Byers T, Colditz GA, Gould MK, Jett JR, Sabichi AL, Smith-Bindman R, Wood DE, Qaseem A, Detterbeck FC. Benefits and harms of CT screening for lung cancer: a systematic review. JAMA. 2012;307(22):2418–29. https://doi.org/10.1001/jama.2012.5521.
5. Bak SH, Lee HY, Kim JH, Um SW, Kwon OJ, Han J, Kim HK, Kim J, Lee KS. Quantitative CT scanning analysis of pure ground-glass opacity nodules predicts further CT scanning change. Chest. 2016;149(1):180–91. https://doi.org/10.1378/chest.15-0034.
6. Chang B, Hwang JH, Choi YH, Chung MP, Kim H, Kwon OJ, Lee HY, Lee KS, Shim YM, Han J, Um SW. Natural history of pure ground-glass opacity lung nodules detected by low-dose CT scan. Chest. 2013;143(1):172–8. https://doi.org/10.1378/chest.11-2501.
7. Cho S, Yang H, Kim K, Jheon S. Pathology and prognosis of persistent stable pure ground-glass opacity nodules after surgical resection. Ann Thorac Surg. 2013;96(4):1190–5. https://doi.org/10.1016/j.athoracsur.2013.05.062.
8. Gaeta M, Barone M, Russi EG, Volta S, Casablanca G, Romeo P, La Spada F, Minutoli A. Carcinomatous solitary pulmonary nodules: evaluation of the tumor-bronchi relationship with thin-section CT. Radiology. 1993;187(2):535–9. https://doi.org/10.1148/radiology.187.2.8475303.
9. Gao F, Li M, Ge X, Zheng X, Ren Q, Chen Y, Lv F, Hua Y. Multi-detector spiral CT study of the relationships between pulmonary ground-glass nodules and blood vessels. Eur Radiol. 2013;23(12):3271–7. https://doi.org/10.1007/s00330-013-2954-3.
10. Hall FM. Fleischner Society glossary of terms: infiltrates. Radiology. 2008;248(3):1083. https://doi.org/10.1148/radiol.2483080610.
11. Hendee WR, O'Connor MK. Radiation risks of medical imaging: separating fact from fantasy. Radiology. 2012;264(2):312–21. https://doi.org/10.1148/radiol.12112678.
12. Henschke CI, Yankelevitz DF, Libby DM, Pasmantier MW, Smith JP, Miettinen OS. Survival of patients with stage I lung cancer detected on CT screening. N Engl J Med. 2006;355(17):1763–71. https://doi.org/10.1056/NEJMoa060476.
13. Ichinose J, Kohno T, Fujimori S, Harano T, Suzuki S, Fujii T. Invasiveness and malignant potential of pulmonary lesions presenting as pure ground-glass opacities. Ann Thorac Cardiovasc Surg. 2014;20(5):347–52.
14. Kaneda H, Nakano T, Taniguchi Y, Saito T, Konobu T, Saito Y. A decrease in the size of ground glass nodules may indicate the optimal timing for curative surgery. Lung Cancer. 2014;85(2):213–7. https://doi.org/10.1016/j.lungcan.2014.05.015.
15. Kitami A, Sano F, Hayashi S, Suzuki K, Uematsu S, Kamio Y, Suzuki T, Kadokura M, Omatsu M, Kunimura T. Correlation between histological invasiveness and the computed tomography value in pure ground-glass nodules. Surg Today. 2016;46(5):593–8. https://doi.org/10.1007/s00595-015-1208-1.
16. Kudo Y, Matsubayashi J, Saji H, Akata S, Shimada Y, Kato Y, Kakihana M, Kajiwara N, Ohira T, Nagao T, Ikeda N. Association between high-resolution computed tomography findings and the IASLC/ATS/ERS classification of small lung adenocarcinomas in Japanese patients. Lung Cancer. 2015;90(1):47–54. https://doi.org/10.1016/j.lungcan.2015.07.007.
17. Lim HJ, Ahn S, Lee KS, Han J, Shim YM, Woo S, Kim JH, Yie M, Lee HY, Yi CA. Persistent pure ground-glass opacity lung nodules ≥10 mm in diameter at CT scan: histopathologic comparisons and prognostic implications. Chest. 2013;144(4):1291–9. https://doi.org/10.1378/chest.12-2987.
18. Mathews JD, Forsythe AV, Brady Z, Butler MW, Goergen SK, Byrnes GB, Giles GG, Wallace AB, Anderson PR, Guiver TA, McGale P, Cain TM, Dowty JG, Bickerstaffe AC, Darby SC. Cancer risk in 680,000 people exposed to computed tomography scans in childhood or adolescence: data linkage study of 11 million Australians. BMJ. 2013;346:f2360. https://doi.org/10.1136/bmj.f2360.

19. McCollough CH. Automated data mining of exposure information for dose management and patient safety initiatives in medical imaging. Radiology. 2012;264(2):322–4. https://doi.org/10.1148/radiol.12121152.
20. Mets OM, de Jong PA, Scholten ET, Chung K, van Ginneken B, Schaefer-Prokop CM. Subsolid pulmonary nodule morphology and associated patient characteristics in a routine clinical population. Eur Radiol. 2017;27(2):689–96. https://doi.org/10.1007/s00330-016-4429-9.
21. Moon Y, Sung SW, Lee KY, Sim SB, Park JK. Pure ground-glass opacity on chest computed tomography: predictive factors for invasive adenocarcinoma. J Thorac Dis. 2016;8(7):1561–70. https://doi.org/10.21037/jtd.2016.06.34.
22. Park CM, Goo JM, Lee HJ, Kim KG, Kang MJ, Shin YH. Persistent pure ground-glass nodules in the lung: interscan variability of semiautomated volume and attenuation measurements. AJR Am J Roentgenol. 2010;195(6):W408–14. https://doi.org/10.2214/ajr.09.4157.
23. Sakai N, Yabuuchi H, Kondo M, Kojima T, Nagatomo K, Kawanami S, Kamitani T, Yonezawa M, Nagao M, Honda H. Volumetric measurement of artificial pure ground-glass nodules at low-dose CT: comparisons between hybrid iterative reconstruction and filtered back projection. Eur J Radiol. 2015;84(12):2654–62. https://doi.org/10.1016/j.ejrad.2015.08.018.
24. Sawada S, Yamashita N, Sugimoto R, Ueno T, Yamashita M. Long-term outcomes of patients with ground-glass opacities detected using CT scanning. Chest. 2017;151(2):308–15. https://doi.org/10.1016/j.chest.2016.07.007.
25. Sim HJ, Choi SH, Chae EJ, Kim HR, Kim YH, Kim DK, Park SI. Surgical management of pulmonary adenocarcinoma presenting as a pure ground-glass nodule. Eur J Cardiothorac Surg. 2014;46(4):632–636.; discussion 636. https://doi.org/10.1093/ejcts/ezu007.
26. Tamura T, Satoh H. Quantitative CT scanning analysis of pure ground-glass opacity nodules predicts further CT change. Chest. 2016;149(6):1586–7. https://doi.org/10.1016/j.chest.2016.03.062.
27. Thrall JH. Radiation exposure in CT scanning and risk: where are we? Radiology. 2012;264(2):325–8. https://doi.org/10.1148/radiol.12121137.
28. van Riel SJ, Sanchez CI, Bankier AA, Naidich DP, Verschakelen J, Scholten ET, de Jong PA, Jacobs C, van Rikxoort E, Peters-Bax L, Snoeren M, Prokop M, van Ginneken B, Schaefer-Prokop C. Observer variability for classification of pulmonary nodules on low-dose CT images and its effect on nodule management. Radiology. 2015;277(3):863–71. https://doi.org/10.1148/radiol.2015142700.
29. Yamaguchi M, Furuya A, Edagawa M, Taguchi K, Shimamatsu S, Toyokawa G, Toyozawa R, Nosaki K, Hirai F, Seto T, Takenoyama M, Ichinose Y. How should we manage small focal pure ground-glass opacity nodules on high-resolution computed tomography? A single institute experience. Surg Oncol. 2015;24(3):258–63. https://doi.org/10.1016/j.suronc.2015.08.004.

Chapter 7
Part-Solid Ground-Glass Nodules

Guozhen Zhang and Xiangpeng Zheng

7.1 CT Findings and Pathological Correlation of Part-Solid Ground-Glass Nodules

Early-stage lung adenocarcinoma can have various imaging manifestations due to heterogeneity in location, developmental stage, and growth rate of parts of the lesion. Anatomically, adenocarcinoma can initially occur in various pulmonary locations, such as alveolar wall, alveolar duct, or respiratory or terminal bronchiole. In SMPLC or MMPLC, multiple nodules can be seen in the same lobe or separate lobes at same or different developmental stages, i.e., AAH, AIS, MIA, or LPA. In a specific nodule, there may exist inhomogeneous areas of active proliferation, growth inertia, regression, or necrosis. All of these factors contribute to the radiological and pathological complex of lung adenocarcinoma at very early stage.

7.1.1 Morphology

On CT imaging, pulmonary pGGNs can have various shapes which have been summarized into ten patterns, including cotton ball-like, filling, piling, granulated, bronchovascular, branching, cavitary, honeycomb, scar-like, and umbilical. Except that cotton ball-like GGNs less than 10 mm are commonly seen in preinvasive lesions, other categories of part-solid or solid GGNs carry substantial risks of invasive adenocarcinomas. In pathologically proven malignant GGNs, solid components with

G. Zhang (✉)
Department of Radiology, Fudan University Huadong Hospital, Shanghai, China
e-mail: cjr.zhangguozhen@vip.163.com

X. Zheng
Department of Radiation Oncology, Fudan University Huadong Hospital, Shanghai, China

X. Zheng et al. (eds.), *Early-stage Lung Cancer*,
https://doi.org/10.1007/978-981-10-7596-4_7

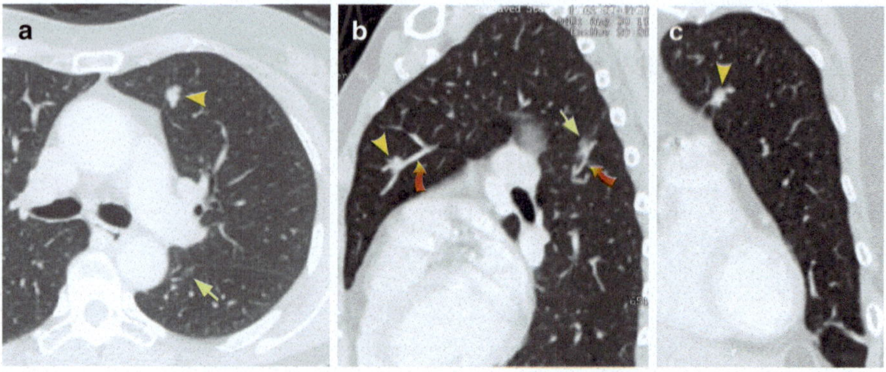

Fig. 7.1 Differential diagnosis of AIS and MIA. (**a**) Female, 55 years old. A 12 mm-diameter GGN (arrowhead) is seen in the anterior segment of left upper lobe and a 4 mm-diameter GGN (yellow arrow) adjacent to the major fissure in the superior segment of left lower lobe. However, the axial images provide inadequate information for assessment of the relationship between nodules and related vessels. (**b**, **c**) The coronal and sagittal reformations show that microvessels of ≥2 mm in diameter (red arrow) migrate into and distribute within both lesions (arrowhead and yellow arrow), indicative of MIA with pathological confirmation. Of note, for ≤5 mm MIAs (yellow arrow), especially those with poor visualization of solid component on nonenhancement images, CT scan with contrast medium can provide valuable information for differential diagnosis

increasing attenuation on follow-up CT scans correspond to invasive portions within lesions. However, the shape is nonspecific for discrimination between benign and malignant nodules, so is the nodule size. Some GGNs up to 20 mm are found to be in the benign preinvasive stage. In contrast, surgical resection has revealed lung adenocarcinoma smaller than 4 mm (Fig. 7.1). Therefore, the notion that nodules less than 5 mm or 8 mm are benign is not justified, and there does not exist a size threshold between benign and malignant nodules.

7.1.2 Attenuation

A persistent GGN with homogenous texture or attenuation tends to be benign or at a benign process. With the development of a solid component, a homogenous pure GGN progresses into an inhomogeneous mixed part-solid lesion with increasing probability of malignancy. Researches have indicated that the absolute of average CT number of GGN (could) can be of value in discrimination between benign and malignant diseases: on follow-up CT scans, constantly increasing average attenuation over −600 HU favors malignancy, while a GGN with average attenuation below −600 HU is less likely to be malignant. Besides the average CT number, a recent quantitative study showed that the peak CT number (PEAK) in CT number histogram of ground-glass opacity in IAC was significantly higher than that in preinvasive lesions and −820.50 HU might be used as a threshold for differentiation between PIA and IAC [1]. In addition, the mean rate of PEAK change of IAC was smaller than that of preinvasive lesions with a threshold of −0.829 HU per day. Correlation has been found between average CT number and nodule size, every 100 HU increment in attenuation corresponding to 10% increase in nodule volume.

To be noted, nodule attenuation and size measurements are subject to various factors, including scanning protocols (kVp, mAs, slice thickness, reconstruction algorithm, etc.), respiration status (free breathing or breathholding), and even patient position (prone or supine). Ferretti et al. presented a case report on the effect of lung volume and gravity on the attenuation and size of a pure ground-glass nodule [2]. A GGN manifested as a 4.7 mm part-solid opacity with attenuation of 27 HU in the supine position and as a 7.8 mm pure ground-glass opacity with attenuation of −406 HU in the prone position. Thus, for accurate measurement and follow-up, reproducibility and consistency should be emphasized on GGN imaging examination: consistency on scanning parameters, consistency on reconstruction algorithm, consistency on ROI setting, and consistency on measurement levels. Some reports indicated that mass measurements could reflect the growth of GGNs earlier and were subject to less variability than were volume or diameter measurements [3].

7.1.3 Internal Imaging Features

Various nodular features can be seen on CT scans, some of which raise the possibility of malignancy, including foci of higher attenuation, CTA-TA sign, air-bronchogram and air-bubble sign, and honeycomb-like change. In particular, if abovementioned signs coexist with typical margin changes, such as lobulation, spiculation, or prominence, MIA should be highly suspected.

Generally, contrast CT scanning facilitates the assessment of suspected nodules. However, for most of pGGNs ≤5 mm, contrast medium administration may fail to provide additional information compared to nonenhancement CT scans due to lack of efficient blood circulation (avascular stage). If GGNs continue developing, adequate blood flow directed to lesions is required for sustainable nutrition supply. Hence, in part-solid and solid nodules of 5–10 mm, direct vascular branches from adjacent pre-existing vessels are commonly seen migrating into nodules, a transformation from avascular stage to vascular stage. In these cases, standard contrast CT scanning is useful for evaluation of solid component, tumor vasculatures, and location relationship between nodules and surrounding vessels. And image post-processing techniques, such as MIP, MPR, and CPR, are of use for better visualization, especially of the CTA-TA sign (Figs. 7.2, 7.3, and 7.4). From our viewpoint and clinical experiences, in cases of nodules larger than 5 mm with adequate suspicion of malignancy, contrast scanning is a mandatory instead of an elective procedure, unless contraindications exist.

With development of advanced imaging acquisition and reconstruction techniques, more sophisticated contrast procedures have been utilized to facilitate lesion

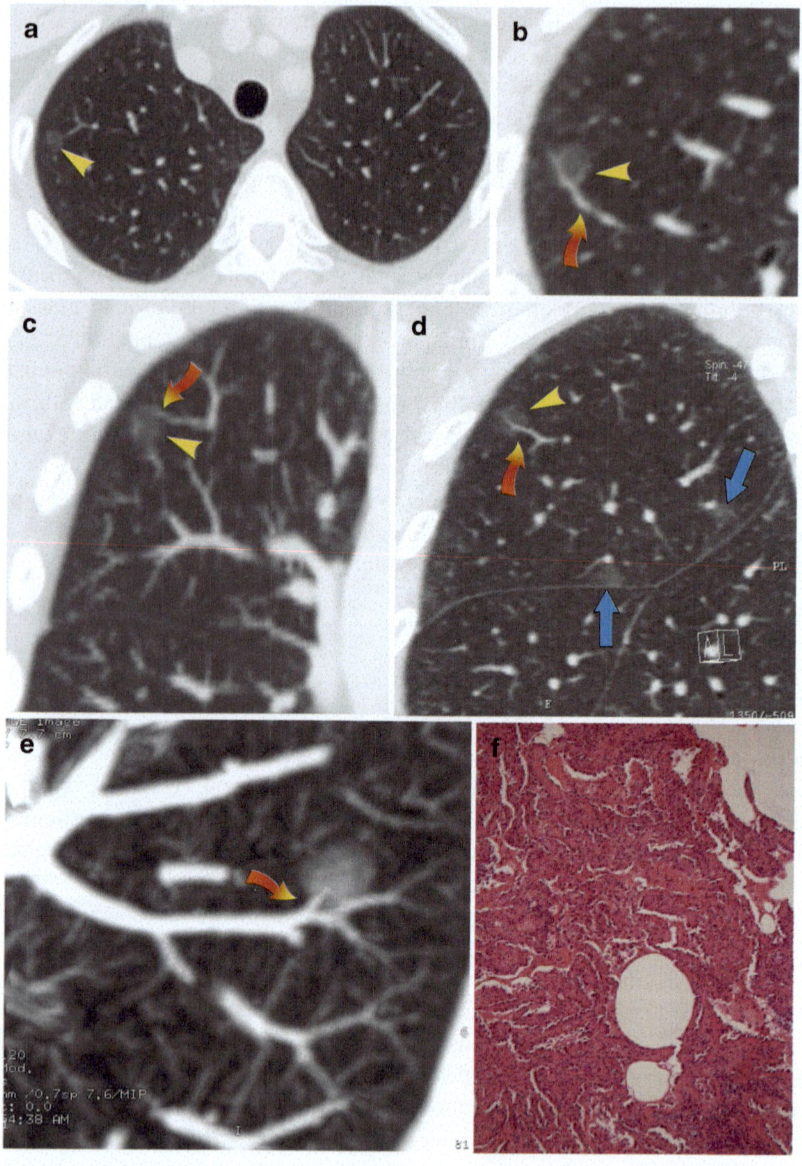

Fig. 7.2 Differential diagnosis of AAH, AIS, and MIA. (**a–d**) In a 40-year-old female, a 7 mm in diameter GGN (arrowhead) is found in the anterior segment of the right upper lobe on axial images. MIP (**c**) and MPR (**d**) images reveal $\leq$2 mm in diameter microvessels into the nodule which is hardly enhanced with contrast medium, indicative of AIS with surgical pathological confirmation. In the same patient, two additional GGNs of about 5 mm in diameter (blue arrow) are found adjacent to major and minor fissures, respectively (**d**). Both nodules without microvessels are resected simultaneously with the AIS nodule and proven to be AAH by surgical pathology. (**e**, **f**) In a 58-year-old male, a 9 mm in diameter GGN is seen in the left lower lobe with typical CTA-TA sign, $\geq$2 mm microvessels migrating into and distributing within the lesion with significant enhancement on contrast images, indicative of MIA with surgical pathological confirmation. (**f**) Microscopically, irregular glandular formation and interstitial fibrosis are observed within the minimally invasive zone with tumor cells growing in a lepidic pattern (H&E stain, 100 × magnification)

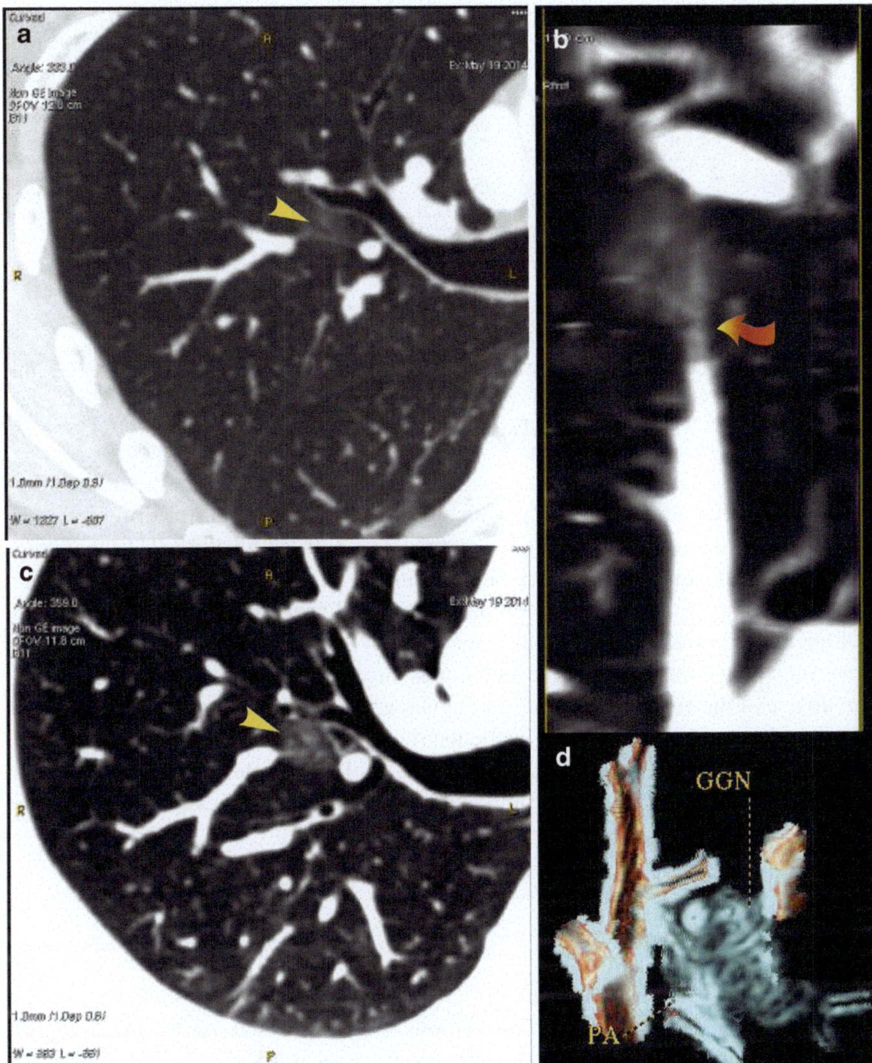

Fig. 7.3 CTA-TA sign in MIA: Contrast-enhanced CT imaging. (**a**) In a 40-year-old otherwise healthy female, conventional CT imaging reveals a GGN with undefined margin. (**b**) With administration of contrast medium, the nodule is significantly enhanced with evident solid component visualized within. (**c**) Typical CTA-TA sign (arrow) is readily observed on CPR views. (**d**) VR imaging shows the nodule is surrounded by microvessels and bronchioles. Based on the imaging feature, MIA is strongly suspected and confirmed by surgical pathology

evaluation. Among them, perfusion study and dual-energy CT-based iodine mapping have shown promising results in a differential diagnosis. Son et al. [4] reported their quantitative CT analysis of pulmonary ground-glass opacity nodules using iodine mapping with the findings that besides common predictors (i.e., mass, uniformity, etc.) of invasive adenocarcinoma, adding the iodine-enhanced imaging parameters improved the diagnostic accuracy from AIS or MIA. CT perfusion

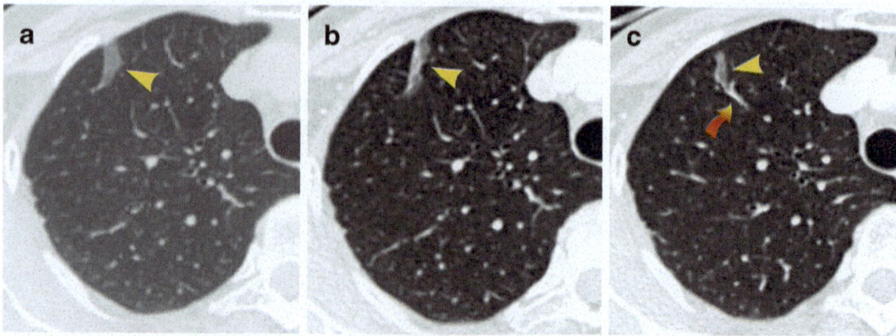

Fig. 7.4 CTA-TA sign in MIA. In a 62-year-old female, a 7 mm GGN (arrowhead) is seen in the right upper lobe on conventional CT images (**a**). On contrast-enhanced images (**b**, **c**), CTA-TA sign is better recognized with enhanced microvessels (arrow) migrating into the nodule (**c**). The surgical pathology confirms the imaging diagnosis of MIA

imaging has been suggested as a promising and feasible method for differentiation of solitary pulmonary nodules [5]. Using first-pass perfusion volume CT technique, Shu et al. found quantitative perfusion parameters closely correlated with tumor angiogenesis and expression of vascular endothelial growth factor (VEGF), typical biological features distinguishing malignancy from nonmalignant diseases. However, some concerns on these techniques have been raised, especially the radiation dose and the risk of secondary malignancy. Undoubtedly, with more advanced imaging procedures performed, patients receive additional radiation exposure, which further emphasizes the importance of following the basic principles of ALARA, AHARA, and ASARA in the practice of radiological examination.

7.1.4 Margins

The margin of part-solid or solid nodules may have some specific features indicative of malignancy, including short spiculation, lobulation, and prominence. In the meanwhile, certain findings in adjacent structures surrounding nodules may have the same indication, such as CTA-TA signs and pleural indentation. The majority of benign nodules lack lobulation but may present irregular margin due to traction from chronic reactive fibrotic tissues, distinct from short spiculation in malignant lesions. The margin of malignant GGNs is commonly clear due to tumor cell invasion, but it tends to be ill-defined in inflammatory GGNs due to edema and infiltration of inflammatory cells.

The incidence of spiculation may be less common in part-solid GGNs than in solid nodules. However, once cluster of spiculation (multiple, nonbranching, length < 2 mm, irradiating linear opacity) is found, the probability of malignancy dramatically increases up to 90%, predominated by adenocarcinoma. The pathological findings corresponding to malignant spiculation are summarized into three components: (1) directional invasion of tumor cells, (2) reactive hyperplasia of connective tissues and fibrosis, and (3) vasculitis, lymphangitis, and bronchiolitis resulting from tumor cell invasion and/or congestion.

All of abovementioned features are not limited in lung adenocarcinoma but shared by other malignancies, including squamous cell carcinoma, small cell lung cancer, and large cell lung cancer. Every single feature is nonspecific in discrimination between malignancy and nonmalignant diseases. More features present, more likely the lesion to be malignant. Some automated algorithms, such as computerized texture analysis, have been developed to integrate as many features as possible in nodule evaluation with an aim to further improve diagnostic accuracy by reducing interobserver and intraobserver variability [6].

7.2 CT Findings, Pathological Correlation, and Differential Diagnosis of Minimally Invasive Adenocarcinoma

The WHO defines MIA of the lung as a small, solitary adenocarcinoma, (≤3 cm), with a predominantly lepidic pattern and 5 mm or less invasion. The invasive component to be measured in MIA is defined as follows: (1) histologic subtypes other than a lepidic pattern (i.e., acinar, papillary, micropapillary, and/or solid) or (2) tumor cells infiltrating myofibroblastic stroma [7]. In a pGGN suspected of AIS, the presence of solid/invasive component (≤5 mm) indicates the disease progression into MIA, while if the invasive component is larger than 5 mm, the lesion should be classified as lepidic-predominant adenocarcinoma (LPA) instead of MIA.

The progression from pGGN-predominant AIS to part-solid GGN-predominant MIA involves numerous intrinsic and extrinsic factors. The former includes activation of specific genes, regulation of signaling pathways, and overexpression of biological factors, such as EGF and VEGF, which provide momentum for disease progression from molecular levels. In contrast, the latter is related to the interaction between tumors and the host or the microenvironment where the tumor resides. One of the most interactions is the construction of blood circulation in tumors, a process known as neoangiogenesis, which has been described in detail in Chap. 5. The characteristic CTA-TA sign is the result of tumor neoangiogenesis. CTA-TA sign can be seen in both AIS and MIA lesions. The difference is that neovasculature in AIS is much more immature and primitive than in MIA, so microvessels of CTA-TA sign in AIS are much smaller and finer (less than 2 mm in diameter) than in MIA on CT imaging.

By definition, the solid component in MIA is less than 5 mm, which may not be readily recognized on nonenhancement CT scan in some cases. In these scenarios, contrast CT has particular diagnostic value on displaying CTA-TA sign and nodule enhancement (Fig. 7.5). An increment of 30 HU on average attenuation of nodules between nonenhanced and enhanced imaging is regarded as a vital sign for malignancy. Therefore, for discrimination between MIA and benign nodules, contrast CT is warranted if no contraindication for intravenous contrast medium exists.

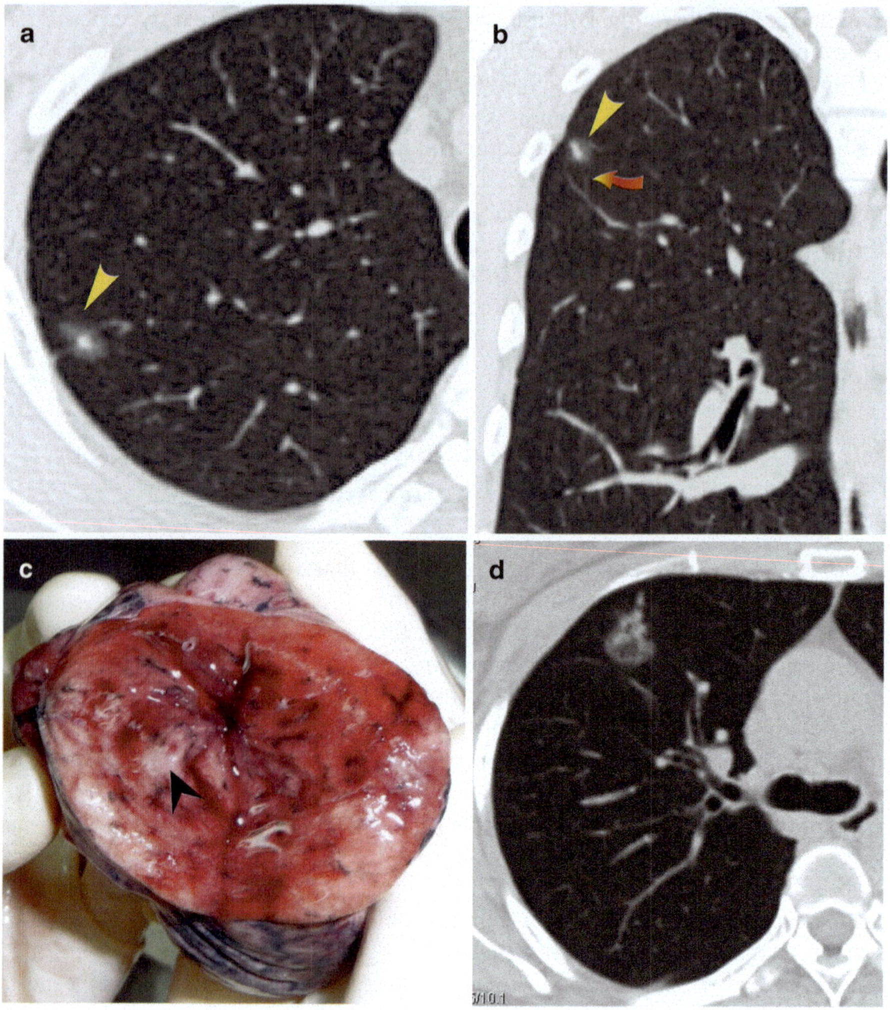

Fig. 7.5 The radiological-pathological correlation in MIA. (**a–c**) In a 38-year-old male, a 10 mm GGN with solid invasive component of ≤5 mm in diameter is seen in right upper lobe (**a**). (**b**) Coronal views show that microvessels (arrow) migrate into nodular lesion (arrowhead), indicative of MIA. (**c**) A whitish nodular lesion (arrowhead) seen in the surgical specimen is proven to be MIA. (**d**) In another MIA case, multiple enhanced microvessels of ≥2 mm in diameter are observed within the lesion, which is one of the imaging features for diagnostic differentiation of MIA and AIS

Pathologically, most MIA is nonmucinous, and mucinous MIA is rare. In the former, differentiated type II pneumocytes and/or Clara cells proliferate in a lepidic pattern along alveolar wall resulting in multiple layers of hyperplastic cells, and in certain part of alveolar wall, proliferating cells invade stromal tissues and generate foci of solid invasive components, producing the typical part-solid/

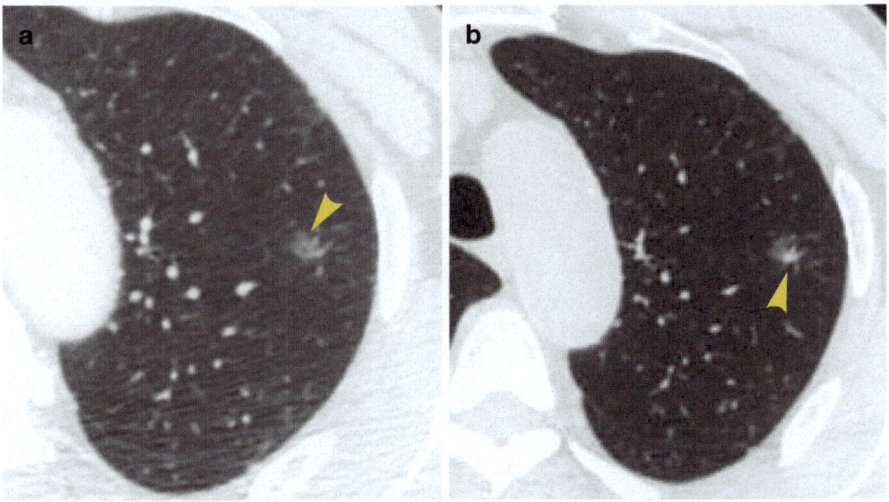

Fig. 7.6 CT findings of MIA. (**a**) An 8 mm GGN (arrowhead) with undefined margin and insignificant solid component is seen in chest CT. The lesion is suspicious of AIS, and routine follow-up is required. (**b**) At 1-year follow-up, ≤5 mm solid component occurred within the lesion, suggestive of disease progression to MIA. Surgical resection is performed, and MIA is pathologically confirmed

mixed ground-glass opacities on CT scans. In the latter, there are an increasing amount of columnar cells with abundant apical mucin and small, often basally oriented nuclei and may show a goblet cell morphologic pattern. Nonmucinous MIA resembles type C adenocarcinoma in Noguchi classification [8]. On CT scan, in addition to internal solid component and CTA-TA signs, spiculation can be seen along the margin of MIA, but no pleural invasion (pleural indentation sign) is observed. The alveolar structures remain intact. Air-bubble and air-bronchogram signs are more likely to be present in part-solid GGNs than in solid nodules. The majority of MIA lesions do not respond to antimicrobial treatment and even grow bigger during the treatment (Fig. 7.6). In a small portion of MIA cases, a temporary size regression may be observed with administration of antibiotics, indicating coexisting of tumors and inflammation. It has been reported that solid components in part-solid GGNs have prognostic value, more solid components, more advanced the disease, higher postoperative recurrence and poorer prognosis.

Air-bubble sign and air-bronchogram sign in ground-glass area of MIA are of diagnostic value. Based on the radiologic-pathological correlation study, air-bubble and air-bronchogram signs can be attributed to (1) air-filled alveolar cavity unoccupied by tumor cells, (2) dilated bronchioles, and (3) alveolar convergence or dilated alveolar cavity (Fig. 7.7). Both signs are distinct from traditional tumor cavitation which mainly results from the excretion of tumor necrotic tissues, commonly seen in tuberculosis, fungal infection, and granulomas (Figs. 7.8 and 7.9).

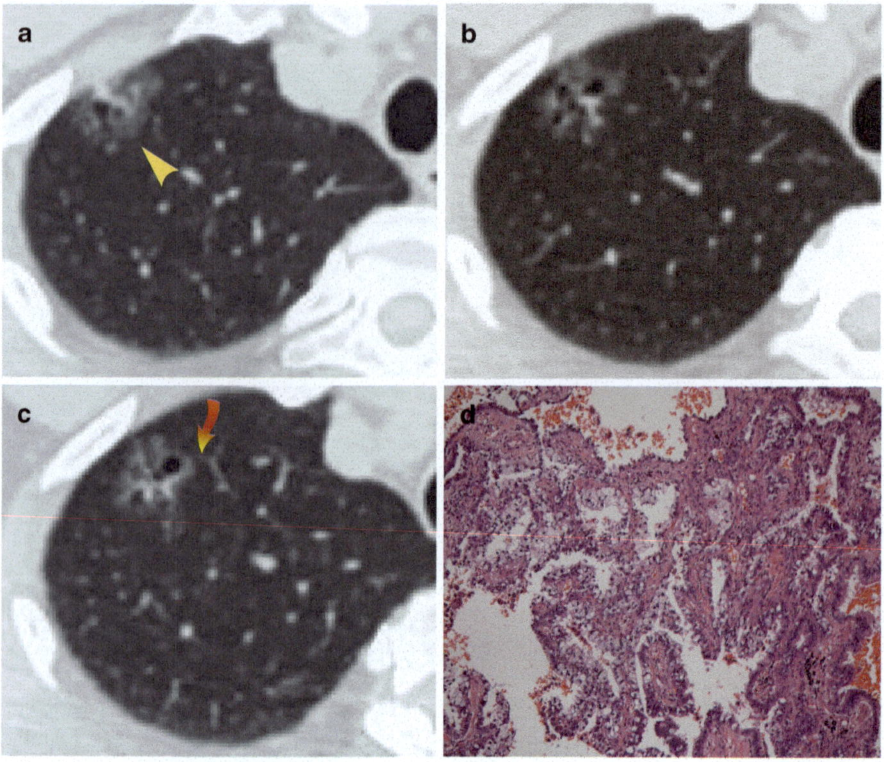

Fig. 7.7 The radiological-pathological correlation in nonmucinous MIA. (**a**) In a 54-year-old male, an approximate 15 mm part-solid GGN (arrowhead) is found in the apical segment of the right upper lobe. (**b**) Multiple air bubbles of less than 5 mm in diameter and air-bronchogram sign are seen within the lesion. (**c**) CTA-TA sign (arrow). (**d**) Surgical pathology confirms a 15 × 7 mm nonmucinous MIA with irregular glandular invasion with AIS seen at the periphery of the lesion (H&E stain, 100 × magnification)

The size of air bubbles can be from 5 mm to several centimeters. Large air bubble is also called pseudocavitation or bubble-like lucencies. For discrimination between pseudocavitation and true cavitation, several imaging features should be scrutinized, including location, size, shape, internal and external walls, enhancement, content, draining bronchi or bronchioles, halo sign, and changes in adjacent tissues or structures.

Most AIS and MIA are nonmucinous, rarely are they mucinous. Patients with both diseases would have a 100% or near-100% disease-free survival, respectively, if these lesions were completely resected [9]. Since with a growing number of published cases no clear recurrences have been reported in patients with AIS and MIA thus far, adjuvant chemotherapy or radiotherapy is not necessarily required [7]. Thus, accurate diagnosis and prompt medical intervention of preinvasive and minimally invasive lesions can significantly improve the overall outcome of lung cancer. According to the seventh TNM

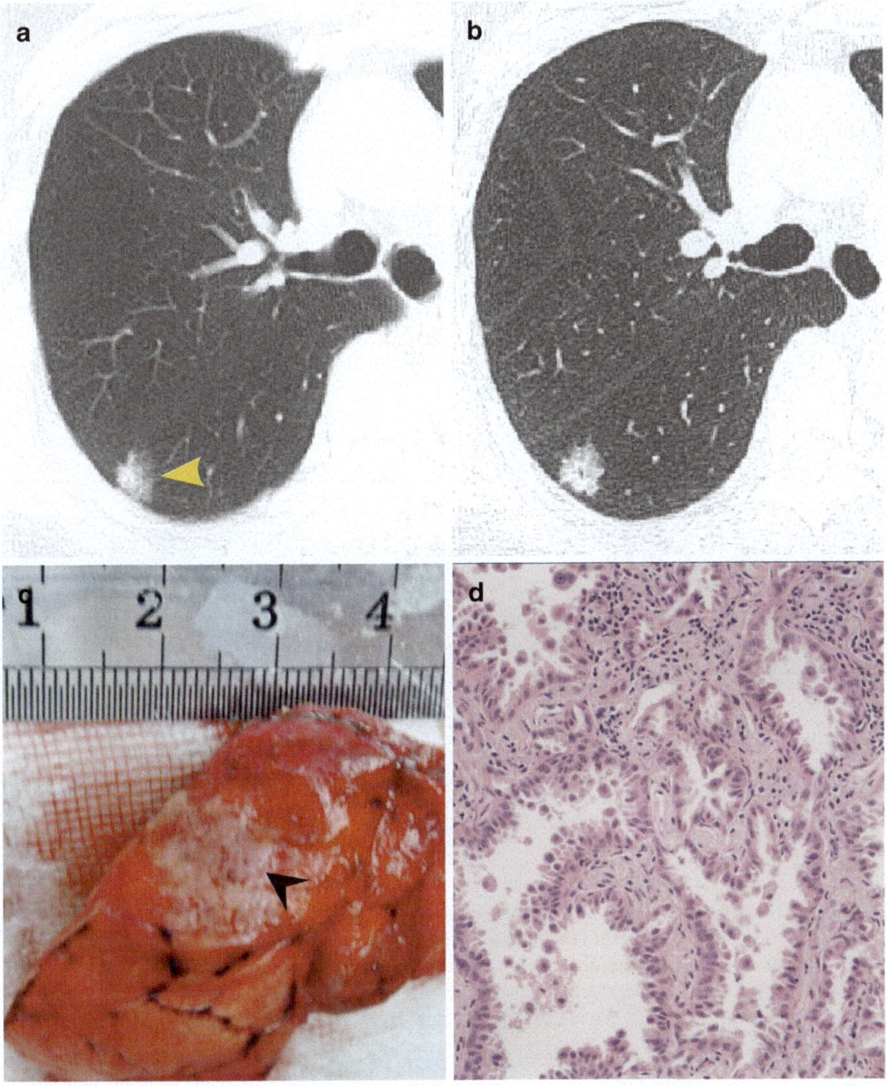

Fig. 7.8 The radiological-pathological correlation in MIA. (**a**) A subpleural semi-solid GGN (arrowhead) of 12 mm in diameter is seen in the superior segment of right lower lobe. Solid component within this lesion is less than 5 mm. (**b**) In the consecutive image, signs of air bubble, spiculation, and lobulation are observed. (**c**) The surgical specimen. (**d**) Pathological examination shows that tumor cells infiltrate within pulmonary interstitium, consistent with MIA

staging, the 5-year overall survival for IA, IB, IIA, IIB, III, and IV is 73%, 58%, 46%, 36%, 20%, and 13%, respectively. In contrast, stage 0 disease (TisN0M0) has a 5-year survival of 100%. Again, early detection, early diagnosis, and early intervention are vital for the reduction of mortality from lung cancer (Fig. 7.10).

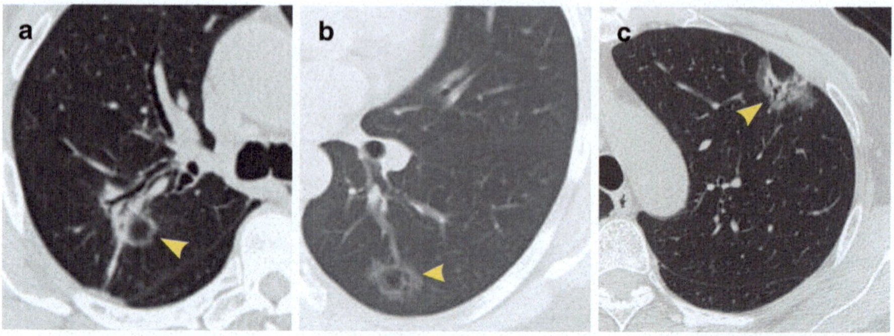

Fig. 7.9 Pseudocavitation, air-bubble sign, and air-bronchogram sign in lung adenocarcinoma. (**a**) In the right upper lobe, an adenocarcinoma (arrowhead) is seen with typical pseudocavitation manifesting as a lesion with central lucency due to tumor cells growing in a circular pattern. (**b**) Pseudocavitation is observed in a lung cancer located in left lower lobe (arrowhead). (**c**) Signs of air bubble and air bronchogram are seen in MIA (arrowhead)

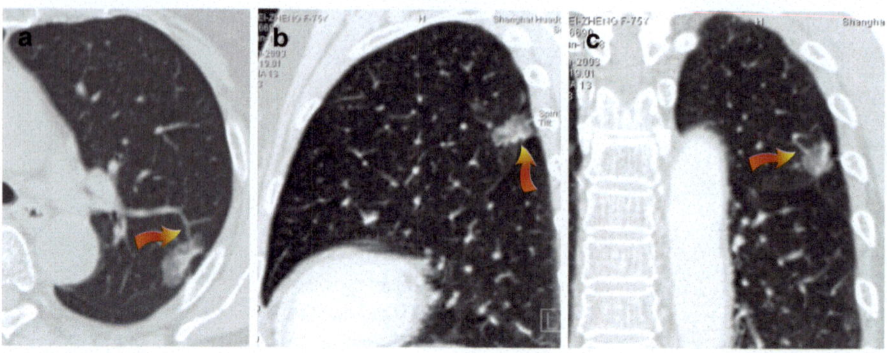

Fig. 7.10 CTA-TA sign in MIA. (**a**) In a 70-year-old male, a mixed GGN with defined margin is seen in the left upper lobe. A 2 mm in diameter vessel migrates into the lesion. (**b**) With administration of contrast medium, the nodule is significantly enhanced, and microvessels (arrow) are visualized within the lesion on the sagittal view. (**c**) Supplying tumor vessels (arrow) can be seen in coronal images

Based on thousands of micronodular lung cancer cases over the past decade, we have proposed an "EAST" principle for the management of MLCs with the goal of detecting and eradicating lung cancer at stage 0/I:

- Early detection of subcentimeter nodules
- Accurate diagnosis of lung cancers in stages 0/I
- Surgical removal of MLCs promptly
- Teamwork for preoperative localization of nodules and postoperative collaboration on pathological assessment

Hasegawa et al. investigated volume-doubling time (VDT) of 61 small lung cancers (<20 mm in diameter) using high-resolution CT [10]. They found that the mean

VDT values for pGGN, mGGN, and solid nodule were 813 days, 457 days, and 149 days, respectively. This study, coupled with some other researches, supports that pGGNs have inert biological behavior, and with solid portion increasing, diseases gradually progress and minimal invasiveness occurs. Therefore, detection and diagnosis at as early stage as possible are of clinical significance.

References

1. Peng M, Li Z, Hu H, Liu S, Xu B, Zhu W, Han Y, Xiong L, Lin Q. Pulmonary ground-glass nodules diagnosis: mean change rate of peak CT number as a discriminative factor of pathology during a follow-up. Br J Radiol. 2016;89(1058):20150556. https://doi.org/10.1259/bjr.20150556.
2. Ferretti GR, Arbib F, Roux JF, Bland V, Lantuejoul S. Effect of lung volume and gravity on the attenuation and size of a pure ground-glass nodule. J Thorac Imaging. 2012;27(1):W15–7. https://doi.org/10.1097/RTI.0b013e31820c7929.
3. de Hoop B, Gietema H, van de Vorst S, Murphy K, van Klaveren RJ, Prokop M. Pulmonary ground-glass nodules: increase in mass as an early indicator of growth. Radiology. 2010;255(1):199–206. https://doi.org/10.1148/radiol.09090571.
4. Son JY, Lee HY, Kim JH, Han J, Jeong JY, Lee KS, Kwon OJ, Shim YM. Quantitative CT analysis of pulmonary ground-glass opacity nodules for distinguishing invasive adenocarcinoma from non-invasive or minimally invasive adenocarcinoma: the added value of using iodine mapping. Eur Radiol. 2016;26(1):43–54. https://doi.org/10.1007/s00330-015-3816-y.
5. Shu SJ, Liu BL, Jiang HJ. Optimization of the scanning technique and diagnosis of pulmonary nodules with first-pass 64-detector-row perfusion VCT. Clin Imaging. 2013;37(2):256–64. https://doi.org/10.1016/j.clinimag.2012.05.004.
6. Chae HD, Park CM, Park SJ, Lee SM, Kim KG, Goo JM. Computerized texture analysis of persistent part-solid ground-glass nodules: differentiation of preinvasive lesions from invasive pulmonary adenocarcinomas. Radiology. 2014;273(1):285–93. https://doi.org/10.1148/radiol.14132187.
7. Travis WD, Asamura H, Bankier AA, Beasley MB, Detterbeck F, Flieder DB, Goo JM, MacMahon H, Naidich D, Nicholson AG, Powell CA, Prokop M, Rami-Porta R, Rusch V, van Schil P, Yatabe Y. The IASLC lung cancer staging project: proposals for coding T categories for subsolid nodules and assessment of tumor size in part-solid tumors in the forthcoming eighth edition of the TNM classification of lung cancer. J Thorac Oncol. 2016;11(8):1204–23. https://doi.org/10.1016/j.jtho.2016.03.025.
8. Noguchi M, Morikawa A, Kawasaki M, Matsuno Y, Yamada T, Hirohashi S, Kondo H, Shimosato Y. Small adenocarcinoma of the lung. Histologic characteristics and prognosis. Cancer. 1995;75(12):2844–52.
9. Travis WD, Brambilla E, Noguchi M, Nicholson AG, Geisinger KR, Yatabe Y, Beer DG, Powell CA, Riely GJ, Van Schil PE, Garg K, Austin JH, Asamura H, Rusch VW, Hirsch FR, Scagliotti G, Mitsudomi T, Huber RM, Ishikawa Y, Jett J, Sanchez-Cespedes M, Sculier JP, Takahashi T, Tsuboi M, Vansteenkiste J, Wistuba I, Yang PC, Aberle D, Brambilla C, Flieder D, Franklin W, Gazdar A, Gould M, Hasleton P, Henderson D, Johnson B, Johnson D, Kerr K, Kuriyama K, Lee JS, Miller VA, Petersen I, Roggli V, Rosell R, Saijo N, Thunnissen E, Tsao M, Yankelewitz D. International association for the study of lung cancer/american thoracic society/european respiratory society international multidisciplinary classification of lung adenocarcinoma. J Thorac Oncol. 2011;6(2):244–85. https://doi.org/10.1097/JTO.0b013e318206a221.
10. Hasegawa M, Sone S, Takashima S, Li F, Yang ZG, Maruyama Y, Watanabe T. Growth rate of small lung cancers detected on mass CT screening. Br J Radiol. 2000;73(876):1252–9. https://doi.org/10.1259/bjr.73.876.11205667.

Suggested Readings

1. Abe H, MacMahon H, Engelmann R, Li Q, Shiraishi J, Katsuragawa S, Aoyama M, Ishida T, Ashizawa K, Metz CE, Doi K. Computer-aided diagnosis in chest radiography: results of large-scale observer tests at the 1996-2001 RSNA scientific assemblies. Radiographics. 2003;23(1):255–65. https://doi.org/10.1148/rg.231025129.
2. Ahn SY, Park CM, Jeon YK, Kim H, Lee JH, Hwang EJ, Goo JM. Predictive CT features of visceral pleural invasion by T1-sized peripheral pulmonary adenocarcinomas manifesting as subsolid nodules. AJR Am J Roentgenol. 2017;209(3):561–6. https://doi.org/10.2214/ajr.16.17280.
3. Asamura H, Suzuki K, Watanabe S, Matsuno Y, Maeshima A, Tsuchiya R. A clinicopathological study of resected subcentimeter lung cancers: a favorable prognosis for ground glass opacity lesions. Ann Thorac Surg. 2003;76(4):1016–22.
4. Benzakoun J, Bommart S, Coste J, Chassagnon G, Lederlin M, Boussouar S, Revel MP. Computer-aided diagnosis (CAD) of subsolid nodules: evaluation of a commercial CAD system. Eur J Radiol. 2016;85(10):1728–34. https://doi.org/10.1016/j.ejrad.2016.07.011.
5. Cha MJ, Lee KS, Kim HS, Lee SW, Jeong CJ, Kim EY, Lee HY. Improvement in imaging diagnosis technique and modalities for solitary pulmonary nodules: from ground-glass opacity nodules to part-solid and solid nodules. Expert Rev Respir Med. 2016;10(3):261–78. https://doi.org/10.1586/17476348.2016.1141053.
6. Cho J, Kim ES, Kim SJ, Lee YJ, Park JS, Cho YJ, Yoon HI, Lee JH, Lee CT. Long-term follow-up of small pulmonary ground-glass nodules stable for 3 years: implications of the proper follow-up period and risk factors for subsequent growth. J Thorac Oncol. 2016;11(9):1453–9. https://doi.org/10.1016/j.jtho.2016.05.026.
7. Cohen JG, Reymond E, Lederlin M, Medici M, Lantuejoul S, Laurent F, Arbib F, Jankowski A, Moreau-Gaudry A, Ferretti GR. Differentiating pre- and minimally invasive from invasive adenocarcinoma using CT-features in persistent pulmonary part-solid nodules in Caucasian patients. Eur J Radiol. 2015;84(4):738–44. https://doi.org/10.1016/j.ejrad.2014.12.031.
8. Fukui M, Suzuki K, Matsunaga T, Oh S, Takamochi K. Surgical intervention for ground glass dominant lesions: observation or outright resection? Jpn J Clin Oncol. 2017;47(8):749–54. https://doi.org/10.1093/jjco/hyx053.
9. Gaeta M, Barone M, Russi EG, Volta S, Casablanca G, Romeo P, La Spada F, Minutoli A. Carcinomatous solitary pulmonary nodules: evaluation of the tumor-bronchi relationship with thin-section CT. Radiology. 1993;187(2):535–9. https://doi.org/10.1148/radiology.187.2.8475303.
10. Godoy MC, Sabloff B, Naidich DP. Subsolid pulmonary nodules: imaging evaluation and strategic management. Curr Opin Pulm Med. 2012;18(4):304–12. https://doi.org/10.1097/MCP.0b013e328354a5f2.
11. Hattori A, Matsunaga T, Hayashi T, Takamochi K, Oh S, Suzuki K. Prognostic impact of the findings on thin-section computed tomography in patients with subcentimeter non-small cell lung cancer. J Thorac Oncol. 2017a;12(6):954–62. https://doi.org/10.1016/j.jtho.2017.02.015.
12. Hattori A, Matsunaga T, Takamochi K, Oh S, Suzuki K. Neither maximum tumor size nor solid component size is prognostic in part-solid lung cancer: impact of tumor size should be applied exclusively to solid lung cancer. Ann Thorac Surg. 2016a;102(2):407–15. https://doi.org/10.1016/j.athoracsur.2016.02.074.
13. Hattori A, Matsunaga T, Takamochi K, Oh S, Suzuki K. Oncological characteristics of radiological invasive adenocarcinoma with additional ground-glass nodules on initial thin-section computed tomography: comparison with solitary invasive adenocarcinoma. J Thorac Oncol. 2016b;11(5):729–36. https://doi.org/10.1016/j.jtho.2016.01.008.
14. Hattori A, Matsunaga T, Takamochi K, Oh S, Suzuki K. Importance of ground glass opacity component in clinical stage IA radiologic invasive lung cancer. Ann Thorac Surg. 2017b;104(1):313–20. https://doi.org/10.1016/j.athoracsur.2017.01.076.

15. Hattori A, Suzuki K, Matsunaga T, Fukui M, Tsushima Y, Takamochi K, Oh S. Tumour standardized uptake value on positron emission tomography is a novel predictor of adenocarcinoma in situ for c-Stage IA lung cancer patients with a part-solid nodule on thin-section computed tomography scan. Interact Cardiovasc Thorac Surg. 2014a;18(3):329–34. https://doi.org/10.1093/icvts/ivt500.
16. Hattori A, Suzuki K, Matsunaga T, Takamochi K, Oh S. Visceral pleural invasion is not a significant prognostic factor in patients with a part-solid lung cancer. Ann Thorac Surg. 2014b;98(2):433–8. https://doi.org/10.1016/j.athoracsur.2014.04.084.
17. Henschke CI, Yankelevitz DF, Mirtcheva R, McGuinness G, McCauley D, Miettinen OS. CT screening for lung cancer: frequency and significance of part-solid and nonsolid nodules. AJR Am J Roentgenol. 2002;178(5):1053–7. https://doi.org/10.2214/ajr.178.5.1781053.
18. Henschke CI, Yip R, Smith JP, Wolf AS, Flores RM, Liang M, Salvatore MM, Liu Y, Xu DM, Yankelevitz DF. CT screening for lung cancer: part-solid nodules in baseline and annual repeat rounds. AJR Am J Roentgenol. 2016;207(6):1176–84. https://doi.org/10.2214/ajr.16.16043.
19. Hiramatsu M, Inagaki T, Inagaki T, Matsui Y, Satoh Y, Okumura S, Ishikawa Y, Miyaoka E, Nakagawa K. Pulmonary ground-glass opacity (GGO) lesions-large size and a history of lung cancer are risk factors for growth. J Thorac Oncol. 2008;3(11):1245–50. https://doi.org/10.1097/JTO.0b013e318189f526.
20. Hwang EJ, Park CM, Kim YT, Kim H, Goo JM. Microscopic invasions, prognoses, and recurrence patterns of stage I adenocarcinomas manifesting as part-solid ground-glass nodules: comparison with adenocarcinomas appearing as solid nodules after matching their solid parts' size. Medicine. 2016;95(15):e3419. https://doi.org/10.1097/md.0000000000003419.
21. Hwang EJ, Park CM, Ryu Y, Lee SM, Kim YT, Kim YW, Goo JM. Pulmonary adenocarcinomas appearing as part-solid ground-glass nodules: is measuring solid component size a better prognostic indicator? Eur Radiol. 2015;25(2):558–67. https://doi.org/10.1007/s00330-014-3441-1.
22. Kakinuma R, Noguchi M, Ashizawa K, Kuriyama K, Maeshima AM, Koizumi N, Kondo T, Matsuguma H, Nitta N, Ohmatsu H, Okami J, Suehisa H, Yamaji T, Kodama K, Mori K, Yamada K, Matsuno Y, Murayama S, Murata K. Natural history of pulmonary subsolid nodules: a prospective multicenter study. J Thorac Oncol. 2016;11(7):1012–28. https://doi.org/10.1016/j.jtho.2016.04.006.
23. Kaneda H, Nakano T, Taniguchi Y, Saito T, Konobu T, Saito Y. A decrease in the size of ground glass nodules may indicate the optimal timing for curative surgery. Lung Cancer. 2014;85(2):213–7. https://doi.org/10.1016/j.lungcan.2014.05.015.
24. Kim H, Park CM, Koh JM, Lee SM, Goo JM. Pulmonary subsolid nodules: what radiologists need to know about the imaging features and management strategy. Diagn Interv Radiol. 2014;20(1):47–57. https://doi.org/10.5152/dir.2013.13223.
25. Kim H, Park CM, Woo S, Lee SM, Lee HJ, Yoo CG, Goo JM. Pure and part-solid pulmonary ground-glass nodules: measurement variability of volume and mass in nodules with a solid portion less than or equal to 5 mm. Radiology. 2013;269(2):585–93. https://doi.org/10.1148/radiol.13121849.
26. Ko JP, Naidich DP. Current readings: radiologic interpretation of the part-solid nodule: clinical relevance and novel technologies. Semin Thorac Cardiovasc Surg. 2014;26(2):145–56. https://doi.org/10.1053/j.semtcvs.2014.07.001.
27. Lee HJ, Ahn MI, Kim YK, Seon HJ, Goo JM, Im JG, Park CS. Notes from the 2010 annual meeting of the Korean Society of Thoracic Radiology: pure ground-glass nodules, part-solid nodules and lung adenocarcinomas. J Thorac Imaging. 2011;26(3):W99–104. https://doi.org/10.1097/RTI.0b013e318219d910.
28. Lee HY, Lee KS. Ground-glass opacity nodules: histopathology, imaging evaluation, and clinical implications. J Thorac Imaging. 2011;26(2):106–18. https://doi.org/10.1097/RTI.0b013e3181fbaa64.
29. Lee JH, Park CM, Lee SM, Kim H, McAdams HP, Goo JM. Persistent pulmonary subsolid nodules with solid portions of 5 mm or smaller: their natural course and predictors of interval growth. Eur Radiol. 2016;26(6):1529–37. https://doi.org/10.1007/s00330-015-4017-4.

30. Lee SM, Goo JM, Lee KH, Chung DH, Koh J, Park CM. CT findings of minimally invasive adenocarcinoma (MIA) of the lung and comparison of solid portion measurement methods at CT in 52 patients. Eur Radiol. 2015;25(8):2318–25. https://doi.org/10.1007/s00330-015-3616-4.
31. Lee SM, Park CM, Goo JM, Lee HJ, Wi JY, Kang CH. Invasive pulmonary adenocarcinomas versus preinvasive lesions appearing as ground-glass nodules: differentiation by using CT features. Radiology. 2013;268(1):265–73. https://doi.org/10.1148/radiol.13120949.
32. Lee SM, Park CM, Song YS, Kim H, Kim YT, Park YS, Goo JM. CT assessment-based direct surgical resection of part-solid nodules with solid component larger than 5 mm without preoperative biopsy: experience at a single tertiary hospital. Eur Radiol. 2017;27(12):5119–26. https://doi.org/10.1007/s00330-017-4917-6.
33. Liao JH, Amin VB, Kadoch MA, Beasley MB, Jacobi AH. Subsolid pulmonary nodules: CT-pathologic correlation using the 2011 IASLC/ATS/ERS classification. Clin Imaging. 2015;39(3):344–51. https://doi.org/10.1016/j.clinimag.2014.12.009.
34. Matsunaga T, Suzuki K, Takamochi K, Oh S. What is the radiological definition of part-solid tumour in lung cancer? dagger. Eur J Cardiothorac Surg. 2017;51(2):242–7. https://doi.org/10.1093/ejcts/ezw344.
35. Mets OM, de Jong PA, Scholten ET, Chung K, van Ginneken B, Schaefer-Prokop CM. Subsolid pulmonary nodule morphology and associated patient characteristics in a routine clinical population. Eur Radiol. 2017;27(2):689–96. https://doi.org/10.1007/s00330-016-4429-9.
36. Miyata N, Endo M, Nakajima T, Kojima H, Maniwa T, Takahashi S, Isaka M, Kameya T, Ohde Y. High-resolution computed tomography findings of early mucinous adenocarcinomas and their pathologic characteristics in 22 surgically resected cases. Eur J Radiol. 2015;84(5):993–7. https://doi.org/10.1016/j.ejrad.2015.01.014.
37. Mori K, Saitou Y, Tominaga K, Yokoi K, Miyazawa N, Okuyama A, Sasagawa M. Small nodular lesions in the lung periphery: new approach to diagnosis with CT. Radiology. 1990;177(3):843–9. https://doi.org/10.1148/radiology.177.3.2243999.
38. Mountain CF, Dresler CM. Regional lymph node classification for lung cancer staging. Chest. 1997;111(6):1718–23.
39. Murray JG, Breatnach E. The American Thoracic Society lymph node map: a CT demonstration. Eur J Radiol. 1993;17(2):61–8.
40. Park CM, Goo JM, Lee HJ, Lee CH, Chun EJ, Im JG. Nodular ground-glass opacity at thin-section CT: histologic correlation and evaluation of change at follow-up. Radiographics. 2007;27(2):391–408. https://doi.org/10.1148/rg.272065061.
41. Seidelman JL, Myers JL, Quint LE. Incidental, subsolid pulmonary nodules at CT: etiology and management. Cancer Imaging. 2013;13(3):365–73. https://doi.org/10.1102/1470-7330.2013.9025.
42. Shimizu K, Ohtaki Y, Nakazawa S, Mogi A, Kuwano H. Neither the maximum tumor size nor solid component size is prognostic in part-solid lung cancer: to be ground-glass opacity or not to be, is that really the question? J Thorac Dis. 2016;8(9):2334–6. https://doi.org/10.21037/jtd.2016.08.32.
43. Silva M, Sverzellati N, Manna C, Negrini G, Marchiano A, Zompatori M, Rossi C, Pastorino U. Long-term surveillance of ground-glass nodules: evidence from the MILD trial. J Thorac Oncol. 2012;7(10):1541–6. https://doi.org/10.1097/JTO.0b013e3182641bba.
44. Song YS, Park CM, Park SJ, Lee SM, Jeon YK, Goo JM. Volume and mass doubling times of persistent pulmonary subsolid nodules detected in patients without known malignancy. Radiology. 2014;273(1):276–84. https://doi.org/10.1148/radiol.14132324.
45. Swensen SJ, Aughenbaugh GL, Douglas WW, Myers JL. High-resolution CT of the lungs: findings in various pulmonary diseases. AJR Am J Roentgenol. 1992;158(5):971–9. https://doi.org/10.2214/ajr.158.5.1566699.
46. Swensen SJ, Viggiano RW, Midthun DE, Muller NL, Sherrick A, Yamashita K, Naidich DP, Patz EF, Hartman TE, Muhm JR, Weaver AL. Lung nodule enhancement at CT: multicenter study. Radiology. 2000;214(1):73–80. https://doi.org/10.1148/radiology.214.1.r00ja1473.

47. Yanagawa M, Johkoh T, Noguchi M, Morii E, Shintani Y, Okumura M, Hata A, Fujiwara M, Honda O, Tomiyama N. Radiological prediction of tumor invasiveness of lung adenocarcinoma on thin-section CT. Medicine. 2017;96(11):e6331. https://doi.org/10.1097/md.0000000000006331.
48. Yang W, Sun Y, Fang W, Qian F, Ye J, Chen Q, Jiang Y, Yu K, Han B. High-resolution computed tomography features distinguishing benign and malignant lesions manifesting as persistent solitary subsolid nodules. Clin Lung Cancer. 2017. https://doi.org/10.1016/j.cllc.2017.05.023.
49. Yip R, Henschke CI, Xu DM, Li K, Jirapatnakul A, Yankelevitz DF. Lung cancers manifesting as part-solid nodules in the National Lung Screening Trial. AJR Am J Roentgenol. 2017;208(5):1011–21. https://doi.org/10.2214/ajr.16.16930.
50. Zhao LL, Xie HK, Zhang LP, Zha JY, Zhou FY, Jiang GN, Chen C. Visceral pleural invasion in lung adenocarcinoma ≤3 cm with ground-glass opacity: a clinical, pathological and radiological study. J Thorac Dis. 2016;8(7):1788–97. https://doi.org/10.21037/jtd.2016.05.90.
51. Zhou QJ, Zheng ZC, Zhu YQ, Lu PJ, Huang J, Ye JD, Zhang J, Lu S, Luo QQ. Tumor invasiveness defined by IASLC/ATS/ERS classification of ground-glass nodules can be predicted by quantitative CT parameters. J Thorac Dis. 2017;9(5):1190–200. https://doi.org/10.21037/jtd.2017.03.170.

Chapter 8
Solid Pulmonary Nodules

Guozhen Zhang and Xiangpeng Zheng

8.1 CT Findings and Pathological Correlation of Solid Pulmonary Nodules

8.1.1 The Peripheral Imaging Features and Pathological Findings of SPNs

8.1.1.1 Shape

The shape of an SPN is a nonspecific imaging feature used in the differential diagnosis to distinguish between benign and malignant nodules. However, irregular polygonal or deeply lobulated formations, for example, might reflect the developmental heterogeneity of the disease. Lobulation is a sign that primarily results from the imbalanced growth of tumor cells in each direction, probably due to clonal diversity or a dysfunctional nutrition supply. In addition, barriers on the tumor-growing pathway such as preexisting fibrotic scars, vessels, or bronchioles can decelerate tumor cell proliferation in a particular direction, causing irregular indentation along the nodular margin. The lobulation sign frequently occurs in lesions with an expansive or bulking growth pattern.

Spiculation is another nonspecific imaging sign. However, spicules in malignant nodules tend to be multiple, short, fine, and rigid, without evident bifurcation. The underlying pathological correlation includes tumor cells infiltrating along bronchovascular bunches, the intratumoral fibrotic component retracting adjacent lobular septa, and connective tissue hyperplasia reactive to peripheral inflammation. Occasionally,

G. Zhang (✉)
Department of Radiology, Fudan University Huadong Hospital, Shanghai, China
e-mail: cjr.zhangguozhen@vip.163.com

X. Zheng
Department of Radiation Oncology, Fudan University Huadong Hospital, Shanghai, China

X. Zheng et al. (eds.), *Early-stage Lung Cancer*,
https://doi.org/10.1007/978-981-10-7596-4_8

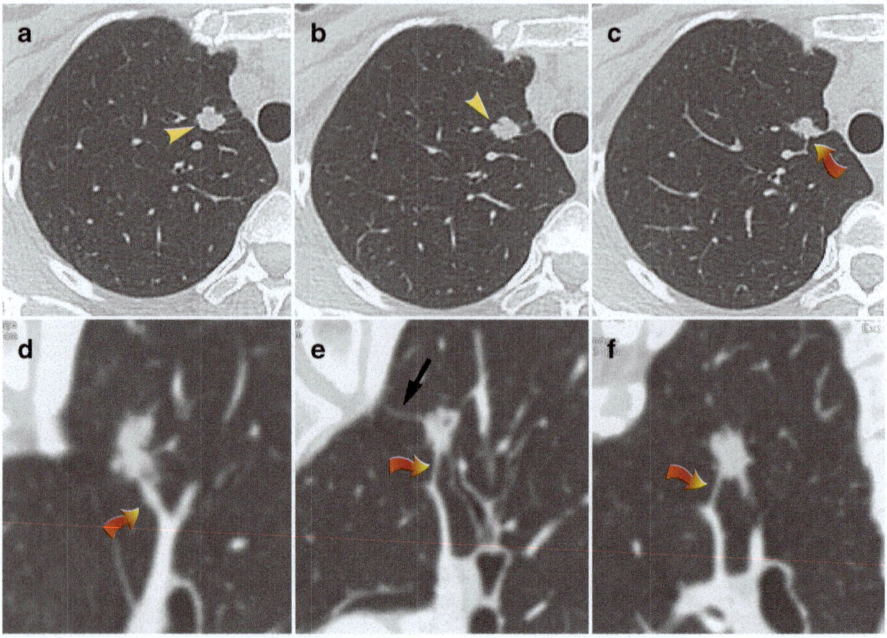

Fig. 8.1 CT findings of solid IAC. A 39-year-old otherwise healthy female presents to the clinic for an imaging consultation. (**a**–**c**) In the axial images, a 10 mm diameter solid nodule is seen in the apical segment of the right upper lobe. This nodule has multiple imaging signs, including spiculation (**a**, arrowhead), deep lobulation (**b**, arrowhead), spinous process sign, pleural indentation, air bubble, and vascular migration (**c**, arrow). (**d**–**f**) Multiplanar reformation imaging provides better visualization of the tumor vasculature (arrow) and pleural indentation (**e**, dark arrow), as well as other features of the nodule. This nodule was surgically resected, and IAC was pathologically confirmed

several dome-like protuberances of 1–2 mm in size (the so-called spinous process sign) may be seen at the margin, and this results from focal fibrotic hyperplasia in alveolar septa. Despite the high incidence of spiculation and spinous process signs in lung adenocarcinoma, both signs can be observed in benign nodules such as tuberculous granuloma. Spicules in tuberculous nodules appear longer and distribute along part of the margin in a comb-like pattern, whereas in lung adenocarcinomas, spicules are shorter and distribute widely along the entire margin in a radial alignment. In contrast to lobulation, spiculation, and spinous process signs, air bubbles and air bronchograms are less likely to be seen in malignant solid nodules, most likely correlated with pathological types and the biological behavior of the nodules (Fig. 8.1).

8.1.1.2 Pleural Involvement

In CT images, pleural involvement by tumors may have various presentations, among which the "pleural indentation sign," also called the "pleural tail sign" or "rabbit's ear sign," is somewhat specific in the differential diagnosis of lung cancer. Pathologically, tumor cells infiltrate visceral pleura and drag them toward the tumor, which creates the characteristic imaging finding: a linear structure seen between the tumor and pleura and a triangular or bell-mouthed indentation in the involved pleural surface due to the retraction from thickening lobular septa, fibrotic hyperplasia, and scar tissues. Earlier studies have shown that there exists a high possibility (50–80%) of pleural invasion or contact with the pleura in small lung cancers with pleural indentation, with the predominance of a low ground-glass opacity (GGO) ratio or Noguchi's type C adenocarcinoma [1]. In some benign nodules (10–30%), this imaging feature can be visualized, and caution and an individualized analysis of this sign in the diagnostic differentiation are therefore warranted.

8.1.1.3 Contrast Enhancement

The administration of contrast media facilitates the assessment of pulmonary nodules. Malignant nodules have immature vasculature with increasing permeability due to the lack of an intact endothelial lining, resulting in contrast media readily penetrating the extravascular space and consequently causing a significant enhancement effect with a comparison to benign nodules. Swensen et al. suggested a 20 HU increment in the threshold value for the differential diagnosis of benign and malignant nodules in contrast imaging, and this was revised to 15 HU after further research. According to Yamashita et al., a nodule with a contrast enhancement of 20–60 HU is highly suspicious for malignancy. In contrast, an inflammatory granuloma may have higher contrast enhancement (over 60 HU), but the enhancement pattern differs, presenting as peripheral enhancement and central nonenhancement. Neither inactive tuberculous granuloma nor inflammatory pseudotumor can be significantly enhanced because the former lacks a supplying circulation due to central caseous necrosis and the latter comprises organizing fibrosis.

As described in previous chapters, the development of blood circulation in malignant nodules can be divided into two stages. In the early or external neoangiogenic stage, proangiogenic factors secreted by tumor cells induce preexisting vessels to sprout and promote vascular buds that migrate toward the tumor; in the late or internal neoangiogenic stage, the tumor continues to generate intratumoral microvasculature which gradually develops connections with the recruited external neovasculature to form the tumor circulation that allows for sustainable development. As the tumor volume reaches 2–3 mm^3, an efficient blood supply is required for maintaining tumor growth; if not, necrosis may occur or some tumor cells may enter a status of dormancy or growth inertia [2].

8.1.2 The Imaging Features and Pathological Findings of SPNs

Thin-sliced CT imaging is favorable in the assessment of SPN calcification, nodular density, fatty components, and so forth. Most benign SPNs are homogeneous in density or comprised of a fatty component determined by a specific CT value of

−40 to −90 HU. In contrast, malignant lesions are heterogeneous, consisting of an air bubble, cavity, or bronchogram sign, fine calcification, or ground-glass opacity. The air bubble sign describes the focal lucency within a lesion. The variants of the air bubble sign include a small air cavity and air bronchograms. Specifically, the size of the lucency in the air bubble sign is less than 5 mm in diameter and is larger than 5 mm in the air cavity sign. Air bronchogram refers to the imaging finding of air-filled bronchi passing through airless parenchyma or solid masses without compressing the airways. Persistent air bronchograms and air bubbles after antimicrobial therapy are more commonly seen in malignant nodules, particularly adenocarcinoma. If a nodular or irregular protuberance exists within the lucency, the possibility of malignancy increases.

Pathologically, the air bubble sign reflects residual airspace in the cancerous lesion with cancer cells growing along alveolar walls in a lepidic pattern. Within the residual airspace, uninvolved pulmonary scaffolding structures include bronchioles and alveoli, and the acinar cavity appears as sac-like dilations due to air and/or mucin congestion. Once the air bubble sign or air bronchogram sign disappears in the follow-up imaging (which suggests that solid components increase and occupy airspace because of disease progression), medical intervention should be initiated as soon as possible.

In contrast to the crescent cavity commonly seen in tuberculosis, most cancerous cavities are irregular, with mural nodules along the inconsistent walls. Calcification can be observed in benign and malignant nodules. In the former, it can appear centric, lamellar, diffuse, or popcorn-like, whereas in the latter, irregular, fine, sand-like calcification is frequently seen with an eccentric distribution. When the fatty component is detected, the nodule is benign, in most cases.

8.1.3 *The Size, Location, and Volume-Doubling Time of Nodules*

Tumor size is one of the most important predictors of outcome in lung cancer, making it a key element of TNM staging. Research has shown it to be an independent predictor of survival. In general, nodule size correlates with the probability of malignancy and with prognosis. The Dutch-Belgian lung cancer screening trial (the NELSON study) is the first randomized lung cancer screening trial based on nodule volume rather than nodule diameter [3]. Based on the NELSON study, the probability of developing lung cancer within 2 years in individuals at high risk of lung cancer was calculated, and the risk was stratified by volume, volume-derived diameter, and volume-doubling time [4]. For an individual with a nodule smaller than 5 mm in diameter (or volume <100 mm^3), the probability of malignancy is approximately 0.6%, which is not significantly different from that in individuals without nodules; for a nodule of 5–10 mm diameter (or volume 100–300 mm^3), the probability increases to 0.9–5.8%, and routine follow-up CT is required; for a nodule larger than 10 mm diameter (or volume >300 mm^3), the probability ranges from 11.1 to 26.2%, and immediate medical intervention is warranted for further assessment and management.

Malignant and benign nodules have distinct biological behavior, which is partly reflected by the growth rate. Volume-doubling time (VDT) is a quantitative parameter for the measurement of the growth rate of nodules, thus providing supplemental information for lung cancer risk assessment. In the same study, the lung cancer probabilities were further stratified according to the VDT: 0.8% (range, 0–0.9%) for VDT ≥600 days, 4.0% for VDT of 400–600 days, and 9.9% (range, 6.7–25.0%) for VDT ≤400 days. As noted, calculation of VDT demands long-term routine follow-up CT imaging. For certain inert nodules, VDY may take 5 years or more.

Some nodular diseases have a specific distribution or location which may be helpful for differentiating pulmonary nodules. For example, tuberculous granuloma is predominantly found in the apicoposterior segment of the upper lobe and superior segment of the lower lobe, whereas pulmonary sequestration is frequently seen in the lower lobe.

Routine follow-up LDCT is critical for the assessment of suspected nodules and for the early diagnosis of small cell lung cancer or AIS. Owing to the inert biological behavior of GGNs, approximately 90% of them may have subtle changes in size, density, or vasculature or none at all, during short-term follow-up. Therefore, an effective follow-up for a pulmonary nodule should last 3 years at minimum; five or more years are better to avoid missing early lung cancer. Overall, the accurate diagnosis and differentiation of GGNs rely on comprehensive analysis of the imaging data and clinical information. For those cases of atypical GGNs for which long-term follow-up imaging may not be adequate to solve the diagnosis puzzle, invasive procedures including transbronchial lung biopsy (TBLB) or CT-guided percutaneous biopsy are required to confirm the diagnosis.

8.2 CT Findings, Pathological Correlation, and Differential Diagnosis of Invasive Adenocarcinoma

In MIA, the solid components gradually accumulate and infiltrate into the pulmonary interstitium, leading to irregular nest-like morphology and alveolar collapse. As the extent of the solid component exceeds 5 mm, the disease progresses from MIA into invasive adenocarcinoma (IAC). Pathologically, the solid components in MIA and IAC have the same formation: hyperplastic tumor cells and fibrotic tissues, as well as collapsed alveoli. The solid components in IAC have a higher density than they do in MIA in CT imaging. The incremental rate of solid components reflects, to some extent, the progression status of the disease. In advanced disease, the solid components grow faster than in very early-stage disease and eventually occupy nonsolid or partly solid areas. Contrast enhancement CT imaging can readily reveal characteristic features, including enhanced solid nodules with lobulation

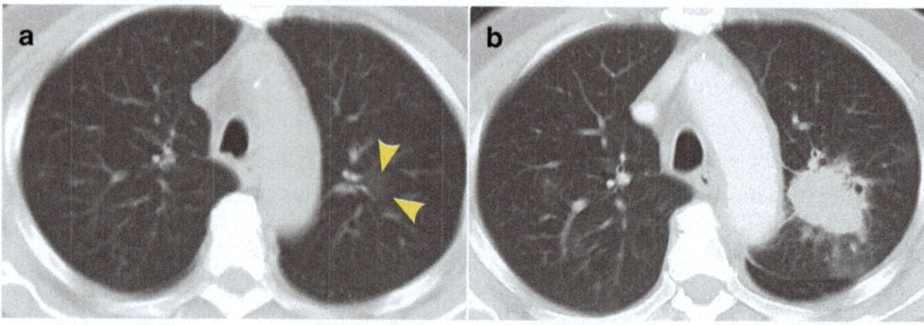

Fig. 8.2 The typical CT findings in IAC. (**a**) Annual LDCT lung cancer screening revealed a 5 mm GGN (arrowhead) in the apicoposterior segment of the left upper lobe, and routine follow-up was advised. (**b**) The patient failed to follow these medical instructions and 4 years later returned to the clinic with complaints of chest pain. Chest CT showed the GGN had progressed into a mass with characteristic fine spiculation and a halo sign, consistent with malignant disease. IAC was confirmed by surgical pathology

and/or the CTA-TA sign along the nodular margin. IAC diseases are potentially invasive. In some cases, the pleural indentation may be observed due to the involvement of the pleura. In addition, fine spiculation or prominence may exist (Fig. 8.2).

IAC carries a high risk of lymphatic and vascular involvement. Lymphatic involvement may cause carcinomatous lymphangitis, pathologically characterized by cancer cells infiltrating the lymphatics and perilymphatic structures, reactive inflammation and hyperplasia, and variable thickening of the lobular septum and bronchovascular branches, which presents as several coarse linear structures running toward the hilum in CT imaging. Therefore, a thorough and cautious interpretation of GGN imaging is needed for accurate assessment of the outcome and prognosis. A GGN with a predominant ground-glass component has a better prognosis than one with a predominant solid component. Microscopically, IAC is categorized into five types according to the predominant component: lepidic, acinar, papillary, micropapillary, and solid with mucin production. This classification system is distinct from the AIS categorization (Fig. 8.3). Ideally, any resected GGN should receive an accurate diagnosis prior to surgical removal. However, it is challenging for pulmonologists to perform a biopsy on these subcentimeter GGNs and even challenging for pathologists to reach a definite pathological diagnosis and classification based on a trace amount of biopsy specimens, which renders imaging analysis more important. As described in previous chapters, once an incidentally detected GGN becomes bigger, denser, and richer in vasculature and enhanced in contrast imaging during routine follow-up CT, the possibility AIS or MIA should be entertained and surgical resection advised.

If a GGN lesion continues growing during routine long-term follow-up and fails to respond to antimicrobial treatment, preinvasive diseases (AAH and AIS) or invasive diseases (MIA and IAC) should be suspected. The notion of human tumor development as a multistep progress has been histologically documented in various organs, including the lungs. Tumor progression is driven by a sequence of randomly

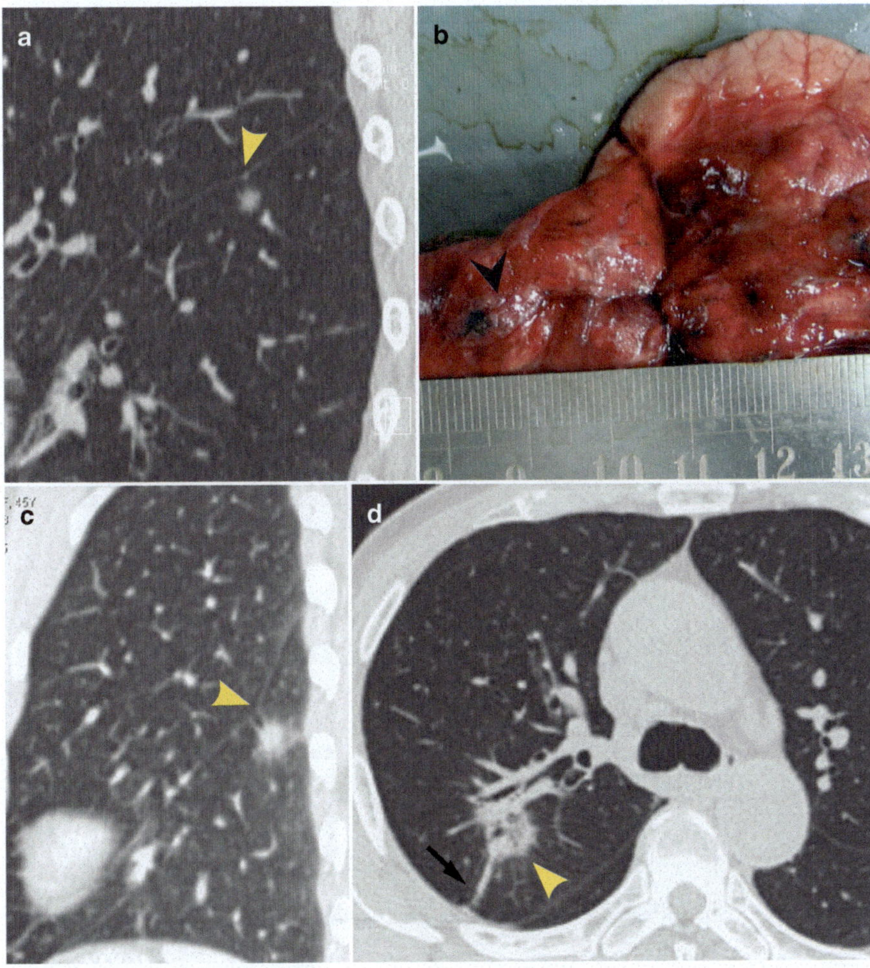

Fig. 8.3 CT findings in IAC: Pleural indentation, fine spiculation, and small prominence. (**a**) A 5 mm solid nodule with pleural involvement was seen in the left lower lobe (arrowhead). (**b**) In the surgical specimens, the nodule was recognized (arrowhead) and pathologically confirmed as IAC. (**c**) A 15 mm, pathologically proven IAC in the superior segment of the left lower lobe had pleural indentation, fine spiculation, and the halo sign (arrow). (**d**) Pleural indentation (arrow), a small prominence, and fine spiculation (arrowhead) were seen in a pathologically proven IAC

occurring mutations and epigenetic alterations of DNA that affect the genes controlling cell proliferation, survival, and other traits associated with malignant cell phenotypes. As tumor progression proceeds, cells accumulate genetic and epigenetic alterations [5]. Most lung adenocarcinomas experience a multistep developmental progress from AAH to AIS, MIA, and finally IAC with gradual accumulation of abnormal molecular events (Fig. 8.4). Furthermore, it is not uncommon to detect multiple GGNs at various steps, particularly when LDCT is replacing chest radiog-

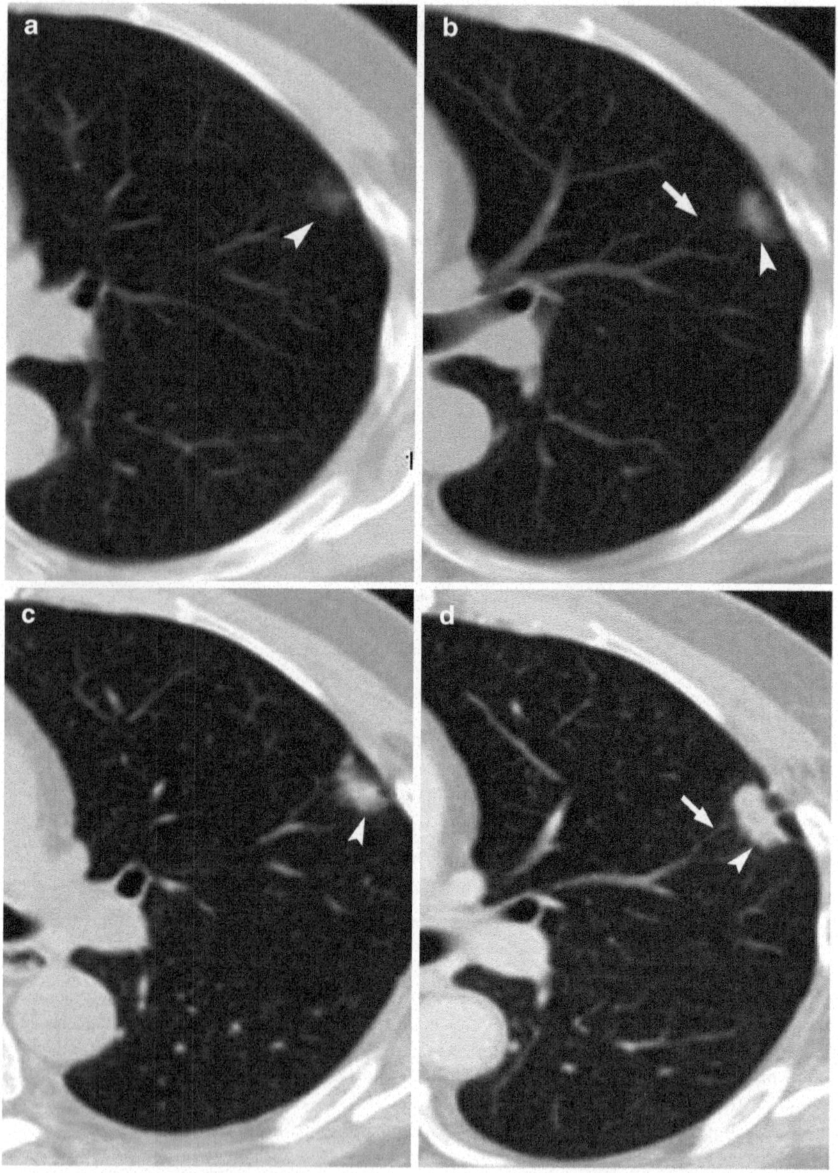

Fig. 8.4 Multistep progression from AAH to lung adenocarcinoma during 4-year follow-up. (**a**) A 5 mm GGN (arrowhead) was found in an otherwise healthy patient for LDCT lung cancer screening. AAH was suspected, and routine follow-up was advised. (**b**) In the second annual follow-up CT, the left upper lobe GGN lesion grew larger and denser, with more solid components than shown on the initial CT. Simultaneously, a small vessel (arrow) began migrating into the nodule. AIS was suspected (arrowhead). (**c**) In the third annual follow-up CT, more solid components were seen within the lesion (arrowhead). Pleural indentation and a small prominence appeared, indicative of MIA. The patient was advised to undergo a biopsy but refused. (**d**) In the fourth annual CT, the nodule continued to grow larger and denser and became enhanced with contrast media. Pleural indentation, a small prominence, and fine spiculation, as well as the characteristic CTA-TA sign, were clear. Lobar resection was performed via VATS, and IAC was pathologically confirmed

raphy for lung cancer screening. In these cases, synchronous multiple primary lung cancer (SMPLC), metachronous multiple primary lung cancer (MMPLC), and multiple metastases should be distinguished to determine the appropriate prognosis (Fig. 8.5) (please refer to Chap. 10 for more details regarding this topic).

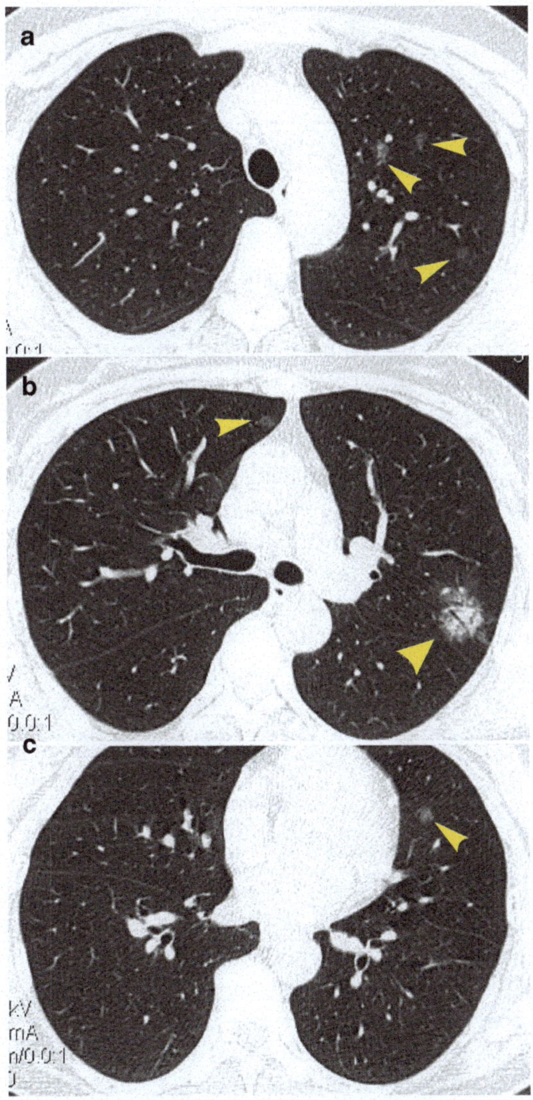

Fig. 8.5 Various imaging presentation of small lung adenocarcinoma. (**a**) Multiple GGNs were seen in the left upper lobe in a 47-year-old, otherwise healthy female patient. At the level of the aortic arch, three pGGNs of 4–5 mm diameter (arrowhead) were seen with pathological confirmation of AAH. (**b**) A 20 mm partly solid nodule with spiculation, prominence, and air bronchograms in the left upper lobe was pathologically proven to be IAC (arrowhead). In the same image, a 3 mm pGGN was seen in the right upper lobe (AAH, probably). (**c**) A mixed GGN in the lingular segment of the left upper lobe was pathologically proven to be AIS (arrowhead)

Research has shown that persistent GGN may represent preinvasive lesions or even early-stage adenocarcinoma. Among 43 pathologically proven persistent focal GGNs (≤2 cm), the proportions of AAH, AIS, and MIA were 20.9%, 53.5%, and 25.6%, respectively [6]. GGNs with solid components were highly associated with adenocarcinoma (malignant rate, 93.3%). This study could be one of the earliest on persistent GGN. In another report from Kim, 53 persistent focal GGNs were found in 49 patients. Surgical pathology showed that besides AAH (6%) and AIS/MIA (75%), ten nodules (19%) represented nonspecific fibrosis or organizing pneumonia, and no significant differences in morphologic findings on thin-section CT scans were found among the three diseases.

8.3 CT Findings and Pathological Correlation of Invasive Adenocarcinoma with Special Imaging Features

Most MIAs are nonmucinous. Without medical intervention, nonmucinous MIA continues progressing to invasive adenocarcinoma with various predominant patterns, including lepidic, acinar, papillary, and micropapillary, while the rarely occurring mucinous MIA/IAC tends to infiltrate adjacent structures, including the pulmonary interstitium and vessels, eventually causing intrapulmonary or distant metastasis (Fig. 8.6). Intrapulmonary metastases forming mucinous MIA/IAC may manifest as multiple nodules or diffuse consolidation. Thus, compared to nonmucinous adenocarcinoma, mucinous adenocarcinoma may involve a more extensive pulmonary portion (frequently an entire lobe). In some cases, miliary distribution in both lungs can be seen, resembling the CT findings in miliary tuberculosis, diffuse pulmonary metastasis, and interstitial pneumonitis. In addition, mucinous IAC frequently has a higher TNM stage and a low mutation rate and is insensitive to EGFR-targeted tyrosine kinase inhibitors, leading to a poor prognosis and low survival.

8.3.1 Multiple Nodule Type

The continuous development and convergence of nodular lesions may partially or totally obstruct segmental or subsegmental bronchi, producing the typical radiological manifestations of post-obstructive pneumonia and atelectasis. The distribution of nodular lesions may be limited to the left or right lung or to a single lobe, or both lungs may show involvement, with a diffuse or spotty distribution. Nodules have a variety of imaging features on CT imaging, including deep lobulation, spiculation, and protuberances along margins (Fig. 8.7). Pathologically, a lobulation, lobulated margin, or notch sign reflects heterogeneous growth rates in different parts of the margin, causing irregular morphology of the nodule. The "spiculation sign" or a spiculated margin refers to short linear structures radiating from the lesion to the pulmonary parenchyma, and it is attributed to direct tumor cell invasion along

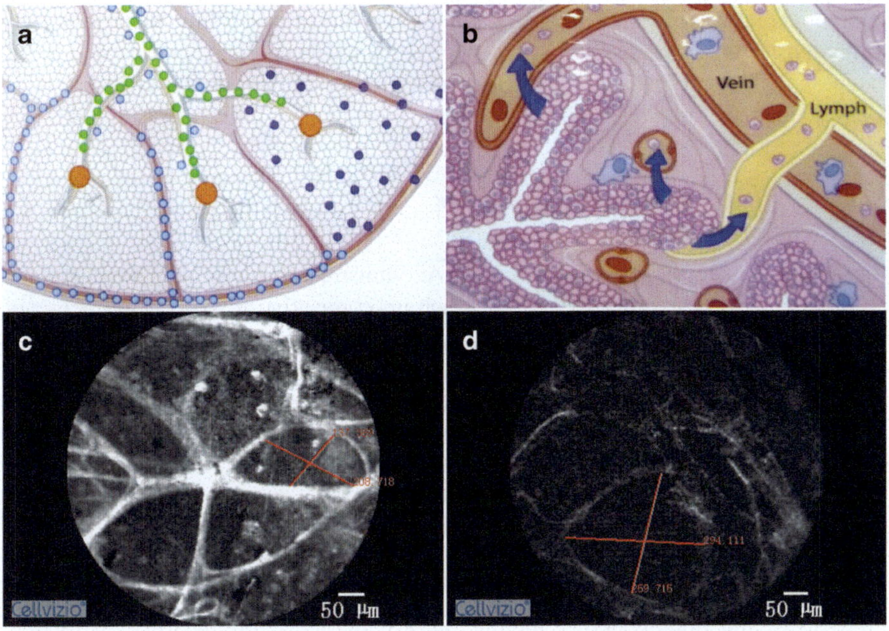

Fig. 8.6 Diagram of lung cancer invasion and metastasis as well as microscopic findings in pulmonary alveolar confocal imaging. (**a**) Diagram of lung cancer cells invading within and spreading through the pulmonary interstitium and pulmonary and lymphatic vessels (centrilobular, red circle; perilymphatic, blue circle; centrilobular, bud-like green circle; intralobar random, purple circle). (**b**) Metastasis of lung cancer cells via the lymphatic system. (**c** and **d**) Transbronchial confocal endoscopy can be used to directly observe and assess changes in pulmonary alveoli and septa due to lung cancer (**c**) and inflammation (**d**). (**c**) In the images of confocal endoscopy of lung cancer, collapsed alveoli, thickening septa, as well as increasing light density from alveoli and septa are observed. (**d**) In contrast, the structures of alveoli and septa remain intact, as does normal light density in the setting of alveolar inflammation (Figs. **c** and **d** courtesy Dawei Yang & Chunxue Bai, Department of Respiratory Diseases, Fudan University Zhongshan Hospital)

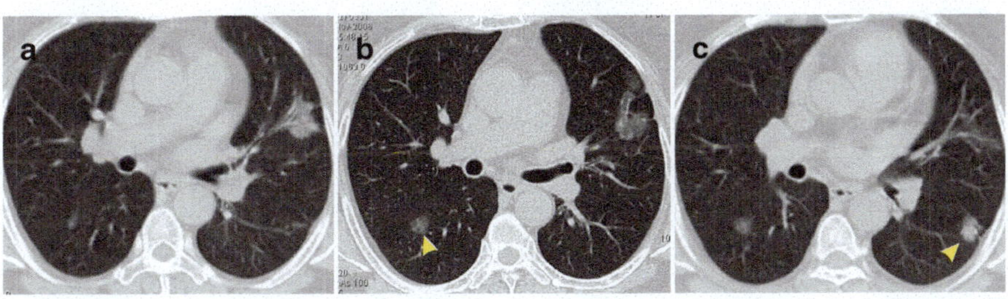

Fig. 8.7 CT findings in IAC with multiple GGNs. (**a**) LDCT lung cancer screening in a 61-year-old female patient showed multiple GGNs in both lungs. The largest nodule was located in the left upper lobe with a deep lobulation sign. (**b**) In the right lower lobe, a mixed GGN was seen (arrowhead), and AIS was suspected. (**c**) In the subpleural area of left lower lobe, a third GGN with clear pleural indentation was seen, suggestive of IAC (confirmed by CT-guided biopsy)

interstitial planes and lymphatic spread in malignancy or is a desmoplastic response in benign lesions. These signs reflect the biological behavior of the lesion, to an extent, and their presence can be viewed as a suggestion of malignancy.

8.3.2 Diffuse Consolidation Type

As the disease progresses from AIS to MIA, clinical and pathological development accelerates. Invasive tumor tissues encroach upon preexisting hyperplastic fibrosis and pulmonary structures and eventually transform into invasive adenocarcinoma. IAC becomes even more heterogeneous than its precursor lesions. As the revised IASLC/ATS/ERS classification of lung adenocarcinoma addresses, most IACs are comprised of a complex heterogeneous mixture of histologic subtypes. It is recommended that individual tumor be classified according to the predominant pattern (lepidic, acinar, papillary, micropapillary, or solid), a factor that plays a crucial role in treatment decision-making and the assessment of prognosis.

If pulmonary airspaces are completely congested with proliferating tumor cells, the involved area may present as irregular or segmental consolidation with increasing density and homogeneous attenuation, a pattern resembling lobar or lobular pneumonia (Fig. 8.8). Occasionally, large, centrally located bronchi can be visualized within the consolidated area (air bronchogram), but peripheral bronchi are rarely seen, creating the sign known as a "withering tree." If the tumor mass is centrally located and is adjacent to a displaced fissure from obstructive atelectasis, this could give rise to the characteristic Golden S sign in conventional radiography.

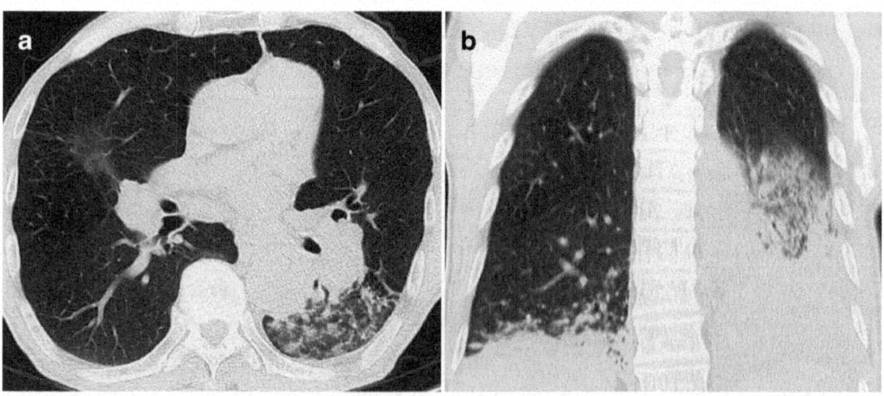

Fig. 8.8 CT findings in IAC with multiple nodules. A 72-year-old male patient came to the clinic complaining of white foamy, occasionally blood-tinged phlegm. Chest CT revealed multiple GGNs in the posterolateral segment of the left lower lobe with diffuse distribution, as well as lymphadenopathy in the left hilum (A). None of the lesions responded to antimicrobial treatment. Eight months later, the disease continued to progress with nodular convergence and pulmonary consolidation. CT-guided percutaneous biopsy confirmed invasive adenocarcinoma

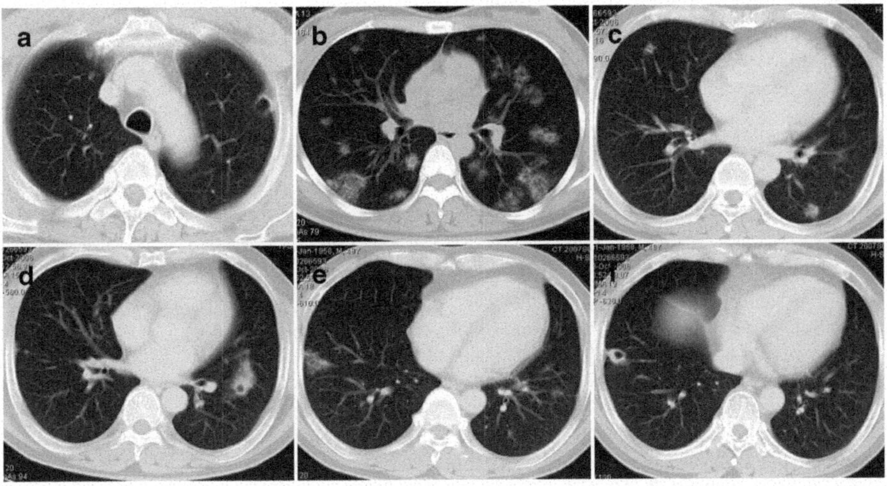

Fig. 8.9 CT findings in IAC with diffuse distribution. The patient was a 45-year-old, non-smoking, nonsymptomatic male. Diffuse multiple heterogeneous GGNs were seen in both lungs and had various morphologies, including ground-glass, partly solid, bubble-like, and cyst-like. A fine-needle biopsy was performed, and IAC was pathologically confirmed

In cases in which airspaces and the bronchi are partially obstructed, various cysts or cavitation may be observed (Fig. 8.9). In diseases with diffuse consolidation, the differential diagnosis of pneumonia remains challenging. Contrast enhancement scanning and/or 18F-DG PET-CT are necessary imaging procedures, and transbronchial biopsy or CT-guided percutaneous biopsy may be required for those patients with equivocal imaging findings.

References

1. Saito H, Oshima M, Kiuchi R, Watanabe K, Kitagawa K, Masuda S. Relationship between pleural indentation on computed tomography scans and pleural invasion in small peripheral lung cancer of 2 cm in size or less. Kyobu Geka. 2009;62(9):767–70. discussion 770-762.
2. Naumov GN, Folkman J, Straume O, Akslen LA. Tumor-vascular interactions and tumor dormancy. APMIS. 2008;116(7–8):569–85. https://doi.org/10.1111/j.1600-0463.2008.01213.x.
3. van Klaveren RJ, Oudkerk M, Prokop M, Scholten ET, Nackaerts K, Vernhout R, van Iersel CA, vanden Bergh KA, van't Westeinde S, vander Aalst C, Thunnissen E, Xu DM, Wang Y, Zhao Y, Gietema HA, de Hoop BJ, Groen HJ, de Bock GH, van Ooijen P, Weenink C, Verschakelen J, Lammers JW, Timens W, Willebrand D, Vink A, Mali W, de Koning HJ. Management of lung nodules detected by volume CT scanning. N Engl J Med. 2009;361(23):2221–9. https://doi.org/10.1056/NEJMoa0906085.
4. Horeweg N, van Rosmalen J, Heuvelmans MA, van der Aalst CM, Vliegenthart R, Scholten ET, ten Haaf K, Nackaerts K, Lammers JW, Weenink C, Groen HJ, van Ooijen P, de Jong PA, de Bock GH, Mali W, de Koning HJ, Oudkerk M. Lung cancer probability in patients with CT-detected pulmonary nodules: a prespecified analysis of data from the NELSON trial of low-dose CT screening. Lancet Oncol. 2014;15(12):1332–41. https://doi.org/10.1016/s1470-2045(14)70389-4.

5. Weinberg RA. The biology of cancer. 2nd ed. New York: Garland Science, Taylor & Francis Group; 2014.
6. Nakata M, Saeki H, Takata I, Segawa Y, Mogami H, Mandai K, Eguchi K. Focal ground-glass opacity detected by low-dose helical CT. Chest. 2002;121(5):1464–7.

Suggested Readings

1. Austin JH, Garg K, Aberle D, Yankelevitz D, Kuriyama K, Lee HJ, Brambilla E, Travis WD. Radiologic implications of the 2011 classification of adenocarcinoma of the lung. Radiology. 2013;266(1):62–71. https://doi.org/10.1148/radiol.12120240.
2. Diederich S, Lenzen H, Windmann R, Puskas Z, Yelbuz TM, Henneken S, Klaiber T, Eameri M, Roos N, Peters PE. Pulmonary nodules: experimental and clinical studies at low-dose CT. Radiology. 1999;213(1):289–98. https://doi.org/10.1148/radiology.213.1.r99oc29289.
3. Edey AJ, Hansell DM. Incidentally detected small pulmonary nodules on CT. Clin Radiol. 2009;64(9):872–84. https://doi.org/10.1016/j.crad.2009.03.006.
4. Godoy MC, Sabloff B, Naidich DP. Subsolid pulmonary nodules: imaging evaluation and strategic management. Curr Opin Pulm Med. 2012;18(4):304–12. https://doi.org/10.1097/MCP.0b013e328354a5f2.
5. Kaneko M, Kusumoto M, Kobayashi T, Moriyama N, Naruke T, Ohmatsu H, Kakinuma R, Eguchi K, Nishiyama H, Matsui E. Computed tomography screening for lung carcinoma in Japan. Cancer. 2000;89(11 Suppl):2485–8.
6. Kawakami S, Sone S, Takashima S, Li F, Yang ZG, Maruyama Y, Honda T, Hasegawa M, Wang JC. Atypical adenomatous hyperplasia of the lung: correlation between high-resolution CT findings and histopathologic features. Eur Radiol. 2001;11(5):811–4. https://doi.org/10.1007/s003300000790.
7. Kim HY, Shim YM, Lee KS, Han J, Yi CA, Kim YK. Persistent pulmonary nodular ground-glass opacity at thin-section CT: histopathologic comparisons. Radiology. 2007;245(1):267–75. https://doi.org/10.1148/radiol.2451061682.
8. Liang M, Yip R, Tang W, Xu D, Reeves A, Henschke CI, Yankelevitz DF. Variation in screening CT-detected nodule Volumetry as a function of size. AJR Am J Roentgenol. 2017;209(2):304–8. https://doi.org/10.2214/ajr.16.17159.
9. Munden RF, Erasmus JJ, Wahba H, Fineberg NS. Follow-up of small (4 mm or less) incidentally detected nodules by computed tomography in oncology patients: a retrospective review. J Thorac Oncol. 2010;5(12):1958–62. https://doi.org/10.1097/JTO.0b013e3181f2636e.
10. Murrmann GB, van Vollenhoven FH, Moodley L. Approach to a solid solitary pulmonary nodule in two different settings-"common is common, rare is rare". J Thorac Dis. 2014;6(3):237–48. https://doi.org/10.3978/j.issn.2072-1439.2013.11.13.
11. Perandini S, Soardi G, Motton M, Oliboni E, Zantedeschi L, Montemezzi S. Distribution of solid solitary pulmonary nodules within the lungs on computed tomography: a review of 208 consecutive lesions of biopsy-proven nature. Polish J Radiol. 2016a;81:146–51. https://doi.org/10.12659/pjr.895417.
12. Perandini S, Soardi GA, Motton M, Rossi A, Signorini M, Montemezzi S. Solid pulmonary nodule risk assessment and decision analysis: comparison of four prediction models in 285 cases. Eur Radiol. 2016;26(9):3071–6. https://doi.org/10.1007/s00330-015-4138-9.
13. Revel MP, Mannes I, Benzakoun J, Guinet C, Leger T, Grenier P, Lupo A, Fournel L, Chassagnon G, Bommart S. Subsolid lung nodule classification: a CT criterion for improving Interobserver agreement. Radiology. 2017;170044. https://doi.org/10.1148/radiol.2017170044.
14. Ridge CA, Yildirim A, Boiselle PM, Franquet T, Schaefer-Prokop CM, Tack D, Gevenois PA, Bankier AA. Differentiating between subsolid and solid pulmonary nodules at CT:

inter- and Intraobserver agreement between experienced thoracic radiologists. Radiology. 2016;278(3):888–96. https://doi.org/10.1148/radiol.2015150714.
15. Slattery MM, Foley C, Kenny D, Costello RW, Logan PM, Lee MJ. Long-term follow-up of non-calcified pulmonary nodules (<10 mm) identified during low-dose CT screening for lung cancer. Eur Radiol. 2012;22(9):1923–8. https://doi.org/10.1007/s00330-012-2443-0.
16. Sone S, Takashima S, Li F, Yang Z, Honda T, Maruyama Y, Hasegawa M, Yamanda T, Kubo K, Hanamura K, Asakura K. Mass screening for lung cancer with mobile spiral computed tomography scanner. Lancet (London, England). 1998;351(9111):1242–5. https://doi.org/10.1016/s0140-6736(97)08229-9.
17. Tamura M, Shimizu Y, Yamamoto T, Yoshikawa J, Hashizume Y. Predictive value of one-dimensional mean computed tomography value of ground-glass opacity on high-resolution images for the possibility of future change. J Thorac Oncol. 2014;9(4):469–72. https://doi.org/10.1097/jto.0000000000000117.
18. Truong MT, Ko JP, Rossi SE, Rossi I, Viswanathan C, Bruzzi JF, Marom EM, Erasmus JJ. Update in the evaluation of the solitary pulmonary nodule. Radiographics. 2014;34(6):1658–79. https://doi.org/10.1148/rg.346130092.
19. Walter JE, Heuvelmans MA, de Jong PA, Vliegenthart R, van Ooijen PMA, Peters RB, Ten Haaf K, Yousaf-Khan U, van der Aalst CM, de Bock GH, Mali W, Groen HJM, de Koning HJ, Oudkerk M. Occurrence and lung cancer probability of new solid nodules at incidence screening with low-dose CT: analysis of data from the randomised, controlled NELSON trial. Lancet Oncol. 2016;17(7):907–16. https://doi.org/10.1016/s1470-2045(16)30069-9.

Chapter 9
CT-Based Categorization of Small Lung Adenocarcinoma

Guozhen Zhang, Xiangpeng Zheng, and Ming Li

Lung adenocarcinoma can originate from various anatomical locations, such as respiratory bronchioles, alveolar ducts, sacs, or alveoli. Within the malignant lesion, the distribution and metabolic status of tumor cells may not be homogeneous, frequently heterogeneous in different zones. For example, those cells in the central zone may appear apoptotic and less active due to the limited blood supply, while those in peripheral zone show more active and aggressive behavior with invasion to adjacent structures. All these factors contribute to the heterogeneous imaging manifestations of small adenocarcinomas, which have been categorized into ten patterns: cotton ball-like, filling, pilling, branching, granulated, bronchovascular, cavitary, honeycomb-like, scar-like, and umbilical.

9.1 Cotton Ball-Like Pattern

On CT, some AIS lesions appear focal ground-glass opacity in a round or oval shape with a resemblance to a cotton ball, well-circumscribed from the adjacent normal pulmonary tissue. Histologically, tumor cells grow along alveolar walls in a sparsely lepidic pattern; mucin production or secretion may be seen in the alveolar cavity, which in combination with residual air creates a ground-glass appearance. The margin of cotton ball-like GGN could be irregular with seriated prominence corresponding to proliferating tumor cell foci (and reactive fibrotic hyperplasia). It is commonly seen that fine vessels penetrate into hazy lesions with predominant distribution in the peripheral area which can be well visualized as CTA-TA sign with

G. Zhang (✉) • M. Li
Department of Radiology, Fudan University Huadong Hospital, Shanghai, China
e-mail: cjr.zhangguozhen@vip.163.com

X. Zheng
Department of Radiation Oncology, Fudan University Huadong Hospital, Shanghai, China

X. Zheng et al. (eds.), *Early-stage Lung Cancer*,
https://doi.org/10.1007/978-981-10-7596-4_9

the administration of contrast medium, the critical differential point between AIS and AAH. In addition, the size is another differential point. For most AIS, the size is larger than 5 mm, while most AAH is smaller than 5 mm.

The attenuation of cotton ball-like GGN is as low as −600 HU. For better visualization and evaluation of the nodule and collateral features, advanced post-processing of CT images may be indispensable (Figs. 9.1, 9.2, 9.3, and 9.4). The

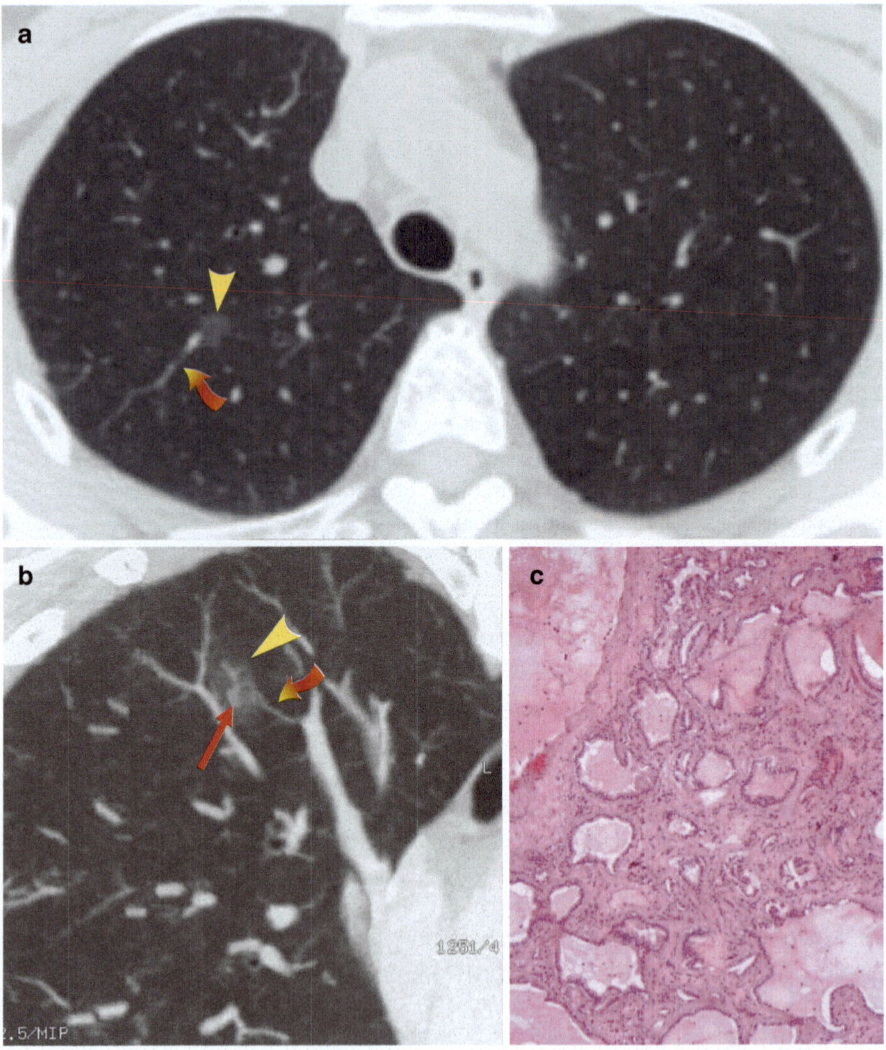

Fig. 9.1 Small adenocarcinoma with cotton ball-like pattern. (**a**) A GGN (arrowhead) is detected in the right upper lobe. Microvessels (arrow) are evident along the margin. (**b**) With administration of contrast medium, typical CTA-TA sign characterized by migration and interconnection of tumor neovessels is seen on MIP images. (**c**) Lobectomy via VATS reveals MIA with tumor cells growing along alveolar wall in lepidic pattern and central invasive component less than 5 mm (H&E stain, 200× magnification)

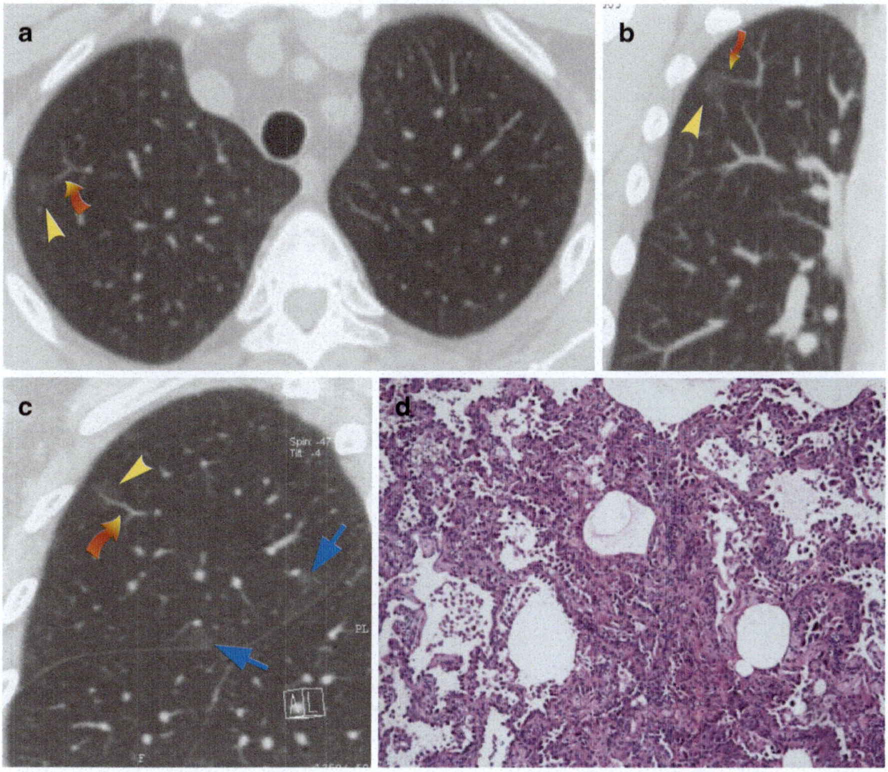

Fig. 9.2 Cotton ball-like adenocarcinoma. In the right upper lobe, a GGN (arrowhead, **a**) is detected with typical CTA-TA sign (red arrows, **a**, **b**, **c**). Surgical pathology confirms MIA with microscopic findings that tumor cells grow in the lepidic pattern, a few cells accumulate in the alveolar cavity, and stromal invasion is observed (H&E stain, 100× magnification). In the same lobe, two additional pure GGNs (blue arrows, **c**) close to the fissure are resected simultaneously with pathological confirmation of AIS (**d**), which makes this patient a victim of synchronous multiple primary lung cancer (SMPLC)

sign of CTA-TA reflects the angiogenesis under the influence of tumor-secreted proangiogenic factors on pre-existing pulmonary vessels and dynamics of novel vessels from sprouting to migrating toward tumors to interconnecting with each other within the tumor. The CTA-TA sign is distinct from vascular convergence sign seen with larger pulmonary tumors.

9.2 Filling Pattern

Numerous studies suggested that the development of lung adenocarcinoma is a stepwise evolution starting from GGN to AAH, to AIS, to MIA, to IAC, reflecting the gradual progression of biological behavior of the disease. Chronologically, this progression may last several years to decades. On imaging, a dynamic change from

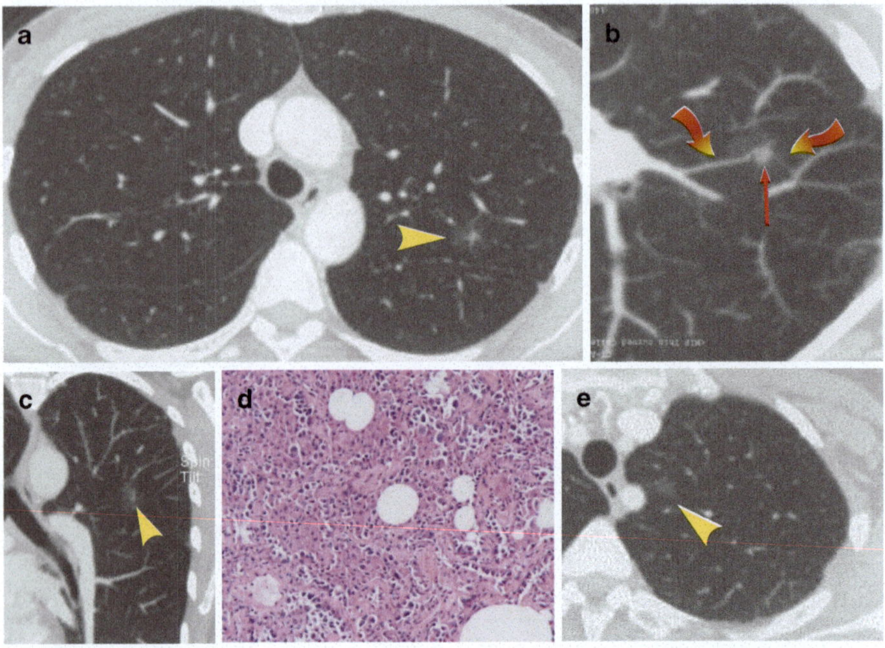

Fig. 9.3 Cotton ball-like adenocarcinoma. (**a**) On thin-sliced CT, an 11 mm subsolid GGN containing solid components of 3 mm in diameter (arrowhead) is seen in left upper lobe. (**b**) The migrating and interconnecting neovessels of typical CTA-TA sign (coarse arrow) as well as the solid component (fine arrow) are evident on MIP imaging. (**c**) Coronal reformation shows CTA-TA sign and the core of solid component with significant enhancement. (**d**) Lobectomy confirms MIA (H&E stain, 200× magnification). (**e**) The pGGN in the apical segment is located in the surgical specimen and proven to be AIS

pure GGN, to subsolid GGN, to solid GGN, is the typical manifestation. However, in some cases, the intermediate stages are transient (for nonmucinous adenocarcinoma) or totally absent (for mucinous adenocarcinoma), and the initial imaging presentations are small nodular opacities, filling with papillary or polyp-like solid components with increasing attenuation of approximately −400 HU.

Lack of peripheral ground-glass component is the hallmark of this imaging pattern. Sometimes the central zone of the lesion appears hypodense with a comparison to peripheral zone, i.e., the central lucency sign or central air-bubble sign, rendering the lesion subsolid. Of note, this subsolid presentation is distinct from the conventional subsolid with the peripheral distribution of ground-glass components. AIS with central lucency sign has inert biological behavior and could remain stable in 5 or even more years without any detectable change in either size, or density, or attenuation (Fig. 9.5). Nevertheless, those lesions with the complete filling pattern, lobulation, spiculation, and void of central lucency may have highly aggressive biological behavior even at the very early stage. Histologically, they may be mucinous AIS/MIA, papillary-predominant adenocarcinoma, or solid-predominant adenocarcinoma with mucin pro-

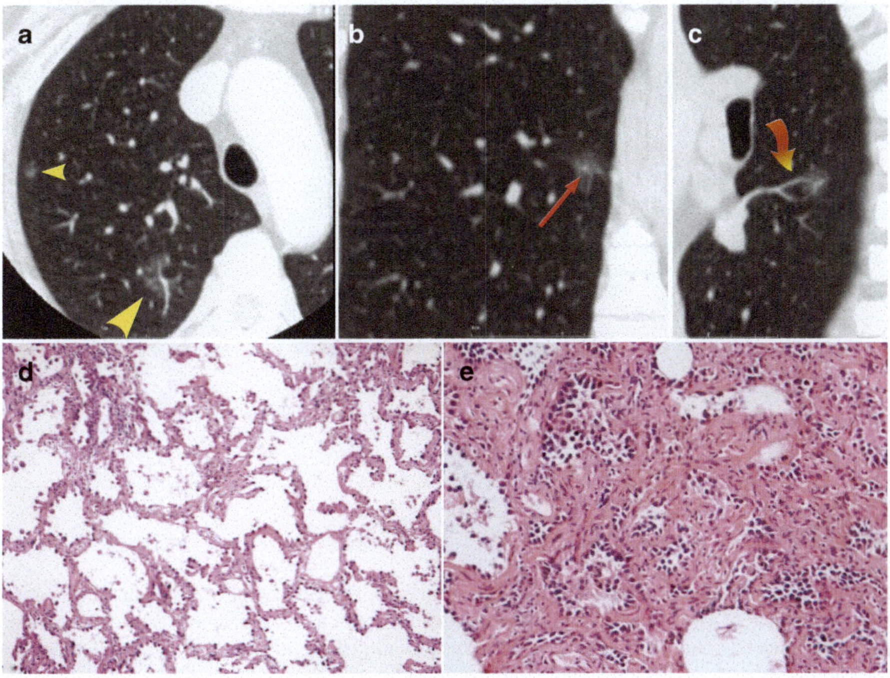

Fig. 9.4 Cotton ball-like adenocarcinoma. (**a**) A 34-year-old otherwise healthy female patient received low-dose CT lung cancer screening. A 10 mm subsolid GGN (large arrow) was found in paravertebral region of the apicoposterior segment in left upper lobe. In addition, a smaller pGGN of 3 mm in diameter was found in the same lobe (small arrow). (**b**) The subsolid GGN contained solid component with a measurement of 3 mm (arrow). (**c**) On contrast CT, characteristic CTA-TA sign was seen with the subsolid lesion. (**d**) Lobectomy via VATS confirmed AAH of the pGGN with intact alveolar structure and mildly to moderately atypical type II pneumocytes lining alveolar walls (H&E, 100× magnification). (**e**) The subsolid GGN was pathologically diagnosed as MIA with coexisting of lepidic growth and stromal invasion of neoplastic cells (H&E stain, 200× magnification)

duction, less than 20 mm in size and intrapulmonary and/or mediastinal metastasis are frequently seen. Therefore, prompt surgical resection instead of routine follow-up is the proper management strategy for such lesions (Figs. 9.6, 9.7, 9.8, and 9.9).

9.3 Granulated Pattern

Anatomically, the pulmonary gaseous exchange between blood and air takes place in respiratory bronchioles and their subdivisions, alveolar ducts, sacs, and grape-like alveoli. The alveolar sacs consist of several alveoli opening into a single chamber. Each alveolus is surrounded by a rich network of blood

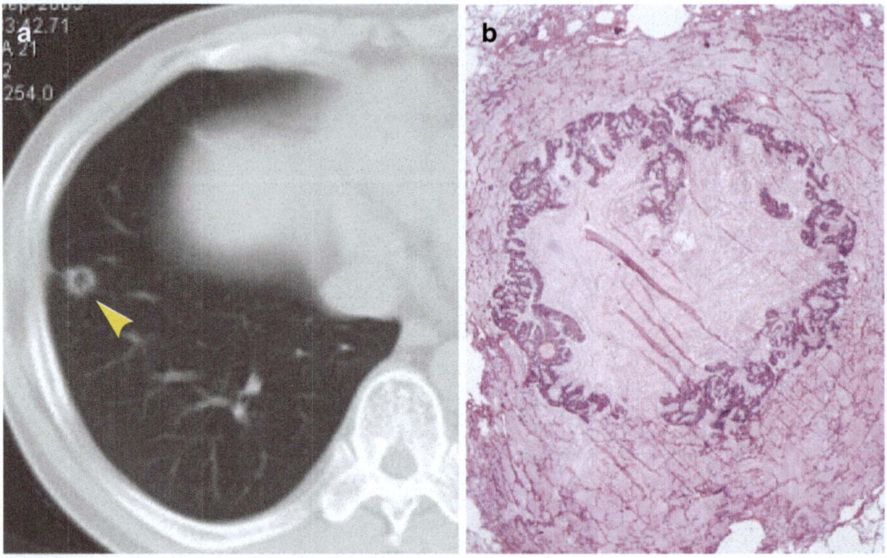

Fig. 9.5 Small adenocarcinoma with filling pattern. (**a**) A subsolid GGN was seen in the postero-lateral segment of right lower lobe with circular distribution of solid component and central hypodense lucency or central air-bubble sign (arrowhead). (**b**) Surgical pathology revealed acinar and papillary abnormal mucinous epithelium within pools of mucin, consistent with primary mucinous adenocarcinoma (H&E stain, 20× magnification)

capillaries as the fundamental structure and primary site for gaseous exchange. Adjacent alveoli are communicated via interalveolar connections, the pores of Kohn, which are the pathways of tumor cell spreading. Lung adenocarcinoma may involve multiple alveoli or alveolar sacs. Through the pores of Kohn and alveolar ducts, more alveoli can be implicated, leading to characteristic imaging manifestations of multiple round or oval granulated opacities in a bead-string alignment (Figs. 9.10 and 9.11).

9.4 Piling Pattern

In contrast to the filling pattern and granulated pattern, lesions with pilling pattern appear convergence of several discrete oval ground-glass opacities with evident or undetectable solid components, resulting in irregular or petaloid lobulated margins. The histological examination may reveal multiple tumor origin centers involving multiple discrete alveoli or alveolar sacs. Each center progresses separately and tends to emerge with others to produce a cluster formation or papillary appearance. Stromal invasion is frequently seen. With lobulation developing, a

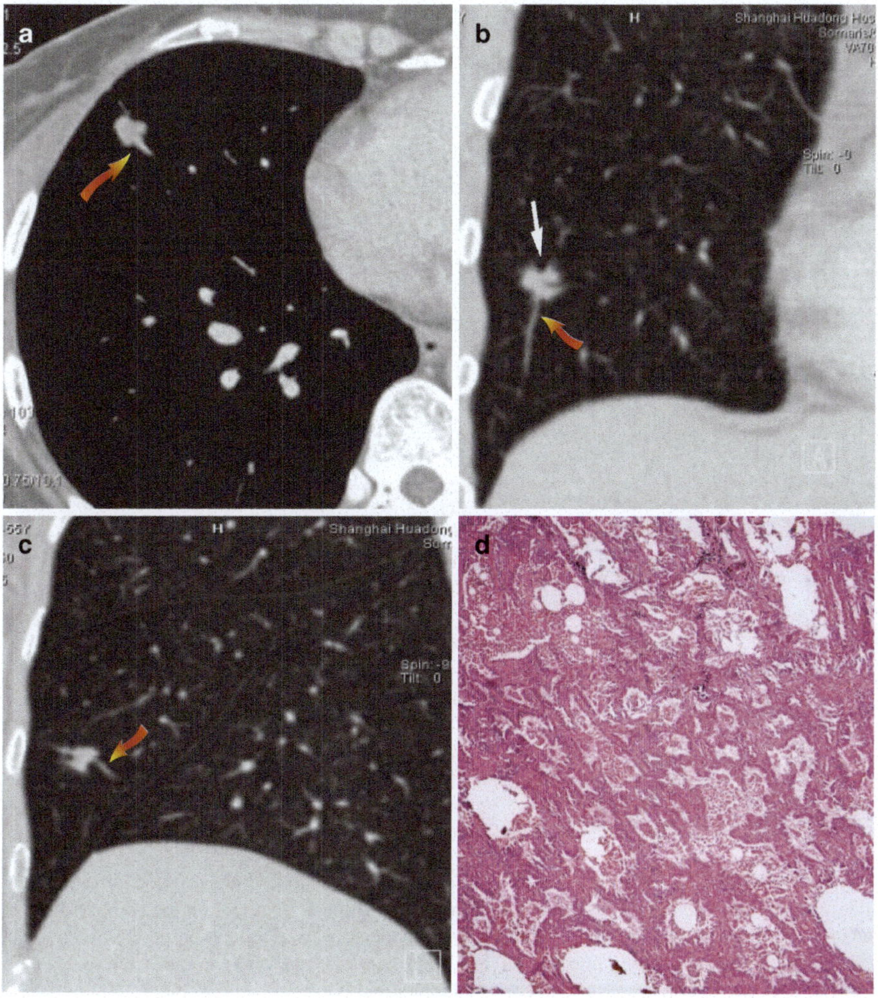

Fig. 9.6 Adenocarcinoma with filling pattern. (**a**) An 8 mm solid nodule was found in the lateral segment of the right middle lobe in a 55-year-old female patient. There were microvessels connecting with the nodule (arrow); on the coronal (**b**) and sagittal reformations (**c**), the nodule had irregular shape with deep lobulation on the margin and CTA-TA sign. (**d**) Microscopic examination revealed the tumor was composed of variously sized acinars with invasive growth, consistent with invasive adenocarcinoma (H&E stain, 40× magnification)

halo sign may be seen along the GGN lesion, which may reflect the collapse of focal pulmonary tissue due to tumor compression, stromal microinvasion, or alveolar hemorrhage due to microvascular embolism (Figs. 9.12 and 9.13). Therefore, halo sign is a nonspecific imaging finding and should be taken into consideration with other imaging features.

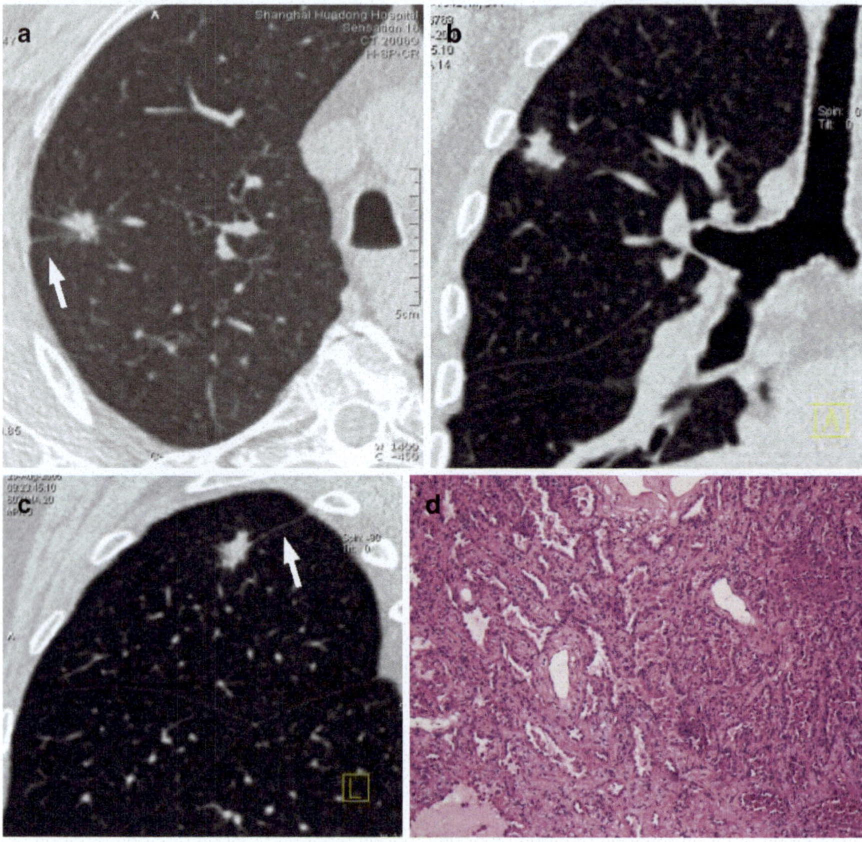

Fig. 9.7 Adenocarcinoma with filling pattern. (**a**) A 12 mm solid nodule was seen in right upper lobe with pleura indentation (white arrow) in a 64-year-old male patient; on the coronal (**b**) and sagittal reformations (**c**), the nodule had irregular shape with deep lobulation on the margin and evident pleural indentation (white arrow). (**d**) Microscopic examination revealed the tumor was composed of heterogeneous invasive acinar and interstitial fibrosis as well as minor inflammation, consistent with invasive adenocarcinoma (H&E stain, 100× magnification)

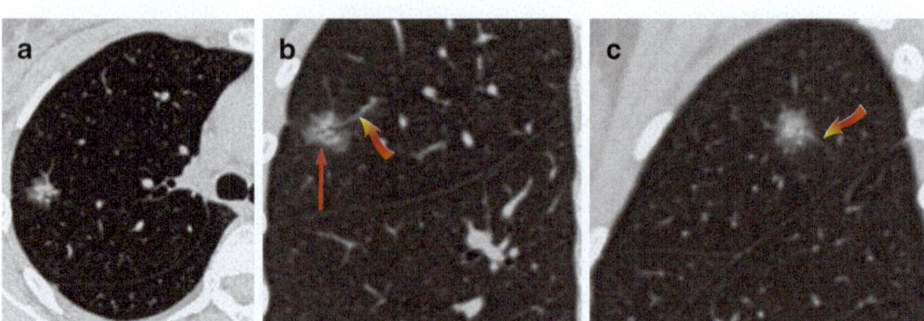

Fig. 9.8 Adenocarcinoma with filling pattern. (**a**) A 13 mm irregular subsolid GGN was seen in right upper lobe in a 54-year-old female patient; the coronal (**b**) and sagittal reformations (**c**) showed the characteristic CTA-TA sign (arrow); surgical pathology confirmed invasive adenocarcinoma

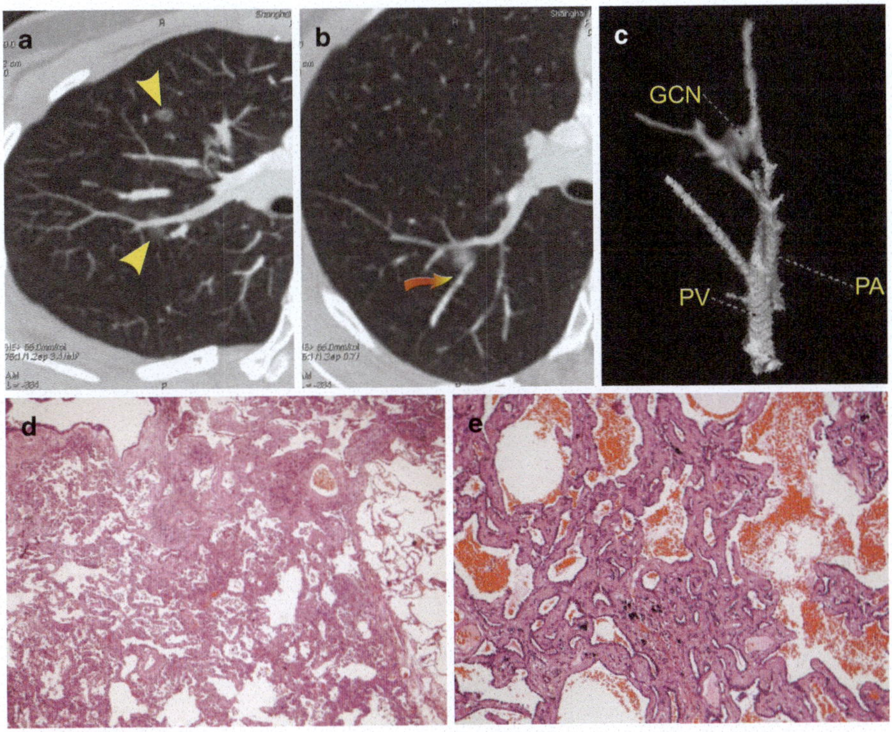

Fig. 9.9 Adenocarcinoma with filling pattern. (**a**) Two subsolid GGNs with measurements of 5 and 8 mm (arrowhead) in diameter were incidentally detected in right upper lobe in a 40-year-old female patient. (**b**) Characteristic CTA-TA sign (arrow) was observed in the 8 mm GGN. (**c**) 3D reconstruction with volume rendering technique clearly showed the relationship between the subsolid GGN (8 mm) and supplying microvessels. Microscopic examination of surgical specimen of the 8 mm GGN revealed lepidic growth of tumor cells with central invasive solid component, consistent with MIA (H&E stain, 40× magnification). (**d**) The smaller GGN was proven to be AIS with monolayers of cuboidal epithelial cells proliferating along alveolar wall in lepidic pattern (H&E stain, 100× magnification)

9.5 Bronchovascular Pattern

The intrapulmonary bronchovascular bundles or structures are composed of bronchi, pulmonary arteries, and surrounding supportive peribronchovascular connective tissues. On chest radiography or CT, the bronchovascular markings present a centrifugal distribution pattern, extending from the hilar regions to the peripheral lungs. If imaged along the main axis, vessels manifest as branching linear opacities progressively tapering toward the periphery, while bronchi appear as tube-like opacities running parallel to arteries, creating the characteristic "railway track" appearance. If imaged in the perpendicular or oblique direction, the characteristic "finger ring" appearance should be observed with the arteries as the diamond and the parallel bronchi as the circular ring [1].

As tumor cells grow along the longitudinal direction of the bronchovascular bundles, a characteristic bronchovascular imaging pattern occurs with manifesta-

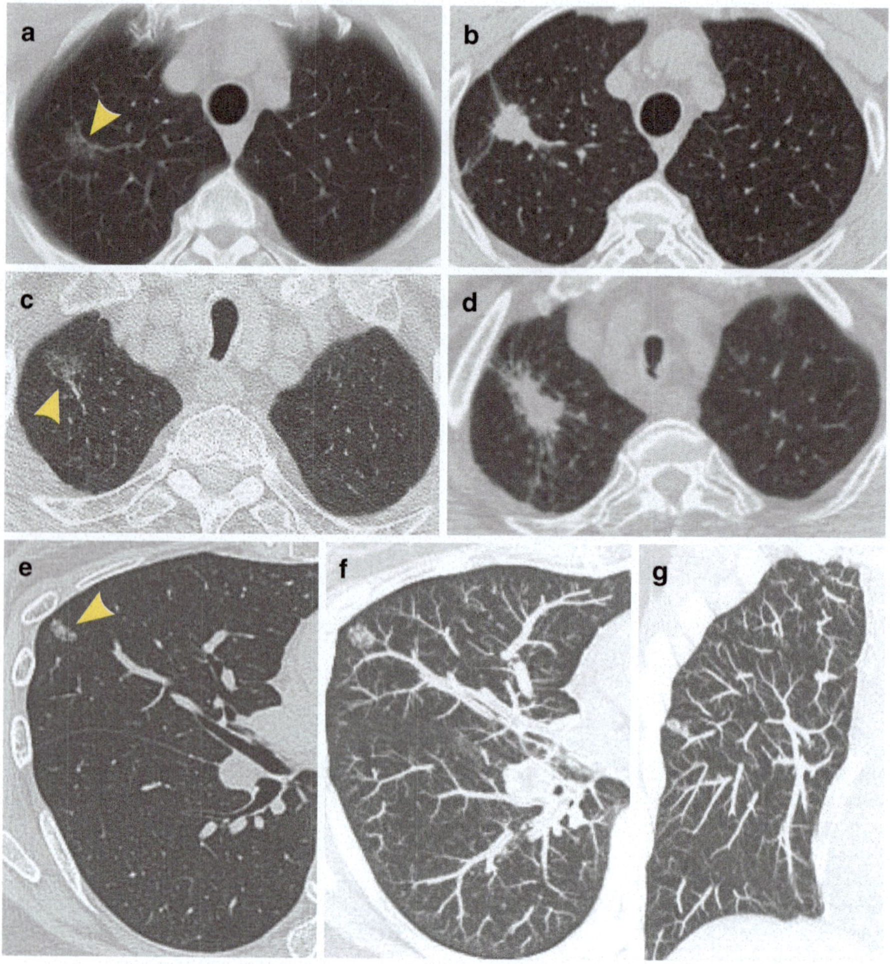

Fig. 9.10 Small adenocarcinoma with granulated pattern. (**a**, **b**) A cluster of granulated lesions were seen in the right upper lobe (**a**). Six years later, granulated lesions converged into a larger and denser nodule with enhancement, vasculatures and pleural indentation (**b**). Invasive adenocarcinoma was confirmed by surgical pathology. (**c**, **d**) A cluster of granulated lesions in the right upper lobe (**c**) converged into a larger, denser and enhanced nodule with spiculation and prominence on the margin during the follow-up period of 4 years (**d**). Invasive adenocarcinoma was confirmed by surgical pathology. (**e**–**g**) In the right middle lobe (was seen), a subsolid GGN containing multiple granulated solid components was seen (**e**). On the axial and coronal MIP images (**f**, **g**), evident microvessels were observed migrating into the nodule. Minimally invasive adenocarcinoma was confirmed by surgical pathology

tions of irregular or distorted "railway track" or "finger ring" appearance, tubular opacities, nodular prominence along bronchiolar walls, and string-of-bead appearance of solid components distributing along the bundles (Figs. 9.14, 9.15, 9.16, and 9.17).

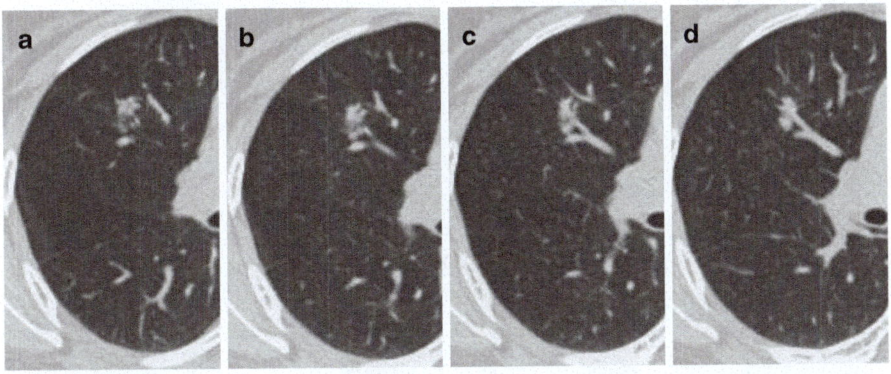

Fig. 9.11 Adenocarcinoma with granulated pattern. (**a**) An irregular subsolid GGN with measurement of 15 mm in diameter was found in the anterior segment of the right upper lobe in an otherwise healthy 54-year-old woman. Multiple granulated solid components in cluster alignment were present within the nodule. (**b–d**) Magnified views of the GGN in consecutive 1 mm slice-thickness images revealed various sizes of granulated solid components with acinar distribution. Invasive adenocarcinoma was definitely diagnosed with pathological confirmation

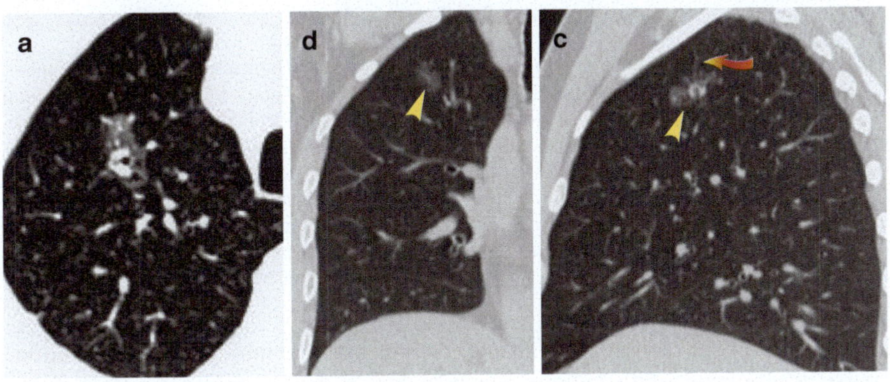

Fig. 9.12 Adenocarcinoma with piling pattern. (**a**) A 14 mm subsolid GGN was seen in the apical segment of the right upper lobe in an otherwise healthy 56-year-old man; the coronal (**b**) and sagittal (**c**) reformations revealed a ground-glass piling pattern on the irregular margin and characteristic CTA-TA sign (arrow). The GGN was resected with confirmation of MIA

9.6 Branching Pattern

If tumor cells spread along pre-existing small airways, for example, from alveolar ducts to respiratory bronchioles, to terminal bronchioles, even to more proximal bronchioles, the lesion may manifest a typical branching pattern on CT imaging, corresponding to the distribution of involved small airways. On a single cross-sectional image, the lesion may be a morphologically regular subsolid nodule with possible central lucencies if bronchiolar lumen is not entirely congested with tumor

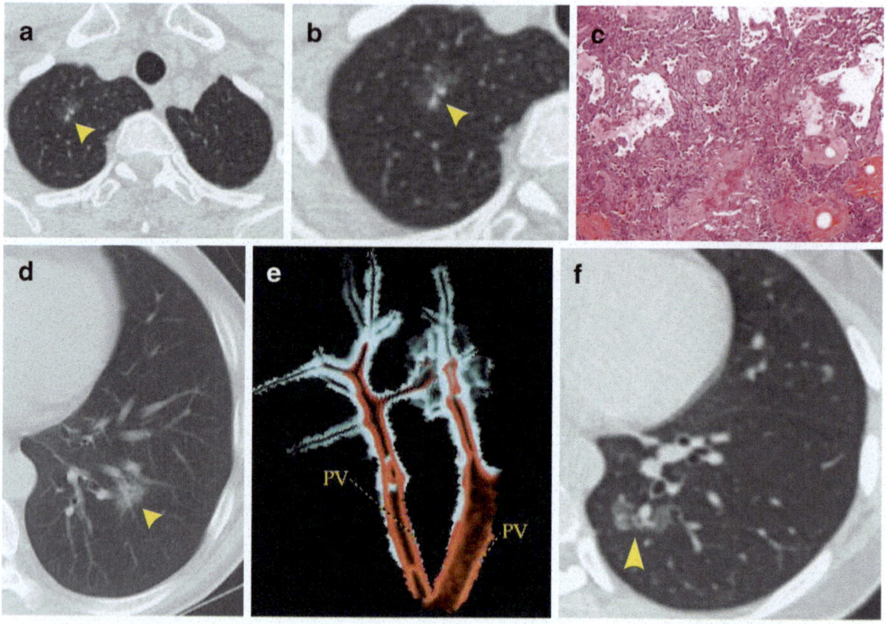

Fig. 9.13 Small adenocarcinoma with piling pattern. (**a–c**) In the apical segment of right upper lobe was seen a 14 mm irregular subsolid GGN (arrowhead) with spotty ≤5 mm solid component in an otherwise healthy 48-year-old woman. (**b**) The magnified view of GGN. (**c**) Microscopic examination showed disorderly distribution of minor stromal invasion of tumor cells, consistent with MIA (H&E stain, 100× magnification). (**d**, **e**) A 12 mm subsolid GGN (D, arrowhead) with piling pattern was seen in the left lower lobe. With volume rendering technique (**e**), the lesion distributed along pulmonary vessels, particularly branches of pulmonary veins. (**f**) A subsolid GGN with piling pattern and interconnecting vessels (arrowhead) was seen in the posterior segment of the left lower lobe, with histological confirmation of MIA

cells. However, on consecutive images or images with multiplanar reformation, coarse linear opacity with dichotomous branching is the typical finding (Figs. 9.18, 9.19, and 9.20). Besides that, various nonspecific manifestations may be seen dependent on the relationships between cross sections and the longitudinal axis of lesions.

9.7 Cavitary Pattern

Pseudocavitation, different from a real cavitation, is characterized by a round or oval low-attenuation area without evident contents or walls. It can be seen in pulmonary nodules or progressive consolidations. And it is reported that approximately 20% of lung adenocarcinomas could have this imaging sign in their early developmental stage [2]. Of note, the frequency of pseudocavitation in preinvasive and

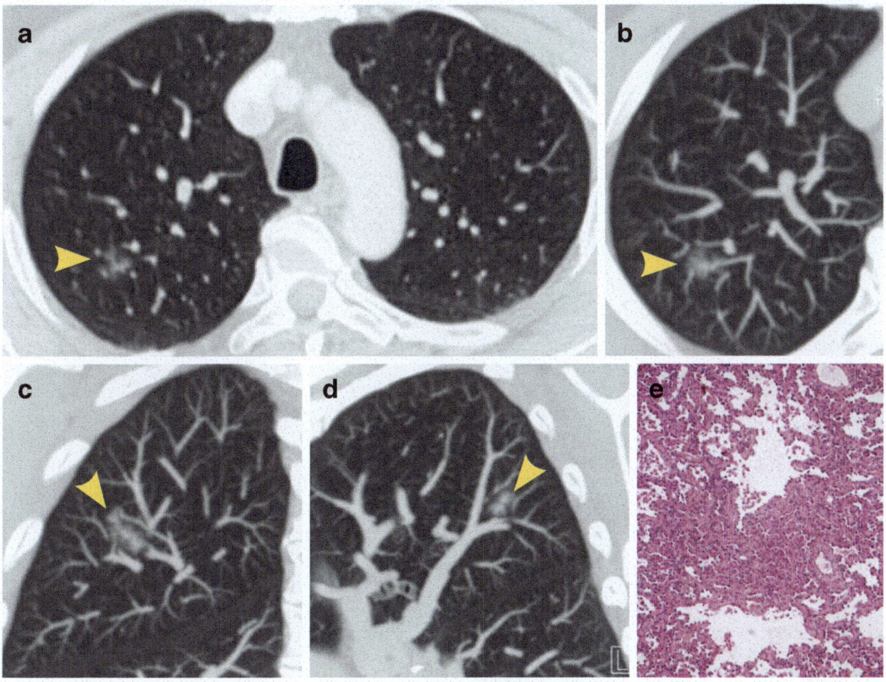

Fig. 9.14 Small adenocarcinoma with bronchovascular pattern. (**a**) In the apical segment of right upper lobe (was seen) a 5 mm subsolid GGN (arrowhead) was seen in a 43-year-old female patient; on the axial (**b**), coronal (**c**) and sagittal (**d**) reformations, the lesion was better visualized with bronchovascular distribution of invasive solid components. (**e**) Microscopic examination showed predominant lepidic growth of tumor cells with formations of papillary and micropapillary invasions, consistent with the diagnosis of MIA (H&E stain, 100× magnification)

minimally invasive adenocarcinomas (formerly bronchioloalveolar carcinoma) is reported as high as 50%. Pathologically, pseudocavitation reflects collective changes due to lepidic growth or infiltration of adenocarcinoma cells, including increasing solid components, thickening alveolar septa, and dilated bronchi in mixture with intact parenchyma. Typically, air-fluid level or necrotic change is absent. Pseudocavities are often multiple, are typically small (<1 cm in diameter), and may be scattered throughout a lesion. Because of these characteristics, pseudocavitation is sometimes referred to as "bubble-like lucencies" or "cystic air spaces" in a lesion (Figs. 9.21 and 9.22) [3].

In comparison to other types of NSCLC, the pseudocavitation sign has preference for adenocarcinomas, especially early-stage diseases. In a report from Tailor et al., the overall incidence of pseudocavitation in lung tumors was approximately 14.6%, and more than four fifths were associated with adenocarcinoma [4]. Obviously, this was reflected in the statistical analysis with a significant difference (*p* value, 0.007). Subgroup analysis by histology validated that adenocarcinoma had higher frequency (about four times) than other types of lung cancer in manifestation

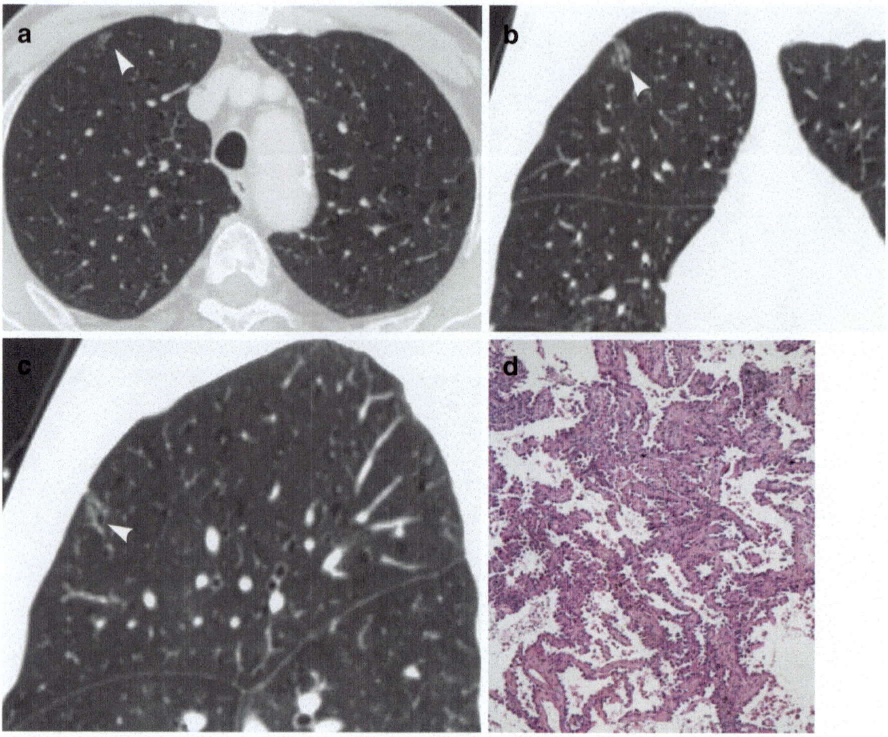

Fig. 9.15 Small adenocarcinoma with bronchovascular pattern. (**a**) In the apicoanterior segment of right upper lobe (was seen) a 4 mm subsolid GGN (arrowhead) was seen; on the coronal (**b**) and sagittal (**c**) reformations, the lesion appeared irregular, thin slab-like and perivascular in distribution. (**d**) Surgical pathology confirmed the diagnosis of AIS with the findings of tumor cells sparsely distributing and proliferating in lepidic pattern (H&E stain, 100× magnification)

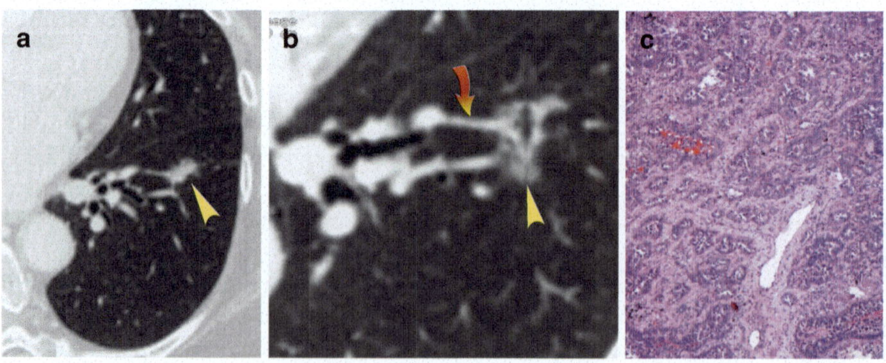

Fig. 9.16 Small adenocarcinoma with bronchovascular pattern. (**a**) An irregular linear subsolid GGN (arrowhead) was found in the anterior segment of left lower lobe in an 82-year-old female patient. (**b**) Curved planar reformations showed perivascular invasion and characteristic CTA-TA sign with two vessels (arrow) migrating into the lesion (arrowhead). (**c**) Invasive adenocarcinoma was histologically confirmed with findings of atypical acinar invasion (H&E stain, 100× magnification)

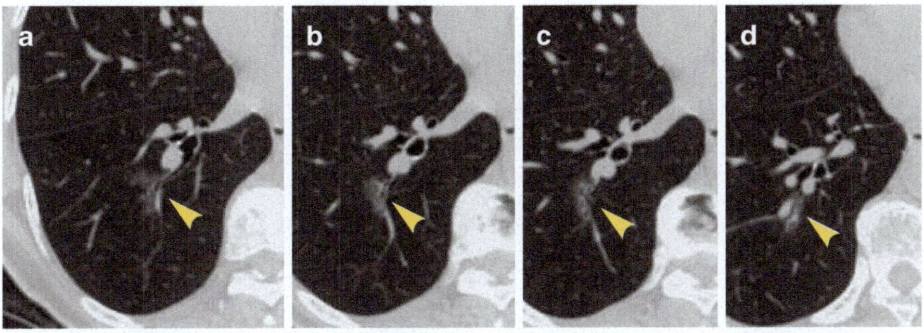

Fig. 9.17 Small adenocarcinoma with bronchovascular pattern. A 12 mm subsolid GGN (arrowhead) was seen in the right lower lobe in a 75-year-old female patient. On consecutive images (**a–d**), the lesion distributed along the longitudinal direction of bronchovascular bundles. The GGN was histologically diagnosed as MIA

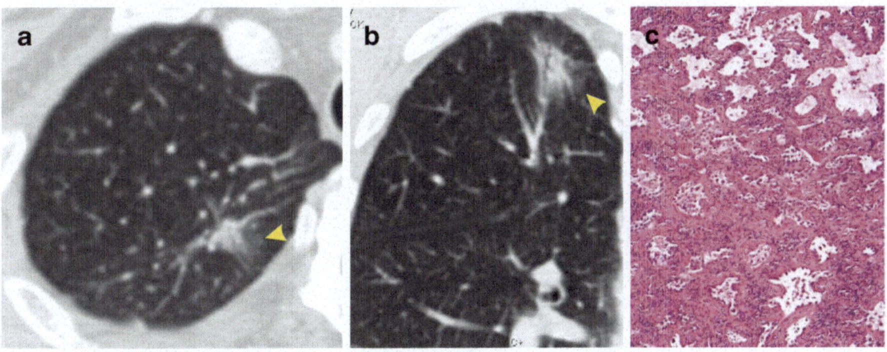

Fig. 9.18 Small adenocarcinoma with branching pattern. A 15 mm subsolid GGN (**a**, arrowhead) was found in the apical segment of the right upper lobe in a 62-year-old female patient. Coronal reformations (**b**) revealed a heterogeneous lesion with branching appearance, spiculation, and halo sign (arrowhead) along the margin. Microscopic examination of surgical specimens showed the disorderly distribution of acinar invasion in the background of fibrosis, suggestive of the histological diagnosis of invasive adenocarcinoma (**c**, H&E stain, 100× magnification)

of pseudocavitation. Hence, a calculated specificity of the pseudocavitation for differential diagnosis of adenocarcinoma was 0.94. Considering the low sensitivity (0.22), radiologists should be aware that the absence of pseudocavitation cannot rule out the diagnosis of adenocarcinoma.

Histologically, pseudocavitation reflects the lepidic growth pattern, i.e., the propensity of tumor cells growing along alveolar walls without disrupting lung architecture and resultant residual air spaces or air bronchograms, which may be accentuated by fibrotic contraction. In contrast, since nonlepidic growth commonly causes compression or obliteration of small airways or airspaces, pseudocavitation in nonlepidic adenocarcinomas is an uncommon finding [5]. Hence, pseudocavitation may be considered as a potential predictor of lepidic growth as well as favorable prognosis correspondingly.

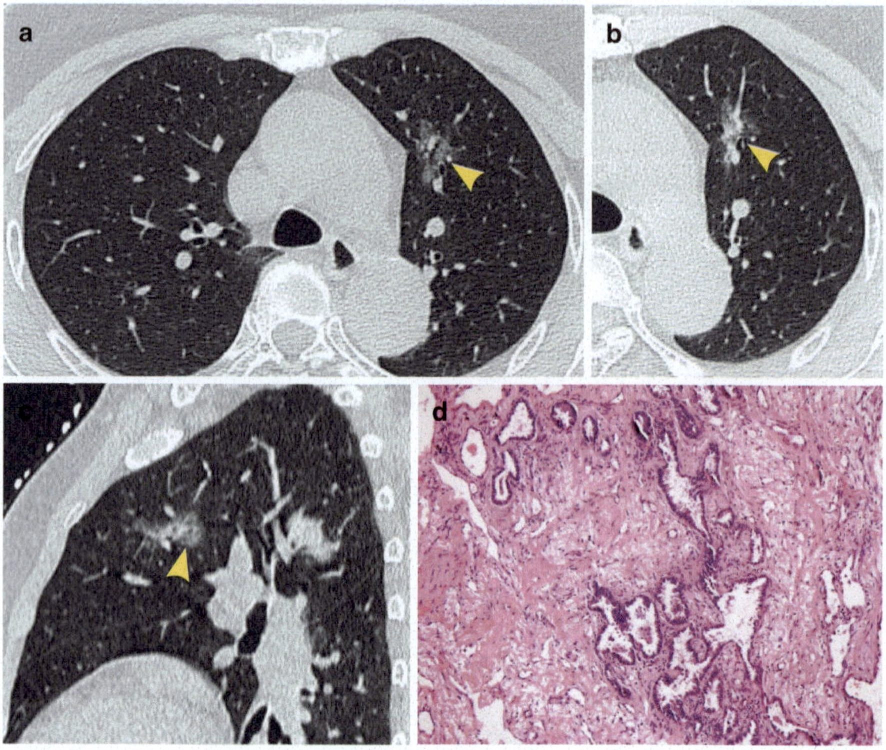

Fig. 9.19 Small adenocarcinoma with branching pattern. A 14 mm long subsolid GGN (**a**, **b**, arrowhead) was found in the anterior segment of the left upper lobe in a 53-year-old female patient. Sagittal reformations (**c**) revealed a branching lesion in correlation with the pathological findings that tumor cells proliferated along the bronchiolar walls in lepidic pattern with minor amount of stromal invasion, suggestive of the histological diagnosis of MIA (D, H&E stain, 100× magnification)

9.8 Honeycombing Pattern

According to the glossary of terms for thoracic imaging published by the Fleischner Society, honeycombing represents destroyed and fibrotic lung tissue containing numerous cystic airspaces with thick fibrous walls, representing the late stage of various lung diseases. The honeycombing pattern in a small adenocarcinoma describes that multiple cystic lucencies are observed within the tumor. On CT scans, the cystic lucencies range in size on the order of 3–8 mm with well-defined walls 1–3 mm in thickness (Figs. 9.23 and 9.24). Pathologically, honeycombing indirectly reflects the lepidic growth of tumor cells along alveolar walls but not entirely occupying alveolar cavities. The residual alveolar airspaces are imaged as cystic lucencies. Occasionally, extensive stromal invasion results in the loss of acinar architecture and deformed alveolar cavities filled with mucin.

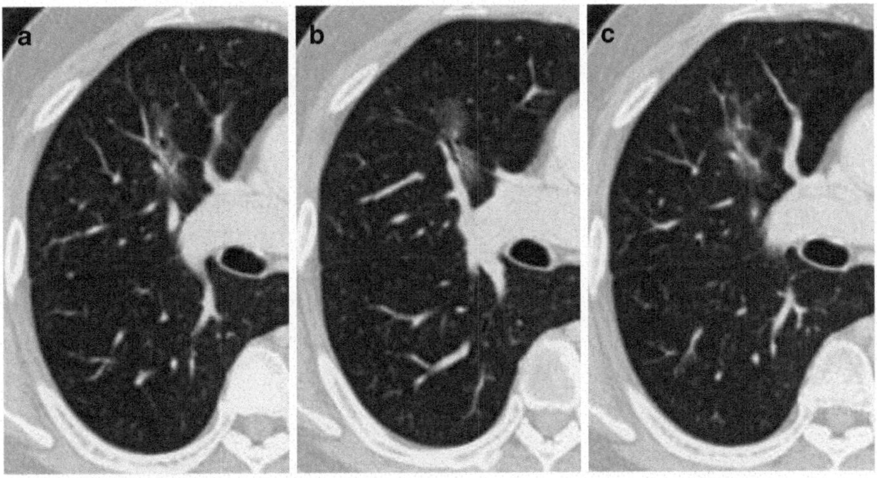

Fig. 9.20 Small adenocarcinoma with branching pattern. (**a**–**c**) In the anterior segment of the right upper lobe (was seen), a subsolid GGN of 20 mm in longitudinal measurement was seen. On consecutive images, the lesion had a branching appearance distributing along the bronchiolar walls. The diagnosis of MIA was histologically confirmed

9.9 Scar-Like Pattern

Pulmonary scars are common findings in chest CT imaging. Scars are chronic organizing fibrotic tissues and traditionally ruled out of possibility of malignancy as well as routine imaging follow-up. However, several studies have reported that lung cancers occasionally present as fibrotic changes or as scar-like lesions or grow on the basis of pre-existing fibrotic scars, hence the scar cancer or scar-cinoma [6]. At the mechanistic level, lung fibrosis is considered to be the result of a dysregulated wound repair response to lung injury characterized by the accumulation and persistence of activated reparative mesenchymal cells. Like fibrosis, tumors have been described as "wounds that do not heal," and an extensive literature supports the overlapping mechanisms of wound repair, chronic inflammation, and cancer. Among these mechanisms are critical roles for tumor stroma and tumor-associated fibroblasts. TGF-β signaling in fibroblasts, for instance, has been identified as a major determinant of the oncogenic potential of adjacent epithelia. In light of these evidences, fibrotic scars should not be completely exempt from routine monitoring.

On consecutive follow-up CT scans, if ground-glass opacities extend from the rigid margin of pre-existing scar tissues or some parts of scar tissues are gradually replaced by ground-glass components, scar-cinoma should be highly suspected (Figs. 9.25 and 9.26). This kind of presentation is usually slow growing, and the volume-doubling time (could) can be up to years; long-term routine follow-up CT scans are mandatory for detecting disease progression and differential diagnosis. In some cases with equivocal findings, empirical antibiotic administration may be given to exclude the possibility of chronic inflammation.

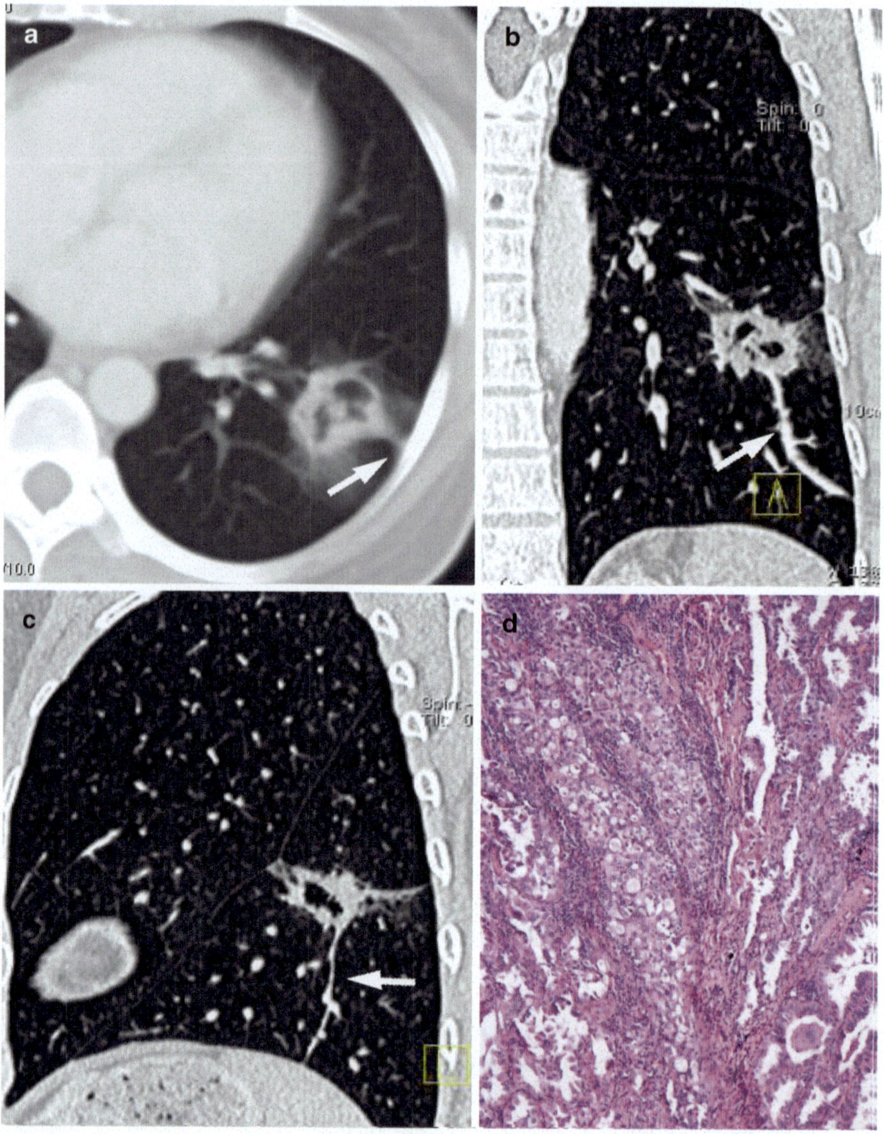

Fig. 9.21 Small adenocarcinoma with cavitary pattern. A 22 mm lesion was seen in the subpleural area in lateral segment of the left lower lobe with signs of cavitation, halo, and pleural indentation (**a**, arrow). The coronal and sagittal images showed irregular cavitation within the solid lesion and pleural involvement (**b**, **c**, arrow). Empirical antifungal treatment was given but failed. CT-guide biopsy found malignant cells, and lobectomy of left lower lobe was performed with pathological confirmation of invasive adenocarcinoma (**d**, H&E stain, 100× magnification)

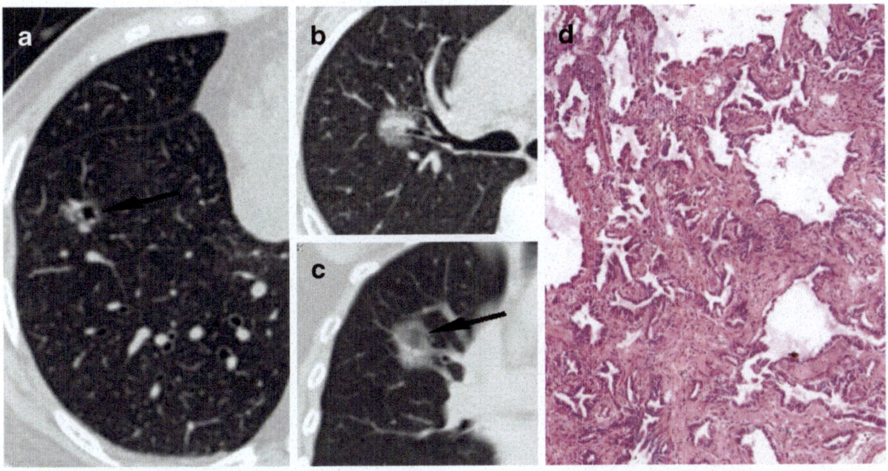

Fig. 9.22 Small adenocarcinoma with cavitary pattern. Pseudocavitation commonly can be well visualized in axial CT images (**a**, arrow). Otherwise, MPR should be utilized for better evaluation (**b**, **c** arrow). This patient received surgery, and microscopic examination revealed irregular acinar invasion with stromal fibrosis (H&E stain, 100× magnification)

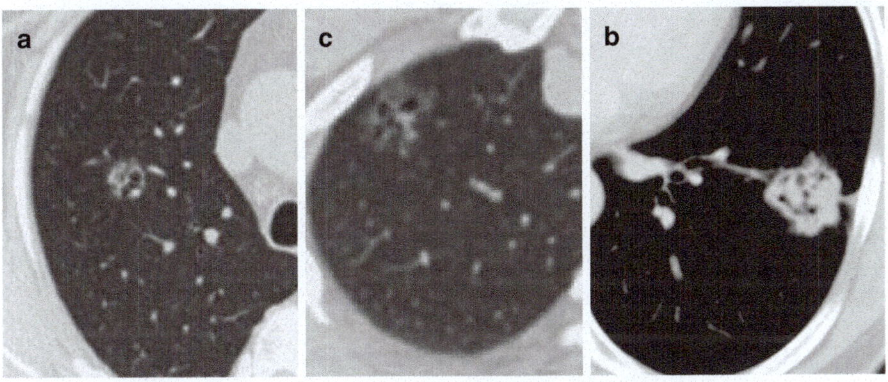

Fig. 9.23 Small adenocarcinoma with honeycombing pattern. Subsolid GGNs were seen in three individual patients (**a**–**c**). These lesions shared common imaging features, including multiple clusters of air-containing cysts, measuring 3 mm in diameter and 1–3 mm in the thickness of cystic walls, generating a honeycomb pattern. All GGNs were surgically resected with histological confirmation of adenocarcinoma

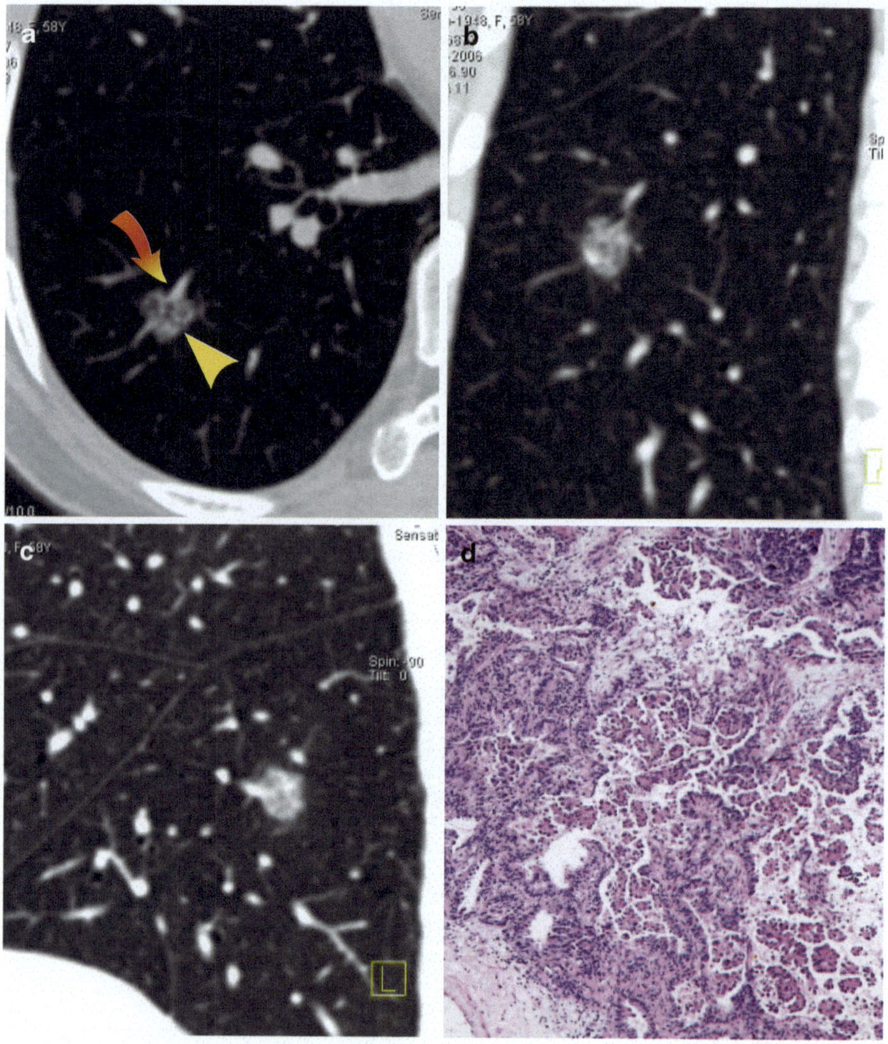

Fig. 9.24 Small adenocarcinoma with honeycombing pattern. In the right lower lobe (was seen), a subsolid GGN (arrowhead) was seen with evident tumor vessels (arrow) and a honeycomb pattern (**a**). In cases with equivocal findings in axial images, multiple planar reformations may be of special use for better visualization of specific features. In the same patient, coronal (**b**) and sagittal (**c**) reformations showed characteristic CTA-TA sign contributing to the diagnosis of adenocarcinoma. Surgical pathology confirmed the diagnosis of mixed adenocarcinoma with papillary, micropapillary, and acinar components (H&E stain, 40× magnification)

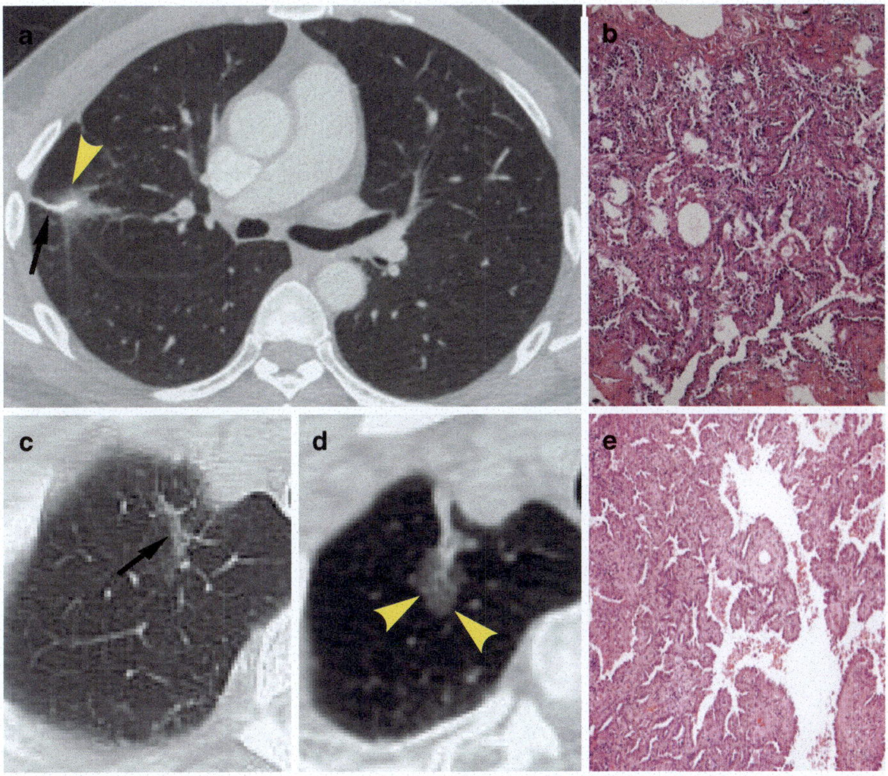

Fig. 9.25 Small adenocarcinoma with scar-like pattern. (**a**, **b**) Ill-defined focal ground-glass opacities (arrowhead, **a**) appeared along the margin of postoperative fibrotic scars (arrow) in the right lung with suspicion of malignancy. Surgical pathology revealed a great amount of irregular acinar invasion (**b**) in the fibrotic background, indicative of invasive adenocarcinoma (H&E stain, 100× magnification). (**c**–**e**) Ground-glass opacities (arrowhead) continuously developed around the tuberculous fibrotic tissues (arrow) in the right upper lobe during the 6-year follow-up of 2005 through 2011. Microscopic examination revealed irregular acinar structures with micropapillary invasion (H&E stain, 40× magnification)

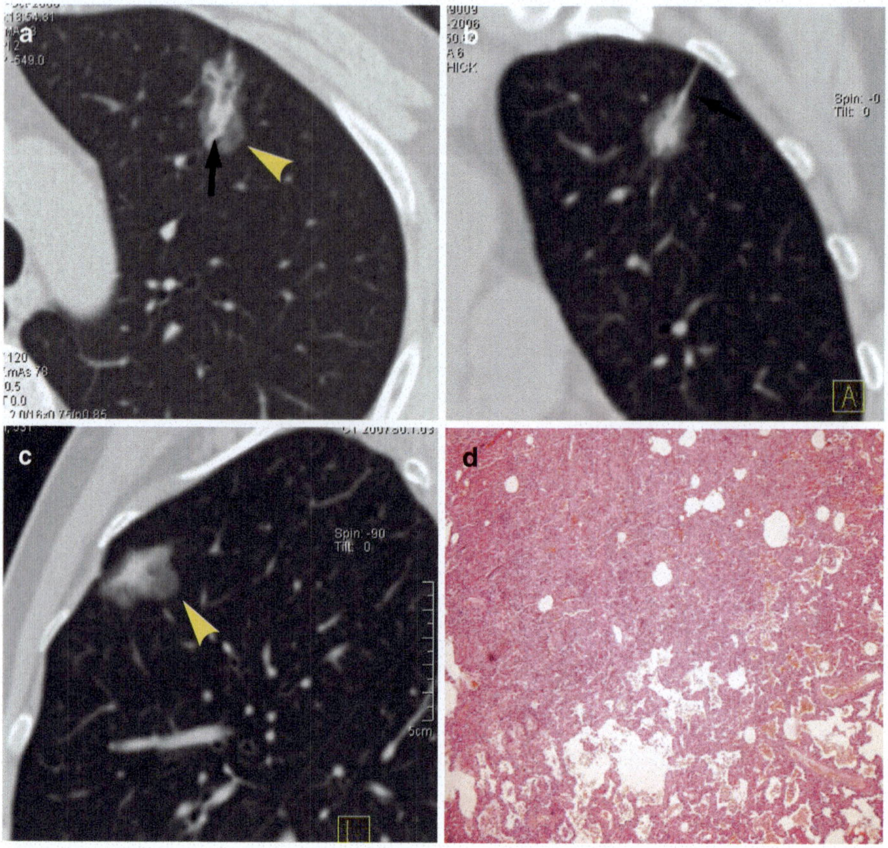

Fig. 9.26 Small adenocarcinoma with scar-like pattern. During the period of 4-year consecutive follow-up, surrounding the pre-existing fibrotic scar (arrow) (were seen), ground-glass opacities (arrowhead) were seen with a slow but persistent growing pattern, pathologically proven to be adenocarcinoma. A, axial view; B, coronal view; C, sagittal view; D, microscopic view (H&E stain, 40× magnification)

9.10 Umbilical Pattern

If a tumor is located by interlobular fissure, the fissure may be invaded and retracted toward the tumor. Histologically, the visceral pleura of the fissure may be irregularly thickening due to nodular microinvasive foci-reactive fibrotic hyperplasia. On CT, the involved pleura is connected to the tumor via a linear, or necklace-like, or Y-shape, or V-shape structure, which produces the pleural indentation sign at the pleural side and the umbilical concave at the tumor side (Figs. 9.27 and 9.28).

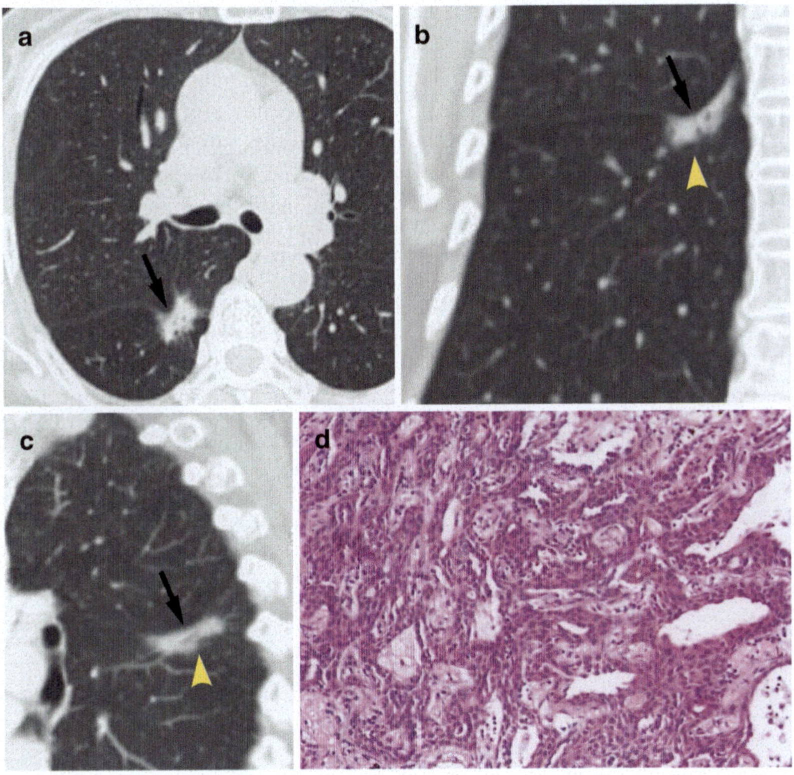

Fig. 9.27 Small adenocarcinoma with umbilical pattern. In the superior segment of the right lower lobe (was seen), a subsolid GGN (arrowhead) with lobulation was seen. The pleural invasion and traction (was) were evident with the appearance of the necklace-like umbilical pattern (arrow). Microscopic examination showed invasive proliferation of tumor cells and acinar structures within the lesion, consistent with invasive adenocarcinoma. A, axial view; B, coronal view; C, sagittal view; D, microscopic view (H&E stain, 200× magnification)

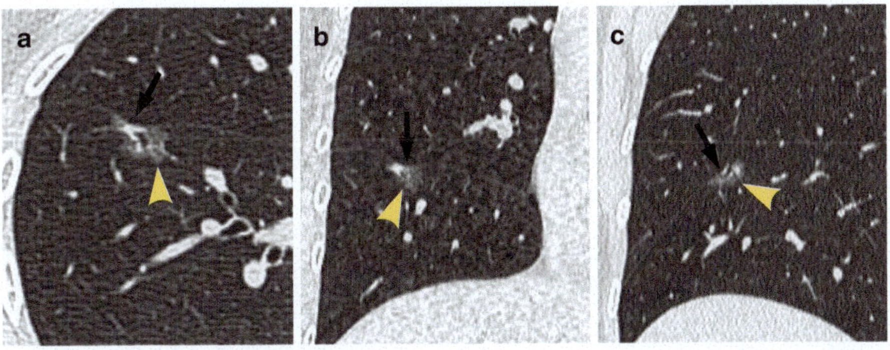

Fig. 9.28 Small adenocarcinoma with umbilical pattern. In the anterior segment of the right lower lobe (was seen), a subsolid GGN (arrowhead) was seen with pseudocavitation and interlobar pleural involvement presenting as an umbilical pattern (arrow). Surgical pathology confirmed the diagnosis of MIA. A, axial view; B, coronal view; C, sagittal view

References

1. Maffessanti M, Dalpiaz G. Diffuse lung diseases: clinical features, pathology, HRCT. 1st ed. Milan: Springer-Verlag Italia; 2004.
2. Hansell DM, Bankier AA, MacMahon H, McLoud TC, Muller NL, Remy J. Fleischner society: glossary of terms for thoracic imaging. Radiology. 2008;246(3):697–722. https://doi.org/10.1148/radiol.2462070712.
3. Kojima Y, Saito H, Sakuma Y, Kondo T, Ito H, Tsuboi M, Oshita F, Nakayama H, Yokose T, Kameda Y, Noda K, Yamada K. Correlations of thin-section computed tomographic, histopathological, and clinical findings of adenocarcinoma with a bubblelike appearance. J Comput Assist Tomogr. 2010;34(3):413–7. https://doi.org/10.1097/RCT.0b013e3181d275b6.
4. Tailor TD, Schmidt RA, Eaton KD, Wood DE, Pipavath SN. The Pseudocavitation sign of lung adenocarcinoma: a distinguishing feature and imaging biomarker of Lepidic growth. J Thorac Imaging. 2015;30(5):308–13. https://doi.org/10.1097/rti.0000000000000168.
5. Nakazono T, Sakao Y, Yamaguchi K, Imai S, Kumazoe H, Kudo S. Subtypes of peripheral adenocarcinoma of the lung: differentiation by thin-section CT. Eur Radiol. 2005;15(8):1563–8. https://doi.org/10.1007/s00330-004-2595-7.
6. Horowitz JC, Osterholzer JJ, Marazioti A, Stathopoulos GT. "scar-cinoma": viewing the fibrotic lung mesenchymal cell in the context of cancer biology. Eur Respir J. 2016;47(6):1842–54. https://doi.org/10.1183/13993003.01201-2015.

Chapter 10
Multiple Primary Early-Stage Lung Cancer

Xiangpeng Zheng

Multiple primary lung cancer (MPLC) describes an entity of two or more lung cancerous lesions with independent origins simultaneously or successively occurred in one patient. Despite that MPLC was firstly described by Billroth and von Winiwarter over 100 years ago, it is Beyreuther who is credited with directing attention to this subgroup of cancer patients with his 1924 report of two primary lung cancers at autopsy in a tuberculosis patient. Since then, more clinical case reports have been published with a reported incidence 3.8%. With the extensive utilization of CT, especially submillimeter high-resolution multidetector spiral CT in the evaluation of lung diseases and lung cancer screening, the detection rate of MPLC rises rapidly and the latest incidence is reported in the range of 5–6%.

The pathogenesis of MPLC remains not fully understood yet. Currently, four underlying theoretical mechanisms have been proposed.

1. *Field cancerization.* This concept initially was introduced to account for the development of oral squamous cell carcinoma by Slaughter et al. in 1953 and then extrapolated to other solid tumors [1]. According to this theory, lung cancer per se can be presumed as a potential multicentric/multifocal disease with spatial and temporal heterogeneity. High-risk factors, such as cigarettes, exert atypia-inducing or carcinogenic effects on epithelial cells along respiratory tracts and provide proliferation momentum for disease progression. And the development of primary lung cancer results from the continuous exposure to carcinogenic stimuli of several areas of the lung with a different risk for cancer development. Therefore, the distribution of cellular mutations and the resulting neoplasms are relatively extensive rather than isolated or solitary, which is described pathologically as field cancerization. Given adequate time, detectable microscopic or macroscopic tumors occur within lungs.

X. Zheng
Department of Radiation Oncology, Fudan University Huadong Hospital, Shanghai, China
e-mail: zhengxp@fudan.edu.cn

X. Zheng et al. (eds.), *Early-stage Lung Cancer*,
https://doi.org/10.1007/978-981-10-7596-4_10

2. *Aging*. Correlations have been reported between the aging and the incidence of MPLC, suggesting that respiratory degeneration and accumulated cellular mutations may have some roles in the development of MPLC. Statistical data revealed that MPLC accounted for 5–12% of lung cancers in patients at the age of 54–64 years old, while the prevalence of MPLC in lung cancer patients over 80 years old could be somewhere between 12 and 26%.
3. *Familial genetic predisposition*. A growing body of evidence has implied the potential link between MPLC and genetic susceptibility. In particular, it seems that the occurrence of MPLC has a familial predisposition. The risk of development of a second even third primary lung cancer in a lung cancer patient with a family history of any cancer is significantly higher than patients without a family history of cancer. This risk could be up to nine times.
4. *Iatrogenic factors*. Chemotherapy or radiotherapy is commonly used to treat the first primary lung cancer, and both treatments have carcinogenic risks. Lung cancers secondary to chemotherapy or radiotherapy have been sporadically reported. In addition, iatrogenic radiation exposure from examinations, for instance, annual low-dose CT screening, mammography, and nuclear medicine examination, increases the risk of tumorigenesis in lungs as well as other parts of the body.

10.1 Clinical Characteristics of Multiple Primary Lung Cancer

The diagnosis of MPLC remains challenging. Pulmonary multifocal nodules may be reflections of many entities, including infectious diseases, advanced stages of primary lung cancer (T3 or T4), and intrapulmonary metastases from other malignancies. Therefore, the diagnosis of MPLC requires a thorough review of medical history, meticulous imaging evaluations, and an exclusion strategy to rule out other possibilities. Table 10.1 briefly lists the diagnostic criteria of MPLC and comparison with common differential diseases according to the guidelines from the American College of Chest Physicians (ACCP) [2, 3].

Generally, MPLC is classified as synchronous MPLC (sMPLC) and metachronous MPLC (mMPLC) mainly depending on whether cancerous lesions are present at the same time or a later time. For diagnosis of sMPLC, two or more lesions are detected or resected simultaneously or sequentially with an interval less than 6 months. If the interval is more than 2 years, mMPLC should be advised. A significant variability in genetic profiles among MPLC has been reported, including somatic mutations in oncogenes or tumor suppressor genes, X-chromosome inactivation, or loss of heterozygosity (LOH) [7]. Among them, mutation analysis of the p53 tumor suppressor gene was reported to be a valid diagnostic tool for a solid diagnosis in 35–66% of synchronous and metachronous cancer cases and hence could be used as a molecular marker for differentiation of MPLC and intrapulmonary metastases. EGFR and K-ras mutations are common genetic events in the pathogen-

Table 10.1 A brief comparison between MPLC, multiple intrapulmonary metastases, and T3 and T4 tumors with multiple nodules

<table>
<tr><th>Disease</th><th colspan="2">Characteristics</th></tr>
<tr><td>MPLC modified from Shen et al. [4]</td><td colspan="2">A: Same histology, in combination with one of the following:
• Different lobes, and no N2, 3 involvement, and no systemic metastases
• Temporarily separated and ≥4-year interval between cancers and no systemic metastases from either cancer
B: Different histology, or different molecular genetic characteristics, or arising separately from focus of carcinoma in situ</td></tr>
<tr><td>MPLC modified from Antakli et al. [5]</td><td colspan="2">A: Different histological conditions
B: Same histological condition with two or more of the following:
• Anatomical distinct
• Associated premalignant lesion
• No systemic metastases
• No mediastinal spread
• Different DNA ploidy</td></tr>
<tr><td>MPLC by Martini Criteria [6]</td><td>Synchronous MPLC (sMPLC):
A. Tumors physically distinct and separate
B. Histological type:
1. Different
2. Same, but in different segment, lobe or lung originally from carcinoma in situ, without carcinoma in common lymphatics and extrapulmonary metastases at the time of diagnosis</td><td>Metachronous MPLC (mMPLC):
A. Histologically different
B. Histologically identical, if The free interval between cancers ≥2 years without carcinoma in common lymphatics and extrapulmonary metastases at the time of diagnosis</td></tr>
<tr><td>Multiple intrapulmonary metastases</td><td colspan="2">Same histology, in combination with one of the following:
• Multiple extrapulmonary metastases
• Different lobes and presence of N2, 3 involvement
• ≤2-year interval</td></tr>
<tr><td>T3 (multiple nodules)</td><td colspan="2">Multiple nodules with same histology and located in the same lobe as the primary tumor</td></tr>
<tr><td>T4 (multiple nodules)</td><td colspan="2">Multiple nodules with same histology but located in anatomically separated and different ipsilateral lobe from primary cancer</td></tr>
</table>

esis of lung adenocarcinoma and in particular the driven force in the early developmental stage, such as AAH. Combinations of K-ras mutations with 3p deletions and p53 alterations and combinations of EGFR and p53 have been suggested as a useful marker of the clonal origin of the multiple neoplastic and preneoplastic lesions with similar histopathological features.

For once MPLC, especially sMPLC, was presumed as a rare entity. However, the advancement in imaging technology has shown that the incidence of this particular lung cancer is underestimated. And histological types found in sMPLC have changed with the predominance of multiple primary adenocarcinomas over squamous cell carcinoma. On resected specimens, the major pattern of MPLC is the coexisting of preinvasive lesions, atypical adenomatous hyperplasia (AAH) and adenocarcinoma in situ (AIS), and invasive lesions, minimally invasive adenocarcinoma (MIA) and invasive adenocarcinoma (IAC). Due to the heterogeneity of coexisting lung cancers in developmental stages, histology, genetic profiles, and locations, the management of patients with sMPLC is complicated with a variable prognosis, which is typically worse than the solitary lung cancer. Thus, patients are suspected of sMPLC should undergo a careful clinical and radiographic assessment for distant and mediastinal node metastases. Approximately one-third of the second foci of cancer are found incidentally at the time of resection.

Metachronous MPLC is much more difficult in diagnosis than sMPLC. The time interval from the first lung cancer and exclusion of intrapulmonary metastases are the key points. According to Martini criteria, the minimum interval between detection of the first primary tumor and the appearance of the second or more primary tumors should be 2 years. In other studies, different interval thresholds have been used from 24 to 48 months. Considering the previous history of lung cancer, intrapulmonary metastases should be excluded prior to the diagnosis of mMPLC, especially in the circumstance of same histology found in primary and second lung cancers, which may require comprehensive evaluation including invasive procedures (percutaneous CT-guided biopsy or transbronchial lung biopsy), imaging (PET/CT, MRI, etc.), and immunohistochemical and genetic analysis. It is reported that the incidence of metachronous second primary lung cancers is estimated to be 0.5% overall, including 2.5% of the surgical patients and 10–32% of long-term survivors. The risk of developing an mMPLC after curative resection of an initial early-stage NSCLC is 0.65 to 5% annually. A review of 346 surgical specimens found mMPLC in 10% of stage I NSCLC patients [8]. As far as location, there appears to be a prevalence for metachronous lesions to develop on the same side as the initial primary lung cancer. Feld et al. reported the metachronous second primary lung cancers in 390 stage I and II NSCLC patients to occur twice as often on the ipsilateral side compared to the contralateral side, 26% and 13%, respectively [9].

10.2 Imaging Features of Multiple Primary Lung Cancer

MPLC can occur in the setting of multiple AAH, AIS, and invasive adenocarcinoma, indicating that the imaging features of either sMPLC or mMPLC are the collective imaging characteristics of each independent lesion. In chest CT imaging, MPLC is commonly described as multifocal nodular opacities, and similarities or differences in attenuation may provide clues regarding the relative percentage of lepidic versus solid histologic components. Of note, subsolid nodules are very rarely metastatic.

Each nodular lesion should be independently analyzed, leading to various imaging features seen in MPLC cases, which from radio-pathological perspective reflects the multicentric origin and dynamic progression of separated lesions. AAH, AIS, MIA, LPA, and IAC may be found simultaneously or by different combinations in a patient. According to the definition of MPLC, there is no correlation among the various lesions in origin. Therefore, imaging features related to the solitary early-stage lung cancer discussed in previous chapters could be found in the case of MPLC.

The high-resolution chest CT imaging is capable of detecting tiny-sized pulmonary nodules, multiple times as many as with conventional chest radiography. Each pulmonary nodule should be meticulously analyzed and recorded for comparison and future follow-up if necessary, including the following:

- Incidentally detected or persistent nodule.
- Sizes in three dimensions, location, and distribution.
- Nodular classification: pure GGN, subsolid GGN, or solid nodule. When a ground-glass component is predominant in nodules, multiple primary cancers are more likely than metastatic nodules which are characterized by solid components.
- If subsolid component exists, evaluate the ratio of solid components.
- Evaluation of microvasculature related to the nodule according to the anatomical relationship proposed in Chap. 5.
- Other possible imaging features described in previous chapters and response to medical interventions (mostly antibiotic use).

In consistency with genetic findings, MPLC has a familial predisposition. The direct clinical implication is that when a patient is suspected of MPLC, the family medical history should be inquired, and the immediate family members are advised for lung cancer screening on a routine basis (Figs. 10.1 and 10.2). And if one family member has been proven to have MPLC, the other family members with persistent multifocal pulmonary GGNs are encountered with higher risks of MPLC than the general population. As stated in the previous section and reported in numerous studies, remarkable heterogeneity, both intertumoral and intratumoral, has been observed in MPLC cases [10]. Liu et al. analyzed genetic profiles of 15 MPLC using whole-genome sequencing (WGS) or whole-exome sequencing in combination with microarray-based comparative genomic hybridization (CGH), suggesting that in the context of identical constitutional genetic background and environmental exposure, different lung cancers in the same individual may have distinct genetic profiles and can be driven by distinct molecular events (Fig. 10.3) [11]. Obviously, the intertumoral heterogeneity complicates the treatment decision and account for the variations in response to treatment observed in MPLC cases.

Despite that it remains unclear whether there exists a certain correlation between tumor imaging presentation and genetic mutation site, a recent genetic growth study on 104 GGNs reported that quadruple-negative GGNs (i.e., negative for EGFR, ALK, HER2, and KRAS mutations) tend to show an indolent biological behavior pattern (significantly long volume-doubling time and mild increase of solid component in a 2-year follow-up period) with significant association with preinvasive diseases (AAH/AIS), whereas EGFR mutation-positive tumors were correlated with growth and invasive diseases (MIA and IAC) [12].

In MPLC cases, each cancer may have same histology or different histology. For the latter, a diagnosis of MPLC is not difficult. But in the former situation,

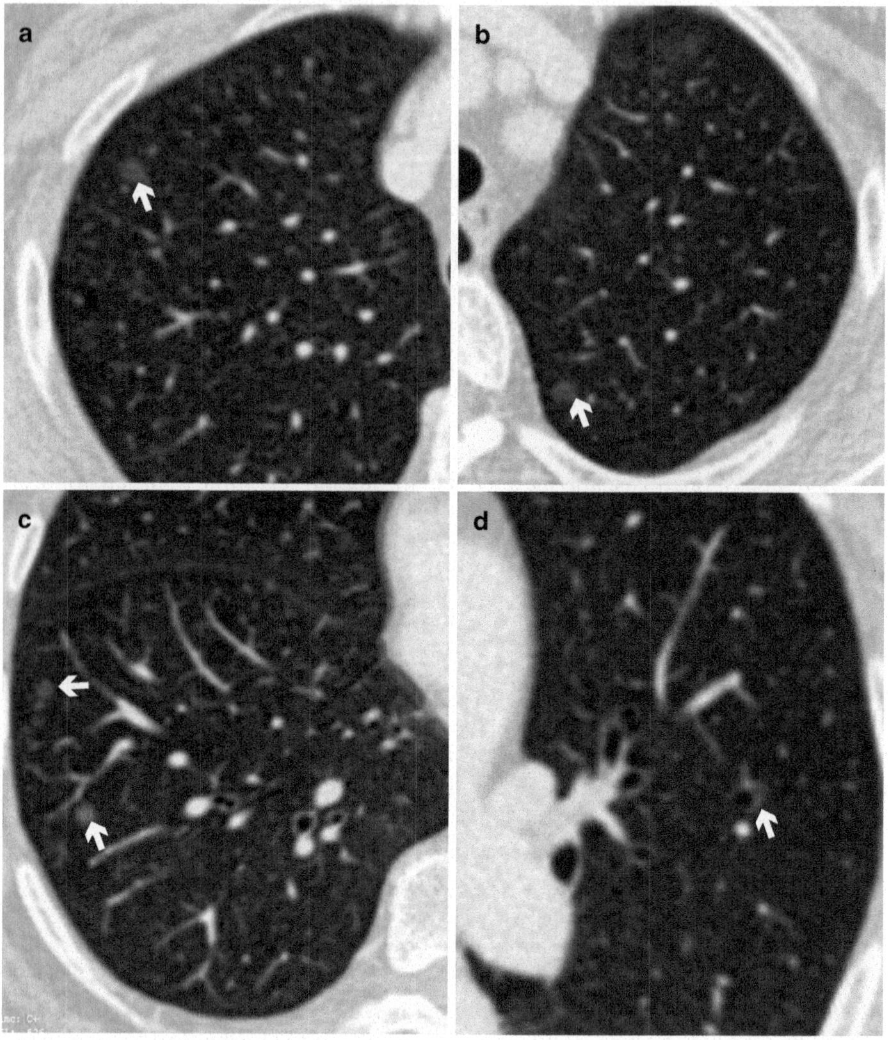

Fig. 10.1 Synchronous MPLC. A 58-year-old female received lung cancer screening. Multiple intrapulmonary pure and subsolid ground-glass nodules (arrowhead) were found. Microvascular formation was visualized in some lesions (C). Despite empirical antibiotic therapy, nodular lesions were persistent without evidential response. During the 2-year follow-up, no significant change was seen in nodular size and density. An imaging diagnosis of synchronous MPLC is suspected with AAHs in images a and d and AISs in images b and c

intrapulmonary metastases should be distinguished and excluded. The following CT imaging features may be helpful for differential diagnosis. (1) Most nodules in MPLC cases possess typical imaging characteristics of primary lung cancer, i.e., isolated round or oval nodules with lobulated and/or spiculated morphology, coarse or irregular edges, heterogeneous attenuation, and probably accompanying by

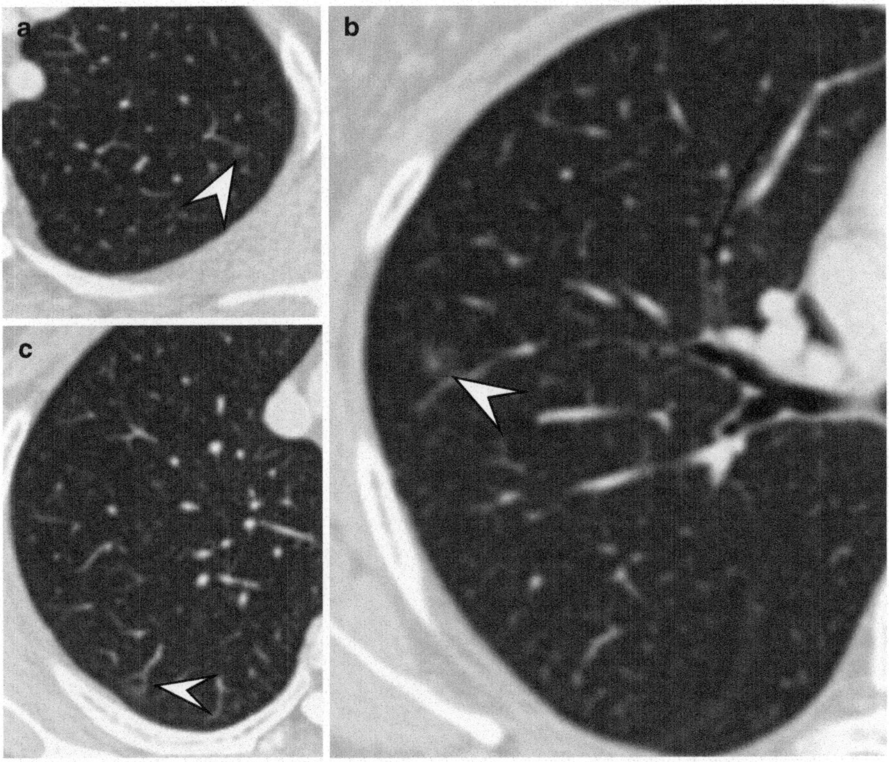

Fig. 10.2 Synchronous MPLC. A 61-year-old female received lung cancer screening with a referral of her family physician due to suspicious sMPLC found in her sister (Fig. 10.1). They lived in separated cities, Guangzhou and Shanghai, for decades. Same as her sister, multiple GGNs (arrowhead) were found in her bilateral lungs with the predominance of upper lobes. In some lesions, feeding blood microvessels (**a** and **c**) and central solid components (**b**) were visible. No response to antibiotic use and no evidential change with 2-year follow-up indicated a persistent nodular disease. Synchronous MPLC was suspected. Imaging diagnosis: AISs in images a and c; AAH in image b

bronchial or vascular stenosis, whereas metastatic nodules commonly present as multiple spherical solid nodules or masses with homogeneous density and well-defined margin. Lobulation sign and lobar or segmental atelectasis are infrequently seen. (2) The majority of nodular lesions in MPLC cases have a sluggish growing pattern with significant volume-doubling time. Patients with MPLC are typically in good physical condition and could be put on active surveillance before a definitive treatment approach is determined. In contrast, most patients with metastatic diseases are unavoidably facing quick progression unless effective systemic therapies are given. (3) Locoregional lymph node involvement or distant metastasis or abnormal tumor biomarker level is seldom found in patients with MPLC at the time of diagnosis while fairly common in metastatic diseases. (4) In cases of multiple nodules with predominantly peripheral distribution, the likelihood of metastatic diseases

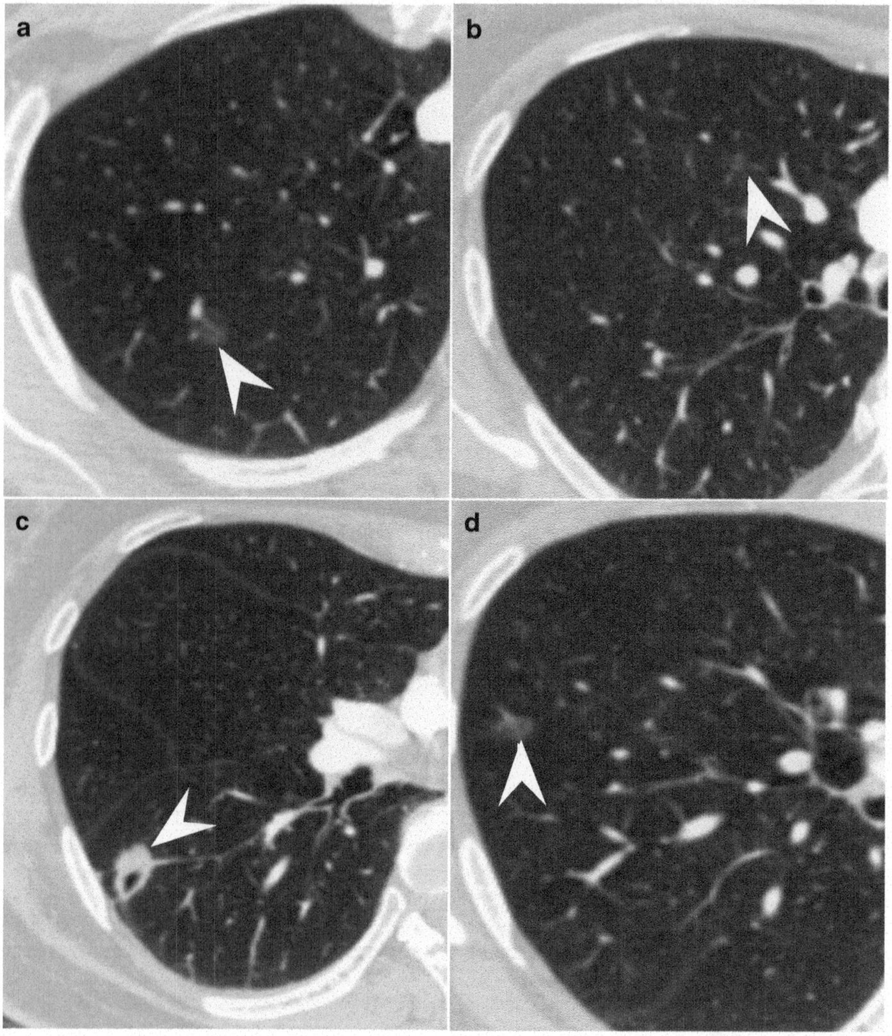

Fig. 10.3 Synchronous MPLC. Multiple solid nodules and subsolid and pure GGNs (arrowhead) with varying sizes were found in the annual chest CT images of a 61-year-old female. All lesions were located in the right lung with the predominance of the upper lobe (**a**, **b**, **d**). Feeding blood microvessels were seen (**a**, **d**). In the dorsal segment of right lower lobe, a solid nodule with air bubble was highly suspected of invasive adenocarcinoma (**c**). This patient was imaging diagnosed of sMPLC and received lobectomy of the right upper lobe and wedge resection of the right lower lobe. Postoperative pathological examinations confirmed the diagnosis of sMPLC with AAH in image B, AIS in images A and D, and IAC in image C. Genetic analysis revealed EGFR mutations of L858R in exon 21 in the lesion of image A and E746–A750 frame deletion in exon 19 in the lesion of image C

is higher than MPLC. (5) Infiltration in common lymphatic tracts in patients with MPLC is less frequently seen than in patients with metastatic diseases.

In addition to the indirect evidence from imaging examination, molecular genetic analysis can provide a direct basis for the differentiation based on numerous advances in tumor biology researches. The method for LOH analysis relies on the comparison between single-nucleotide polymorphism or microsatellite genotypes or between tumor DNA samples and patient-matched control (germ-line) DNA samples obtained from normal (non-tumor) tissue. Huang et al. [7] reported that synchronous and metachronous MPLC with identical histology could be successfully distinguished from intrapulmonary metastases using this methodology. And the combination of LOH analysis with p53 mutation profiling increases specificity and sensitivity in the diagnosis of independent primary lung cancers [13]. The homology of DNA ploidy type also can be used to distinguish primary carcinoma, metastatic carcinoma, recurrent carcinoma, and multiple primary carcinomas.

Overall, the diagnosis of MPLC should be based on comprehensive evaluation of patient's medical history, chest CT imaging from multiple examinations, response to empirical treatment, and even molecular or genetic profiles of tumor tissues for differentiation of other diseases with multifocal nodules, including metastases and coexisting of metastases and MPLC.

10.3 Management and Prognosis of Multiple Primary Lung Cancer

Besides diagnosis, numerous controversies exist related to the staging and management of MPLC. In the 7th edition of the AJCC lung cancer staging system, MPLC with separate nodules in a contralateral lobe is classified as the M1a disease. However, amounting survival data have shown that the prognosis of MPLC is far better than the M1a disease and the current staging has been required for revision [14]. The upcoming 8th edition has answered the call by recognizing multifocal adenocarcinoma as a unique disease entity and using the size of the largest nodule for staging with a letter "m" in parentheses denoting the multifocal nature of the disease, which apparently will facilitate future researches and guide clinical practice [15].

In the setting of MPLC, surgical resection remains a viable option unless involvement of mediastinal lymph nodes or metastatic diseases is suspected. However, consensus on the standard management strategy in multiple lesions has not yet been established. In most cases, individualized treatment is performed by taking into consideration of the following factors: number, size, and distribution of nodules, synchronous versus metachronous lesions, the predicted reserve of pulmonary function after resections, and the specific nature of each nodule (AAH, AIS, and MIA). Typically, the 5-year survival rate of patients with MPLC was significantly lower than that of single primary lung cancer patients. The lower survival rates may be explained by an overall greater probability of recurrent disease given two independent cancers, more aggressive biologic behavior and an inherent increased risk of developing a neoplastic process. Inadequate resectional margins due to the simultaneous or sequential operation are another major factor accounting for an unfavorable prognosis. For resection of multiple lesions, standard lobectomy may not be technically feasible. Alternatively, limited resections, wedge or segmental resection, are more frequently adopted in these patients. Numerous studies have shown that these sublobar procedures are associated with an increased incidence of locoregional recurrence and lower survival. However, compared to other treatment methods (i.e., radiation therapy, ablative procedures, chemotherapy), surgery remains the first-line treatment choice in MPLC patients with allowed physical conditions.

The 5-year overall survival rate in clinical stage I patients of sMPLC treated with surgical resection is reported only 25 and 40% in pathological stage I patients. In dealing with sMPLC, management strategies should vary with different clinical situations. (1) In patients with double or multiple primary cancers in the same lobe, standard lobectomy is certainly the preferred treatment option. (2) In patients with ipsilateral nodules in separated lobes, synchronous resection is advised if pulmonary function permits. Generally, lobectomy for the large lesion and wedge resection for smaller lesions are recommended. Wedge resection can be performed for multiple subcentimeter lesions with a predominance of ground-glass components. (3) For patients with bilateral sMPLC, sequential surgical resections with an interval of longer than 1 month are advised for safety consideration. And those lesions with centrally location, or rapid growth pattern, or large size, or potential hilar or mediastinal involvement, should be surgically removed in the first operation. (4) In patients with multiple bilateral pulmonary lesions unamendable to surgical approaches, medical treatment with chemotherapy or targeted therapy should be considered. Prior to medical treatment, pathological and genetic evaluation of lesions (as many as possible due to intertumoral heterogeneity) should be performed either on samples from biopsy or obtained by thoracotomy. Hence, patients with targetable mutations (such as EGFR mutations) could be treated with targeted therapy, whereas those without targetable mutations are given chemotherapy.

Approximately 75% of second primary lung cancers in mMPLC are stage I, and approximately 80% are incidentally detected during routine imaging follow-up for the first primary lung cancer. According to data of ACCP, the 5-year survival of all patients with metachronous MPLC is approximately 30%, and the survival of patients undergoing resection of the second primary is 40%. Since most patients received surgical treatment (and adjuvant therapy) for the first lung cancer, re-operation for new cancerous lesions is challenging with increased postoperative complication rate and mortality. Patients who are unfit for re-operation may be treated with nonsurgical approaches, such as stereotactic radiotherapy or radiofrequency ablation.

References

1. Slaughter DP, Southwick HW, Smejkal W. Field cancerization in oral stratified squamous epithelium; clinical implications of multicentric origin. Cancer. 1953;6(5):963–8.
2. Kozower BD, Larner JM, Detterbeck FC, Jones DR. Special treatment issues in non-small cell lung cancer: diagnosis and management of lung cancer, 3rd ed: American College of Chest Physicians evidence-based clinical practice guidelines. Chest. 2013;143(5 Suppl):e369S–99S. https://doi.org/10.1378/chest.12-2362.

3. Loukeri AA, Kampolis CF, Ntokou A, Tsoukalas G, Syrigos K. Metachronous and synchronous primary lung cancers: diagnostic aspects, surgical treatment, and prognosis. Clin Lung Cancer. 2015;16(1):15–23. https://doi.org/10.1016/j.cllc.2014.07.001.
4. Shen KR, Meyers BF, Larner JM, Jones DR. Special treatment issues in lung cancer: ACCP evidence-based clinical practice guidelines (2nd edition). Chest. 2007;132(3 Suppl):290s–305s. https://doi.org/10.1378/chest.07-1382.
5. Antakli T, Schaefer RF, Rutherford JE, Read RC. Second primary lung cancer. Ann Thorac Surg. 1995;59(4):863–6. discussion 867.
6. Martini N, Melamed MR. Multiple primary lung cancers. J Thorac Cardiovasc Surg. 1975;70(4):606–12.
7. Huang J, Behrens C, Wistuba I, Gazdar AF, Jagirdar J. Molecular analysis of synchronous and metachronous tumors of the lung: impact on management and prognosis. Ann Diagn Pathol. 2001;5(6):321–9. https://doi.org/10.1053/adpa.2001.29338.
8. Pairolero PC, Williams DE, Bergstralh EJ, Piehler JM, Bernatz PE, Payne WS. Postsurgical stage I bronchogenic carcinoma: morbid implications of recurrent disease. Ann Thorac Surg. 1984;38(4):331–8.
9. Feld R, Rubinstein LV, Weisenberger TH. Sites of recurrence in resected stage I non-small-cell lung cancer: a guide for future studies. J Clin Oncol. 1984;2(12):1352–8. https://doi.org/10.1200/jco.1984.2.12.1352.
10. Bonanno L, Calabrese F, Nardo G, Calistri D, Tebaldi M, Tedaldi G, Polo V, Vuljan S, Favaretto A, Conte P, Amadori A, Rea F, Indraccolo S. Morphological and genetic heterogeneity in multifocal lung adenocarcinoma: the case of a never-smoker woman. Lung Cancer. 2016;96:52–5. https://doi.org/10.1016/j.lungcan.2016.03.009.
11. Liu Y, Zhang J, Li L, Yin G, Zhang J, Zheng S, Cheung H, Wu N, Lu N, Mao X, Yang L, Zhang J, Zhang L, Seth S, Chen H, Song X, Liu K, Xie Y, Zhou L, Zhao C, Han N, Chen W, Zhang S, Chen L, Cai W, Li L, Shen M, Xu N, Cheng S, Yang H, Lee JJ, Correa A, Fujimoto J, Behrens C, Chow CW, William WN, Heymach JV, Hong WK, Swisher S, Wistuba II, Wang J, Lin D, Liu X, Futreal PA, Gao Y. Genomic heterogeneity of multiple synchronous lung cancer. Nat Commun. 2016;7:13200. https://doi.org/10.1038/ncomms13200.
12. Kobayashi Y, Mitsudomi T, Sakao Y, Yatabe Y. Genetic features of pulmonary adenocarcinoma presenting with ground-glass nodules: the differences between nodules with and without growth. Annals of oncology : official journal of the European society for. Med Oncol. 2015;26(1):156–61. https://doi.org/10.1093/annonc/mdu505.
13. Shimizu S, Yatabe Y, Koshikawa T, Haruki N, Hatooka S, Shinoda M, Suyama M, Ogawa M, Hamajima N, Ueda R, Takahashi T, Mitsudomi T. High frequency of clonally related tumors in cases of multiple synchronous lung cancers as revealed by molecular diagnosis. Clin Cancer Res. 2000;6(10):3994–9.
14. Kocaturk CI, Cansever L, Kanmaz DZ, Bedirhan MA. Metachronous lung cancer that presented as bilateral synchronous lung cancer. J Thorac Dis. 2013;5(3):E87–9. https://doi.org/10.3978/j.issn.2072-1439.2013.04.16.
15. Detterbeck FC, Marom EM, Arenberg DA, Franklin WA, Nicholson AG, Travis WD, Girard N, Mazzone PJ, Donington JS, Tanoue LT, Rusch VW, Asamura H, Rami-Porta R. The IASLC lung cancer staging project: background data and proposals for the application of TNM staging rules to lung cancer presenting as multiple nodules with ground glass or Lepidic features or a pneumonic type of involvement in the forthcoming eighth edition of the TNM classification. J Thorac Oncol. 2016;11(5):666–80. https://doi.org/10.1016/j.jtho.2015.12.113.

Suggested Readings

1. Dai C, Ren Y, Xie H, Jiang S, Fei K, Jiang G, Chen C. Clinical and radiological features of synchronous pure ground-glass nodules observed along with operable non-small cell lung cancer. J Surg Oncol. 2016;113(7):738–44. https://doi.org/10.1002/jso.24235.

2. Derlin T, Clauditz TS, Quaas A, Habermann CR. Synchronous bronchioloalveolar and squamous cell lung cancer with different 18F-FDG avidity on PET/CT. Clin Nucl Med. 2012;37(10):e255–6. https://doi.org/10.1097/RLU.0b013e31824440f9.
3. Hattori A, Matsunaga T, Takamochi K, Oh S, Suzuki K. Surgical management of multifocal ground-glass opacities of the lung: correlation of Clinicopathologic and radiologic findings. Thorac Cardiovasc Surg. 2017;65(2):142–9. https://doi.org/10.1055/s-0036-1572437.
4. Hattori A, Suzuki K, Matsunaga T, Takamochi K, Oh S. Prognostic significance of the standardized uptake value on positron emission tomography in patients with multiple clinical-N0 lung cancers. Thorac Cardiovasc Surg. 2015;63(7):597–603. https://doi.org/10.1055/s-0034-1395392.
5. Hiroshima K, Toyozaki T, Kohno H, Ohwada H, Fujisawa T. Synchronous and metachronous lung carcinomas: molecular evidence for multicentricity. Pathol Int. 1998;48(11):869–76.
6. Hsu HH, Ko KH, Chou YC, Lin LF, Tsai WC, Lee SC, Chang H, Huang TW. SUVmax and tumor size predict surgical outcome of synchronous multiple primary lung cancers. Medicine. 2016;95(6):e2351. https://doi.org/10.1097/md.0000000000002351.
7. Isaka T, Yokose T, Ito H, Imamura N, Watanabe M, Imai K, Nishii T, Yamada K, Nakayama H, Masuda M. Diagnosis of metachronous multiple lung adenocarcinoma at the cut-end by epidermal growth factor receptor mutation status discordance 4 years after sublobar resection for adenocarcinoma in situ: report of a case. Surg Today. 2015;45(10):1330–4. https://doi.org/10.1007/s00595-014-1077-z.
8. Linhas R, Tente D, Dias M, Barroso A. Synchronous mucinous and non-mucinous lung adenocarcinomas with different epidermal growth mutational status. Respir Med Case Rep. 2017;22:15–8. https://doi.org/10.1016/j.rmcr.2017.06.001.
9. Scialpi M, Franzini C, Piscioli I, Barberini F, Pusiol T, Rondelli F, Nicolanti V, Rulli A, Izzo P, Merlin G, Forcione AR, Pugliese F, Di Cello P, Paliotta A, Izzo L. Synchronous primary lung cancer. Critical review of diagnostic criteria. Ann Ital Chir. 2013;84(1):33–40.
10. Stella GM, Cemmi F, Inghilleri S, Zorzetto M, Luisetti M, Pozzi E. Synchronous lung cancers: when same histological types feature different molecular profiles and response phenotypes. J Cancer. 2011;2:474–7.
11. Stiles BM, Schulster M, Nasar A, Paul S, Lee PC, Port JL, Altorki NK. Characteristics and outcomes of secondary nodules identified on initial computed tomography scan for patients undergoing resection for primary non-small cell lung cancer. J Thorac Cardiovasc Surg. 2015;149(1):19–24. https://doi.org/10.1016/j.jtcvs.2014.10.057.
12. Taira N, Kawabata T, Ichi T, Kushi K, Yohena T, Kawasaki H, Ishikawa K, Kato S. A case of synchronous double primary lung cancer presenting with pleomorphic carcinoma and adenocarcinoma. Am J Case Rep. 2014;15:576–9. https://doi.org/10.12659/ajcr.892339.
13. Xue X, Xue Q, Wang N, Zhang L, Guo L, Li X, Sun J, Wang J. Early clinical diagnosis of synchronous multiple primary lung cancer. Oncol Lett. 2012;3(1):234–7. https://doi.org/10.3892/ol.2011.452.
14. Yasuda M, Nagashima A, Haro A, Saitoh G. How should synchronous multiple primary adenocarcinomas of the lung be resected? Ann Thorac Surg. 2014;97(5):e151–3. https://doi.org/10.1016/j.athoracsur.2014.02.057.
15. Zhao H, Yang H, Han K, Xu J, Yao F, Zhao Y, Fan L, Gu H, Shen Z. Clinical outcomes of patients with metachronous second primary lung adenocarcinomas. Onco Targets Ther. 2017;10:295–302. https://doi.org/10.2147/ott.s122908.

Part III
Management Strategies for Early-Stage Lung Cancer

Chapter 11
Management Strategies for Subcentimeter Lung Cancer: Surgery

Huilin Zhang, Huibiao Zhang, and Fanzhen Lv

With the development and extensive use of high-resolution computed tomography (CT), an increasing number of ground glass opacities (GGOs) are detected. Studies have shown that persistent GGOs have a high risk of malignancy, and almost of these nodules were adenocarcinoma. In general, the treatment of lung cancer requires multidisciplinary collaboration, including surgery, radiotherapy, chemotherapy and molecular-targeted therapy, and so forth. For early-stage NSCLC, surgery remains the first choice of option. Among various surgical techniques, conventional lobectomy in combination with complete mediastinal lymphadenectomy is considered the gold standard. But for a small, subcentimeter GGN with suspicion of preinvasive diseases or minimally invasive adenocarcinoma (MIA), whether the conventional lobectomy is the best surgical option has received increasing debate.

11.1 Preoperative Evaluation

11.1.1 Imaging Assessment

Currently, there lacks consensus or guideline regarding the timing, i.e., when a newly detected GGO in CT images should be surgically removed. However, according to NCCN guidelines on lung cancer screening, routine follow-ups with CT examinations are necessary for assessment of nodular lesions, especially those mixed GGO with higher possibility than other GGOs. The volume doubling time (VDT) of GGO may be variable, and other imaging features including internal density and neovasculature should be taken into consideration in discrimination of

H. Zhang • H. Zhang • F. Lv (✉)
Department of Thoracic Surgery, Fudan University Huadong Hospital, Shanghai, China
e-mail: lvfzh@sohu.com

X. Zheng et al. (eds.), *Early-stage Lung Cancer*,
https://doi.org/10.1007/978-981-10-7596-4_11

nodular benignancy or malignancy. Studies have confirmed that solid transformation of GGO is strongly indicative of malignancy. The increment of more than 2 mm in maximal diameter, development of a solid component in a pure GGO, or progressive growth of a pre-existing solid component in a part-solid GGO has predictive value of the invasiveness of a preinvasive disease. As a result, the occurrence of these features may mark the proper timing for surgical intervention.

11.1.2 Pathologic Diagnosis

Preoperative pathologic diagnosis should be well established. The pathologic diagnosis of lung cancer requires biopsied tissue which can be obtained by percutaneous CT-guided needle biopsy, transbronchial lung biopsy (TBLB), or surgical biopsy. However, for GGOs, considering the small size, location, loose cellular distribution, and vague radiographic appearance, percutaneous needle aspiration or biopsy (PCNA or PCNB) has been reported a high false-negative ratio, which may require multiple repeated biopsies. The same situation occurs to TBLB. Moreover, those peripheral GGOs may inaccessible for TBLB. Therefore, in many cases, surgery has dual intents, diagnostic and curative. Patients with GGOs are typically suspected of stage 1A (T1N0M0) disease. Currently, there is no strong evidence supporting the preoperative staging of the mediastinum.

11.1.3 Cardiopulmonary Evaluation

Pulmonary and cardiac risk assessment is an essential part of the preoperative evaluations, including complete pulmonary function test and transthoracic echocardiography. Any evidence of risks should be comprehensively evaluated and well controlled by specialties. Otherwise, patients may face increasing risks of perioperative complications and even mortality.

11.2 Surgical Options and Approaches

For a patient with very early-stage NSCLC (in particular, stage IA), surgical resection is the first-line treatment option unless this patient is considered as inoperable. Technically, a small, subcentimeter GGO can be readily surgically removed. The challenge in the surgical management of small-sized GGOs is how to balance the maximal resection of the suspected lesion and minimal resection of normal lungs to preserve pulmonary function and quality of life maximally. In a situation that a subcentimeter GGO could be resected with lobectomy, segmentectomy, or wedge resection, via open surgery or thoracoscopic surgery, the decision-making could be a challenging process.

11.2.1 Open Surgery or Minimally Invasive Surgery (MIS)

Open thoracic surgery has been used in the treatment of lung cancer for over a century. Over the last two decades, with the advances in optical and endoscopic instrumentation, thoracic surgery has proceeded at a slow but steady pace to minimally invasive surgery, characterized by the assistance from camera/video imaging, small incisions (<1 cm), an access and/or extraction incision measuring less than 5 cm, and sparing of rib removal.

The implementation of MIS requires supports from technical platforms, which basically can be divided into three categories, video-assisted thoracic surgery (VATS), robotic-assisted thoracic surgery (RATS), and uniportal VATS. Despite previous debate on the advantage and disadvantage of MIS over open approach, with mounting cases and maturing surgical skills under thoracoscopy, the debate has gradually abated, and MIS has been accepted as the mainstream treatment approach. It has been reported approximately of 75% of patient with early-stage NSCLC in a tertiary hospital received surgical treatment via MIS. The indications for MIS are similar to those for the open approach.

In comparison to open procedures, the MIS procedures have evident advantages, including decreased acute postoperative pain, reduced cytokine release, less impairment in pulmonary function, shorter chest tube duration, and consequently, shorter hospital stay and faster returning to usual activities of daily living. Yan et al. [1] conducted a meta-analysis to assess the safety and efficacy of VATS lobectomy in comparison with open lobectomy. In this study, 21 studies including 2641 patients were included. VATS did not demonstrate any significant difference in locoregional recurrence, as compared with the open lobectomy arm. Furthermore, a reduced systemic recurrence rate and an improved 5-year mortality rate were observed in the VATS arm. These results are confirmed by subsequent numerous randomized and nonrandomized studies.

11.2.2 Lobectomy

Lobectomy is defined as the anatomic resection of an entire lobe of the lung (Fig. 11.1). Lobectomy and complete nodal dissection achieve the maximum survival benefit in patients with stage IA disease. Hence, this surgical has been accepted as the gold standard for resection of early-stage NSCLC for more than two decades. In this procedure, the anatomic resection includes individual dissection and stapling of the involved pulmonary vein, pulmonary artery, and bronchus and appropriate management of the mediastinal lymph nodes. Lobectomy could be performed via

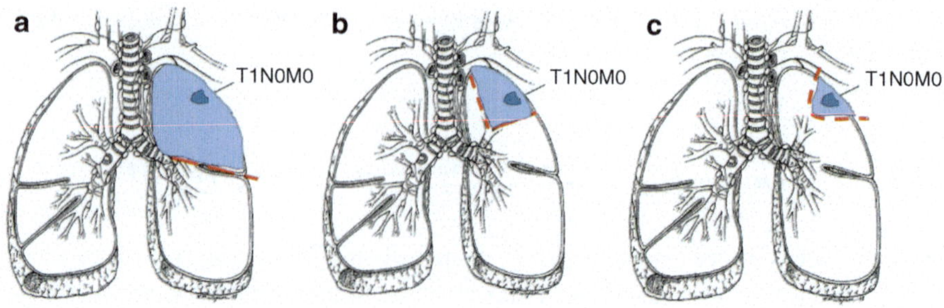

Fig. 11.1 Comparative diagram for common surgical approaches for early-stage NSCLC. (**a**), lobectomy; (**b**), segmentectomy; (**c**), wedge resection (From http://cancergrace.org. Reprinted with permission)

open thoracotomy or videoscopes. As discussed previously, VATS has gained popularity in lobectomy in the majority of patients.

However, the cost-effectiveness of lobectomy has been challenged. In the context of increasing incidence of small-sized GGOs, is it necessary or worthwhile to remove an entire lobe for a subcentimeter nodule or a lobectomy is an overtreatment? On the other hand, considering the increasing incidence of multiple lung tumors, either primary or metastatic, a previous lobectomy may leave no room for another lung surgery, which could be devastating to the prognosis. Therefore, a shared decision-making process may be proper to the patient and thoracic surgeons not only for a successful operation but also for preservation of pulmonary function and preparation for possible forthcoming events. When having these considerations in mind, surgeons may not take lobectomy for granted in patients with early-stage NSCLC. A risk stratification and comprehensive assessment of patient status and imaging would be helpful to make an individualized surgical approach benefitting the patient most. The surgical approach may be lobectomy, or sublobectomy, such as segmentectomy and wedge resection.

11.2.3 Segmentectomy

Despite that lobectomy with complete mediastinal lymphonodus dissection is the first choice for patients with stage I NSCLC, certain patients with compromised cardiopulmonary status or other severe comorbidities who cannot tolerate the loss of an entire lobe may be treated with segmentectomy. Segmentectomy refers to removing a section of a lobe along the anatomical boundary. Anatomical segmentectomy may offer a lung-preserving alternative to lobectomy, much as lobectomy did to pneumonectomy. This approach was first described by Churchill and Belsey in 1939 for resection of bronchiectasis and tuberculosis. The major concern on this procedure in the treatment of lung cancer is the perceived higher risk of local recurrence as shown in the 1995 report of Lung Cancer Study Group [2].

However, recent evidence, in particular a large meta-analysis, supports the use of intentional limited resection for small (≤2 cm in size), peripheral stage I NSCLC, especially those confined to an anatomic segment without detectable hilar or mediastinal nodal involvement [3]. Such operations are safe and carry a similar risk profile and survival outcomes compared to that of lobectomy. Patients with pure GGOs on preoperative imaging or those with noninvasive adenocarcinoma diagnosed by intraoperative pathologic examination may be particularly good candidates for limited resection. Thoracoscopic and open segmentectomy have similar risk profiles and long-term clinical outcomes.

11.2.4 Wedge Resection

Wedge resection is another sublobectomy, by removing a triangle-shaped slice of lung tissue containing the tumor and a small amount of normal tissue around it. This is a more limited resection than segmentectomy, and the cutting edge is not the natural anatomical boundary, leading to an unfavorable oncological outcome with higher local recurrence rates. Therefore, wedge resections are reserved for small peripheral lesions in patients with an impaired cardiopulmonary reserve that are not candidates for lobectomy or segmentectomy. Another indication of wedge resection is surgical biopsy in patients with multiple pulmonary nodules (primary or metastatic) for pathologic diagnosis to facilitate subsequent systemic therapies.

Wedge resection margin distance is associated with local recurrence and survival rate, so a sufficient margin distance is considered as no less than 2 cm or tumor diameter. Possible criteria for wedge resection include (1) tumors less than 2 cm in diameter (T1a lesion), (2) tumors located in the outer third of lung and approachable, (3) no endobronchial extension, (4) frozen section evidence of negative pathological resection margins, and (5) intraoperative mediastinal and hilar nodal staging.

11.3 Localization Techniques

Accurate localization of the tumor is critically important for effective resection with adequate margin. For those solid or large-sized NSCLC, localization could be successfully performed by visual inspection and/or palpation during surgical procedures. However, for small-sized tumors or tumors with few solid components, traditional techniques may be futile. Currently, several localization methods have been developed to increase localization and diagnostic accuracy during thoracoscopy, such as percutaneous wire placement, injection of dye, intraoperative imaging with ultrasound, fluoroscopy, or molecular imaging devices [4].

As the most common and convenient preoperative localization approach, percutaneous needle localization technique places a guidewire nearby the tumor under

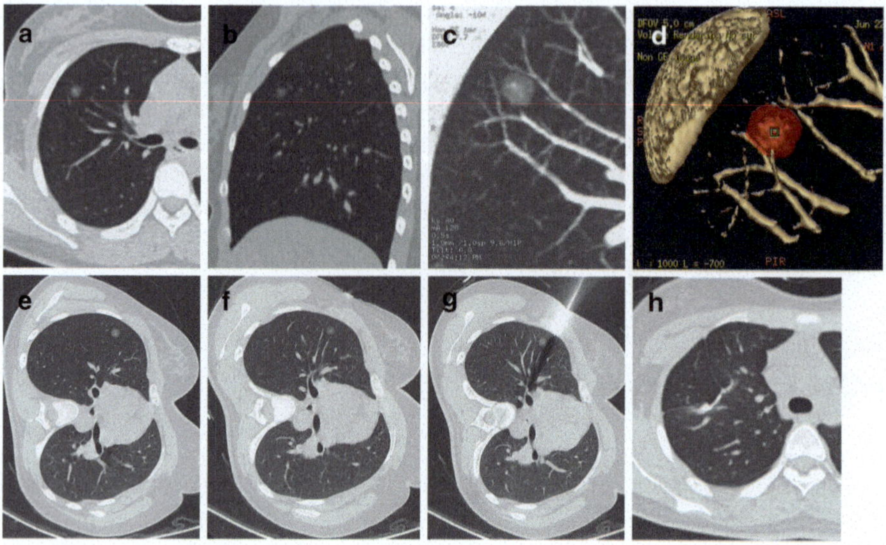

Fig. 11.2 Needle localization of a semisolid GGN for wedge resection. A 15-year-old girl received chest CT scan due to a dry cough for 2 weeks. A semisolid 9 mm nodule was found in the right upper lobe. This nodule was considered irrelevant with her symptoms and undetermined. She was prescribed antibiotics for possible occult infection and follow-up CT was performed 2 months later. In the follow-up CT, the nodule did not show any change with characteristic CTA-TA sign, indicative of preinvasive AIS (**a**–**d**. **a**, axial view; **b**, sagittal view; **c**, MIP image; **d**, volume rendering image). After discussion with her family and multidisciplinary assessment, VATS wedge resection was recommended for both diagnostic and curative purposes. The patient received preoperative needle localization under CT guidance. (**e**), the patient was immobilized at the left lateral position; (**f**), a skin marker was placed to guide the needle biopsy under CT guidance; (**g**), the localization needle was inserted along the planned angle and route; (**h**), the nodule was successful resected with a pathologic diagnosis of AIS

the guidance of CT immediately before the surgery. Commonly used guidewires include microcoils, hookwires, and spiral wires (Fig. 11.2).

Besides, dye injection is another localization strategy by injecting certain dye or radioisotope into tumor area by using guidance by CT or bronchoscopy. Those dyes could be methylene blue, lioplo, cyanoacrylate, India ink, and technetium-99 m (^{99m}Tc). During the operation, the dye could be directly visualized or detected with imaging detector for localization. Methylene blue staining is an earlier established technique and has shown to produce high sensitivity for nodule localization in small sample sizes. Likewise, it is less costly than wire-related techniques and obviates wire-related complications. However, the efficacy of dye injection technique is compromised by the diffusion of the injected materials. In comparison to robust localization from needle localization, the robustness of localization from this approach is greatly affected by the interval between dye injection and the operation. Intraoperative localization using ultrasound, fluoroscopy, and molecular imaging devices is time-consuming and not routinely utilized in clinical practices.

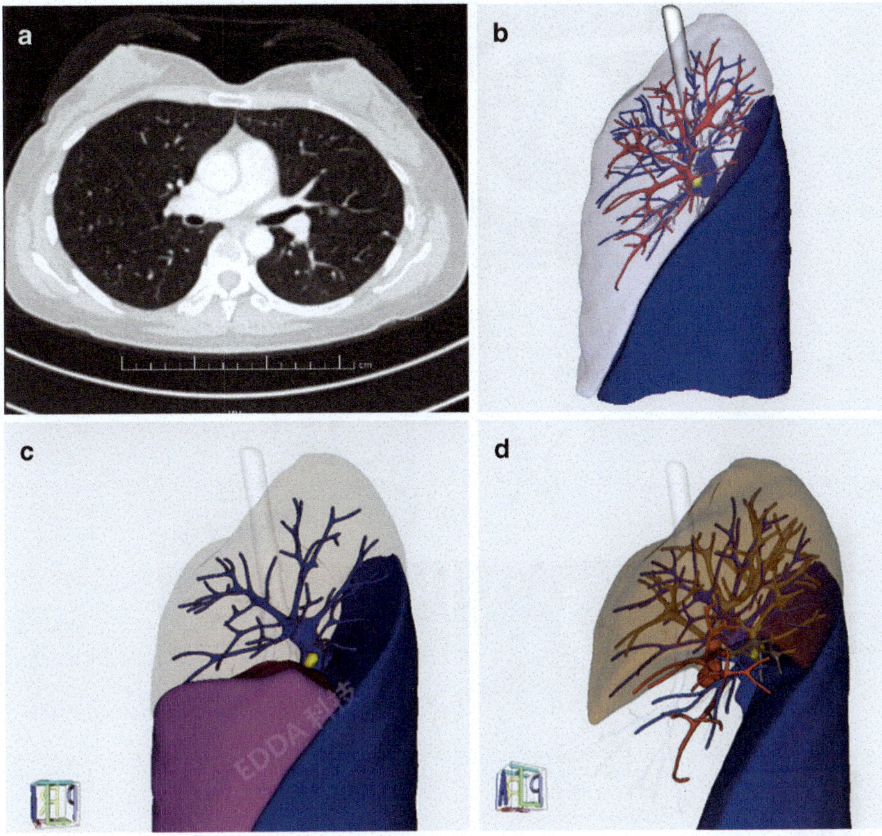

Fig. 11.3 Preoperative localization and evaluation. (**a**) Axial view of a 9-mm nodule in the left upper lobe. (**b**) Segmentation of lobe in the left lung, showing the lesion (yellow), bronchi (gray), veins (blue), and arteries (red). (**c, d**) Segmentation of segments in the left upper lobe

Currently, artificial intelligence (AI)-based preoperative localization, evaluation, and planning system has been increasingly adopted in the surgical treatment of various diseases, such as renal cancer, liver cancer, and transplant, as well as early-stage lung cancer. At Huadong Hospital, we have been using such a system (IQQA-3D, EDDA Technology, Inc., FDA, and CFDA cleared) in assisting preoperative planning for several years (Fig. 11.3). The system takes CT images as input and provides fast 3D quantification of the lung, including pulmonary nodules, airways, arteries, veins, and lung lobes. Furthermore, the system can facilitate the evaluation of bronchopulmonary segments as well as vascular territories, with instant volumetric measurements, spatial occupation and relationship analysis, etc., which are desirable and critical for assessment and management of pulmonary nodules.

Additionally, the IQQA system is utilized for the precision surgery planning (Fig. 11.4). First, a comprehensive 3D evaluation is performed to assess the size and location of the pulmonary nodule, boundaries and volumes of each bron-

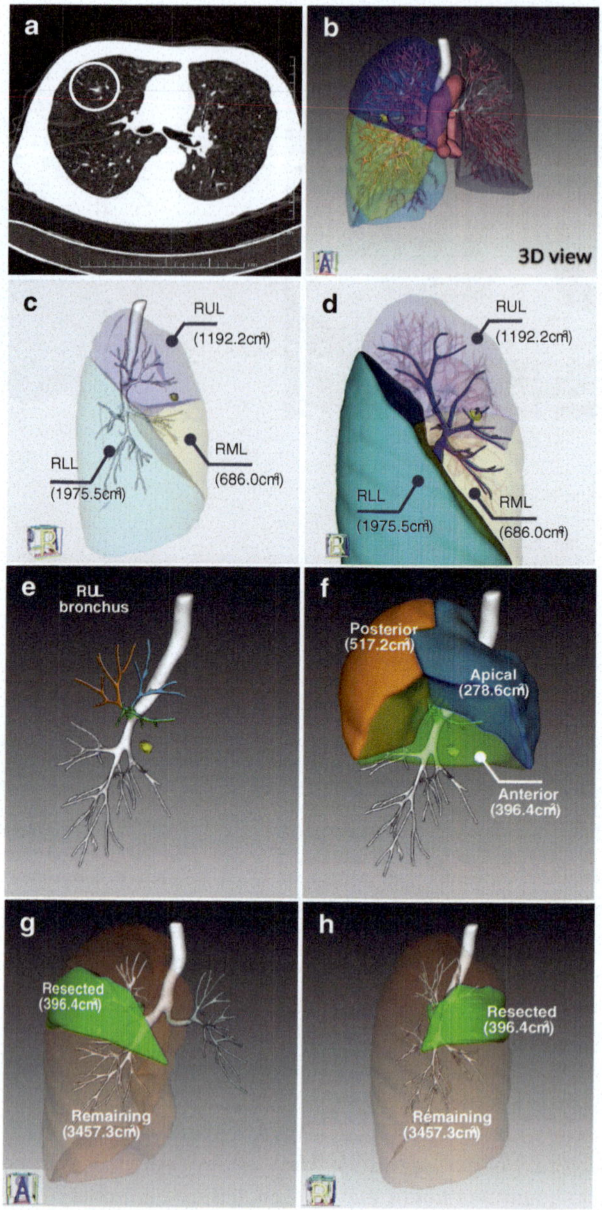

Fig. 11.4 Preoperative planning. (**a**) Axial view of an 8-mm nodule (circle) in the right upper lobe. (**b**) 3D view of bilateral lungs with manifestation of the nodule (yellow) in the right upper lobe. (**c**, **d**) Quantitative analysis of lobes in the right lung. The volumes of RUL, RML, and RLL are 1192.2 cm^3, 686.0 cm^3, and 1975.5 cm^3, respectively. (**e**) Reformatted right bronchial tree and the spatial relationship of the nodule (yellow). (**f**) Quantitative analysis of segments in the right upper lung. The volumes of the apical segment, anterior segment, and posterior segment are 278.6 cm^3, 396.4 cm^3, and 517.2 cm^3, respectively. (**g**, **h**) The simulated segmentectomy of the anterior segment. The remaining lung volume will be 3457.3 cm^3 once the segmentectomy is performed (Courtesy of Drs. Li Fan and Xiaolan Zeng, EDDA Technology, Inc.)

chopulmonary segments that are of interest, pulmonary arteries/veins and abnormalities (if any), and spatial relationship of major anatomies. Based upon the segmental review, the bronchopulmonary segments to be resected are chosen and an optimal surgical plan determined, in a real-time interactive manner with instant volumetric measurements updated. Our experience indicates that quantitative 3D imaging assessment and planning approach can positively assist precision VATS segmentectomy.

In addition, to facilitate the postoperative localization of small-sized tumor within a bulk of lung specimens (much like searching for a needle in a haystack), our team developed a postoperative localization strategy which is the CT-guided fine-needle localization in reaerated lung specimens [5]. This strategy has been proven to be highly effective in finding out single and multiple pure GGO as small as 4 mm. For more information regarding this technique, please refer to Chap. 1.

11.4 Other Issues Related to Surgical Treatment

11.4.1 Mediastinal Lymph Node Dissection

For many decades, mediastinal lymph node dissection (MLND) has been deemed an indispensable step for a standard surgical treatment for early-stage NSCLC. A meta-analysis evaluated impacts of different mediastinal lymph node evaluations (MLND vs. mediastinal lymph node sampling, MLNS) on the overall survival, local recurrence, distant metastasis, and complications. No significant difference in all measured parameters was seen between MLND and MLNS in early-stage NSCLC patients, indicating that a limited mediastinal lymph node evaluation (MLE) may be sufficient [6]. Furthermore, in the context of GGO-predominant nodules, Park et al. found MLE was not an essential procedure for clinical N0 NSCLC presenting as a 3 cm or smaller GGO-predominant nodule, but MLE was a significant risk factor for recurrence in solid-predominant tumors. The incidence of mediastinal lymph node metastasis is extremely rare in GGO-predominant lung cancer. In particular, postoperative lymph nodal upstaging seldom occurs in GGO-predominant lung cancer. Whether MLE can be safely spared in GGO-predominant nodules requires more studies, especially well-designed randomized clinical trials.

11.4.2 Adjuvant Therapy

Since most GGO-predominant tumors are histologically diagnosed as preinvasive diseases or minimally invasive adenocarcinoma (the former bronchioloalveolar carcinoma), the long-term prognosis after standard surgical treatment is pretty optimistic with a 5-year survival rate of close to 100% even in some cases treated with sublobar resection. For the majority of stage I diseases, particularly stage Ia diseases, adjuvant chemotherapy is not required. However, for those with micropapillary component, adjuvant therapy is recommended due to a relatively poor biological behavior by frequent vascular and stromal invasion. Sumiyoshi et al. also revealed that pulmonary adenocarcinomas with micropapillary component significantly correlated with recurrence but could be well controlled with EGFR tyrosine kinase inhibitors in patients with EGFR mutation. In Kobayashi et al. study, poor differentiation of tumor cells was regarded as the only risk factor for recurrence and an unfavorable prognosis in patients with stage I NSCLC and a tumor diameter of ≤20 mm; thus, histologic grade should be routinely assessed for assisting decision-making for further management [7]. Overall, the postoperative management of early-stage NSCLC should be established based on comprehensive assessment of histopathologic findings.

References

1. Yan TD, Black D, Bannon PG, McCaughan BC. Systematic review and meta-analysis of randomized and nonrandomized trials on safety and efficacy of video-assisted thoracic surgery lobectomy for early-stage non-small-cell lung cancer. J Clin Oncol. 2009;27(15):2553–62. https://doi.org/10.1200/jco.2008.18.2733.
2. Ginsberg RJ, Rubinstein LV. Randomized trial of lobectomy versus limited resection for T1 N0 non-small cell lung cancer. Lung cancer study group. Ann Thorac Surg. 1995;60(3): 615–22; discussion 622-613.
3. Liu Y, Huang C, Liu H, Chen Y, Li S. Sublobectomy versus lobectomy for stage IA (T1a) non-small-cell lung cancer: a meta-analysis study. World J Surg Oncol. 2014;12:138. https://doi.org/10.1186/1477-7819-12-138.
4. Keating J, Singhal S. Novel methods of intraoperative localization and margin assessment of pulmonary nodules. Semin Thorac Cardiovasc Surg. 2016;28(1):127–36. https://doi.org/10.1053/j.semtcvs.2016.01.006.
5. Li M, Shen G, Gao F, Zheng X, Hua Y, Xiao L. CT-guided fine-needle localization of ground-glass nodules in re-aerated lung specimens: localization of solitary small nodules or multiple nodules within the same lobe. Diagn Interv Radiol. 2015;21(5):391–6. https://doi.org/10.5152/dir.2015.14516.
6. Moon Y, Sung SW, Lee KY, Park JK. Clinicopathological characteristics and prognosis of non-lepidic invasive adenocarcinoma presenting as ground glass opacity nodule. J Thorac Dis. 2016;8(9):2562–70. https://doi.org/10.21037/jtd.2016.08.46.
7. Kobayashi N, Toyooka S, Soh J, Ichimura K, Yanai H, Suehisa H, Ichihara S, Yamane M, Aoe M, Sano Y, Date H. Risk factors for recurrence and unfavorable prognosis in patients with stage I non-small cell lung cancer and a tumor diameter of 20 mm or less. J Thorac Oncol. 2007;2(9):808–12. https://doi.org/10.1097/JTO.0b013e31814617c7.

Suggested Readings

1. Agarwal M, Brahmanday G, Chmielewski GW, Welsh RJ, Ravikrishnan KP. Age, tumor size, type of surgery, and gender predict survival in early stage (stage I and II) non-small cell lung cancer after surgical resection. Lung Cancer. 2010;68(3):398–402. https://doi.org/10.1016/j.lungcan.2009.08.008.

2. Colonias A, Betler J, Trombetta M, Bigdeli G, Gayou O, Keenan R, Werts ED, Parda DS. Mature follow-up for high-risk stage I non-small-cell lung carcinoma treated with sublobar resection and intraoperative iodine-125 brachytherapy. Int J Radiat Oncol Biol Phys. 2011;79(1):105–9. https://doi.org/10.1016/j.ijrobp.2009.10.030.
3. Echavarria MF, Cheng AM, Velez-Cubian FO, Ng EP, Moodie CC, Garrett JR, Fontaine JP, Robinson LA, Toloza EM. Comparison of pulmonary function tests and perioperative outcomes after robotic-assisted pulmonary lobectomy vs segmentectomy. Am J Surg. 2016;212(6):1175–82. https://doi.org/10.1016/j.amjsurg.2016.09.017.
4. El-Sherif A, Gooding WE, Santos R, Pettiford B, Ferson PF, Fernando HC, Urda SJ, Luketich JD, Landreneau RJ. Outcomes of sublobar resection versus lobectomy for stage I non-small cell lung cancer: a 13-year analysis. Ann Thorac Surg. 2006;82(2):408–415; discussion 415-406. https://doi.org/10.1016/j.athoracsur.2006.02.029.
5. Gharagozloo F, Tempesta B, Margolis M, Alexander EP. Video-assisted thoracic surgery lobectomy for stage I lung cancer. Ann Thorac Surg. 2003;76(4):1009–15. https://doi.org/10.1016/s0003-4975(03)00267-4.
6. Hasegawa M, Sone S, Takashima S, Li F, Yang ZG, Maruyama Y, Watanabe T. Growth rate of small lung cancers detected on mass CT screening. Br J Radiol. 2000;73(876):1252–9. https://doi.org/10.1259/bjr.73.876.11205667.
7. Iwasaki A, Shirakusa T, Shiraishi T, Yamamoto S. Results of video-assisted thoracic surgery for stage I/II non-small cell lung cancer. Eur J Cardiothorac Surg. 2004;26(1):158–64. https://doi.org/10.1016/j.ejcts.2004.02.033.
8. Keenan RJ, Landreneau RJ, Maley RH Jr, Singh D, Macherey R, Bartley S, Santucci T. Segmental resection spares pulmonary function in patients with stage I lung cancer. Ann Thorac Surg. 2004;78(1):228–233; discussion 228-233. https://doi.org/10.1016/j.athoracsur.2004.01.024.
9. Kelsey CR, Marks LB, Hollis D, Hubbs JL, Ready NE, D'Amico TA, Boyd JA. Local recurrence after surgery for early stage lung cancer: an 11-year experience with 975 patients. Cancer. 2009;115(22):5218–27. https://doi.org/10.1002/cncr.24625.
10. Kilic A, Schuchert MJ, Pettiford BL, Pennathur A, Landreneau JR, Landreneau JP, Luketich JD, Landreneau RJ. Anatomic segmentectomy for stage I non-small cell lung cancer in the elderly. Ann Thorac Surg. 2009;87(6):1662–8. https://doi.org/10.1016/j.athoracsur.2009.02.097.
11. Kim HY, Shim YM, Lee KS, Han J, Yi CA, Kim YK. Persistent pulmonary nodular ground-glass opacity at thin-section CT: histopathologic comparisons. Radiology. 2007;245(1):267–75. https://doi.org/10.1148/radiol.2451061682.
12. Kim K, Kim HK, Park JS, Chang SW, Choi YS, Kim J, Shim YM. Video-assisted thoracic surgery lobectomy: single institutional experience with 704 cases. Ann Thorac Surg. 2010;89(6):S2118–22. https://doi.org/10.1016/j.athoracsur.2010.03.017.
13. Landreneau RJ, Sugarbaker DJ, Mack MJ, Hazelrigg SR, Luketich JD, Fetterman L, Liptay MJ, Bartley S, Boley TM, Keenan RJ, Ferson PF, Weyant RJ, Naunheim KS. Wedge resection versus lobectomy for stage I (T1 N0 M0) non-small-cell lung cancer. J Thorac Cardiovasc Surg. 1997;113(4):691–698; discussion 698-700. https://doi.org/10.1016/s0022-5223(97)70226-5.
14. Mery CM, Pappas AN, Bueno R, Colson YL, Linden P, Sugarbaker DJ, Jaklitsch MT. Similar long-term survival of elderly patients with non-small cell lung cancer treated with lobectomy or wedge resection within the surveillance, epidemiology, and end results database. Chest. 2005;128(1):237–45. https://doi.org/10.1378/chest.128.1.237.
15. Moon Y, Sung SW, Namkoong M, Park JK. The effectiveness of mediastinal lymph node evaluation in a patient with ground glass opacity tumor. J Thorac Dis. 2016;8(9):2617–25. https://doi.org/10.21037/jtd.2016.08.75.
16. Okada M, Koike T, Higashiyama M, Yamato Y, Kodama K, Tsubota N. Radical sublobar resection for small-sized non-small cell lung cancer: a multicenter study. J Thorac Cardiovasc Surg. 2006;132(4):769–75. https://doi.org/10.1016/j.jtcvs.2006.02.063.

17. Okami J, Ito Y, Higashiyama M, Nakayama T, Tokunaga T, Maeda J, Kodama K. Sublobar resection provides an equivalent survival after lobectomy in elderly patients with early lung cancer. Ann Thorac Surg. 2010;90(5):1651–6. https://doi.org/10.1016/j.athoracsur.2010.06.090.
18. Port JL, Kent MS, Korst RJ, Libby D, Pasmantier M, Altorki NK. Tumor size predicts survival within stage IA non-small cell lung cancer *. Chest. 2003;124(5):1828–33. https://doi.org/10.1378/chest.124.5.1828.
19. Puri V, Garg N, Engelhardt EE, Kreisel D, Crabtree TD, Meyers BF, Patterson GA, Krupnick AS. Tumor location is not an independent prognostic factor in early stage non-small cell lung cancer. Ann Thorac Surg. 2010;89(4):1053–9. https://doi.org/10.1016/j.athoracsur.2010.01.020.
20. Sawada S, Komori E, Yamashita M, Nakata M, Nishimura R, Teramoto N, Segawa Y, Shinkai T. Comparison in prognosis after VATS lobectomy and open lobectomy for stage I lung cancer: retrospective analysis focused on a histological subgroup. Surg Endosc. 2007;21(9):1607–11. https://doi.org/10.1007/s00464-007-9200-5.
21. Saynak M, Hubbs J, Nam J, Marks LB, Feins RH, Haithcock BE, Veeramachaneni NK. Variability in defining T1N0 non-small cell lung cancer impacts locoregional failure and survival. Ann Thorac Surg. 2010;90(5):1645–1649; discussion 1649-1650. https://doi.org/10.1016/j.athoracsur.2010.06.033.
22. Schuchert MJ, Abbas G, Pennathur A, Nason KS, Wilson DO, Luketich JD, Landreneau RJ. Sublobar resection for early-stage lung cancer. Semin Thorac Cardiovasc Surg. 2010;22(1):22–31. https://doi.org/10.1053/j.semtcvs.2010.04.004.
23. Schuchert MJ, Pettiford BL, Keeley S, D'Amato TA, Kilic A, Close J, Pennathur A, Santos R, Fernando HC, Landreneau JR, Luketich JD, Landreneau RJ. Anatomic segmentectomy in the treatment of stage I non-small cell lung cancer. Ann Thorac Surg. 2007;84(3):926–932. ; discussion 932-923. https://doi.org/10.1016/j.athoracsur.2007.05.007.
24. Schuchert MJ, Pettiford BL, Pennathur A, Abbas G, Awais O, Close J, Kilic A, Jack R, Landreneau JR, Landreneau JP, Wilson DO, Luketich JD, Landreneau RJ. Anatomic segmentectomy for stage I non-small-cell lung cancer: comparison of video-assisted thoracic surgery versus open approach. J Thorac Cardiovasc Surg. 2009;138(6):1318–1325. e1311. https://doi.org/10.1016/j.jtcvs.2009.08.028.
25. Shaw JP, Dembitzer FR, Wisnivesky JP, Litle VR, Weiser TS, Yun J, Chin C, Swanson SJ. Video-assisted thoracoscopic lobectomy: state of the art and future directions. Ann Thorac Surg. 2008;85(2):S705–9. https://doi.org/10.1016/j.athoracsur.2007.11.048.
26. Tsukada H, Satou T, Iwashima A, Souma T. Diagnostic accuracy of CT-guided automated needle biopsy of lung nodules. AJR Am J Roentgenol. 2000;175(1):239–43. https://doi.org/10.2214/ajr.175.1.1750239.
27. Whitson BA, Andrade RS, Boettcher A, Bardales R, Kratzke RA, Dahlberg PS, Maddaus MA. Video-assisted thoracoscopic surgery is more favorable than thoracotomy for resection of clinical stage I non-small cell lung cancer. Ann Thorac Surg. 2007;83(6):1965–70. https://doi.org/10.1016/j.athoracsur.2007.01.049.
28. Yamashita S, Chujo M, Kawano Y, Miyawaki M, Tokuishi K, Anami K, Yamamoto S, Kawahara K. Clinical impact of segmentectomy compared with lobectomy under complete video-assisted thoracic surgery in the treatment of stage I non-small cell lung cancer. J Surg Res. 2011;166(1):46–51. https://doi.org/10.1016/j.jss.2009.04.006.

Chapter 12
Management Strategies for Early-Stage Lung Cancer: Stereotactic Ablative Radiotherapy

Xiangpeng Zheng, Yanping Ren, and Yuxin Jiao

According to the statistics of the World Health Organization (WHO), an estimated 1.8 million new cases of lung cancer and 1.6 million lung cancer-related deaths occurred in 2012. In the coming decades, lung cancer will continually be the major malignancy with top incidence and mortality rates, and it deserves the most priority in treatment and research globally as well as in China. According to the AJCC 7th edition of the TNM Classification of Malignant Tumors, the 5-year OS rates for stage IA, IB, IIA, IIB, III, and IV lung cancer are 73%, 58%, 46%, 36%, 20%, and 13%, respectively. The National Lung Screening Trial (NLST) showed an evident value of low-dose CT screening in early detection and diagnosis of lung cancer: compared to conventional screening using chest radiography, low-dose CT screening detected more (nearly 10 times) and smaller (<5 mm) early-stage lung cancer, and the rate of positive results for stage IA lung cancer increased from 35.1 to 93%, which were ultimately translated into a 20.0% decrease in cancer-specific mortality and a 6.7% decrease in overall mortality. With increasing application of low-dose CT as lung cancer screening tool, it is predictable that the incidence and prevalence of early-stage lung cancer would rise significantly.

Currently, lobectomy is still the standard treatment for early-stage lung cancer. However, due to some comorbidities such as severe diabetes, severe hypertension, chronic obstructive pulmonary disease (COPD), seriously impaired pulmonary function, or medical history of thoracic surgery, more than 20% patients may not be suitable for surgical treatment. For these patients, treatment options other than lobectomy, such as sublobar resections (segmental resection and wedge resection), radiation therapy, and radiofrequency ablation, have been extensively explored. In this chapter, the clinical efficacy of and advances in radiotherapy, especially stereotactic ablative radiotherapy (SABR), in the treatment of early-stage lung cancer are summarized.

X. Zheng (✉) • Y. Ren • Y. Jiao
Department of Radiation Oncology, Fudan University Huadong Hospital, Shanghai, China
e-mail: zhengxp@fudan.edu.cn

X. Zheng et al. (eds.), *Early-stage Lung Cancer*,
https://doi.org/10.1007/978-981-10-7596-4_12

Radiotherapy is one of the mainstay treatments for inoperable early-stage lung cancer. However, with the 3-year OS of 16–57% and 5-year OS of only 18%, the efficacy of the conventional radiotherapy regimen (typically 60 Gy in 30 fractions) was far from satisfying. Local recurrence (LR) was the major failure pattern with reported 3-year LR rate ranging from 19 to 70%. In addition to patients' poor performance status, the total radiation dose and overall treatment time were significantly related to the poor efficacy of conventional radiotherapy.

In general, the higher radiation dose is delivered in higher precision; the better tumor control could be obtained. The total dose cannot be increased without limitation in a living body. Moreover, considering the uncertainties of immobilization and equipment performance within the conventional radiotherapy, the radiation dose should be limited to a reasonable value to avoid any severe radiation-related adverse effects in irradiated surrounding normal tissues. For example, if the radiation dose was too high or delivered improperly, severe radiation pneumonitis or esophagitis could occur, and even fatal in occasional cases. Additionally, a prolonged course of radiotherapy (6 weeks) has negative impacts on patient compliance as well as tumor control. Therefore, a shortened and compact treatment course has advantages in terms of patient compliance and outcome. With the rapid development of computer technology, accelerator technology, and imaging equipment, real-time image-guided high-precision radiation techniques with radical high dose and fewer fractions become widely available. Among them, SABR has been applied to deliver radical treatment to various malignancies, including lung cancer, prostate cancer, liver cancer, and metastatic lesions to bones or brain. Mounting evidence from retrospective clinical studies and prospective trials has shown that with SABR treatment, high local control (LC) and overall survival (OS) could be achieved in early-stage NSCLC patients who were unable to receive standard lobectomy, and even in those operable patients, SABR could produce comparable outcomes to surgical resections.

12.1 SABR Versus Conventional Radiotherapy

Stereotactic ablative radiotherapy (SABR), also known as stereotactic body radiation therapy (SABR), was firstly introduced into clinical application at Catalina University Hospital in Sweden in the 1990s, where liver and lung tumors were treated using a linear accelerator with stereotactic frame and abdominal compression technique to assure positioning reproducibility and reduce intrafractional tumor motion within 5–10 mm. With a single fractional dose ranging from 7.7 to 30 Gy (median: 14.2 Gy) given in 1–4 fractions, a good response (partial and complete regression) was observed in approximately 50% of treated tumors. Since then, SABR has attracted extensive attentions of clinicians and researchers. In contrast to conventional radiotherapy, SABR has some unique characteristics: extremely high biological effective dose (BED) to the tumor in only a few fractions, ablative biological effects to both tumor cells and tumor supporting components, limited expansion from tumor margin to treatment margin, highly conformal dose distribution around treatment margin, sharp dose fall-off outside of treatment margin, robust immobilization and breathing movement management, real-time image-guided treatment delivery, and adaptive plan adjustment. In comparison to more than 20 fractions in conventional radiotherapy, treatment fraction is usually less than 10, delivered once a day or every other day, and completed within 2 weeks. Due to single fractional dose in SABR at least four times as high as in conventional radiotherapy, the treatment time for each fraction is longer, approximately ranging from 20 to 60 min depending on selected imaging guidance strategy. The majority of patients can immediately return to normal life after the treatment. Table 12.1 briefly lists major differentiating points between SABR and conventional radiotherapy.

The safety and efficacy of SABR for stage I NSCLC have been investigated in various scenarios, including elderly patients, inoperable patients, patients with borderline comorbidities, as well as operable patients. With sufficient supports from high-level evidence, the role of SABR in elderly and inoperable patients is solid and steadfast. The NCCN guideline on NSCLC has recommended SABR as an alternative treatment for those patients since the version V.2.2010. By 2012, 68 clinical trials and more than 4000 patients were conducted related to lung cancer SABR treatment, and results suggested that in early-stage lung cancer, SABR could achieve an OS rate twice as high

Table 12.1 Comparison of conventional radiotherapy (CRT) and SABR

Characteristics	CRT	SABR
Dose per fraction (fractional dose)	1.8–3 Gy	6–30 Gy
Total fractions	30–35	1–10
Target definition	GTV, CTV, PTV Tumor may not have a sharp boundary	GTV, CTV, ITV, PTV Well-defined tumors: GTV = CTV
Margin expansion for PTV	Centimeters (cm)	Millimeters (mm)
Physics/dosimetry monitoring	Indirect	Direct
Required setup accuracy (protocols)	TG40, TG142	TG40, TG142
Primary imaging used for TPS	CT	CT, MRI, PET/CT
Redundancy in geometric verification	No	Yes
Treatment accuracy	Moderately enforced	Strictly enforced
Need for respiratory motion management	Moderate—must be at least considered	Highest
Special training requirement	Highest	Highest + Special SABR training
Technology implementation	Highest	Highest
Radiobiology	Defined	Not well understood
Combination with systemic therapy	Yes	No

CTV, clinical target volume, *GTV* gross tumor volume, *ITV* internal target volume, *PTV* planning treatment volume, *TG* AAPM task group report as conventional radiotherapy. However, most of the previous studies were retrospectively designed, and most of the prospective studies were single-arm phase II trials. Multicenter, randomized, double-blind, phase III trials are still needed.

12.2 Effects of Ablative Dose on Normal Tissues

SABR and surgery share some strategic commons in dealing with lung cancers. Surgical treatment of a lung cancer intends to remove not only the tumor itself but also pulmonary tissues distal to the tumor in order to reduce potential serious postoperative complications secondary to necrosis of residual tissues. Similarly, as one of parallel functioning tissues, the airways in the lung follow a branching tubular structure. Radiation injury to a branch will primarily cause dysfunction downstream from the injury with imaging manifestations of pneumonitis and/or atelectasis, not the organ as a whole unless the major trunk itself (i.e., main bronchus) is damaged. So, the pulmonary toxicity after SABR treatment mostly depends on injured pulmonary volume. Therefore, compared with the centrally located lesions, the radiation-induced toxicity in peripheral lesions tends to be mild and readily tolerated (Fig. 12.1).

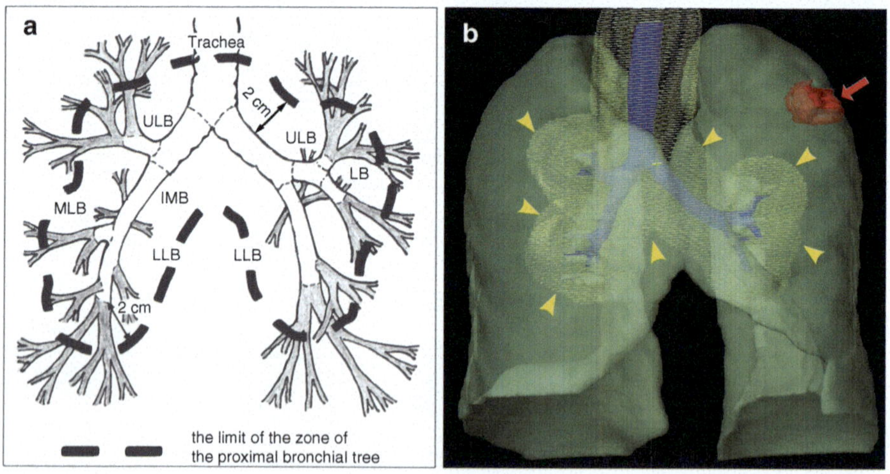

Fig. 12.1 SABR for centrally and peripherally located lung cancer. (**a**) Centrally located lung cancer is a tumor within or touching the zone of the proximal bronchial tree, defined as a volume 2 cm in all directions around the proximal bronchial tree (carina, right and left main bronchi, right and left upper lobe bronchi, intermediate bronchus, right middle lobe bronchus, lingular bronchus right, and left lower lobe bronchi). *IMB* intermediate bronchus, *LB* lingular bronchus, *LLB* lower lobe bronchus, *MLB* middle lobe bronchus, *ULB* upper lobe bronchus. (**b**) Three-dimensional reconstruction of lung images in a treatment planning system: the green circle and arrow indicate a centrally located mass. Special attention should be paid to dose distribution; the red circle and arrow indicate a peripheral lung cancer; the blue represents airways, including the trachea, main bronchi, and segmental bronchi

Tolerance doses of normal tissues in SABR remain poorly understood. High fractional dose and total biological effective dose increase the incidence of both acute reactions and late toxicity. Some toxicities may be life-threatening. It has been reported that fatal bronchial necrosis occurred in a patient receiving SABR treatment of centrally located lung cancer. As in conventional radiotherapy, acute reactions occur and are evaluated within 6 months after SABR. However, the assessment of late toxicity requires long-term follow-up. Currently, late toxicity data are insufficient and still should be collected continually in order to facilitate quantitative studies of risk factors and to determine tolerance dose of individual normal tissues related to lung SABR. Based on limited data available and expert consensus, Radiation Therapy Oncology Group (RTOG) has provided a guideline for a maximum dose-volume limit of critical normal tissues in the protocol of RTOG-0236 for inoperable lung cancer. Certainly, this guideline will be further modified and refined with more data coming up.

12.3 Advancements in SABR Regimens

Generally, the total fractions of SABR are less than 10 times. Each radiotherapy center or each radiation oncologist may have the preference or adjust fractional numbers by disease conditions. For comparison of various SABR regimens, prescribed dose is usually converted to biological effective dose (BED) based on linear quadratic cell survival in radiobiology. BED is intended to measure or compare quantitatively the biological effect of radiotherapy treatment with varying fractionation, taking account of dose-per-fraction or dose rate, total dose, and overall time. The calculation formula for lung cancer BED is $BED_{10} = nd\,[1 + d/10]$, where n is fraction number, d is fractional dose, and 10 is the α/β value for lung cancer cells. In order to optimize dose prescription and determine the maximum tolerable dose (MTD) for centrally and peripherally located lung cancers, prospective studies have been performed. Figure 12.1 shows the distinction between centrally and peripherally located lung cancers. The first prospective phase I clinical trial on SABR dose escalation was conducted at Indiana University. This trial recruited 37 patients with IA or IB peripheral lung cancer, showing that a relatively high-treatment dose (20 Gy × 3, BED_{10} = 180 Gy) was safe and tolerable. Due to the branching tubular structure, proximal tissues are dose-limiting and should be protected from potential severe toxicities. For those centrally located lung cancers, increasing fractions at the expense of a smaller fractional dose is a feasible strategy to reduce risks of serious reactions. Hence, RTOG has launched a series of clinical trials (RTOG0813 phase I/II trial) on SABR for central lung cancer to determine the maximally tolerated dose (MTD) of SABR for centrally located NSCLC and the efficacy of that dose in patients who are not operative candidates. Patients received five fractions of radiation on an every 2-day basis so that the SABR schedule is completed within 1.5–2 weeks. Nine dose levels were investigated starting from 50 Gy/5 Fx to 60 Gy/5 Fx. This trial has completed recruitment, and final results remain yet to be reported.

In 2004, Onishi et al. reported that better local control and survival rates were associated with BED >100 Gy compared with <100 Gy and subgroup analysis showed that survival rates in patients with medically operable diseases and receiving radiation dose of BED >100 Gy were potentially comparable to those treated with surgery [1]. Later on, a series of RTOG phase I/II studies further confirmed that high dose could generate survival benefit. The representative dose regimens are 48 Gy/4 Fx in Japan and 60 Gy/3 Fx in the United States. However, the 48 Gy/4 Fx may not be adequate for larger tumors according to Onimaru et al., which leads to the ongoing JCOG0702 trial designed to investigate dose escalation for T2N0M0 NSCLC. Zhang et al. conducted a meta-analysis to assess the relationship between biologically effective dose (BED) and efficacy of stereotactic body radiation therapy (SABR) and to explore the optimal BED range for stage I non-small cell lung cancer (NSCLC) [2]. They found that in comparison to the low BED group (<83.2 Gy) or high BED group (>146 Gy), the medium or medium to high BED (range, 83.2–146 Gy) may be more beneficial and reasonable in stage I NSCLC. Despite that higher dose could produce a better local tumor control, a trend toward more adverse events of grades 3–5 with higher dose was observed, which may ultimately generate a negative impact on overall survival. Thus, both local control and treatment-related complications should be taken into consideration before SABR regimens. RTOG 0915 is a randomized phase II clinical trials with an aim to compare the efficacy and toxicity of two commonly used SABR regimens (48 Gy/4 Fx and 30 Gy/1 Fx). Considering that the standard regimen of RTOG 0236 resulted in a 3-year local control of 98%, it is difficult that the RTOG 0915 regimen could achieve further improvement but may be more beneficial to the sick patients due to relatively low BED.

Based on previous reviews and meta-analysis, a basic consensus is that regardless of the SABR treatment fraction (3 fractions, 5 fractions, or 8 fractions), BED_{10} for the tumor target should not be less than 100 Gy in order to obtain a good local tumor control rate. However, individualization should be kept in mind, and it is strongly suggested to select fractionation regimen based on tumor location and size. For example, for those peripherally located tumors, a regimen of 60 Gy in 3–4 fractions has been the common practice pattern, while for those centrally located tumors, a relative conservative regimen such as 60 Gy in 7–8 fractions would be safer and tolerable as well as equivalently effective in tumor control. For more information, readers are suggested to refer the guideline of dose regimens for SABR in various scenarios by the National Comprehensive Cancer Network (NCCN).

12.4 Clinical Results of SABR in Early-Stage NSCLC

Carolina University hospital reported the earliest retrospective clinical results of SABR in early-stage non-small cell lung cancer, while RTOG 0236 is the first prospective, multicenter clinical trial for inoperable early-stage NSCLC treated with SABR. Despite that the nominal dose prescription in RTOG 0236 was 60 Gy (in 3 fractions), the actual dose was equivalent to 54 Gy due to the tissue heterogeneity. In addition, the significance of RTOG 0236 is that it developed strict technical protocols for SABR implementation, including the maximum dose constraints for normal tissues, a quality assurance system, and qualification of candidate treatment centers. Starting in 2004, this trial recruited a total of 57 patients. The reported 3-year local control, local-regional control, disease-free survival (DFS), and OS were 90.6%, 87.2%, 48.3%, and 55.8%, respectively, and the median survival was 48.1 months. Nagata reported 45 cases of early-stage NSCLC treated with SABR (48 Gy/4 Fx). After a median follow-up of 30 months, the 3-year DFS and OS were 72% and 83% in patients with stage IA lung cancer and 71% and 72% in stage IB diseases, respectively. The image-guided SABR study (50 Gy/4 Fx) for central lung cancer at the MD Anderson Cancer Center showed that after a median follow-up of 17 months, the local control rate could be as high as 100%. Timmerman [3] reported a phase II study of 70 cases of T1 and T2 central lung cancers treated with dose regimens of 60–66 Gy/3 Fx. The 2-year LC and OS were 95% and 54.7% with a median OS of 32.6 months. Grade 3–5 toxicities occurred in 14 cases, and the median duration was 10.5 months. Both studies showed SABR is effective in the treatment of central lung cancer. However, considering increasing risks of serious side effects with dose escalation, more work should be conducted to optimize dose regimens.

12.4.1 SABR in Pathologically Confirmed Early-Stage Lung Cancer

Without any cancer-specific treatment, the prognosis of early-stage lung cancer with pathological confirmation is poor. Raz et al. [4] analyzed 1432 patients with stage I NSCLC not receiving surgical resection or chemotherapy or radiation, and found that only 42 patients were alive 5 years after diagnosis and median survival was 9 months overall, generating the 5-year OS 6% for stage I NSCLC, 9% for T1 tumors and 11% for patients declining surgical treatment. Wao et al. from Morsani Medical College published a meta-analysis of NSCLS without treatment based on 7 cohort studies (4418 patients) and 15 randomized controlled trials (1031 patients), revealing that untreated lung cancer patients live on average for 7.15 months [5]. Although limited by study design, these findings provide the basis for future trials to explore optimal interventions to improve prognosis with innovative treatments. Murai et al. [6] investigate the relationship between waiting time and disease progression in patients undergoing SABR for lung adenocarcinoma or squamous cell carcinoma, finding that there was a correlation between waiting time and rate of increase in volume in both types of lung cancer but with more impact on squamous cell carcinoma and a waiting time of fewer than 4 weeks seems to be acceptable. Moreover, it is important to note that there exists a close relationship between tumor size and both radiotherapy sensitivity and prognosis. Allibhai et al. [7] examined the influence of tumor size on SABR treatment outcomes in 185 medically inoperable patients with early (T1-T2N0M0) NSCLC [8]. No significant relationship was found between tumor size and local failure. However, tumor size had significant impacts on regional and distant failure as well as survival rates, including overall survival, disease-free survival, and cause-specific survival, suggesting that patients with large tumors may benefit from additional adjuvant therapy. In addition, it appeared that tumor volume was better and more sensitive than diameter to reflect the tumor size. The impact of introducing SABR in patients 75 years of age or older was studied using a population-based cancer registry, showing that SABR introduction was associated with a 16% absolute increase in RT use, a decline in the proportion of untreated elderly patients, and an improvement in OS [9]. In conclusion, SABR should be provided to patients with pathologically confirmed early-stage lung cancer as early as possible, especially to those who are not physically fit for invasive resection or systematic cytotoxic therapy.

12.4.2 Efficacy of SABR in Clinically Diagnosed Early-Stage Lung Cancer

Despite that for patients referred to SABR treatment, definitive pathological evidence is expected not only for medical records but also for treatment outcome evaluation and researches, in the real-world practice, a significant portion of SABR patients lack pathological confirmation due to refusal to invasive biopsy procedures or presence of contraindications for such procedures. As a consensus, a strictly clinical diagnosis is accepted for SABR treatment. To meet the strictly clinical diagnosis, the pulmonary tumor should be (1) evaluated by a multidisciplinary team including pulmonologists, thoracic surgeons, radiation oncologists, radiologists, and pathologists; (2) followed up for more than 1 year using two imaging modalities, CT and PET; (3) treated with antibiotics to exclude possible pneumonia or granuloma; and (4) continuously growing with increasing metabolic activity. In our meta-analysis of 106 SABR studies involving 7105 patients, less than one-half of patients had definitive pathology. Using the absence of pathological confirmation as an excuse to decline SABR treatment, to us and many radiation oncologists globally, is against ethics [10]. Apparently, the low rate of pathological diagnosis is one of the major pitfalls when comparing the efficacy of SABR and surgery in early-stage NSCLC (Figs. 12.2 and 12.3).

According to Inoue et al., the 5-year OS of clinically diagnosed early-stage lung cancer (58 patients) treated with SABR was 89.8% for tumors smaller than 2 cm, and 53.1% for those larger than 2 cm, again reflecting the impact of tumor size on the SABR outcome. Verstegen et al. compared 209 patients with clinically diagnosed early-stage of lung cancer to 382 patients with pathologically confirmed early-stage NSCLC treated with SABR, revealing that there was no significant difference in OS. Atsuya et al. also published a retrospective study of the multicenter data in Japan involving 298 patients with pathologically confirmed or clinically diagnosed early-stage lung cancer. The results showed that no significant difference was seen in 3-year loco-regional control, distant metastasis-free survival (DMFS),

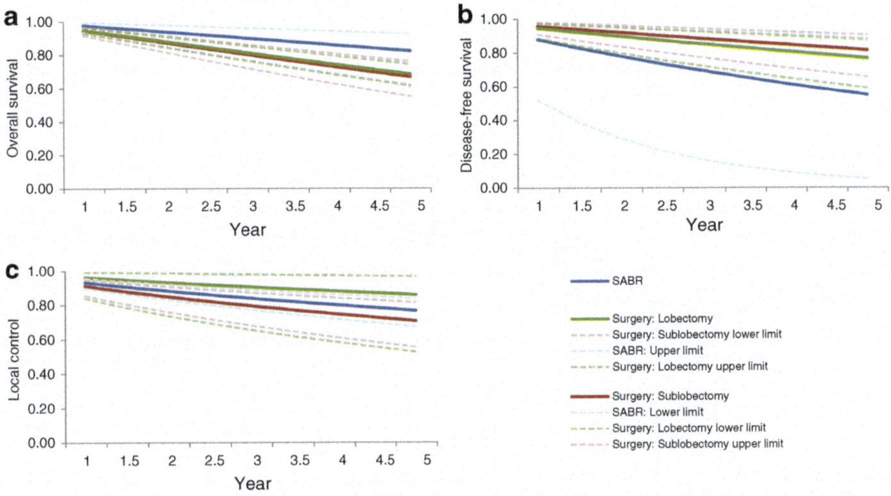

Fig. 12.2 Estimated overall survival (**a**), disease-free survival (**b**), and local control (**c**) by treatments (SABR vs. limited lung resection [LLR] vs. lobectomy [LR]) in patients with median age of 70 and 100% operability

progression-free survival (PFS), DFS, and OS. The above reports plus many others indicate that SABR was suitable and reliable for patients with strictly clinically diagnosed early-stage lung cancer.

12.4.3 Efficacy of SABR in the Treatment of Ground-Glass NSCLC

With the increasing utilization of low-dose CT for lung cancer screening, the detection rate of early-stage lung cancer dramatically rises. Among newly detected small lung cancer, some manifest as ground-glass lesions with or without solid components, which changes the traditional imaging patterns of early-stage lung cancer with solid-component predominance. Currently, numerous controversies remain on the management of ground-glass predominant early-stage lung cancers. Certainly, surgical removal is the first-line treatment. Most researches focused on optimization of surgical procedures based on the amount of solid component, distribution of vascular and bronchial, and doubling time of tumors. As one of the major local treatment options for lung cancer, radiotherapy (including SABR) was seldom used to deal with such lesions. Pathologically, GGO-predominant lesions are formerly bronchioloalveolar adenocarcinoma and now could be adenocarcinoma in situ (AIS) and minimally invasive adenocarcinoma (MIA). No special report is found in SEER database on radiotherapy for GGO or early BAC, and it was mainly due to (1) the cytology of GGO is difficult to obtain, (2) image guidance of radiotherapy in the past is not of precision enough to target beams on these fuzzy lesions, and (3) the

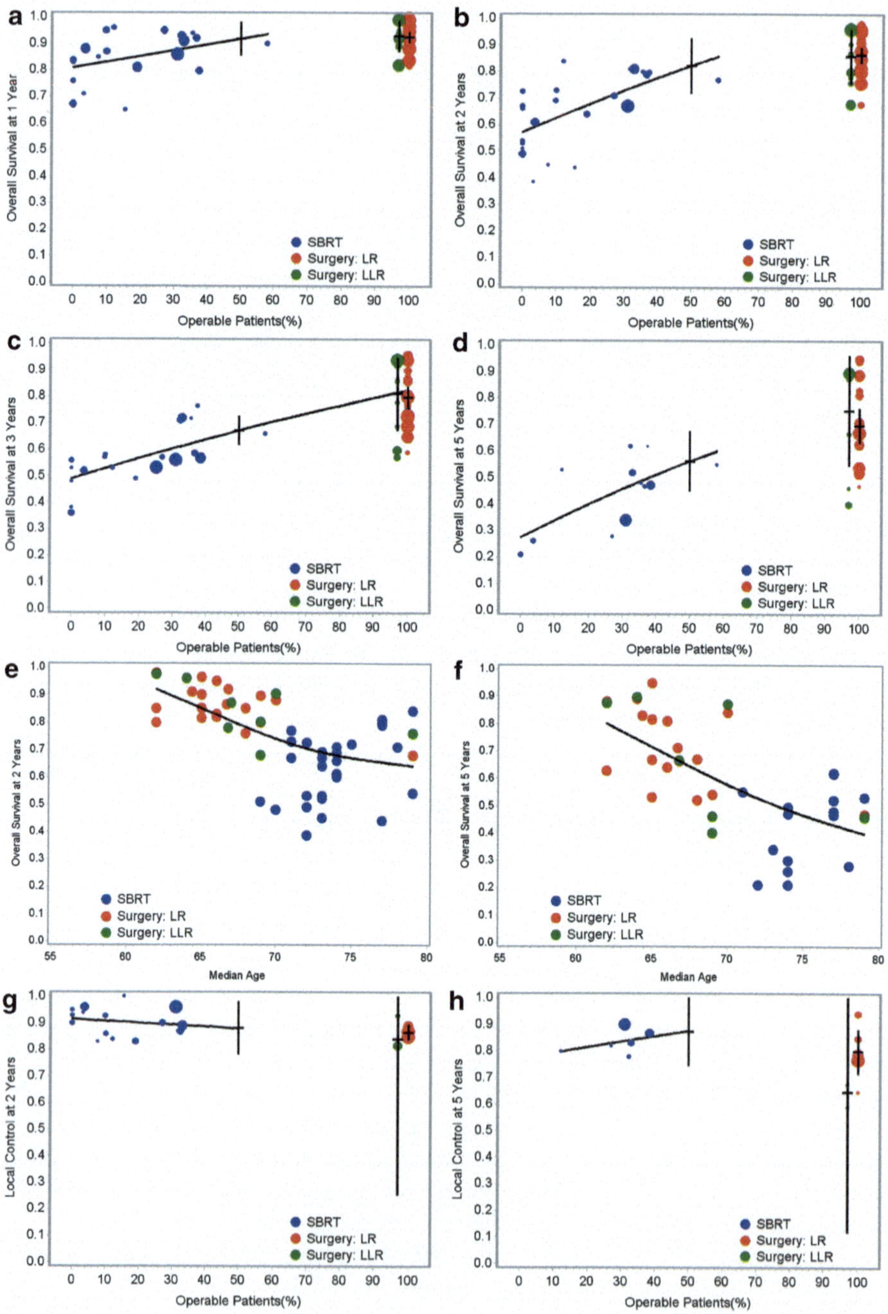

Fig. 12.3 Operability and age-dependent overall survival (OS) in SABR, lobectomy (LR), and limited lung resection (LLR). (**a–d**) Estimated 1-, 2-, 3-, and 5-year OS for surgery versus SABR by the proportion of operable patients in the trial. (**e, f**) Estimated 2- and 5-year OS rates by median trial age. (**g, h**) Estimated 2- and 5-year local control rates by the proportion of operable patients in the trial. (**a–d** and **g, h**) Dot sizes are proportional to the number of patients in specific studies

efficacy of SABR on GGO-like lung cancers is not well established. Many ongoing or completed prospective trials of SABR for early-stage NSCLC, including RTOG 0618, RTOG 0813, RTOG 0915, and RTOG 3502, clearly put BAC diseases into conditions for patient ineligibility.

The improvement of radiotherapy techniques, especially in imaging guidance, may refine radiotherapy roles in dealing with GGO-like lung cancer. In 2012, Urban examined the roles of radiotherapy in unresected, nonmetastatic bronchoalveolar carcinoma by performing a population-based analysis within the Surveillance, Epidemiology, and End Results (SEER) registry [11]. A total of 6933 patients of BAC were included: 74% patients were stage I and 968 patients were inoperable, of whom 300 patients received radiotherapy. Prognosis analysis showed that radiotherapy significantly improved overall survival in patients with BAC who were unable to receive surgery. There was a significant difference in the median survival between patients who received radiotherapy and who did not (for stage I NSCLC, 33 months vs. 28 months). However, less than a third of patients who could have potentially benefited from radiotherapy received it, suggesting that the medical specialists involved in the care of these patients underappreciate the importance of radiotherapy. The JCOG 0403 recruited some patients with BAC, and the 3-year OS was close to surgery. Badiyan et al. [12] performed a pattern of failure analysis to compare SABR outcomes between BAC and other NSCLC subtypes. In their study, 13 patients had radiographically diagnosed BAC and 5 patients had biopsy confirmed BAC. The 3-year local control for BAC overall was 100% and 86% for all other NSCLC subtypes (102 patients), and no significant difference was observed in the 3-year local failure rate, progression-free survival rate, and OS. Surprisingly, there may be an increased risk of distant metastases with BAC, which might be related to uncertainty in the determination of target margin.

Again, in contrast to numerous SABR studies on solid early-stage NSCLC, the evidence of SABR efficacy in GGO-like NSCLC is far from maturity, and more perspective trials with larger patient samples are required to investigate comparative effectiveness of SABR over surgical resections, especially limited sublobar resection.

12.5 Indications of SABR in Lung Cancers

Numerous high-level evidences support that inoperable patients with early-stage lung cancer are the perfect candidate for SABR treatment and SABR is also their first-line treatment option. Technically, a patient is deemed inoperable if the following conditions exist:

1. Severely impaired cardiopulmonary functions which put patients in high risks of perioperative mortality, including:
   (a) Base FEV1 < 40% predicted, postoperative FEV1 < 30% predicted
   (b) Pulmonary diffusing capacity decreased significantly (<40% predictive value)

(c) Presence of hypoxemia (less than or equal to 70 mmHg) and/or oxygen carbon retention (>50 mmHg)
(d) Exercise oxygen consumption <50% predicted
(e) Severe pulmonary hypertension
(f) Diabetes mellitus with severe end-organ damage
(g) Serious cardiovascular, cerebrovascular, and peripheral vascular diseases
(h) Severe chronic heart disease

2. Patients cannot tolerate surgery again because of previous pneumonectomy or lobectomy.
3. Patients refused to surgical treatment due to old age or other factors.

For marginally operable lung cancers, including multiple primary lung cancers (synchronous or metachronous multiple primary lung cancer), the best management strategy may be a multidisciplinary discussion between physicians and patients to balance the benefits and potential risks. Regarding operable early-stage lung cancers, surgical resection is the standard of care, and the efficacy of SABR should be further examined in well-designed trials. Hence, any patient who chooses SABR for his/her operable early-stage lung cancer should be advised and recruited into clinical trials for rigorous evaluation and monitoring.

Besides patients mentioned above with early-stage lung cancers, those with advanced or late-stage lung cancers could benefit from the improvement of local tumor control of SABR treatment. Such conditions include solitary pulmonary metastasis or oligometastasis from other primary sites, local consolidative therapy to the solitary lesion with disease progression after first-line chemotherapy or targeted therapy, and focal boost therapy after conventional radiotherapy in stage III disease and salvage therapy for localized recurrent diseases.

12.6 SABR Protocol

As discussed previously, the characteristic feature that distinguishes SABR from conventional radiation treatment is the delivery of large fractional doses in a few fractions with precise image guidance. For safety consideration, high conformation of prescribed doses to the target and steep dose fall-off beyond the target should be strictly implemented in order to minimize toxicities in surrounding normal tissues [13]. Therefore, the implementation of SABR has high demands on the accuracy of the entire treatment delivery process, which has been accomplished due to the advances in imaging and optimization in simulation, treatment planning, and delivery technologies. Major related international organizations including the American Society for Therapeutic Radiology and Oncology (ASTRO), American College of Radiology (ACR), American Association of Physicists in Medicine (AAPM), European Organization for Research and Treatment of Cancer (EORTC), and International Atomic Energy Agency (IAEA) released specific practice guidelines, reports, and recommendations for planning and delivery of high-dose, high-precision SABR for lung cancer. Among them, AAPM made tremendous contributions by publishing practical series of authoritative reports of AAPM Task Group (TG), TG42, TG76, and TG142, which have been the instructive documents for establishment of SABR program.

12.6.1 Patient Immobilization

SABR requires longer time from positioning patient to treatment completion than conventional radiotherapy. Typically, each fractional treatment takes 10–30 min depending on the radiotherapy platform. Therefore, reliable immobilization of patients is critically important to ensure that rigid body motion of the treatment region is minimized. A variety of immobilization systems may be used, including a vacuum bag, thorax board with alpha cradle, or alpha cradle with customized supporting devices. Regardless of which immobilization device to be used, patients should be maintained at a comfortable position for the whole treatment, and the position must be readily reproducible, which helps to avoid geometrical errors and uncertainties during treatment delivery. The immobilization should ideally be indexed to the treatment couch.

12.6.2 Simulation and Breathing Motion Management

SABR requires high precision and accuracy in target contouring and treatment planning. For such purpose, thoracic computed tomography with a big bore for immobilization devices is the mandatory imaging platform for simulation and treatment planning. Unless there exist contraindications for intravenous administration of iodinated contrast agent (e.g., allergy, severe renal insufficiency, or severe asthma), the planning CT should be acquired with the use of contrast agent to facilitate structure contouring, especially in cases with tumors adjoining to the mediastinum or obstructive atelectasis. Typically imaging acquisition is performed using 5 mm slice thickness and 5 mm interval. For better contouring, the reconstructed slice thickness should be less than 3 mm. The image series used for planning should be acquired at free breathing. If a three-phase CT scanning is conducted to assess the target motion, the patient should be coached to hold breath in the end of inspiration and expiration for the other two imaging acquisitions. Once reconstructed, all images are transferred to the treatment planning system for contouring by radiation oncologists and planning by radiation physicists.

The positions of thoracic tumors are subject to the involuntary respiratory movement. For accurate positioning and intrafractional reproducibility, certain measures should be taken to evaluate and compensate such impacts from respiratory movement. Target motion should be assessed using 3-phase CT scanning or optimally 4D-CT. If the target motion range is more than 5 mm, certain maneuvers should be utilized to reduce motion amplitude. Widely acceptable maneuvers include reliable abdominal compression, accelerator beam gating with the respiratory cycle, fiducial-based tumor tracking, and active breathing control techniques.

12.6.3 Treatment Planning

Treatment planning guidelines for SABR patients are very strict. Once a patient is classified as a candidate for SABR, the treating physician must identify the clinical guideline used to guide the patient's dose fractionation and planning, such as a RTOG protocol or published peer-reviewed study. Representative RTOG protocols are RTOG 0813 for centrally located NSCLC, RTOG 0915 for stage I inoperable peripheral NSCLC, and RTOG 0618 for operable NSCLC.

On pulmonary CT windows, the radiation oncologist carefully contours the target lesion, designated as the gross tumor volume (GTV). If PET-CT imaging is available, image fusion is preferred to better define the GTV by exclusion of adjacent vessels, atelectasis, pneumonitis, or mediastinal or chest wall structures. For patients with pneumonitis or obstructive atelectasis, PET-CT should be performed not only for accurate contouring but also for safety. In SABR, GTV is typically not expanded for prophylactic coverage of presumed microscopic diseases. Hence, the GTV is identical to or very close to the clinical target volume (CTV). The internal target volume (ITV) is generated based on the breathing-related target motion pattern from three-phase CT or 4D-CT. Finally, additional margins (3–5 mm in the axial and 5–8 mm in the longitudinal planes) are added to the ITV to constitute the planning treatment volume (PTV) for compensating treatment uncertainties such as setup errors and intrafractional involuntary body motion.

To deliver highly conformal prescription dose distributions, three-dimensional coplanar or noncoplanar beam arrangements are allowed if the dose distribution and restraints are satisfied. Hence, modern linear accelerators with sophisticated image guidance systems, TomoTherapy and CyberKnife system, are acceptable treatment platforms for SABR. Typically, more than seven radiation beams should be deployed to generate a good-quality SABR plan. Non-opposing, noncoplanar beams with roughly equal weighting are preferable. In comparison to static beams, arc therapy is highly efficient in treatment delivery. With this technique, at least a full arc or multiple partial arcs should be utilized. For dose calculation, the treatment plan should be normalized to a defined point located closely to the PTV center. Typically, this normalization point is the treatment isocenter. Regarding the impact of tissue heterogeneity on dose calculation, there are controversies on this issue. Different dose heterogeneity correction algorithm may generate different results with error variations of 10–20%, and currently there lacks consensus on correction algorithm. In this context, current clinical trials do not recommend correction for tissue heterogeneity but assume all tissues within the body to have unit (water) density.

Specifically, a successful treatment planning should meet all of the following criteria: (1) a minimum of seven non-opposing beams should be used and noncoplanar fields are preferred; (2) the prescription isodose surface is chosen such that 95% of the PTV is conformally covered by the prescription isodose surface and 99% of the PTV receives a minimum of 90% of the prescription dose; (3) prescription lines covering the PTV are typically the 60–90% line (where the maximum dose is 100%); (4) the cumulative volume of all tissue outside the PTV receiving a dose >105% of prescription dose should be no more than 15% of the PTV volume; and (5) conformality of PTV coverage will be judged such that the ratio of the volume of the prescription isodose to the volume of the PTV is ideally <1.2 and respect all critical organ dose-volume limits.

12.6.4 *Critical Organ Dose-Volume Limits*

Tumor ablation and normal tissue protection hold the same weight in SABR. In order to ensure that the dose distribution of SABR is safe and reliable, reasonable and objective dose limits should be established and respected for all critical organs. Although dose constraints for major tissues have been established and validated in conventional radiotherapy, they are not yet well established for SABR treatment partly due to inadequate understanding of SABR-related radiobiology and various fractionations. For parallel functioning tissues, the risk of developing complications is mainly dependent on the irradiated volume rather than the maximum dose received. Hence, the planning goal is to ensure that the dose of a critical volume is below the threshold and to maintain the functional integrity of tissues. In contrast, the risk of complications in serial functioning tissue, such as the esophagus, nerves, and trachea, is strongly associated with the maximum dose. Injury of a small segment may potentially destroy the function of the whole organ. Thus, the most secure treatment plan involving serial functioning tissues is to minimize radiation dose to them. NCCN guidelines for NSCLCT and RTOG protocols have defined maximum tolerable dose limits in terms of point dose or volume dose corresponding to critical serially functioning or parallel functioning organs. Treatment plans that violate these limits should be re-optimized. These limits are established using known tolerance data, radiobiological conversion models, and the clinical experience. In order to evaluate actual received dose, these organs should be carefully contoured such that appropriate dose-volume histograms can be generated.

Representative critical organs in lung SABR include the spinal cord, esophagus, ipsilateral brachial plexus, heart and pericardium, trachea and ipsilateral bronchus, ipsilateral lung, and ribs adjacent to tumors.

12.6.5 *Treatment Verification and Delivery*

Once the treatment planning is validated and approved by physicists and physicians, the final step is to verify the accuracy of target fields and treatment delivery. There are a variety of dosimetric devices, such as MapCHECK and Matrix, to conduct dose verification. It is very important to understand the deformation and displacement of treatment target and the surrounding structures in real-time imaging during treatment delivery. Most SABR-capable equipment, including linear accelerators, TomoTherapy and CyberKnife, is assembled with the real-time imaging system to precisely guide treatment. Among them, kilovoltage-based cone beam CT (CBCT) provides the best image quality. Using CBCT images acquired prior to treatment delivery, physicians will be able to directly observe treatment target and its adjacent structures and make an adjustment to correct any location errors if necessary. By adjusting the treatment couch according to image match between simulation images and CBCT images, it is helpful to eliminate the error of interfraction and intrafraction.

12.7 Outcome Assessment and Follow-Up

After SABR treatment, routine follow-up should be performed for outcome assessment and toxicity monitoring. Usually, patients are recommended for follow-up at 1, 3, 6, and 12 months in the first year, then every half year for the next year, and then every year after. The most common follow-up tool is chest CT. In cases with atypical or equivocal findings such as differentiation between tumor recurrence and reactive consolidation, PET/CT may be a necessary supplement. Typically, the outcome can be evaluated using Response Evaluation Criteria in Solid Tumors (RECIST 1.1): (1) complete response (CR), defined as disappearance of lesions; (2) partial response (PR), defined as decrease in target lesion diameter sum ≥30%; (3) stable disease (SD), defined as diameter change within the range of +30%––20%; and (4) progressive disease (PD), defined as increase in target lesion diameter sum ≥20%. Different from conventional radiotherapy, the local control rate of SABR treatment was high, and distant metastasis is the most common failure pattern, and the local recurrence is reported only 10%.

Radiation-induced toxicities are graded according to Common Terminology Criteria for Adverse Events (CTCAE). Table 12.2 listed radiographic presentations after lung SABR treatment in CT imaging (Figs. 12.4, 12.5, and 12.6). As shown in the table, treatment-related pulmonary reaction may mimic tumor recurrence with imaging presentations of mass-like consolidation or scar-like change. It is important to differentiate reactive changes from tumor recurrence, which has a huge impact on further management [14]. Kato et al. performed a study characterize CT manifestations of local recurrence after SABR for stage I NSCLC [15]. Local recurrence should be suspected when any of the following CT features is observed, including (1) a bulging margin, (2) disappearance of air bronchograms, (3) appearance of pleural effusion, or (4) increase in the abnormal opacity after 12 months. However, radiation fibrosis, which may occur 1 year or longer after completion of SABR, is difficult to distinguish from tumor recurrence. Even when opacities increase on follow-up radiologic scans, recurrence cannot be diagnosed conclusively based on image findings; biopsy occasionally is warranted [16]. FDG-PET/CT provides met-

Table 12.2 Radiographic presentations after lung SABR treatment in CT imaging

Early-stage CT findings (≤6 months)	
Diffuse consolidation	Diffuse and homogeneous increase in pulmonary parenchymal attenuation corresponding to high-dose region. The original tumor may be obscured. Air bronchogram may be seen within the area of consolidation
Patchy consolidation	Similar to diffuse consolidation but limited in the extent with patchy distribution
Diffuse GGO	Extensively increasing attenuation of pulmonary tissues adjacent to the target, probably corresponding to areas receiving moderate and high dose. The pulmonary structures are intact
Patchy GGO	Similar to diffuse GGO but limited in the extent with patchy distribution
Late-stage CT findings (>6 months)	
Modified focal consolidation pattern	Chronic consolidation with contraction changes, such as bronchiectasis and interstitial fibrosis
Mass-like pattern	Focal consolidation with resemblance to a mass
Scar-like pattern	Linear opacity in the region of the tumor
No evident change	No evidence of abnormal density within the irradiated area

From *reference: Linda A, Trovo M, Bradley JD (2011) Radiation injury of the lung after stereotactic body radiation therapy (SBRT) for lung cancer: a timeline and pattern of CT changes. Eur J Radiol 79 (1):147–154*. Reprinted with permission

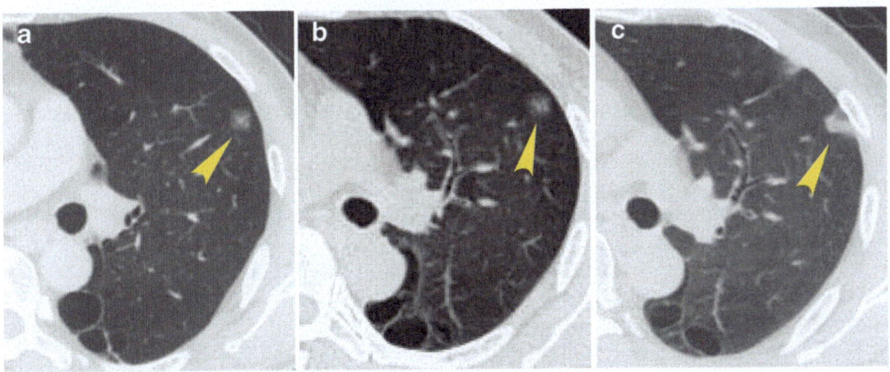

Fig. 12.4 A 60-year-old man received upper lobe resection for lung adenocarcinoma (T1N0M0, Ia) 2 years ago. (**a**) Postoperative follow-up chest CT in May 2013 revealed a 6 mm GGO in the left upper lobe. Five months later, the size of GGO increased to about 10 mm. Second primary lung cancer was highly suspected after a multidisciplinary discussion. Considering the patient's medical history and impaired pulmonary function, SABR was advised to this inoperable lesion; (**b**) Simulated CT image. A regimen of 50 Gy/5 Fx (BED_{10} = 100 Gy) was prescribed; (**c**) One month after SABR, focal consolidation was observed in previous GGO site, suggesting that SABR implementation was precise, and imaging presentations reflected early radiographic changes

abolic information of suspicious lesions and could be helpful in differential diagnosis. FDG uptake tends to be intense and well-defined early after SABR (commonly within 6 months), and in the long term, metabolic intensity decreases and the margin becomes poorly defined. Moderate to intense FDG uptake observed soon after

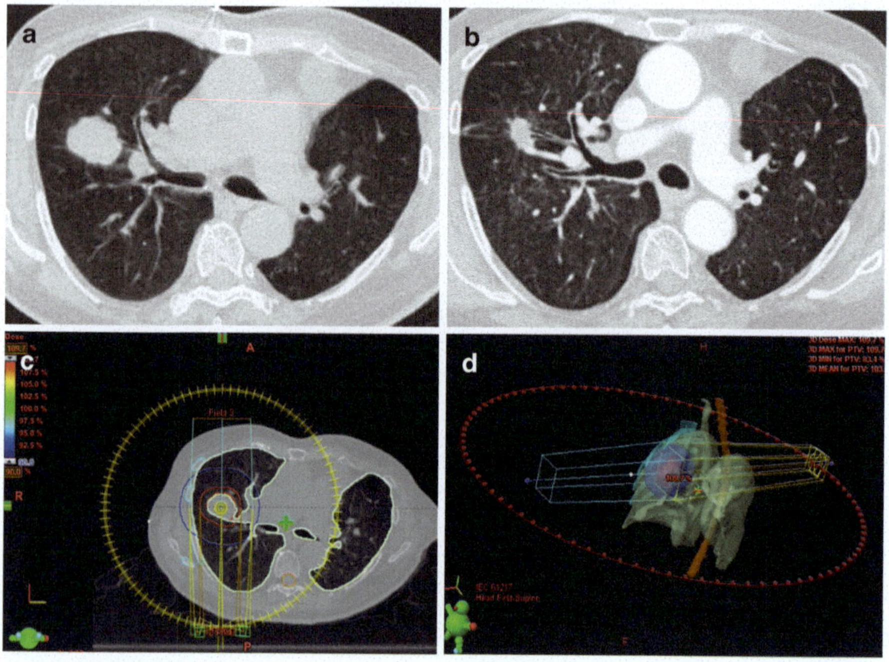

Fig. 12.5 A 79-year-old woman was admitted for a pulmonary nodule. (**a**) CT images showed a 30 mm × 22 mm nodular lesion in the lateral segment of the right middle lobe, with suspicion of peripheral lung adenocarcinoma. The patient was fragile due to severe cardiopulmonary diseases. Invasive procedures including biopsy via bronchoscopy or CT-guided percutaneous biopsy as well as surgery were excluded. She was referred for SABR treatment; (**b**) Two months after SABR delivery, chest CT imaging showed that the lesion significantly regressed to about 16 mm × 15 mm. No evident radiation pneumonitis was observed; (**c**, **d**) SABR treatment planning using arc technique with dose prescription of 50 Gy/5 Fx (BED_{10} = 100 Gy)

SABR does not always indicate a residual tumor, which should be comprehensively analyzed with findings in other imaging modalities, such as CT and physical examinations.

12.8 SABR-Related Adverse Events

Despite that SABR has been proven to be comparably safe and tolerable in patients, especially those with severe comorbidities, various adverse events could occur if it is not properly used or in good quality control. Due to individual susceptibility to radiation exposure, every patient should be consulted on SABR-induced complications.

Considering the short course of SABR, the vast majority of patients do not experience any treatment-related adverse effects during the entire treatment period. The most common adverse is radiation pneumonitis (RP). Typically, it occurs weeks to

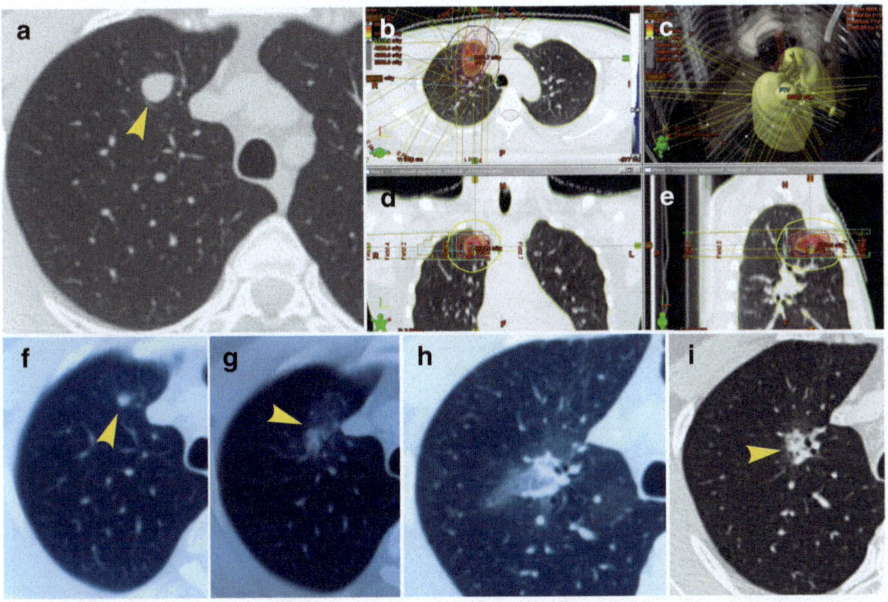

Fig. 12.6 A 43-year-old man was diagnosed nasopharyngeal carcinoma in 2009 and received radiotherapy to nasopharynx and neck. Good local control was achieved. In December 2011, chest CT revealed a solid nodule in the right upper lobe. Follow-up imaging in 2012 showed the lesion grew bigger to 12 mm in diameter. Solitary metastasis was strongly suspected (**a**). The lesion was treated with SABR. (**b–e**) Showed the treatment planning with dose prescription of 60 Gy/8 Fx (BED_{10} = 102 Gy). (**f–i**) Showed follow-up images 2, 7, 12, and 15 months after SABR treatment. The lesion was completely absorbed 7 months later, with only fibrous scars in the previous site

months from treatment, reflecting subacute inflammatory changes in the terminal bronchioles and alveoli. It is reported that the incidence of grade 2–4 pneumonia was about 9.4%, and grade 3–4 severe pneumonia was about 0–15%. The incidence of symptomatic radiation pneumonia was related to V20 and mean lung dose (MLD). Therefore, the incidence and severity can be decreased by limiting the V20 to 20% and MLD < 15 Gy. If a patient undergoes tumor recurrence in the site of previous radiotherapy and re-irradiation using SABR is under consideration, the risk of symptomatic RP will be significantly increased, and the incidence of grade 3 and life-threatening grade 5 pneumonitis could be 18.9% and 1.4%, respectively. The predictive factors for re-irradiation-related RP include ECOG score (2–3), FEV1 (less than or equal to 65%), PTV volume in the previous radiotherapy, and accumulated V20 (≥30%).

Clinically, RP may be very similar to subacute or chronic bacterial pneumonia. The patients may complain fatigue, low-temperature fever, shortness of breath or nonproductive cough, and scattered pulmonary infiltrate on chest X-ray. Chest CT may better reveal the characteristic features of RP, infiltrates or exudates highly matching the radiation fields, known as geometric distribution, instead of following a lobar or segmental distribution. In some cases, the RP may extend outside of radiation fields and ill-defined (Fig. 12.7). If pneumonitis occurs during the treat-

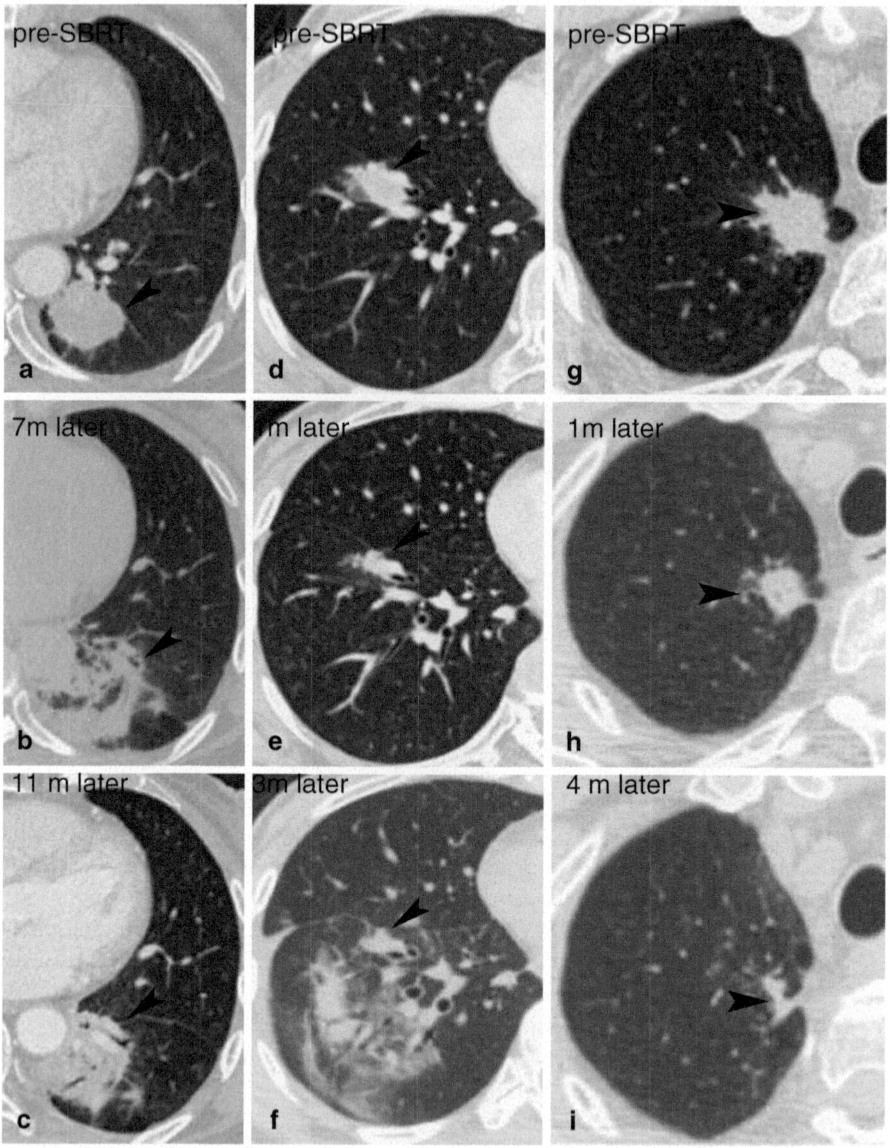

Fig. 12.7 Radiation-induced pneumonitis after SABR. (**a**) A 66-year-old female with lung cancer in the left lower lobe received SABR (48 Gy/8 Fx). Seven months later, the lesion shrank and reactive inflammation scattered around the lesion. Four more months later, the lesion regressed, and pneumonitis was partly dissolved. (**b**) A 38-year-old female with lung adenocarcinoma in the right lower lobe was treated with SABR (50 Gy/5 Fx). The follow-up imaging at 1 month and 3 months after treatment showed the lesion continuously shrank with mild radiation pneumonitis. (**c**) A 62-year-old male with peripheral lung cancer in the right upper lobe received SABR treatment (50 Gy/5 Fx). The follow-up imaging at 1 month and 4 months after treatment showed the lesion continuously shrank without evident reactive pneumonitis

ment, radiation therapy should be interrupted. In the meanwhile, corticosteroids and prophylactic antibiotics should be administered. These patients with intra-treatment RP should be carefully monitored even after radiotherapy since they have increasing risks for severe RP. Nonsteroidal anti-inflammatory agents or steroid inhalers could be used to alleviate mild RP, while in cases of severe pneumonitis comprehensive approaches, including systemic steroids and bronchodilators are required.

Nerve injury could happen if the tumor is located on the apex of the lung, close to the brachial plexus, and at the same time, dose constraint of brachial plexus is not well respected. According to a study reporting 36 cases of apical NSCLC treated with SABR (57 Gy/3 Fx), the incidence of brachial plexopathy was 19.4%. The median of the maximum brachial plexus doses of patients developing brachial plexopathy was 30 Gy. Two-year Kaplan–Meier risk of brachial plexopathy for maximum brachial plexus dose >26 Gy was 46% vs. 8% for doses ≤26 Gy. Clinical symptoms include ipsilateral shoulder/arm neuropathic pain, upper extremity weakness, numbness of the upper extremity, or even paralysis of hand and wrist. For avoid severe injury to brachial plexus, accurate delineation of this structure is important, and RTOG has released a guideline for brachial plexus contouring.

If a tumor is close to the chest wall, pleural pain and rib fracture may occur due to high dose to chest wall and ribs. A study based on 265 patients with tumors located less than 2.5 cm from the chest wall showed that the incidence of chronic chest pain was 17%, and obesity and diabetes are independent risk factors besides dose. Practically, dose limit of the chest wall is usually recommended as V30 < 30 cc (for regimens with 3–5 fractions). Both dose and volume have impacts on ribs. For a 3-fraction SABR regimen (60 Gy/3 Fx), if 2cc rib receives 21 Gy, 27 Gy, and 48 Gy, the risk of rib fractures is 50%, 5%, and 0%, respectively.

Other potential SABR-related adverse events include hemoptysis, interstitial pneumonia, bacterial pneumonia, pulmonary fibrosis, pulmonary embolism, bronchial stenosis, bronchial and pulmonary venous fistula, trachea and esophagus fistula, esophagitis, esophageal ulcer, pleural effusion, pericardial effusion and dermatitis, etc. Well-designed treatment planning with respect to dose constraints of critical organs is the best strategy of minimizing risks of any treatment-related adverse events. After treatment, close monitoring at routine basis is necessary to detect and follow up the development of adverse events, and if necessary to initiate a medical intervention to improve the quality of life of patients.

References

1. Onishi H, Araki T, Shirato H, Nagata Y, Hiraoka M, Gomi K, Yamashita T, Niibe Y, Karasawa K, Hayakawa K, Takai Y, Kimura T, Hirokawa Y, Takeda A, Ouchi A, Hareyama M, Kokubo M, Hara R, Itami J, Yamada K. Stereotactic hypofractionated high-dose irradiation for stage I nonsmall cell lung carcinoma: clinical outcomes in 245 subjects in a Japanese multiinstitutional study. Cancer. 2004;101(7):1623–31. https://doi.org/10.1002/cncr.20539.
2. Zhang J, Yang F, Li B, Li H, Liu J, Huang W, Wang D, Yi Y, Wang J. Which is the optimal biologically effective dose of stereotactic body radiotherapy for stage I non-small-cell

lung cancer? A meta-analysis. Int J Radiat Oncol Biol Phys. 2011;81(4):e305–16. https://doi.org/10.1016/j.ijrobp.2011.04.034.
3. Timmerman RD. Surgery versus stereotactic body radiation therapy for early-stage lung cancer: who's down for the count? J Clin Oncol. 2010;28(6):907–9. https://doi.org/10.1200/jco.2009.26.5165.
4. Raz DJ, Zell JA, Ou SH, Gandara DR, Anton-Culver H, Jablons DM. Natural history of stage I non-small cell lung cancer: implications for early detection. Chest. 2007;132(1):193–9. https://doi.org/10.1378/chest.06-3096.
5. Wao H, Mhaskar R, Kumar A, Miladinovic B, Djulbegovic B. Survival of patients with non-small cell lung cancer without treatment: a systematic review and meta-analysis. Syst Rev. 2013;2:10. https://doi.org/10.1186/2046-4053-2-10.
6. Murai T, Shibamoto Y, Baba F, Hashizume C, Mori Y, Ayakawa S, Kawai T, Takemoto S, Sugie C, Ogino H. Progression of non-small-cell lung cancer during the interval before stereotactic body radiotherapy. Int J Radiat Oncol Biol Phys. 2012;82(1):463–7. https://doi.org/10.1016/j.ijrobp.2010.10.001.
7. Allibhai Z, Taremi M, Bezjak A, Brade A, Hope AJ, Sun A, Cho BC. The impact of tumor size on outcomes after stereotactic body radiation therapy for medically inoperable early-stage non-small cell lung cancer. Int J Radiat Oncol Biol Phys. 2013;87(5):1064–70. https://doi.org/10.1016/j.ijrobp.2013.08.020.
8. Palma DA, Nguyen TK, Kwan K, Gaede S, Landis M, Malthaner R, Fortin D, Louie AV, Frechette E, Rodrigues GB, Yaremko B, Yu E, Dar AR, Lee TY, Gratton A, Warner A, Ward A, Inculet R. Short report: interim safety results for a phase II trial measuring the integration of stereotactic ablative radiotherapy (SABR) plus surgery for early stage non-small cell lung cancer (MISSILE-NSCLC). Radiat Oncol. 2017;12(1):30. https://doi.org/10.1186/s13014-017-0770-7.
9. Palma D, Visser O, Lagerwaard FJ, Belderbos J, Slotman BJ, Senan S. Impact of introducing stereotactic lung radiotherapy for elderly patients with stage I non-small-cell lung cancer: a population-based time-trend analysis. J Clin Oncol. 2010;28(35):5153–9. https://doi.org/10.1200/JCO.2010.30.0731.
10. Zheng X, Schipper M, Kidwell K, Lin J, Reddy R, Ren Y, Chang A, Lv F, Orringer M, Spring Kong FM. Survival outcome after stereotactic body radiation therapy and surgery for stage I non-small cell lung cancer: a meta-analysis. Int J Radiat Oncol Biol Phys. 2014;90(3):603–11. https://doi.org/10.1016/j.ijrobp.2014.05.055.
11. Urban D, Mishra M, Onn A, Dicker AP, Symon Z, Pfeffer MR, Lawrence YR. Radiotherapy improves survival in unresected stage I-III bronchoalveolar carcinoma. Int J Radiat Oncol Biol Phys. 2012;84(3):780–5. https://doi.org/10.1016/j.ijrobp.2012.01.007.
12. Badiyan SN, Bierhals AJ, Olsen JR, Creach KM, Garsa AA, Dewees T, Bradley JD, Robinson CG. Stereotactic body radiation therapy for the treatment of early-stage minimally invasive adenocarcinoma or adenocarcinoma in situ (formerly bronchioloalveolar carcinoma): a patterns of failure analysis. Radiat Oncol. 2013;8:4. https://doi.org/10.1186/1748-717X-8-4.
13. Benedict SH, Yenice KM, Followill D, Galvin JM, Hinson W, Kavanagh B, Keall P, Lovelock M, Meeks S, Papiez L, Purdie T, Sadagopan R, Schell MC, Salter B, Schlesinger DJ, Shiu AS, Solberg T, Song DY, Stieber V, Timmerman R, Tome WA, Verellen D, Wang L, Yin FF. Stereotactic body radiation therapy: the report of AAPM Task Group 101. Med Phys. 2010;37(8):4078–101. https://doi.org/10.1118/1.3438081.
14. Linda A, Trovo M, Bradley JD. Radiation injury of the lung after stereotactic body radiation therapy (SBRT) for lung cancer: a timeline and pattern of CT changes. Eur J Radiol. 2011;79(1):147–54. https://doi.org/10.1016/j.ejrad.2009.10.029.
15. Kato S, Nambu A, Onishi H, Saito A, Kuriyama K, Komiyama T, Marino K, Araki T. Computed tomography appearances of local recurrence after stereotactic body radiation therapy for stage I non-small-cell lung carcinoma. Jpn J Radiol. 2010;28(4):259–65. https://doi.org/10.1007/s11604-009-0415-3.

16. Takeda A, Kunieda E, Takeda T, Tanaka M, Sanuki N, Fujii H, Shigematsu N, Kubo A. Possible misinterpretation of demarcated solid patterns of radiation fibrosis on CT scans as tumor recurrence in patients receiving hypofractionated stereotactic radiotherapy for lung cancer. Int J Radiat Oncol Biol Phys. 2008;70(4):1057–65. https://doi.org/10.1016/j.ijrobp.2007.07.2383.

Suggested Readings

1. Baumann M, Krause M, Overgaard J, Debus J, Bentzen SM, Daartz J, Richter C, Zips D, Bortfeld T. Radiation oncology in the era of precision medicine. Nat Rev Cancer. 2016;16(4):234–49. https://doi.org/10.1038/nrc.2016.18.
2. Bradley JD, El Naqa I, Drzymala RE, Trovo M, Jones G, Denning MD. Stereotactic body radiation therapy for early-stage non-small-cell lung cancer: the pattern of failure is distant. Int J Radiat Oncol Biol Phys. 2010;77(4):1146–50. https://doi.org/10.1016/j.ijrobp.2009.06.017.
3. Buyyounouski MK, Balter P, Lewis B, D'Ambrosio DJ, Dilling TJ, Miller RC, Schefter T, Tome W, Harris EE, Price RA Jr, Konski AA, Wallner PE. Stereotactic body radiotherapy for early-stage non-small-cell lung cancer: report of the ASTRO Emerging Technology Committee. Int J Radiat Oncol Biol Phys. 2010;78(1):3–10. https://doi.org/10.1016/j.ijrobp.2010.04.010.
4. Chang JY, Senan S, Paul MA, Mehran RJ, Louie AV, Balter P, Groen HJ, McRae SE, Widder J, Feng L, van den Borne BE, Munsell MF, Hurkmans C, Berry DA, van Werkhoven E, Kresl JJ, Dingemans AM, Dawood O, Haasbeek CJ, Carpenter LS, De Jaeger K, Komaki R, Slotman BJ, Smit EF, Roth JA. Stereotactic ablative radiotherapy versus lobectomy for operable stage I non-small-cell lung cancer: a pooled analysis of two randomised trials. Lancet Oncol. 2015;16(6):630–7. https://doi.org/10.1016/s1470-2045(15)70168-3.
5. Chen F, Matsuo Y, Yoshizawa A, Sato T, Sakai H, Bando T, Okubo K, Shibuya K, Date H. Salvage lung resection for non-small cell lung cancer after stereotactic body radiotherapy in initially operable patients. J Thorac Oncol. 2010;5(12):1999–2002. https://doi.org/10.1097/JTO.0b013e3181f260f9.
6. Crabtree T, Puri V, Timmerman R, Fernando H, Bradley J, Decker PA, Paulus R, Putnum JB Jr, Dupuy DE, Meyers B. Treatment of stage I lung cancer in high-risk and inoperable patients: comparison of prospective clinical trials using stereotactic body radiotherapy (RTOG 0236), sublobar resection (ACOSOG Z4032), and radiofrequency ablation (ACOSOG Z4033). J Thorac Cardiovasc Surg. 2013;145(3):692–9. https://doi.org/10.1016/j.jtcvs.2012.10.038.
7. De Ruysscher D, Faivre-Finn C, Nestle U, Hurkmans CW, Le Pechoux C, Price A, Senan S. European Organisation for Research and Treatment of Cancer recommendations for planning and delivery of high-dose, high-precision radiotherapy for lung cancer. J Clin Oncol. 2010;28(36):5301–10. https://doi.org/10.1200/JCO.2010.30.3271.
8. Dunlap NE, Larner JM, Read PW, Kozower BD, Lau CL, Sheng K, Jones DR. Size matters: a comparison of T1 and T2 peripheral non-small-cell lung cancers treated with stereotactic body radiation therapy (SBRT). J Thorac Cardiovasc Surg. 2010;140(3):583–9. https://doi.org/10.1016/j.jtcvs.2010.01.046.
9. Forquer JA, Fakiris AJ, Timmerman RD, Lo SS, Perkins SM, McGarry RC, Johnstone PA. Brachial plexopathy from stereotactic body radiotherapy in early-stage NSCLC: dose-limiting toxicity in apical tumor sites. Radiother Oncol. 2009;93(3):408–13. https://doi.org/10.1016/j.radonc.2009.04.018.
10. Jumeau R, Bahig H, Filion E, Campeau MP, Lambert L, Roberge D, Gorgos AB, Vu T. Assessing the need for adjuvant chemotherapy after stereotactic body radiation therapy in early-stage non-small cell lung carcinoma. Cureus. 2016;8(11):e901. https://doi.org/10.7759/cureus.901.
11. Louie AV, Senan S, Dahele M, Slotman BJ, Verbakel WF. Stereotactic ablative radiation therapy for subcentimeter lung tumors: clinical, dosimetric, and image guidance considerations. Int J Radiat Oncol Biol Phys. 2014;90(4):843–9. https://doi.org/10.1016/j.ijrobp.2014.06.064.

12. Love SM, Hardman G, Mashar R, Shah RD. Is it time for SABR to overtake surgery as the treatment of choice for stage I non-small cell lung cancer? Ann Transl Med. 2016;4(24):535. https://doi.org/10.21037/atm.2016.11.69.
13. Matsuo Y, Nakamoto Y, Nagata Y, Shibuya K, Takayama K, Norihisa Y, Narabayashi M, Mizowaki T, Saga T, Higashi T, Togashi K, Hiraoka M. Characterization of FDG-PET images after stereotactic body radiation therapy for lung cancer. Radiother Oncol. 2010;97(2):200–4. https://doi.org/10.1016/j.radonc.2010.04.011.
14. Moghanaki D, Chang JY. Is surgery still the optimal treatment for stage I non-small cell lung cancer? Transl Lung Cancer Res. 2016;5(2):183–9. https://doi.org/10.21037/tlcr.2016.04.05.
15. Nagata Y, Wulf J, Lax I, Timmerman R, Zimmermann F, Stojkovski I, Jeremic B. Stereotactic radiotherapy of primary lung cancer and other targets: results of consultant meeting of the International Atomic Energy Agency. Int J Radiat Oncol Biol Phys. 2011;79(3):660–9. https://doi.org/10.1016/j.ijrobp.2010.10.004.
16. National Comprehensive Cancer Network Non-small cell lung cancer. https://www.nccn.org/professionals/physician_gls/pdf/nscl.pdf. Accessed 20 Aug 2017.
17. Neri S, Takahashi Y, Terashi T, Hamakawa H, Tomii K, Katakami N, Kokubo M. Surgical treatment of local recurrence after stereotactic body radiotherapy for primary and metastatic lung cancers. J Thorac Oncol. 2010;5(12):2003–7. https://doi.org/10.1097/JTO.0b013e3181f8a785.
18. Nguyen TK, Palma DA. Pros: after stereotactic ablative radiotherapy for a peripheral early-stage non-small cell lung cancer, radiological suspicion of a local recurrence can be sufficient indication to proceed to salvage therapy. Transl Lung Cancer Res. 2016;5(6):647–50. https://doi.org/10.21037/tlcr.2016.12.07.
19. Pan H, Simpson DR, Mell LK, Mundt AJ, Lawson JD. A survey of stereotactic body radiotherapy use in the United States. Cancer. 2011;117(19):4566–72. https://doi.org/10.1002/cncr.26067.
20. Paul S, Lee PC, Mao J, Isaacs AJ, Sedrakyan A. Long term survival with stereotactic ablative radiotherapy (SABR) versus thoracoscopic sublobar lung resection in elderly people: national population based study with propensity matched comparative analysis. BMJ. 2016;354:i3570. https://doi.org/10.1136/bmj.i3570.
21. Radiation Therapy Oncology Group RTOG 0236: A Phase II Trial of Stereotactic Body Radiation Therapy (SBRT) in the Treatment of Patients with Medically Inoperable Stage I/II Non-Small Cell Lung Cancer. https://www.rtog.org/ClinicalTrials/ProtocolTable/StudyDetails.aspx?study=0236. Accessed 20 Aug 2017.
22. Radiation Therapy Oncology Group RTOG 0618: A Phase II Trial of Stereotactic Body Radiation Therapy (SBRT) in the Treatment of Patients with Operable Stage I/II Non-Small Cell Lung Cancer. https://www.rtog.org/ClinicalTrials/ProtocolTable/StudyDetails.aspx?study=0618. Accessed 20 Aug 2017.
23. Radiation Therapy Oncology Group RTOG 0813: Seamless Phase I/II Study of Stereotactic Lung Radiotherapy (SBRT) for Early Stage, Centrally Located, Non-Small Cell Lung Cancer (NSCLC) in Medically Inoperable Patients. https://www.rtog.org/ClinicalTrials/ProtocolTable/StudyDetails.aspx?study=0813. Accessed 20 Aug 2017.
24. Radiation Therapy Oncology Group RTOG 0915: A Randomized Phase II Study Comparing 2 Stereotactic Body Radiation Therapy (SBRT) Schedules for Medically Inoperable Patients with Stage I Peripheral Non-Small Cell Lung Cancer. https://www.rtog.org/ClinicalTrials/ProtocolTable/StudyDetails.aspx?study=0915. Accessed 20 Aug 2017.
25. Rosen JE, Salazar MC, Wang Z, Yu JB, Decker RH, Kim AW, Detterbeck FC, Boffa DJ. Lobectomy versus stereotactic body radiotherapy in healthy patients with stage I lung cancer. J Thorac Cardiovasc Surg. 2016;152(1):44–54.e49. https://doi.org/10.1016/j.jtcvs.2016.03.060.
26. Scott JG, Berglund A, Schell MJ, Mihaylov I, Fulp WJ, Yue B, Welsh E, Caudell JJ, Ahmed K, Strom TS, Mellon E, Venkat P, Johnstone P, Foekens J, Lee J, Moros E, Dalton WS, Eschrich SA, McLeod H, Harrison LB, Torres-Roca JF. A genome-based model for adjusting radiotherapy dose (GARD): a retrospective, cohort-based study. Lancet Oncol. 2017;18(2):202–11. https://doi.org/10.1016/s1470-2045(16)30648-9.

27. Senthi S, Lagerwaard FJ, Haasbeek CJ, Slotman BJ, Senan S. Patterns of disease recurrence after stereotactic ablative radiotherapy for early stage non-small-cell lung cancer: a retrospective analysis. Lancet Oncol. 2012;13(8):802–9. https://doi.org/10.1016/s1470-2045(12)70242-5.
28. Shultz DB, Trakul N, Abelson JA, Murphy JD, Maxim PG, Le QT, Loo BW Jr, Diehn M. Imaging features associated with disease progression after stereotactic ablative radiotherapy for stage I non-small-cell lung cancer. Clin Lung Cancer. 2014;15(4):294–301.e293. https://doi.org/10.1016/j.cllc.2013.12.011.
29. Stanic S, Paulus R, Timmerman RD, Michalski JM, Barriger RB, Bezjak A, Videtic GM, Bradley J. No clinically significant changes in pulmonary function following stereotactic body radiation therapy for early- stage peripheral non-small cell lung cancer: an analysis of RTOG 0236. Int J Radiat Oncol Biol Phys. 2014;88(5):1092–9. https://doi.org/10.1016/j.ijrobp.2013.12.050.
30. Subramanian SV, Subramani V, Swamy ST, Gandhi A, Chilukuri S, Kathirvel M. Is 5 mm MMLC suitable for VMAT-based lung SBRT? A dosimetric comparison with 2.5 mm HDMLC using RTOG-0813 treatment planning criteria for both conventional and high-dose flattening filter-free photon beams. J Appl Clin Med Phys. 2015a;16(4):112–24. https://doi.org/10.1120/jacmp.v16i4.5415.
31. Travis WD, Asamura H, Bankier AA, Beasley MB, Detterbeck F, Flieder DB, Goo JM, MacMahon H, Naidich D, Nicholson AG, Powell CA, Prokop M, Rami-Porta R, Rusch V, van Schil P, Yatabe Y, International Association for the Study of Lung Cancer S, Prognostic Factors C, Advisory Board M. The IASLC lung cancer staging project: proposals for coding T categories for subsolid nodules and assessment of tumor size in part-solid tumors in the forthcoming eighth edition of the TNM classification of lung cancer. J Thorac Oncol. 2016;11(8):1204–1223. doi:https://doi.org/10.1016/j.jtho.2016.03.025.
32. Travis WD, Brambilla E, Noguchi M, Nicholson AG, Geisinger KR, Yatabe Y, Beer DG, Powell CA, Riely GJ, Van Schil PE, Garg K, Austin JH, Asamura H, Rusch VW, Hirsch FR, Scagliotti G, Mitsudomi T, Huber RM, Ishikawa Y, Jett J, Sanchez-Cespedes M, Sculier JP, Takahashi T, Tsuboi M, Vansteenkiste J, Wistuba I, Yang PC, Aberle D, Brambilla C, Flieder D, Franklin W, Gazdar A, Gould M, Hasleton P, Henderson D, Johnson B, Johnson D, Kerr K, Kuriyama K, Lee JS, Miller VA, Petersen I, Roggli V, Rosell R, Saijo N, Thunnissen E, Tsao M, Yankelewitz D. International association for the study of lung cancer/american thoracic society/european respiratory society international multidisciplinary classification of lung adenocarcinoma. J Thorac Oncol. 2011;6(2):244–85. https://doi.org/10.1097/JTO.0b013e318206a221.

Chapter 13
Management Strategies for Early-Stage Lung Cancer: Non-SABR Ablative Therapy

Hailiang Li and Lin Zheng

Surgery remains the standard of treatment in early-stage lung cancer. Currently, the 5-year survival rate for stage I NSCLC with standard surgical treatment is approximately 60–80%. As discussed in the previous chapter, about 20% of patients with stage I NSCLC may not tolerate surgical resection due to comorbidities or potentially high risk of severe perioperative complications. For them, nonsurgical approaches should be pursued. Since early-stage NSCLC is localized disease, localized approaches with ablative capability are desirable. Besides radiation-based noninvasive stereotactic ablative radiotherapy (SABR), minimally invasive percutaneous ablative approaches have been proven to be effective. The commonly used percutaneous ablative techniques include radiofrequency ablation (RFA), microwave ablation, and argon-helium cryoablation. These approaches destroy tumor tissues irreversibly by thermal damage of either hyperthermia or hypothermia.

13.1 Radiofrequency Ablative Therapy

13.1.1 Outcomes of RFA in NSCLC

Of note, in most RFA studies, the patient population is heterogeneous, including patients with early-stage NSCLC and those with oligometastatic lung tumors. Therefore, this heterogeneity should be taken into consideration when discussing RFA outcomes in early-stage NSCLC. In 2008, Zhu et al. assessed systemically the safety and efficacy of RFA based on outcome reports of 707 patients from 17 institutions [1]. The lesion number and size were heterogenous, ranging from 1 to 2.8 and 1.7 cm to

H. Li (✉) • L. Zheng
Department of Interventional Radiology, Zhengzhou University Cancer Hospital, Zhengzhou, China
e-mail: cjr.lihailiang@vip.163.com

X. Zheng et al. (eds.), *Early-stage Lung Cancer*,
https://doi.org/10.1007/978-981-10-7596-4_13

5.2 cm, respectively. The progression-free interval was reported between 15 months and 26.7 months. The 1- and 3-year survival rates ranged from 63% to 85% and 15% to 46%, respectively. Complete ablation of tumor varies in the range of 39–97% of lesions after the initial treatment. The local recurrence after RFA was reported between 3 and 38.1%. The overall procedure-related morbidity rate was reported between 15.2 and 55.6%, and the mortality rate could be as high as 5.6%. Pneumothorax was the most commonly reported complication with an incidence ranging from 4.5 to 61.1%. Among them, approximately 11% (ranging from 3.3 to 38.9%) of patients required hospitalization for management, such as chest drain insertion.

It appears to be a strong correlation between tumor size and treatment results, better tumor controls being achieved in smaller tumors. Satisfactory treatment response had been reported in tumors smaller than 5 cm and more frequently in tumors smaller than 3 cm [2]. Based on follow-up imaging assessment, for tumor ≤3 cm, the complete ablation rate was 78–100%, significantly higher than tumors >3 cm. In the study from De Baère et al., the estimated rate of incomplete local treatment per tumor at 18 months was 5% for tumors measuring 2 cm or smaller in their largest diameter and 13% for tumors larger than 2 cm [3]. This difference was not statistically significant, but a trend was noted.

Ablation range is vital to the success of RFA treatment. In the same study from De Baère et al., the association between ablation completeness and the ablation range (measured by the ratio between the area of ground glass and the tumor area before treatment) was analyzed. The results revealed that in the 73 tumors with a ratio ≥ 4, the rate of incomplete local treatment was 4%, which is significantly lower than when this ratio was <4, with a 19% incomplete local treatment rate [3]. Anderson et al. [4] retrospectively reviewed the post-RFA imaging with a purpose to discover early indicators of treatment success. They found that there was substantial consistency between the site without ground-glass opacification (GGO) margin and tumor relapse, implying that a circumferential GGO margin of >5 mm should be recommended as the minimal margin to ensure complete tumor ablation, which is pretty much in consistency with studies on microscopic tumor extension in NSCLC for radiotherapy. Giraud et al. [5] investigated the degree of local microscopic extension based on histological types and found the microscopic extension was different for adenocarcinoma and squamous cell carcinoma. To cover 95% of the microscopic extension in radiotherapy, the expanded distance from detectable tumor margin (gross tumor margin) should be 8 mm and 6 mm for adenocarcinoma and squamous cell carcinoma, respectively.

In contrast to technical specifications of RFA, pathological features have few impacts on outcomes as well as local progression after treatment. In a study conducted by Hiraki et al., 35 primary lung cancers and 217 metastatic lung tumors originally from colorectal cancer, renal cell carcinoma, and hepatocellular carcinoma received RFA treatment [6]. Local control rates appeared subject to tumor histology. In comparison to other four tumor types, metastatic colorectal cancer had the best response to RFA treatment with significantly higher local control rate. However, multivariate analysis showed conflicting results, and all tumor types had the similar relative risk of local progression after RFA treatment.

Vessel proximity, defined as the presence of large vessels (>3 mm diameter) in direct contact with any part of the tumor, has been shown as one of the dominant factors in recurrence after RFA treatment. Vessel proximity creates difficulty of achieving complete ablation in tumors. Simon et al. reported residual tumor enhancement post-ablation when tumors were in close proximity to major pulmonary arteries or veins [7]. Experimental results showed that percutaneous balloon occlusion of the pulmonary artery could improve the shape and volume of ablation in the RFA treatment of lung cancer. However, this procedure has poor clinical performance based on a case report including five patients.

13.1.1.1 Survival

Simon et al. reported long-term outcomes of RFA in primary NSCLC in 2007 [8]. Among 75 patients, 75% was stage IA disease, and the rest was stage IB disease. The overall median survival period was 29 months with 30 months for stage IA and 25 months for stage IB. The 1-, 2-, 3-, 4-, and 5-year overall survival rates were 78%, 57%, 36%, 27%, and 27%, respectively. Smaller tumor (diameter ≤ 3 cm) had a better outcome, and the 5-year survival rate was close to 50%. The same group also reported the outcomes of radiofrequency ablation in combination with brachytherapy treatment in 14 NSCLC with diameter < 3 cm, showing that the 3-year survival rate was 57% with a median survival period of 44.4 months.

With accumulation of clinical experience, technical and equipment development and the safety and efficacy of RFA treatment significantly improved in lung tumors, including recurrent tumors as salvage treatment. Kodama et al. [9] reported RFA treatment to 51 recurrent lesions in 44 patients. In this study, the mean diameter of lesions was 1.7 cm. The 1-, 3-, and 5-year overall survival rates were 97.7%, 72.9%, and 55.7%. Grouped by tumor size, the 1-, 3-, and 5-year survival rates for patients with smaller tumors (diameter ≤ 3 cm) were 100%, 79.8%, and 60.5%, while the 1- and 3-year survival in patients with larger tumors (diameter in a range of 3.1–4.0 cm) were 83.3% and 31.3%, respectively. Palussière et al. reported similar results. Numerous studies have shown that tumor size was one of the major influential factors of disease-free survival.

The milestone prospective RAPTURE study recruited 183 lung tumors that were 3.5 cm in diameter or smaller to identify the feasibility, safety, and effectiveness of RFA of malignant lung tumors [10]. All patients were considered by the treating physician to be unsuitable for surgery and unfit for radiotherapy or chemotherapy. A confirmed complete response of target tumors lasting at least 1 year was shown in 88% of assessable patients. No differences in response were noted among patients with NSCLC or lung metastases. The 1- and 2-year overall survival was 70% and 48% in patients with NSCLC, 89% and 66% with colorectal metastases, and 92% and 64% with other metastases. The 1- and 2-year cancer-specific survival was 92% and 73% in patients with NSCLC, 91% and 68% with colorectal metastases, and 93% and 67% (48–84%) with other metastases. Patients with stage I NSCLC had a 2-year overall survival of 75% and a 2-year cancer-specific survival of 92%.

Charlson comorbidity index (CCI) has been widely used for clinical evaluation of preexisting comorbidities. And studies have shown that CCI could be used to predict RFA treatment outcome. Simon et al. retrospectively analyzed a group of 82 RFA cases using the CCI index. The 3-year overall survival rate was 50.6%. Single-factor comparison revealed that gender, disease stage, histological type, and CCI score were significantly related to survival. After covarying for age, tumor stage > IB, squamous histology, and gender, multiple Cox regressions showed that an increasing CCI score was significantly associated with an increased risk of death. Compared with groups with CCI score of 1–2 points (OS, 55.5 months) or CCI score of 3–4 points (OS, 36.6 months), the group with CCI of 5 points had a poor prognosis with overall survival period of only 10.43 months. Additionally, no significant difference in OS was observed between patient groups with CCI 1–2 points and CCI 3–4 points.

Regarding the comparative efficacy between RFA and other ablative approaches (SABR, mainly), head-to-head clinical trials are absent. Bi et al. performed a systemic review and meta-analysis to provide a comparison between RFA and SABR, for treatment of medically inoperable stage I NSCLC, with a focus on LCR, OS, and treatment-related toxicities [11]. This analysis included 13 studies on RFA (328 patients) and 31 studies on SABR (2767 patients). Local control rate at 1, 2, 3, and 5 years for RFA was 77%, 48%, 55%, and 42%, respectively, which was significantly lower than that for SABR: 97%, 92%, 88%, and 86%. These differences remained significant after correcting for stage IA and age. The effect of RFA was not different from that of SABR on OS. The most frequent complication of RFA is pneumothorax, occurring in 30.9% of patients, while that for SABR (≥grade 3) is radiation pneumonitis, occurring in 2.2% of patients.

13.1.1.2 Post-RFA Follow-Up

In most cases, the ablative operation is CT-guided, and the ablative changes could be real-time monitored. In addition, chest CT imaging is the preferable imaging modality for post-RFA follow-up. A variety of imaging features could be observed in follow-up CT imaging, including ground-glass opacities surrounding and within ablation zone, wrinkled tumor margin edge, vaporization, and "cockade phenomenon" (characterized by concentric rings with various attenuation).

During the course of ablation, the tumor may shrink or remain unchanged. The incidence of cavitation can be up to 25%. In CT images acquired 1 month after RFA, preexisting nodular lesion in ablation zone may appear much larger than before, frequently accompanied by cavitation or translucent bubbles. Six months later, unless a complete response to treatment occurs, the nodular size may not change or increase on the opposite. Jin et al. evaluated the RFA-related imaging changes and their correlation to therapeutic efficacy on consecutive follow-up CT images [12]. In the complete ablation group, no contrast enhancement was observed, and the lesion size gradually decreased by 5.7%, 11.4%, 14.3%, 40%, and 40% at 3, 6, 9, 12, and 15 months, respectively. In contrast, those lesions with partial ablation showed various degrees of enhancement, and more importantly, the lesion size rebounded after a 6-month decrease, indicative of the tumor recurrence. Hence, the enhancement pattern and dynamic size change could be used to determine whether a complete ablation has been achieved or there exist residual tumors. Three months after RFA treatment, pleural thickening may be seen along the trajectory of the ablation electrode puncture due to heating injury from the electrode, but reactive pleural effusion is relatively rare.

Measurement of CT attenuation (CT value) of nodular lesions is helpful to distinguish post-RFA nodular change from residual tumors or local recurrence. With a successful and complete ablation, a dramatic reduction in CT attenuation is commonly observed, and the residual tissues cannot be enhanced with the administration of contrast medium. If the size of soft tissue in ablation region is 1.25 times as large as that in pre-RFA imaging with remarkable heterogeneous enhancement, partial progress should be strongly suspected. However, soft tissues with relatively homogeneous enhancement are located close to ablation zone margin (<5 mm), so the likelihood of reactive pneumonitis is higher than tumor relapse.

Positron emission tomography (PET) is another valuable imaging tool for assessment of RFA treatment. In comparison to baseline pre-RFA PET imaging, decreasing FDG uptake in post-RFA imaging indicates a response, and complete absence of metabolic activity may hint a complete metabolic response. Yoo et al. evaluated initial PET/CT imaging after RFA of stage IA NSCLC to determine whether treatment success or residual disease can be predicted with early post-RFA PET scanning [13]. They found that patients with a complete metabolic response at early PET/CT (within 4 days of RFA) had a 1-year event rate of 43%, whereas those with partial or no response had a 1-year event rate of 67%. In contrast, patients with a complete metabolic response at late post-RFA PET/CT (at 6 months of RFA) had a 1-year event rate of 0%, whereas those with a partial response had an overall event rate of 75%, indicating that 6-month post-RFA PET/CT findings correlate better with clinical outcome at 1 year. Certainly, PET imaging is also useful for the detection of residual or recurrent tumor, which commonly occurs along the periphery of the tumor with increased metabolic activity.

13.1.2 Indications and Contraindications of RFA in NSCLC

13.1.2.1 Indications

Biopsy-proven localized lung tumors are the preferable candidate for RFA treatment, including (a) inoperable early-stage primary lung cancer due to severe comorbidities, such as poor pulmonary function reserve or existing anatomical restrictions for effective surgical resection; (b) tumor recurrence after previous surgery, radiotherapy, or chemotherapy; and (c) solitary metastatic or oligometastatic lung tumors.

13.1.2.2 Contraindications

RFA has good safety profile but risks should be cautioned. This procedure should be avoided or postponed if the following conditions exist, including (a) uncorrected coagulopathy and laboratory abnormalities, for instance, international normalized ratio > 1.5, platelet less than 50,000/mm^3, (b) uncontrolled hemophilia and von Willebrand disease (von Willebrand disease), and (c) bacteremia or active infection.

This procedure should be performed with extreme caution if the following conditions exist, including (a) tumors adjacent to critical structures, such as mediastinal structure, large vessels (aorta and pulmonary trunk), esophagus, and chest wall and (b) adjacent pulmonary vessels diameter greater than 3 mm. Many studies have shown that large vessels have significantly negative impacts on RFA outcomes probably due to a heat sink effect.

13.1.3 RFA Procedures

13.1.3.1 Preoperative Preparation

1. Initial patient evaluation by inquiry of medical history and physical examinations. Inquire about the history of bleeding diathesis, heart, and pulmonary disease. These conditions may influence the choice of anesthesia approaches. Radiofrequency ablation can be used to treat lesions in the contralateral lung of patients receiving pulmonary surgery. For safety, pulmonary function test should be routinely performed as well as cardiac function. Check whether patients have cardiac pacemakers and metal implants. It has been reported that patients with pacemaker may proceed with RFA treatment (especially liver tumor RFA), but as recommended, during the course of RFA of lung tumors, the pacemaker should be disabled, and radiofrequency electrode is at least more than 5 cm away from the pacemaker leads. Metal implants are one of the contraindications for RFA unless implants can be safely removed during the operation since conductive loops between the RF electrode and the grounding pads will heat metal implants causing unexpected thermal damage to tissues surrounding implants.
2. Multidisciplinary discussion is desirable for each potential RFA case. A typical multidisciplinary team includes pulmonologists, thoracic surgeons, medical oncologists, radiation oncologists, diagnostic radiologists, interventional radiologists, and pathologists. For an effective multidisciplinary discussion, information related to the patient subject to RFA should be well prepared and provided, including but not limited to medical history, clinical staging, pathological diagnosis, genetic analysis, and radiographic imaging.
3. If allowed, preoperative biopsy of lesions should be performed. The biopsy results are favorable to optimize the treatment plan. Occasionally, the treatment plan may be completely changed due to biopsy findings, for instance, a benign

hematoma. Biopsy-related intratumoral bleeding may affect the subsequent treatment by interfering thermal conduction and accumulation. Typically, the amount of bleeding is small. Before and after the biopsy procedure, prophylactic administration of hemostatic medicine is advised to prevent bleeding. Additionally, the interval between biopsy and RFA procedure should be as short as possible to minimize the impact of bleeding as well as potential biopsy-related metastasis.

4. Pre-RFA imaging and image guidance. Preoperative imaging, including CT or PET/CT, should be acquired as baseline data for disease staging, RFA planning, and post-RFA follow-up evaluation. The image-guidance approach should be decided and optimized. Several imaging modalities could be used to guide RFA, and each has advantages as well as disadvantages. CT is the most commonly used guidance tool due to high anatomical resolution and operator independence at the expense of radiation exposure. CT-based specific techniques, such as CT fluoroscopy and four-dimensional electromagnetic navigation, may be useful in certain cases. Ultrasound is only applied to cases with peripheral lesions touching or infiltrating pleura or chest wall.

13.1.3.2 Surgical Procedure

1. Anesthesia. RFA may be performed under epidural anesthesia or general anesthesia, but the anesthetic approach has no impact on the outcome. Advantages of general anesthesia include airway control, controlled ventilation (respiratory rate and tidal volume), limited patient movement, and absolute sedation during the procedure. If a patient cannot tolerate general anesthesia, local anesthesia plus sedation method is used instead.
2. Tumor localization and determination of needle puncturing site. Chest CT images are acquired to localize the tumor. These images reflect the current status of the lesion, and any change in its size or location may have impacts on the selection of electrodes and subsequent procedures. Once tumor location is reconfirmed in CT images, the proper site for placement of the needle electrode is determined and marked on the patient's skin. According to manufacturer's recommendations, grounding pads are assembled to complete the electrical circuit during RFA and prevent skin burns. Then, the marked skin site is draped using sterile technique, and a local anesthetic is administered. Supporting pads may be used to avoid potential injury to neurovascular structures (such as brachial plexus) from patient positioning during the RFA procedure.
3. RFA devices. Currently, there are three types of RFA devices commercially available as shown in Fig. 13.1a–c: (a) post-parachute type, such as LeVeen electrode system (Boston Scientific, Watertown, MA, USA), (b) pre-parachute type represented by StarBurst equipment (AngioDynamics, Queensbury, NY, USA), and (c) cool-tip radiofrequency ablation system (Covidien. Boulder, CO, USA).

   Selection of proper RFA needle should take into consideration the tumor size and location and physician's experience. For a larger tumor, pre-parachute, post-

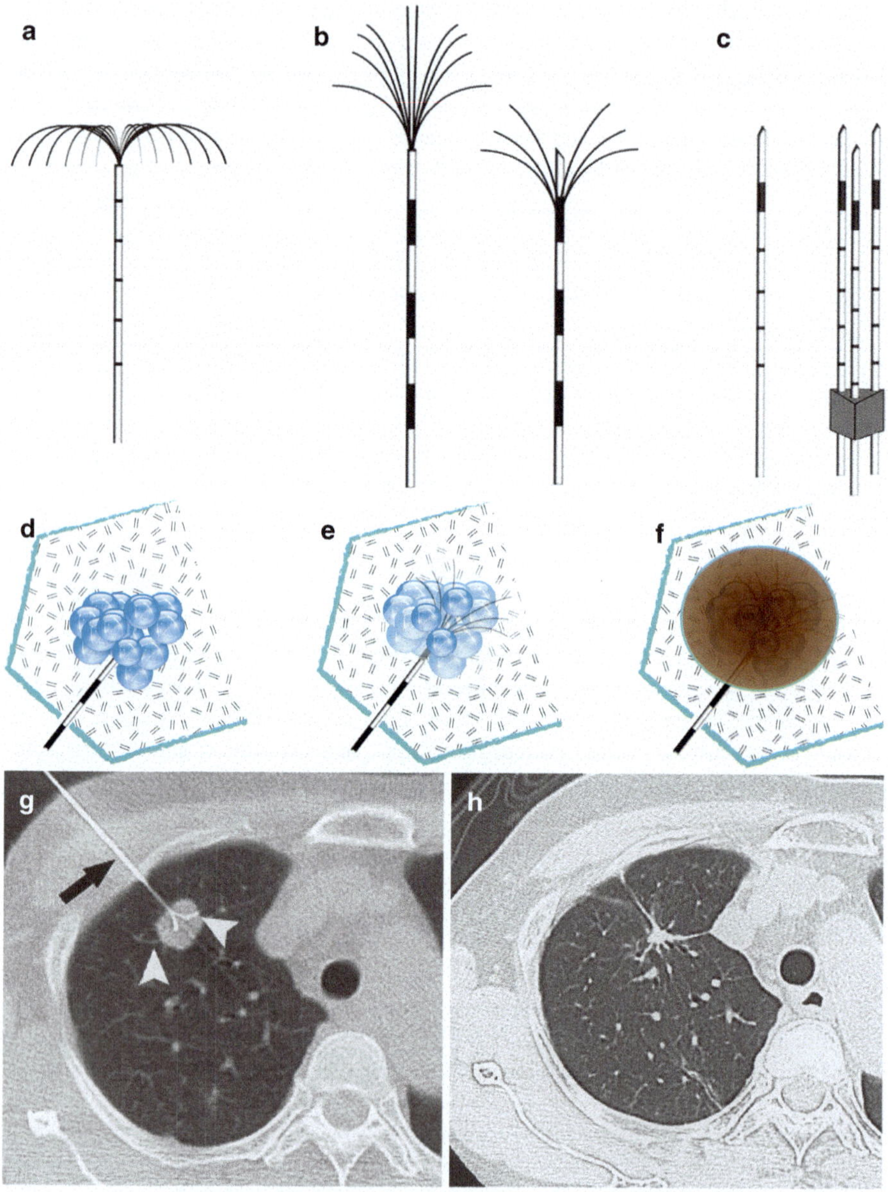

Fig. 13.1 Radiofrequency ablation needles and procedures. (**a**–**c**) RFA needles. (**a**) post-open *umbrella-shaped* RF electrode with multiple warheads; (**b**) front-open *umbrella-shaped* RF electrode with multiple warheads; (**c**) single needle and cluster-type RF electrode A multiple warheads post-parachute-type LeVeen ablation needle. (**d**–**f**) RFA diagram. (**d**) apply RFA needle into the tumor; (**e**) release RF electrode; (**f**) conduct ablation to the entire tumor area. (**g**–**h**) RFA for a peripheral lung cancer. (**g**) RF electrodes via a catheter (arrow) are expanded within the tumor (arrowhead); (**h**) the tumor completely regressed after ablation

parachute, cluster needles, and three-pin combination may be appropriate, while for a smaller tumor or a tumor adjacent to critical structures, a cool-tip single needle may be a better choice than others.

4. Placement of needle electrode. In comparison to the placement of the biopsy needle, the placement of needle electrode has distinct requirements, the electrode passing through the whole tumor to the distal edge or slightly beyond to ensure that the entire tumor could be covered by the treatment field without any missing. During the procedure, image guidance is preferred to real-time monitor the position of the electrode to avoid any unexpected injury to vital structures, especially when lesions are located adjacent to large vessels or bronchus. As the needle electrode reaches into the target lesion, thin-sliced CT images should be acquired to evaluate carefully its position relative to the tumor margins from multiple views for fine adjustments of electrode position (Fig. 13.1d–h).
5. Ablation. When the position of the needle electrode is approved, the ablation process proceeds. The treatment protocol depends on the device's manufacturer. During the ablation, the tumor temperature, tissue impedance, or both will be used to monitor the treatment. Compared to the liver, lung parenchymal thermal and electrical conductivity is poor, so lung RFA requires longer ablation time. Electrode energy usually starts with small wattage (35 W) and then gradually increases to targeting energy. Once the target temperature (e.g., 50 °C) is reached, the tines could be progressively deployed to achieve the planned diameter for the coverage of the entire tumor. The adequacy of tumor ablation can be estimated on the basis of the location of electrode passes and sites where RFA was performed. For large tumors or tumors with irregular shapes, multiple applications may be necessary for adequate ablation. Once the ablation reaches the presetting times, the needle electrode can be removed. Immediately after the RFA procedure, thoracic CT examination should be performed for inspection of any complications such as pneumothorax, hemothorax, or pulmonary hemorrhage.
6. Ablation range. Similar to surgery and radiotherapy, ablation range should be larger than the visible tumor margin to cover microscopic extension, typically 1 cm beyond the tumor margin. On CT imaging, a ground-glass opacity is commonly observed surrounding the target lesion, reflecting the thermal damage to adjacent pulmonary tissues. However, in case of the absence of thermal damage-related imaging changes around the tumors, inadequacy of RFA is usually indicated, and retreatment with higher temperature or longer time should be conducted to minimize the potential risk of tumor relapse. A margin of at least 5 mm of ground-glass opacity is reported to be necessary for an adequate ablation.
7. Prophylactic use of antibiotics. Indeed, necrotic tissue caused by RFA increases the risks of pulmonary infection. Currently, no clinical evidence supports the prophylactic use of antibiotics after RFA procedure. Hence, antibiotics may be suspended and patients are closely monitored. If clinical symptoms indicative of infection occur such as continuous high fever and increasing white blood cell count, a prompt and adequate use of antibiotics for the infection should be prescribed.

8. Protective pneumothorax. For peripheral lesions adjacent to the chest wall or pleura, a maneuver of protective pneumothorax may be necessary by creating an insulating layer of air between the lesion and the chest wall or mediastinum to minimize the likelihood of RFA-induced intolerable pain or nerve injury.

13.1.3.3 Post-RFA Management

Once RFA is completed, immediate chest CT imaging should be acquired for evaluation of complications such as pneumothorax, hemothorax, and pulmonary hemorrhage. If there is a significant pneumothorax, it is readily to be managed before the puncture tube pulled out or insertion of the thoracic drainage tube. Patients should be hospitalized for at least overnight observation. If no immediate adverse effects by thoracic CT imaging and physical examinations exist, the patient may be discharged after a short while of observation on the same day as the procedure. Typically, patients only have mild pain, and nonsteroidal anti-inflammatory drugs could be given to alleviate the symptom. The next day to RFA, patients could be discharged from hospital if vital signs are stable and no additional symptoms occur.

In the longer term, response evaluation should be conducted at a regular basis. Multiple imaging modalities could be applied for this purpose. Contrast-enhanced CT is advised to be performed at 3, 6, and 12 months after RFA and annually thereafter. Due to the acute reaction to thermal damage, the treated lesion may appear larger than its original size in the first follow-up CT. And cavitation may be present. With the acute reaction regressing, the real treatment efficacy is visualized, characterized by focal contracting organization and fibrosis. Increasing metabolic activity may be seen in FDG-PET imaging early after therapy, but the uptake should gradually decline in subsequent examinations. Okuma et al. found that FDG-PET was useful for predicting tumor recurrence at 2 months after RFA [14]. If the measured SUV at the treatment site is higher than 1.8, or the ratio of post-RFA SUV and pre-RFA SUV is less than 0.6, residual tumor should be highly suspected. Any CT or PET findings suspicious of tumor relapse warrant needle biopsy so that retreatment to the residual tumors can be undertaken without delay.

13.1.3.4 RFA-Related Complications

An international survey reported that the mortality rate of lung RFA is 0.4%. Although most of these complications are minor, complications can be severe and even fatal.

1. Pneumothorax.

   Pneumothorax is a common complication, with a reported incidence of 9–63%. It could be an acute event in onset, delayed, or even prolonged. Of note, delayed pneumothorax is reported to occur in 10% of patients. Subcutaneous emphysema may coexist with pneumothorax. Risk factors for pneumothorax included male gender, advanced age, small tumors, multiple tumors ablated simultaneously, lower lobe-located tumors, prolonged or repeated needling procedures, and pulmonary emphysema. For 6–29% of patients, hospitalized management is required with chest tube placement for drainage. The risk factors for chest tube placement for pneumothorax include no history of pulmonary surgery, the use of a cluster electrode, and involvement of the upper lobe [15].

2. Bronchopleural fistula.

   Most pneumothorax cases can be treated conservatively or via the placement of a chest tube. However, pneumothorax occasionally becomes intractable because of the development of a bronchopleural fistula. A literature reported that the incidence of bronchopleural fistula is 0.6%. The underlying mechanism was that RFA treatment caused necrosis of peripheral lung tissues located between pleural space and bronchi or bronchioles [15]. Management of the bronchopleural fistula is challenging. Pleurodesis, endobronchial management, and/or surgical repair may be required (Fig. 13.2).

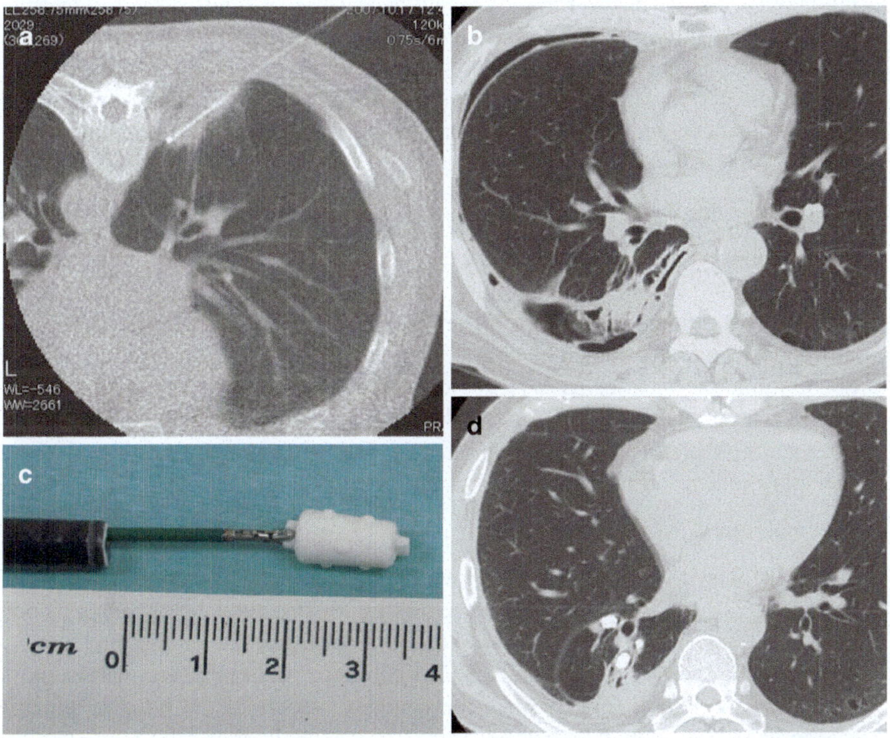

Fig. 13.2 RFA-induced pneumothorax. (**a**) CT images during RFA showed a 17-gauge internally cooled electrode was inserted into a lobulated mass in the right lower lobe. (**b**) Pneumothorax occurred and lasted 1 month despite continuous chest drainage due to the presence of bronchopleural fistula. (**c**) Silicone embolic material was applied to seal the fistula. (**d**) Three months after fistula occlusion, CT images showed pneumothorax completely resolved

3. Pleural effusion.

   The incidence of pleural effusion is reported in the range of 6–19%. Risk factors include the use of a cluster electrode, decreased distance to the nearest pleura, and a decrease in the length of the aerated lung that is traversed by the electrode. Additionally, the occurrence of pleural effusion is reported to be associated with increased pleural temperatures during the procedure, indicating the relationship between pleural effusion and pleuritis induced by thermal injury. Different from regular pleural effusion due to tuberculosis or other infectious reasons, the RFA-induced pleural effusion is aseptic and usually treated conservatively.

4. Hemorrhage.

   Pulmonary hemorrhage can be massive and even life-threatening if a pulmonary artery is mechanically injured by the needle electrode. Fortunately, massive hemorrhage is very rare, but hemoptysis after RFA is common with a reported incidence of 3–9%. Patients with predisposing risk factors, such as treated lesions smaller than 1.5 cm, intrapulmonary needle track longer than 2.5 cm, presence of pulmonary vessels in the track of ablation, and use of multi-tined electrodes, should be carefully monitored for hemorrhage during and after RFA procedures [15]. The vast majority of parenchymal hemorrhages are self-limiting and do not require specific management. For hemothorax secondary to ablation in peripheral lung cancer mainly caused by intercostal artery injury, intercostal artery embolization may be necessary to effectively control the hemorrhage (Fig. 13.3).

5. Needle tract seeding.

   It was reported that the incidence of RFA-associated needle tract seeding is in the range of 0.3–0.7% in cases of lung cancer. This event is mainly related to improper operations, such as biopsy prior to RFA, absence of tract ablation, use of a single internally cooled electrode, and electrode tip temperature lower than 60 °C immediately after RFA [15]. Additionally, it is reported that poorly differentiated tumors have increasingly likelihood of seed via needle tract. To minimize the risk of this complication, strictly following protocols is mandatory, including cauterization of the electrode tract (Fig. 13.4).

6. Thermal injury.

   Thermal injury to the tumor is the underlying therapeutic mechanism of RFA treatment. In contrast, thermal injury to non-tumor structures belongs to adverse events. Among numerous structures likely surrounding tumors, peripheral nerves appear highly heat-sensitive. Thus, RFA operations near peripheral nerves may cause thermal neural injury. Since the caudal elements of the brachial plexus (comprising the C8 and T1 nerves) course immediately above the lung apex, it was reported that the incidence of brachial nerve injury was 15% during RFA treatment of apical lung tumors. The common symptoms related to injury of the caudal brachial plexus include sensory dysfunction and motor dysfunction at the

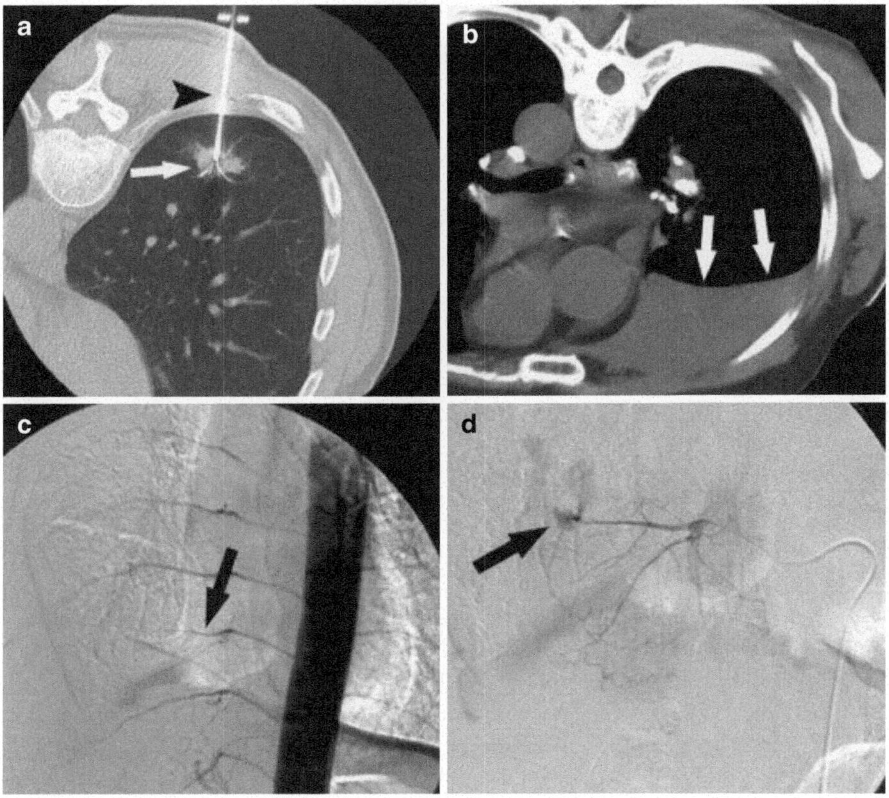

Fig. 13.3 RFA-related hemothorax. (**a**) CT images during RFA showed a multi-tined expandable electrode (arrowhead) was introduced into a tumor (arrow) in the right lower lobe. (**b**) CT image immediately after RFA revealed massive hemothorax (arrows). (**c**) Thoracic aortography showed truncation of an intercostal artery (arrow). (**d**) Intercostal arteriography demonstrated extravasation of contrast medium (arrow), in consistency with active hemorrhage

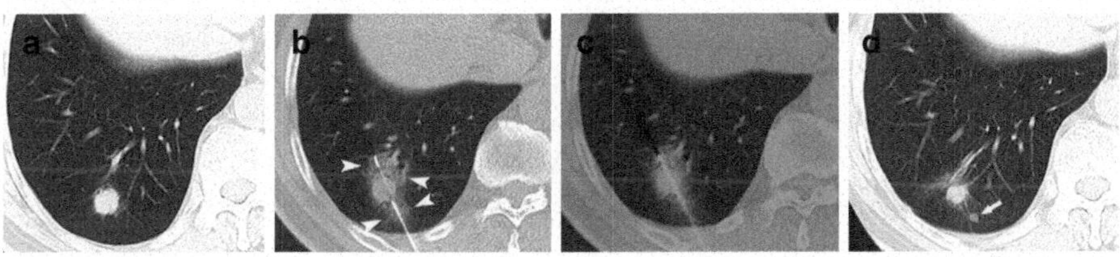

Fig. 13.4 Needle tract seeding. (**a**) Pre-RFA CT images showed a 1.5 cm tumor in the right laterobasal segment. (**b**) CT-guided biopsy. Arrowheads indicated biopsy-induced bleeding. (**c**) Immediately after biopsy, RFA was performed under CT guidance. CT images showed the electrode into the tumor along the same route to that of the biopsy needle. (**d**) In chest CT images 4 months after RFA, a small solitary seeding metastatic nodule (arrow) measured 6 mm in diameter was seen in the needle tract

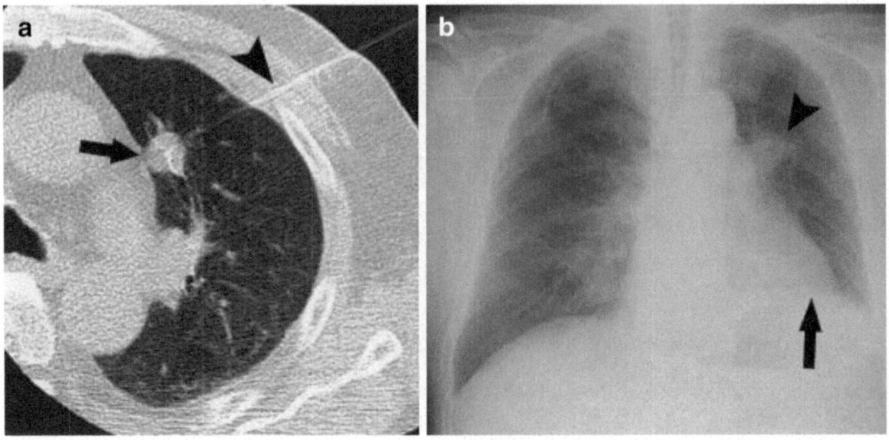

Fig. 13.5 Phrenic nerve injury. (**a**) CT image during RFA procedure showed a multi-tined expandable electrode (arrowhead) into a tumor (arrow) close to the pulmonary trunk. (**b**) Chest radiography after RFA demonstrated abnormal elevation of the left diaphragm (arrow). The arrowhead denotes the ablation zone

medial side of the forearm and upper arm and in the fourth and fifth fingers, which may partially recover over time [15].

The phrenic nerve may be injured in RFA treatment of tumors in lower lobes or close to the mediastinum. The incidence is reported to be approximately 1.3%. If the distance between the phrenic nerve and tumor is less than 10 mm, the nerve is at a high stake of thermal injury. Serious phrenic nerve injury may cause an average of 20% reduction of vital capacity and forced expiratory volume in 1 s. During the procedure, if patients have complaints of pains irradiating to shoulders, teeth, or jaw bone, phrenic nerve injury may occur (Fig. 13.5).

If a tumor is located close to the lung surface or adjoining the pleura, thermal injury to the adjacent chest wall is nearly inevitable. The common symptom is pain along the rib, resulting from injury to the intercostal nerve. For a tumor having a wide base with pleura, rib osteonecrosis may occur after RFA. Some operational techniques have been developed to expand the space between the tumor and the chest wall, for instance, administration of air or artificial pleural effusion or use of thoracoscopic guidance instead of the percutaneous approach. For tumors close to the diaphragm, the RFA-induced hernia is a common complication with a reported incidence of 0.1%.

7. Pneumonitis.

For patients receiving previous radiation therapy prior to RFA, the risk of severe interstitial pneumonia after RFA is higher than those without radiotherapy history. Hence, in cases with previous radiation therapy, use of RFA should be cautioned with comprehensive evaluation prior to the procedure. Bronchiolitis obliterans organizing pneumonia (BOOP)-like reactive pneumonitis has been reported following RFA for lung cancer [6]. Among the reported cohort of RFA-

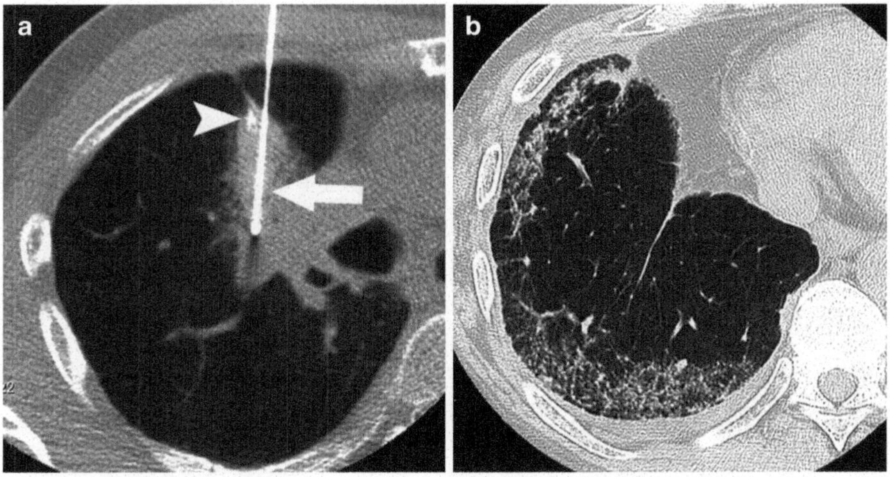

Fig. 13.6 RFA-related pneumonitis. (**a**) CT images during RFA showed an electrode (arrow) within the tumor. Arrowhead indicated a surgical stapler. (**b**) CT images 2 days after RFA showed peripheral ground-glass opacities with reticulonodular changes, indicative of interstitial pneumonitis in the right lower lobe

treated patients, the incidence of BOOP was approximately 0.4%. Clinical symptoms are nonspecific. In thoracic CT images, peripheral consolidation or ground-glass opacity may be seen as well as patchy airspace opacities (Fig. 13.6). Generally, the disease responded poorly to antibiotics, but pulse steroid therapy was reported useful to alleviate symptoms. Acute respiratory distress syndrome and acute exacerbation of interstitial pneumonia have been sporadically reported with RFA.

8. Systemic air embolism.

   As in lung biopsy, systemic air embolism is a rare but potentially fatal complication. The incidence is reported in a range from 0.01% to 0.16%. Positive pressure ventilation could be a predisposing factor for this complication. In some cases, it may be asymptomatic but only found in the post-RFA follow-up CT scanning (Fig. 13.7). Occasionally, it presents an acute onset. In the case reported by Okuma et al., the patient developed acute respiratory arrest and unresponsive following a coughing episode. Successful resuscitation without any neurologic deficit was performed [16]. Once systemic air embolism occurs, the mainstay of therapy is immediate administration of hyperbaric oxygen therapy using 100% oxygen to reduce gas volume substantially and promote the replacement of nitrogen within the embolized air by oxygen.

9. Cavitation.

   The incidence of cavitation after lung RFA treatment is reported to be approximately 14%. Most patients are asymptomatic. Risk factors include tumor adjoin-

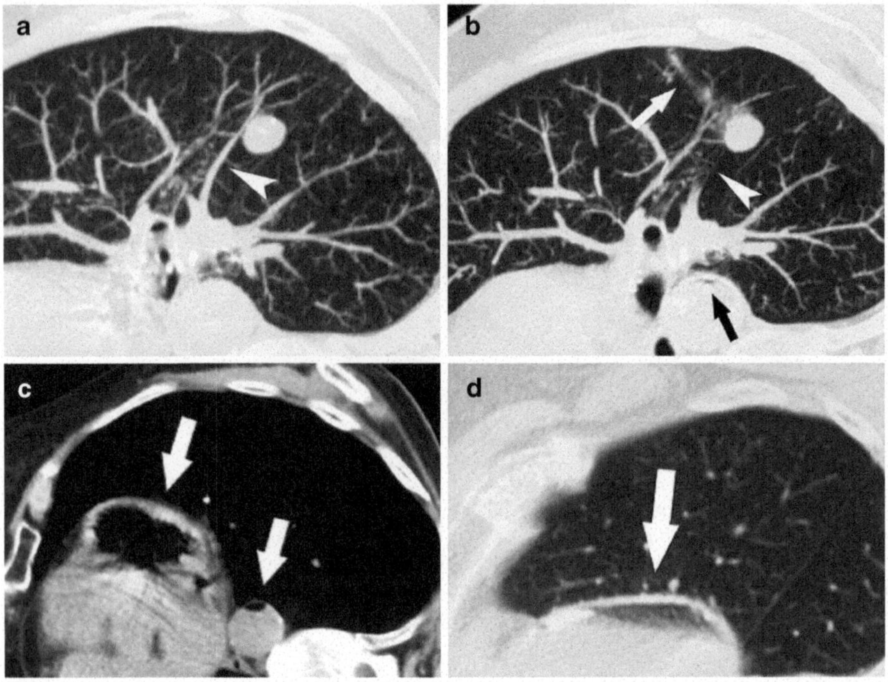

Fig. 13.7 Systemic air embolism. (**a**) Pre-RFA CT images showed a nodule in the left upper lobe. The nodule adjoined a pulmonary vein (arrowhead). No evidence of emphysema or interstitial lung diseases was seen. (**b**) After RFA procedure, air was seen in the pulmonary vein (arrowhead) and the descending aorta (black arrow). Additionally, bleeding (white arrow) was shown along the needle tract. (**c**) Air accumulated within the left atrium (arrow), left ventricle, and the descending aorta (arrow). (**d**) With axial CT reconstruction, air was seen within aortic arch (arrow)

ing chest wall, primary lung cancer, and preexisting emphysema. In most cases, cavitation does not cause clinically relevant adverse events. However, occasionally cavities may increase with time and then rupture resulting in pneumothorax and/or bleeding. In addition, this cavitary lesion is subject to *Aspergillus* infection (Fig. 13.8).

Besides complications above mentioned, other serious complications including lung abscess, empyema, and skin burns have been reported. While these complications are serious, the incidence is extremely low.

13.2 Microwave Ablation

In contrast to the most commonly and widely used radiofrequency ablation, microwave ablation (MWA) is an emerging ablative technique. The first large clinical study on MWA was published in 2008 [17]. Both thermal ablations, RFA and MWA,

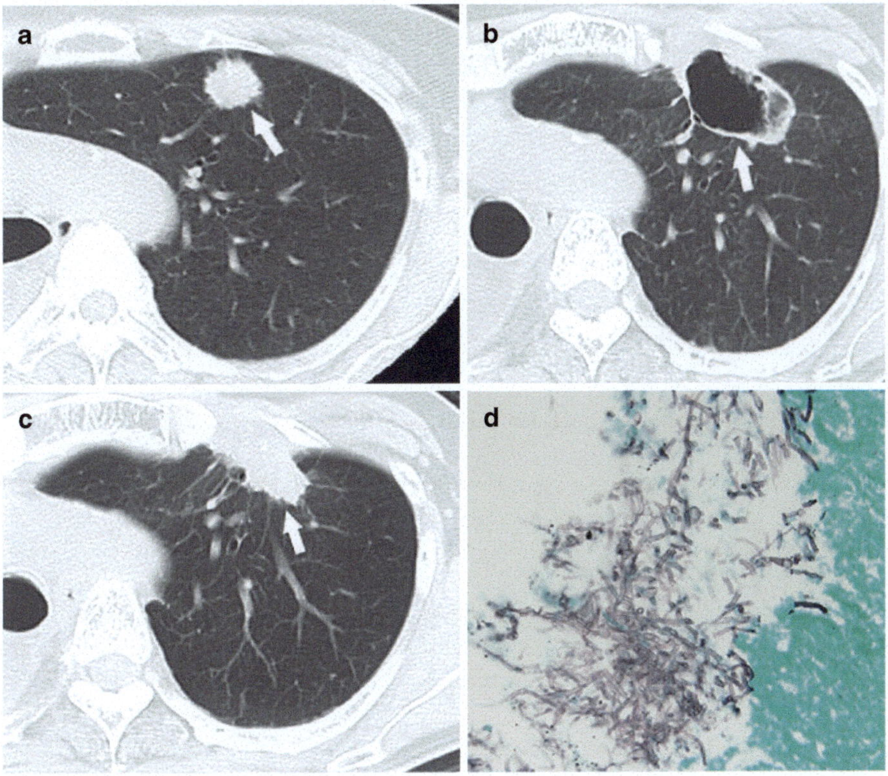

Fig. 13.8 Cavitation. (**a**) Pre-RFA CT image revealed a 2 cm tumor in the left upper lobe (arrow). (**b**) CT images 1 month after RFA showed a large thin-walled cavitary ablation zone (arrow). (**c**) Eight months after RFA cavity disappeared, filling with solid component in CT images (arrow). (**d**) CT-guided percutaneous biopsy confirmed the presence of *Aspergillus* hyphae, indicating *Aspergillus* infection (Grocott stain, magnification 40×)

share similar indications and are conducted in a very similar fashion. In MWA, a needlelike applicator is introduced into the target lesion, and an ellipsoidal microwave field is generated around the applicator with an extent covering the lesion. Microwaves are electromagnetic radiation with frequencies ranging from 300 MHz to 300 GHz. The water molecule has positively and negatively charged poles which tend to align with the electromagnetic waves in the microwave field. Microwave ablation produces heat to injure tumors through a mechanism of dielectric hysteresis. Dielectric hysteresis describes a phenomenon that polar molecules (primarily water) are forced to continuously realign billions of times per second within an oscillating electromagnetic field, resulting in increasing kinetic energy and temperature by friction. The frequencies used in the current MW manufacturers are 915 MHz or 2450MHz, partially matching the resonance frequency of the water molecules to achieve a balance between efficient energy-heat conversion and tissue penetrability.

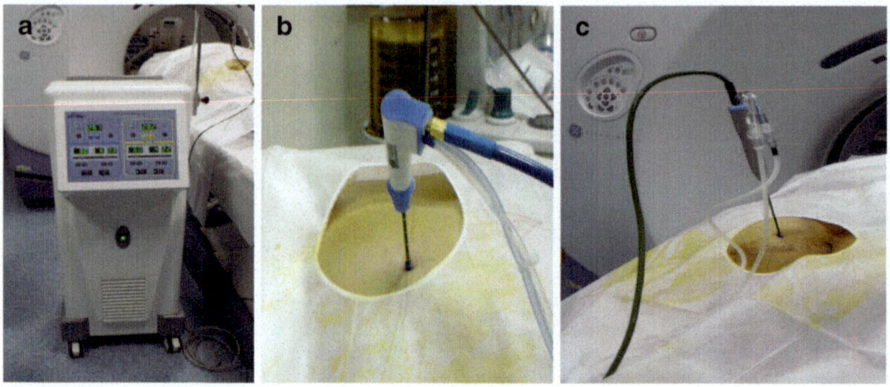

Fig. 13.9 Devices for microwave ablation. (**a**) Microwave ablation machine. (**b**) Microwave electrode. (**c**) Microwave electrode

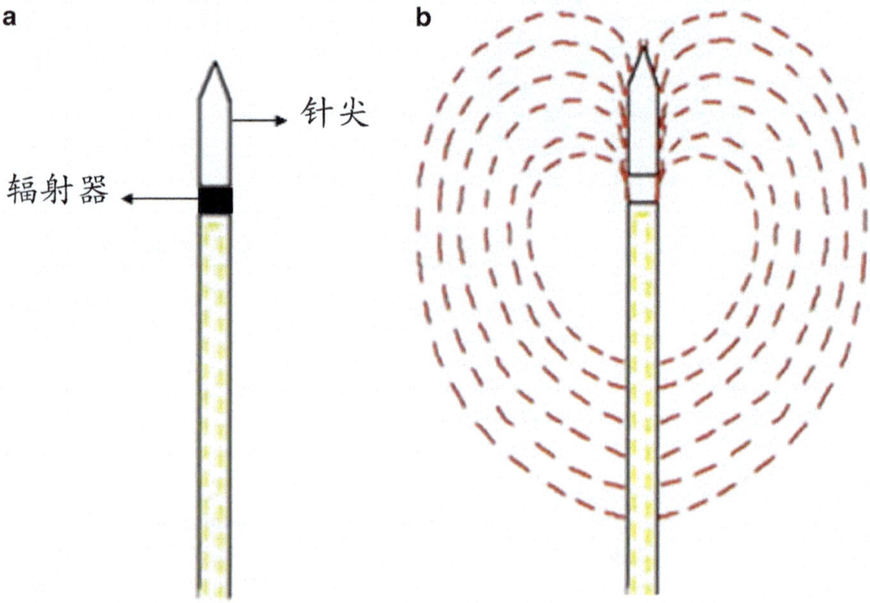

Fig. 13.10 Schematic diagram of microwave ablation. (**a**) The ablation needle. (**b**) The energy distribution around ablation needle

MWA generally produces larger, more spherical, and predictable ablation zones because the microwave field uniformly penetrates the tissue. In vivo, the conduction of microwave is not dependent on the conductivity of the tissue and is little influenced by carbonation and dehydration, so the microwave ablation range is larger. Moreover, the achievable temperature within the target tumor is high enough, leading to a short ablation time and high efficiency. Additionally, MWA is less affected by the cooling effect from blood circulation, which is favorable to tumors near large

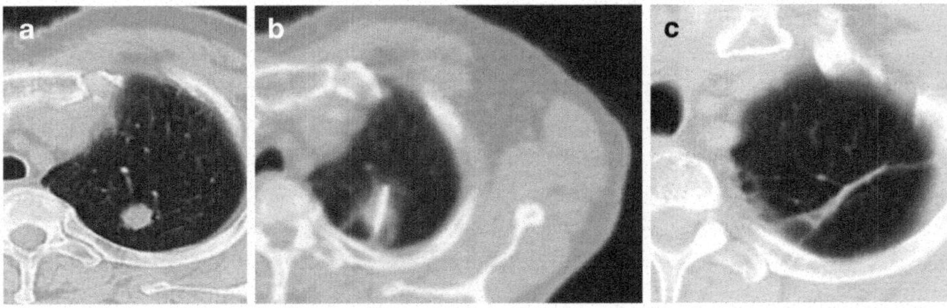

Fig. 13.11 Microwave ablation for a peripheral lung cancer. (**a**) CT images showed a peripheral lung cancer located in the left upper lobe of the lung. (**b**) During microwave ablation, the needle has been inserted into the tumor. (**c**) Eighteen months after ablation, follow-up CT images showed the tumor completely regressed with replacement of fibrotic scars (CR by RECIST criterion)

vessels. Multiple microwave energy sources can be applied at the same time without mutual interference (Figs. 13.9, 13.10, and 13.11).

13.2.1 Curative Effect and Study Progress of Microwave Ablation

Peripheral lung cancer is the preferred lesion of MWA. Many studies have reported good outcomes of MWA for peripheral lung cancer. Feng et al. treated 28 peripheral lesions (8 primary lung cancer, 12 metastatic lung cancer) in 20 patients with single-pole microwave ablation needles under CT guidance. The microwave frequency was 2450 MHz, and the ablation power was 65 W. Patients were followed up for 3–24 months. By the last follow-up, 16 patients were alive, and all lesions showed a response to treatment with 13 recorded as PR and 3 as CR. Guo et al. reported results on 31 peripheral lung cancers in 23 patients treated by CT-guided MWA with a frequency of 2450 MHz and power of 50–70 W. Within the median follow-up period of 33 months, the overall response rate was 78.3%, the 1-year local control rate was 65.2%, the median progression-free survival time was 14.6 months, and the 1- and 2-year survival rates were 91.3% and 82.6%, respectively. These results validated the safety and efficacy of CT-guided MWA in the treatment of peripheral lung cancer.

As observed in RFA treatment, ablation effectiveness is subject to tumor size. For a tumor ≤3 cm in diameter, a single electrode would be adequate to cover the entire lesion with sufficient thermal injury. However, for a tumor larger than 3 cm, there will be an increasing likelihood of inadequate and inhomogeneous thermal coverage, leading to tumor residue and consequent local recurrence after MWA. Wolf et al. reported 82 primary and metastatic lung cancers in 50 patients treated by CT-guided MWA [17]. The mean follow-up period was 10 months. Residual disease at the ablation site was seen in 26% of patients, predicted by using index size of larger than 3 cm. Another 22% of patients had recurrent disease resulting in a 1-year local control rate of 67%, with a mean time to first recurrence of 16.2 months. The actuarial 1-, 2-, and 3-year survival rates were 65%, 55%, and 45%, respectively. The 1-, 2-, and 3-year cancer-specific survival (CSS) rates were 83%, 73%, and 61%, respectively. However, CSS was not significantly affected by tumor size. In another retrospective study conducted by Lu et al., the 1-, 2-, and 3-year overall survival rates were 66.7%, 44.9%, and 24.6%, respectively. Of note, primary NSCLC had better outcomes than metastatic tumors in terms of overall survival and recurrence-free survival with a numerical difference of 20% approximately.

13.2.2 MWA-Associated Complications

Basically, MWA is a safe procedure with minimal invasion, which makes it particularly suitable for patients with technically operable diseases but inoperable conditions. However, as discussed in RFA, physicians should be fully aware of procedure-associated adverse events.

Pneumothorax is reported to be the most frequent complication and occurred in 24.64% (range of 8.5–63%) of patients after ablation. The high variability is more likely attributed to the report bias from the investigators. The occurrence of pneumothorax has more association with the insertion of the antenna than with collateral thermal damage to the pleura. Generally, the MWA-induced pneumothorax is mild, asymptomatic, and self-limiting. In approximately 0.8–15% of cases, pneumothorax may be progressive and unable to be spontaneously absorbed. Hence, interventional management is required, primarily placement of chest tube. Occasionally, a delayed pneumothorax may occur.

Pain and chest wall damage are frequent complications after MWA. In cases of subpleural tumors, part of chest wall may be located within the ablation field which causes chest wall burns and pain in various degrees. Treatment-related pain is common and could be lasting for weeks but mild to moderate in severity. Severe chest pain is reported in 2–27.6% of cases probably due to intercostal neuralgia or pathologic rib fractures. Pain usually responds well to analgesics.

Other complications, such as hemorrhage, pleural effusion, infection, cavitation, air embolisms, needle tract seeding, and pneumonitis, could be encountered in MWA cases. Overall, the complication profile in MWA is similar to RFA, and readers are advised to refer to RFA complication session for further information.

13.3 Cryoablation

Cryoablation started in the 1960s when Cooper and Lee developed liquid nitrogen-containing cryoprobes to freeze deep tissues. With recent development of argon-based cryoablation systems, cryoablation probe diameters have decreased substantially, making percutaneous cryoablation more feasible. The first clinical application of cryoablation in lung tumors is reported in 2005. Since then, more investigations have been conducted, and mounting evidence shows cryoablation is feasible as an alternative treatment approach for inoperable lung tumors.

Technically, pressurized argon gas can cool to temperatures as low as −140 °C, utilizing the Joule-Thomson effect. It has been commonly stated that −20 °C is lethal for cells and that this temperature should be produced in the tissue to achieve a destructive effect; however, no in vivo experiments have been done to support the view that −20 °C is an appropriate goal in cryoablation. The ablation process lasts 25–30 min and consists of successive freezing-thawing cycles to induce cell death due to protein denaturation, membrane disruption, and microvascular thrombosis. High-pressure helium gas is typically used for the thawing process to increase the needle tip temperature up to 45 °C in tens of seconds, hence the argon-helium cryoablation. The main advantage of cryoablation is better real-time CT monitoring of the ablation zone in comparison to the other techniques.

Cryoablation is usually carried out under local anesthesia under CT guidance. For secure cryoablation, the margins of the ice ball should extend 3–10 mm beyond the tumor margins to assure adequate coverage of microscopic diseases as does in RFA and radiotherapy. In the solid organ, the ice ball can be clearly visualized on CT images. However, due to the low water content in the lung, the ablation edge may not be well recognized, which may cause difficulty in determining the adequacy of treatment margins. Argon-helium cryoablation usually uses 17 G frozen needles, and the space between each needle tip is 2 cm, so that there is a slight overlap between each ice ball to form a seamless ablation coverage. When there was the potential risk of position shift during puncture, a 21 G anchor needle was first used to fix the focus, and then two or three needles were inserted symmetrically into the edges of a tumor. Generally, two freeze-thaw cycles are needed, and each cycle includes 10–15 min of freezing phase and 2–4 min of thawing phase (specific time with reference to different manufacturers). If the distance from the tumor to the heart and large vessels is less than 10 mm, a third freeze-thaw cycle is needed (Figs. 13.12 and 13.13).

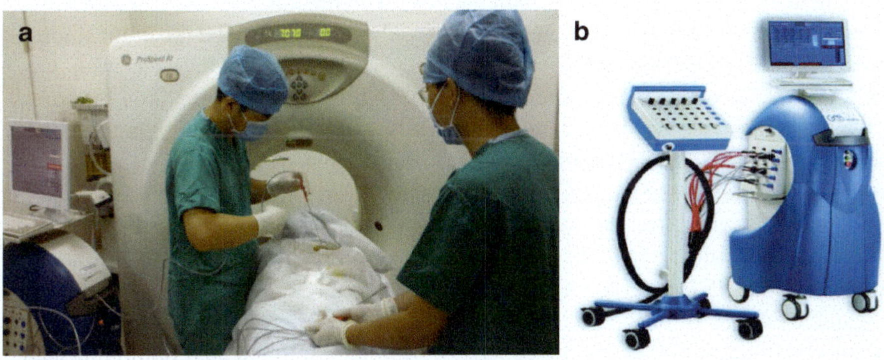

Fig. 13.12 Argon-helium cryoablation system. (**a**) Cryoablation under CT guidance. (**b**) Israel Galileo cryoablation machine

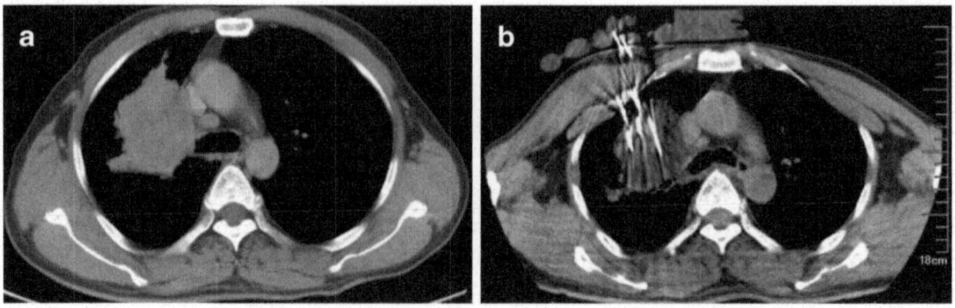

Fig. 13.13 Cryoablation procedure. (**a**) There was no obvious boundary between the right lung cancer and adjacent trachea and vessels. (**b**) The ice hockey formed by cryoablation completely covered the lesion

In comparison to RFA and MWA, cryoablation possesses several unique properties: (a) good visualization under CT guidance, which allows real-time imaging evaluation of therapeutic effects; (b) preservation of collagenous architecture, which as a special tumor-associated antigen could stimulate systemic immune reaction to resist tumors; and (c) the operational convenience and capability under local anesthesia. Certainly, the effects of cryoablation are subject to achievable cryoablation size, thermal sink effect from blood circulation, and tumor size. These inherent pitfalls of cryoablation should be taken into full consideration prior to choosing this approach over other ablations for lung tumors.

13.3.1 Outcomes

Due to a short history of cryoablation in lung cancer, only a small number of retrospective studies with limited sample size could be retrieved. Yamauchi et al. reported midterm results of percutaneous cryoablation for 34 medically inoperable stage I non-small cell lung cancer in 22 patients [18]. The median observation period was 23 months. Local control failure was seen in only one tumor. The mean local tumor progression-free interval was 69 months. The overall 2- and 3-year survivals were 88% and 88%, respectively. The results were superior to the previous reports of RFA, probably due to the recruitment of smaller tumor ($\leq$3 cm) in this study, whereas the previous RFA study included tumors that were 3–4 cm. Zhang et al. dynamically monitored the outcomes of percutaneous conformal cryoablation on 46 patients [19]. After treatment, tumor density and size continuously decreased at follow-up imaging at 1, 3, 6, 12, and 24 months. By the last follow-up at 24th month, by RECIST criteria, CR and PR rates were 83.7% and 16.3%, respectively. No stable disease or progressive disease was recorded, resulting in the 2-year overall survival rate of 100%. Moore et al. [20] evaluated retrospectively the long-term survival of patients with early-stage NSCLC treated with cryoablation. Cryoablation was performed on 47 T1N0M0 NSCLCs in 45 consecutive patients. The 5-year survival rate was 67.8%, the cancer-specific survival rate at 5 years was 56.6%, and the 5-year progression-free survival rate was 87.9%. The combined local and regional recurrence rate was 36.2%. Major complications occurred in 6.4% of patients, including two cases of hemoptysis and a prolonged placement of a chest tube requiring mechanical sclerosis in one patient. There were no deaths in the first 30 days after treatment. This is the first report of long-term outcomes of cryoablation in early-stage NSCLC by now.

Zemlyak et al. conducted a comparative study to evaluate the efficacy of sublobar resections (SLR), radiofrequency ablation (RFA), and percutaneous cryoablation therapy (PCT) for high-risk patients with stage I NSCLC unfit for standard resection [21]. The probability of 3-year survival for the SLR, RFA, and PCT groups was 87.1%, 87.5%, and 77%, respectively. The 3-year cancer-specific survival was 90.6%, 87.5%, and 90.2%, and 3-year cancer-free survival was 60.8%, 50%, and 45.6%, respectively. They concluded that ablative therapies could achieve comparable survival to sublobar resections at 3 years. However, this study is limited by small sample size in each group, 25 in SLR, 27 in cryoablation, and 12 in RFA.

13.3.2 Complications

Generally, cryoablation is a safe procedure, and procedure-related death is rare with a reported mortality rate of 1%. The reported causes of death were pulmonary embolism and acute respiratory distress syndrome. As in MWA, the most common complication in cryoablation is pneumothorax due to using multiple frozen probes and the diameters of frozen needles. The incidence of pneumothorax is reported somewhere between 12% and 62%, and chest tube insertion is needed in only a few of these patients (less than 12%). With the application of 17G probes, the incidence of pneumothorax decreases. Another common complication is pleural effusion associated with hemoptysis, which in most cases is self-limited and can be managed with conservative approaches. Other reported complications include cough, skin frostbite, arm paralysis, phrenic nerve paralysis, empyema, tumor implantation, and subcutaneous emphysema.

References

1. Zhu JC, Yan TD, Morris DL. A systematic review of radiofrequency ablation for lung tumors. Ann Surg Oncol. 2008;15(6):1765–74. https://doi.org/10.1245/s10434-008-9848-7.
2. Herrera LJ, Fernando HC, Perry Y, Gooding WE, Buenaventura PO, Christie NA, Luketich JD. Radiofrequency ablation of pulmonary malignant tumors in nonsurgical candidates. J Thorac Cardiovasc Surg. 2003;125(4):929–37. https://doi.org/10.1067/mtc.2003.18.
3. de Baere T, Palussiere J, Auperin A, Hakime A, Abdel-Rehim M, Kind M, Dromain C, Ravaud A, Tebboune N, Boige V, Malka D, Lafont C, Ducreux M. Midterm local efficacy and survival after radiofrequency ablation of lung tumors with minimum follow-up of 1 year: prospective evaluation. Radiology. 2006;240(2):587–96. https://doi.org/10.1148/radiol.2402050807.

4. Anderson EM, Lees WR, Gillams AR. Early indicators of treatment success after percutaneous radiofrequency of pulmonary tumors. Cardiovasc Intervent Radiol. 2009;32(3):478–83. https://doi.org/10.1007/s00270-008-9482-6.
5. Giraud P, Antoine M, Larrouy A, Milleron B, Callard P, De Rycke Y, Carette MF, Rosenwald JC, Cosset JM, Housset M, Touboul E. Evaluation of microscopic tumor extension in non-small-cell lung cancer for three-dimensional conformal radiotherapy planning. Int J Radiat Oncol Biol Phys. 2000;48(4):1015–24.
6. Hiraki T, Gobara H, Kato K, Toyooka S, Mimura H, Kanazawa S. Bronchiolitis obliterans organizing pneumonia after radiofrequency ablation of lung cancer: report of three cases. J Vasc Interv Radiol. 2012;23(1):126–30. https://doi.org/10.1016/j.jvir.2011.09.011.
7. Simon TG, Beland MD, Machan JT, Dipetrillo T, Dupuy DE. Charlson Comorbidity Index predicts patient outcome, in cases of inoperable non-small cell lung cancer treated with radiofrequency ablation. Eur J Radiol. 2012;81(12):4167–72. https://doi.org/10.1016/j.ejrad.2012.06.007.
8. Simon CJ, Dupuy DE, DiPetrillo TA, Safran HP, Grieco CA, Ng T, Mayo-Smith WW. Pulmonary radiofrequency ablation: long-term safety and efficacy in 153 patients. Radiology. 2007;243(1):268–75. https://doi.org/10.1148/radiol.2431060088.
9. Kodama H, Yamakado K, Murashima S, Takaki H, Uraki J, Nakatsuka A, Shoumura S, Tarukawa T, Shimamoto A, Takao M, Takeda K. Intractable bronchopleural fistula caused by radiofrequency ablation: endoscopic bronchial occlusion with silicone embolic material. Br J Radiol. 2009;82(983):e225–7. https://doi.org/10.1259/bjr/23975691.
10. Lencioni R, Crocetti L, Cioni R, Suh R, Glenn D, Regge D, Helmberger T, Gillams AR, Frilling A, Ambrogi M, Bartolozzi C, Mussi A. Response to radiofrequency ablation of pulmonary tumours: a prospective, intention-to-treat, multicentre clinical trial (the RAPTURE study). Lancet Oncol. 2008;9(7):621–8. https://doi.org/10.1016/s1470-2045(08)70155-4.
11. Bi N, Shedden K, Zheng X, Kong FM. Comparison of the effectiveness of radiofrequency ablation with stereotactic body radiation therapy in inoperable stage I non-small cell lung cancer: a systemic review and pooled analysis. Int J Radiat Oncol Biol Phys. 2016;95(5):1378–90. https://doi.org/10.1016/j.ijrobp.2016.04.016.
12. Jin GY, Lee JM, Lee YC, Han YM, Lim YS. Primary and secondary lung malignancies treated with percutaneous radiofrequency ablation: evaluation with follow-up helical CT. AJR Am J Roentgenol. 2004;183(4):1013–20. https://doi.org/10.2214/ajr.183.4.1831013.
13. Yoo DC, Dupuy DE, Hillman SL, Fernando HC, Rilling WS, Shepard JA, Siegel BA. Radiofrequency ablation of medically inoperable stage IA non-small cell lung cancer: are early posttreatment PET findings predictive of treatment outcome? AJR Am J Roentgenol. 2011;197(2):334–40. https://doi.org/10.2214/ajr.10.6108.
14. Okuma T, Okamura T, Matsuoka T, Yamamoto A, Oyama Y, Toyoshima M, Koyama K, Inoue K, Nakamura K, Inoue Y. Fluorine-18-fluorodeoxyglucose positron emission tomography for assessment of patients with unresectable recurrent or metastatic lung cancers after CT-guided radiofrequency ablation: preliminary results. Ann Nucl Med. 2006;20(2):115–21.
15. Hiraki T, Gobara H, Fujiwara H, Ishii H, Tomita K, Uka M, Makimoto S, Kanazawa S. Lung cancer ablation: complications. Semin Interv Radiol. 2013;30(2):169–75. https://doi.org/10.1055/s-0033-1342958.
16. Okuma T, Matsuoka T, Tutumi S, Nakmura K, Inoue Y. Air embolism during needle placement for CT-guided radiofrequency ablation of an unresectable metastatic lung lesion. J Vasc Interv Radiol. 2007;18(12):1592–4. https://doi.org/10.1016/j.jvir.2007.06.038.
17. Wolf FJ, Grand DJ, Machan JT, Dipetrillo TA, Mayo-Smith WW, Dupuy DE. Microwave ablation of lung malignancies: effectiveness, CT findings, and safety in 50 patients. Radiology. 2008;247(3):871–9. https://doi.org/10.1148/radiol.2473070996.
18. Yamauchi Y, Izumi Y, Hashimoto K, Yashiro H, Inoue M, Nakatsuka S, Goto T, Anraku M, Ohtsuka T, Kohno M, Kawamura M, Nomori H. Percutaneous cryoablation for the treatment of medically inoperable stage I non-small cell lung cancer. PLoS One. 2012;7(3):e33223. https://doi.org/10.1371/journal.pone.0033223.
19. Zhang X, Tian J, Zhao L, Wu B, Kacher DS, Ma X, Liu S, Ren C, Xiao YY. CT-guided conformal cryoablation for peripheral NSCLC: initial experience. Eur J Radiol. 2012;81(11):3354–62. https://doi.org/10.1016/j.ejrad.2012.04.035.

20. Moore W, Talati R, Bhattacharji P, Bilfinger T. Five-year survival after cryoablation of stage I non-small cell lung cancer in medically inoperable patients. J Vasc Interv Radiol. 2015;26(3):312–9. https://doi.org/10.1016/j.jvir.2014.12.006.
21. Zemlyak A, Moore WH, Bilfinger TV. Comparison of survival after sublobar resections and ablative therapies for stage I non-small cell lung cancer. J Am Coll Surg. 2010;211(1):68–72. https://doi.org/10.1016/j.jamcollsurg.2010.03.020.

Suggested Readings

1. Akeboshi M, Yamakado K, Nakatsuka A, Hataji O, Taguchi O, Takao M, Takeda K. Percutaneous radiofrequency ablation of lung neoplasms: initial therapeutic response. J Vasc Interv Radiol. 2004;15(5):463–70.
2. Alberti N, Buy X, Desjardin M, Al Ammari S, Cazzato RL, Bechade D, Desolneux G, Michot A, Palussiere J. Diaphragmatic hernia after lung percutaneous radiofrequency ablation: incidence and risk factors-reply. Cardiovasc Intervent Radiol. 2016;39(2):318–9. https://doi.org/10.1007/s00270-015-1231-z.
3. Ambrogi MC, Lucchi M, Dini P, Melfi F, Fontanini G, Faviana P, Fanucchi O, Mussi A. Percutaneous radiofrequency ablation of lung tumours: results in the mid-term. Eur J Cardiothorac Surg. 2006;30(1):177–83. https://doi.org/10.1016/j.ejcts.2006.03.067.
4. Carrafiello G, Mangini M, Fontana F, Lagana D, Cotta E, Di Massa A, Piacentino F, Ianniello A, Floridi C, Ierardi AM, Fugazzola C. Radiofrequency ablation for single lung tumours not suitable for surgery: seven years' experience. Radiol Med. 2012;117(8):1320–32. https://doi.org/10.1007/s11547-012-0849-z.
5. Christian C, Erica S, Morandi U. The prognostic impact of tumor size in resected stage I non-small cell lung cancer: evidence for a two thresholds tumor diameters classification. Lung Cancer. 2006;54(2):185–91. https://doi.org/10.1016/j.lungcan.2006.08.003.
6. Donohoo JH, Anderson MT, Mayo-Smith WW. Pacemaker reprogramming after radiofrequency ablation of a lung neoplasm. AJR Am J Roentgenol. 2007;189(4):890–2. https://doi.org/10.2214/ajr.05.1399.
7. Egashira Y, Singh S, Bandula S, Illing R. Percutaneous high-energy microwave ablation for the treatment of pulmonary tumors: a retrospective single-center experience. J Vasc Interv Radiol. 2016;27(4):474–9. https://doi.org/10.1016/j.jvir.2016.01.001.
8. Ghaye B, Bruyere PJ, Dondelinger RF. Nonfatal systemic air embolism during percutaneous radiofrequency ablation of a pulmonary metastasis. AJR Am J Roentgenol. 2006;187(3):W327–8. https://doi.org/10.2214/ajr.06.0179.
9. Gillams AR, Lees WR. Radiofrequency ablation of lung metastases: factors influencing success. Eur Radiol. 2008;18(4):672–7. https://doi.org/10.1007/s00330-007-0811-y.
10. Higaki F, Okumura Y, Sato S, Hiraki T, Gobara H, Mimura H, Akaki S, Tsuda T, Kanazawa S. Preliminary retrospective investigation of FDG-PET/CT timing in follow-up of ablated lung tumor. Ann Nucl Med. 2008;22(3):157–63. https://doi.org/10.1007/s12149-007-0113-0.
11. Hinshaw JL, Littrup PJ, Durick N, Leung W, Lee FT Jr, Sampson L, Brace CL. Optimizing the protocol for pulmonary cryoablation: a comparison of a dual- and triple-freeze protocol. Cardiovasc Intervent Radiol. 2010;33(6):1180–5. https://doi.org/10.1007/s00270-010-9868-0.
12. Hiraki T, Gobara H, Mimura H, Sano Y, Takigawa N, Tanaka T, Kanazawa S. Aspergilloma in a cavity formed after percutaneous radiofrequency ablation for lung cancer. J Vasc Interv Radiol. 2009a;20(11):1499–500. https://doi.org/10.1016/j.jvir.2009.07.029.
13. Hiraki T, Gobara H, Mimura H, Sano Y, Tsuda T, Iguchi T, Fujiwara H, Kishi R, Matsui Y, Kanazawa S. Does tumor type affect local control by radiofrequency ablation in the lungs? Eur J Radiol. 2010;74(1):136–41. https://doi.org/10.1016/j.ejrad.2009.01.026.
14. Hiraki T, Gobara H, Shibamoto K, Mimura H, Soda Y, Uka M, Masaoka Y, Toyooka S, Kanazawa S. Technique for creation of artificial pneumothorax for pain relief during radiofrequency ablation of peripheral lung tumors: report of seven cases. J Vasc Interv Radiol. 2011;22(4):503–6. https://doi.org/10.1016/j.jvir.2010.12.018.

15. Hiraki T, Mimura H, Gobara H, Sano Y, Fujiwara H, Iguchi T, Sakurai J, Kishi R, Kanazawa S. Two cases of needle-tract seeding after percutaneous radiofrequency ablation for lung cancer. J Vasc Interv Radiol. 2009b;20(3):415–8. https://doi.org/10.1016/j.jvir.2008.12.411.
16. Hiraki T, Tajiri N, Mimura H, Yasui K, Gobara H, Mukai T, Hase S, Fujiwara H, Iguchi T, Sano Y, Shimizu N, Kanazawa S. Pneumothorax, pleural effusion, and chest tube placement after radiofrequency ablation of lung tumors: incidence and risk factors. Radiology. 2006;241(1):275–83. https://doi.org/10.1148/radiol.2411051087.
17. Kang S, Luo R, Liao W, Wu H, Zhang X, Meng Y. Single group study to evaluate the feasibility and complications of radiofrequency ablation and usefulness of post treatment position emission tomography in lung tumours. World J Surg Oncol. 2004;2:30. https://doi.org/10.1186/1477-7819-2-30.
18. Lee EW, Suh RD, Zeidler MR, Tsai IS, Cameron RB, Abtin FG, Goldin JG. Radiofrequency ablation of subpleural lung malignancy: reduced pain using an artificially created pneumothorax. Cardiovasc Intervent Radiol. 2009;32(4):833–6. https://doi.org/10.1007/s00270-009-9513-y.
19. Lee JM, Jin GY, Goldberg SN, Lee YC, Chung GH, Han YM, Lee SY, Kim CS. Percutaneous radiofrequency ablation for inoperable non-small cell lung cancer and metastases: preliminary report. Radiology. 2004;230(1):125–34. https://doi.org/10.1148/radiol.2301020934.
20. Matsui Y, Hiraki T, Gobara H, Uka M, Masaoka Y, Tada A, Toyooka S, Mitsuhashi T, Mimura H, Kanazawa S. Phrenic nerve injury after radiofrequency ablation of lung tumors: retrospective evaluation of the incidence and risk factors. J Vasc Interv Radiol. 2012;23(6):780–5. https://doi.org/10.1016/j.jvir.2012.02.014.
21. Nakatsuka S, Yashiro H, Inoue M, Kuribayashi S, Kawamura M, Izumi Y, Tsukada N, Yamauchi Y, Hashimoto K, Iwata K, Nagasawa T, Lin YS. On freeze-thaw sequence of vital organ of assuming the cryoablation for malignant lung tumors by using cryoprobe as heat source. Cryobiology. 2010;61(3):317–26. https://doi.org/10.1016/j.cryobiol.2010.10.157.
22. Nour-Eldin NE, Naguib NN, Mack M, Abskharon JE, Vogl TJ. Pulmonary hemorrhage complicating radiofrequency ablation, from mild hemoptysis to life-threatening pattern. Eur Radiol. 2011;21(1):197–204. https://doi.org/10.1007/s00330-010-1889-1.
23. Nour-Eldin NE, Naguib NN, Saeed AS, Ackermann H, Lehnert T, Korkusuz H, Vogl TJ. Risk factors involved in the development of pneumothorax during radiofrequency ablation of lung neoplasms. AJR Am J Roentgenol. 2009;193(1):W43–8. https://doi.org/10.2214/ajr.08.1457.
24. Pastorino U, Buyse M, Friedel G, Ginsberg RJ, Girard P, Goldstraw P, Johnston M, McCormack P, Pass H, Putnam JB Jr. Long-term results of lung metastasectomy: prognostic analyses based on 5206 cases. J Thorac Cardiovasc Surg. 1997;113(1):37–49.
25. Sakurai J, Hiraki T, Mukai T, Mimura H, Yasui K, Gobara H, Hase S, Fujiwara H, Iguchi T, Tajiri N, Aoe M, Sano Y, Date H, Kanazawa S. Intractable pneumothorax due to bronchopleural fistula after radiofrequency ablation of lung tumors. J Vasc Interv Radiol. 2007;18(1 Pt 1):141–5. https://doi.org/10.1016/j.jvir.2006.10.011.
26. Sakurai J, Mimura H, Gobara H, Hiraki T, Kanazawa S. Pulmonary artery pseudoaneurysm related to radiofrequency ablation of lung tumor. Cardiovasc Intervent Radiol. 2010;33(2):413–6. https://doi.org/10.1007/s00270-009-9565-z.
27. Steinke K, Haghighi KS, Wulf S, Morris DL. Effect of vessel diameter on the creation of ovine lung radiofrequency lesions in vivo: preliminary results. J Surg Res. 2005;124(1):85–91. https://doi.org/10.1016/j.jss.2004.09.008.
28. Tong NY, HJ R, Ling HY, Cheung YC, Meng LW, Chung PC. Extracardiac radiofrequency ablation interferes with pacemaker function but does not damage the device. Anesthesiology. 2004;100(4):1041.
29. Yan TD, King J, Sjarif A, Glenn D, Steinke K, Morris DL. Percutaneous radiofrequency ablation of pulmonary metastases from colorectal carcinoma: prognostic determinants for survival. Ann Surg Oncol. 2006;13(11):1529–37. https://doi.org/10.1245/s10434-006-9101-1.
30. Yashiro H, Nakatsuka S, Inoue M, Kawamura M, Tsukada N, Asakura K, Yamauchi Y, Hashimoto K, Kuribayashi S. Factors affecting local progression after percutaneous cryoablation of lung tumors. J Vasc Interv Radiol. 2013;24(6):813–21. https://doi.org/10.1016/j.jvir.2012.12.026.

Part IV
Case Discussion

Chapter 14
Case Discussion

Guozhen Zhang, Ming Li, and Xiangpeng Zheng

Practicability is one of the features of this book. In this part, 50 clinical cases are provided. Each case includes four sections of Clinical History, CT Findings, Pathological Diagnosis, and Discussions and Comments, which is convenient for our readers to do self-tests. Besides lung cancers, cases of benign nodular diseases are added as differential diagnosis not only as a complement to the former chapters but also as a reminder to readers that the majority of micronodules are benign and a comprehensive evaluation is crucial. At last, two cases of inoperable early-stage lung cancer treated with stereotactic radiotherapy and radiofrequency ablation are described in details as references for interested readers.

14.1 Case 1: Atypical Adenomatous Hyperplasia

14.1.1 Clinical History

A 51-year-old male presented to the clinic with an over 1-month history of chest congestion and shortness of breath. The patient was otherwise healthy without bloody sputum, fever/night sweating, nausea/vomiting, dizziness/headache, bone pain, or choking/hoarseness. A chest CT was ordered, and a ground-glass nodule (GGN) was reported in the left lower lobe (LLL).

G. Zhang • M. Li
Department of Radiology, Fudan University Huadong Hospital, Shanghai, China

X. Zheng (✉)
Department of Radiation Oncology, Fudan University Huadong Hospital, Shanghai, China
e-mail: zhengxp@fudan.edu.cn

X. Zheng et al. (eds.), *Early-stage Lung Cancer*,
https://doi.org/10.1007/978-981-10-7596-4_14

14.1.2 CT Findings

Chest CT: A subcentimeter GGN with central solid component was seen in the superior segment of the left lower lobe (Fig. 14.1).

14.1.3 Pathological Diagnosis

Atypical adenomatous hyperplasia.

14.1.4 Discussions and Comments

Despite a small size (6 mm in diameter), a solid component has been found within the lesion, and a fine vessel (less than 2 mm in diameter) connects the micronodule and intrapulmonary vein. Initially, this nodule was classified as a semisolid GGN with CTA-TA sign. Based on that, a preinvasive lesion, most likely adenocarcinoma in situ (AIS), was suspected. Postoperative pathological diagnosis

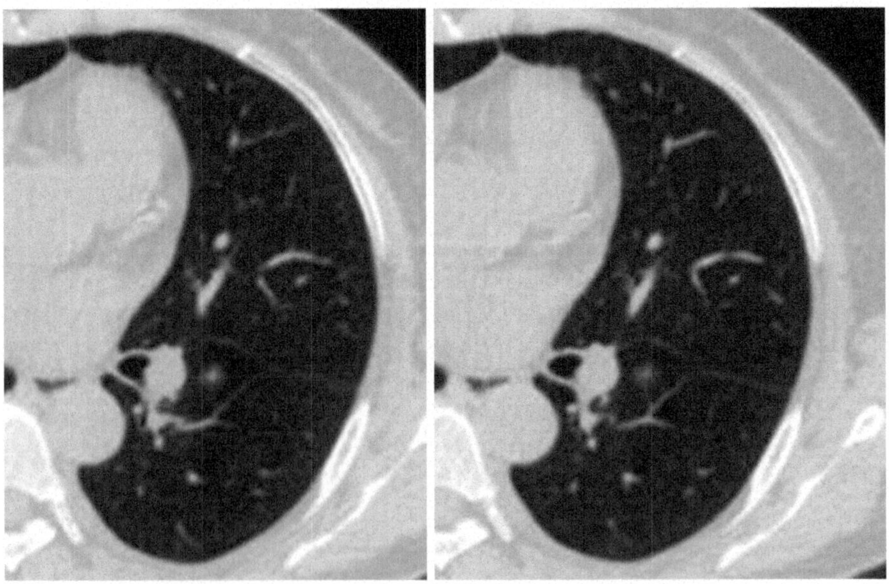

Fig. 14.1 Atypical adenomatous hyperplasia. (**a**, **b**) Consecutive images showed a poorly defined part-solid GGN measuring about 6 mm in diameter in the superior segment of LLL. A fine vessel was seen connecting the nodule and adjacent intrapulmonary vein

confirmed preinvasive disease of atypical adenomatous hyperplasia (AAH) rather than AIS.

Both AAH and AIS are preinvasive diseases and could be imaging differentiated according to the following features:

1. *Size*. A typical AAH is less than 5 mm in diameter, but occasionally the size could be up to 12 mm.
2. *Density and solid component*. In chest CT imaging, the typical feature of AHH is a low-density pure GGO without detectable solid component. However, a solid component is not the absolute exclusion criterion for AAH. Pathological-radiological correlation studies have reported that some AAH lesions may have solid components resulting from fibrotic hyperplasia instead of neoplastic proliferation. The fibrotic hyperplasia (or fibrotic scar) may be a reactive proliferation or pre-existing chronic pulmonary injury, indicating that solid components observed in a GGN lesion do not necessarily reflect neoplastic proliferation. Therefore, dynamic evaluation in follow-up imaging, particularly with contrast medium, is favorable to differentiate the nature of solid components. In comparison with solid components frequently seen in AIS or minimally invasive adenocarcinoma (MIA), the solid components in AAH are very limited in size (a large ratio of the ground-glass component to solid component) and irregular and multiple in distribution, in consistency with fibrotic proliferation.
3. *Tumor margin*. In AAH, neoplastic cells of AAH proliferate discontinuously lining along the alveolar cavity, creating a partially clear margin between the lesion and pulmonary parenchyma. Hence in CT images, most AAH lesions have an incomplete or poorly defined margin. In contrast, most AIS and invasive lesions possess a well-defined contour.
4. *Differentiation of true CTA-TA sign and false CTA-TA sign*. As discussed in previous chapters, CTA-TA sign is a well-proven and characteristic sign for imaging diagnosis of AIS and minimally invasive adenocarcinoma. Basically, CTA-TA sign includes two components, i.e., one or more abnormal connecting vessel between lesions and pre-existing pulmonary vessels and vascular proliferation within lesions (reflected by increasing attenuation with contrast medium). In this case, a fine connecting vessel was seen, but this vessel appears normal without unusual features such as distortion and dilation. So, the so-called CTA-TA sign related to this nodule is not a true CTA-TA sign.

Pathologically, as the early stage of preinvasive disease, AAH does not have direct feeding vessels or does not have the capability of recruiting neovasculature. Nutrients reach to neoplastic cells via diffusion. Unless located nearby a vessel, AAH appears a solitary GGN without connection with surrounding pulmonary tissues.

(Xiaohua Zhu, Ming Li)

14.2 Case 2: Atypical Adenomatous Hyperplasia

14.2.1 Clinical History

A 55-year-old otherwise healthy heavy smoker received an annual chest CT scanning for lung cancer screening. Physical examination did not reveal concerned signs. Blood test on tumor biomarkers was negative.

14.2.2 CT Findings

A 10-mm pure ground-glass nodule with poorly defined margin and homogeneous attenuation is seen in the right upper lobe (Fig. 14.2). A fine vessel is passing through the lesion. In the contrast-enhanced CT imaging, the vessel is clearly visualized with nodular dilation. Early-stage lung cancer, specifically most likely a transition state from AIS to MIA, is highly suspected. The patient is referred to a thoracic surgeon for a further consultation.

14.2.3 Pathological Diagnosis

This patient received lobectomy of RUL via VATS. Pathological examination confirmed AAH, measuring 10 mm in diameter. Within the lung tissues surrounding the lesion, telangiectasia and fibrous proliferation were found, resulting in irregular widening of alveolar septa.

14.2.4 Discussions and Comments

In AAH, mild to moderate proliferation of atypical type II pneumocytes and/or Clara cells is commonly seen in alveoli and sometimes respiratory bronchioles. On CT images, most AAHs present as a pure GGN with poorly defined margin and homogeneous density. A solid component is an infrequent finding. Normal vessels may be seen passing through the lesion.

Characteristically AAH is ≤5 mm but in a minority of cases may be up to 12 mm. In this case, the nodule is 10 mm. Histopathologically, AAH is atypical hyperplasia of alveolar epithelial cells along the alveolar walls in rounded, cuboidal, low columnar, or "peg" morphology. These cells have microscopic and ultrastructural features of Clara cells or type II alveolar epithelial cells.

AAH is the initial stage of the multistep developmental process of lung adenocarcinoma. And it has been reported that AAH is a reversible process, indicating that it

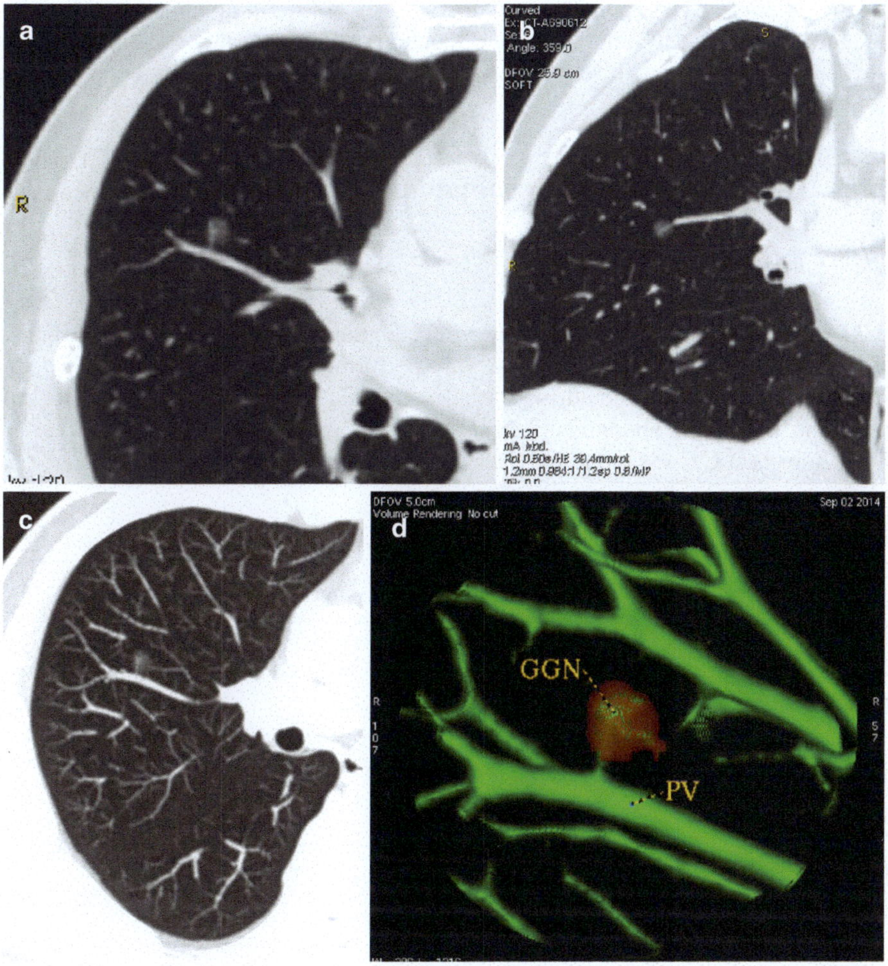

Fig. 14.2 (**a**, **b**) CPR images: A fine vessel connects the semi-GGN and a branch of pulmonary vein. (**c**) MIP image shows a vessel sprouting from the pulmonary vein and entering into the nodular lesion. (**d**) VR image provides a clear relationship between the lesion and pulmonary vein

could progress to irreversible AIS or regress and disappear completely. The apoptosis of epithelial cells with atypical hyperplasia in the alveolar walls affects the stability of alveolar structures, leading to alveolar atrophy and interstitial fibrous proliferation, widening of alveolar septa, and ultimately the formation of fibrous scars and capillary dilation, which causes difficulty in imaging differentiation and overestimation of the disease severity as in this case. In addition, the observed abnormal morphology of fine connecting vessel results from the fibrous proliferation and contraction, which is difficult for imaging differentiation from tumor-related angiogenesis. Again, the CTA-TA sign is not the sole and absolute sign for AIS and invasive diseases. The application of this sign should be in combination of other imaging findings for a comprehensive evaluation of any suspected nodular lesions.

(Xiaojun Ge, Ming Li)

14.3 Case 3: Atypical Adenomatous Hyperplasia

14.3.1 Clinical History

A 39-year-old female came to the clinic with complaints of fever, chest pain, fatigue, and night sweats. A chest CT scan was performed with pneumonia reported. Antibiotics were administered for 2 weeks. Clinical symptoms improved without headache, bone pain, abdominal distention, or other symptoms. Six months later, a follow-up chest CT was requested. Her father and grandfather died of lung cancer.

14.3.2 CT Findings

A faint ground-glass nodule is seen in the RML with slightly inhomogeneous in density. There is another part-solid nodule in the subpleural area of the left upper lobe (Fig. 14.3).

14.3.3 Pathological Diagnosis

Per patient's request, both lesions were resected via VATS.

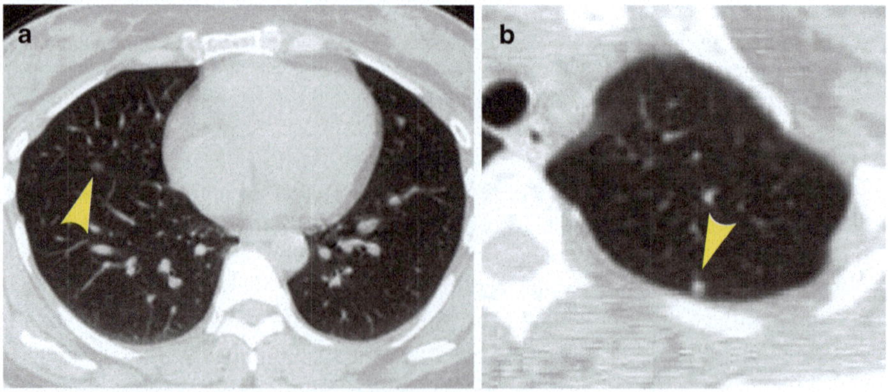

Fig. 14.3 There is a pure ground-glass nodule measuring 4 mm in diameter in the right middle lobe (**a**). A 5-mm part-solid nodule was found in the apical segment of the left upper lobe

Pathological examination confirmed AAH in the right middle lobe and an intrapulmonary lymph node in the left upper lobe.

14.3.4 Discussions and Comments

The nodule located in the RML meets the imaging diagnostic criterion for AAH: pure GGN, less than 5 mm without solid component and CTA-TA sign. In the meanwhile, the nodule in the LUL has a high probability of being benign. However, this is a very concerned patient. Despite that the risk-benefit has been fully consulted, she requested surgical removal of both nodules considering her family history of lung cancer.

(Xiaohua Zhu, Ming Li)

14.4 Case 4: Occult Lung Cancer

14.4.1 Clinical History

A 45-year-old male engineer has a 22-year smoking history. Malignant cells were found in his sputum. A chest CT was ordered for further evaluation and localizing primary disease.

14.4.2 CT Findings

In the axial high-resolution multislice CT images and reformatted images (multiplanar reformation, MPR and CT virtual endoscopy, CTVE), no obvious nodular lesion or mass is visualized. The only suspicious finding is abnormal tracheobronchial stenosis in the right upper lobe (Fig. 14.4).

14.4.3 Pathological Diagnosis

Transbronchial lung biopsy (TBLB) was performed to the suspicious nodular lesion and small-cell lung cancer was confirmed.

14.4.4 Discussions and Comments

According to the 7th IASLC lung cancer TNM staging system, primary tumor cannot be assessed, or tumor proven by the presence of malignant cells in sputum or bronchial washings but not visualized by imaging or bronchoscopy is classified as occult lung cancer, denoted by Tx.

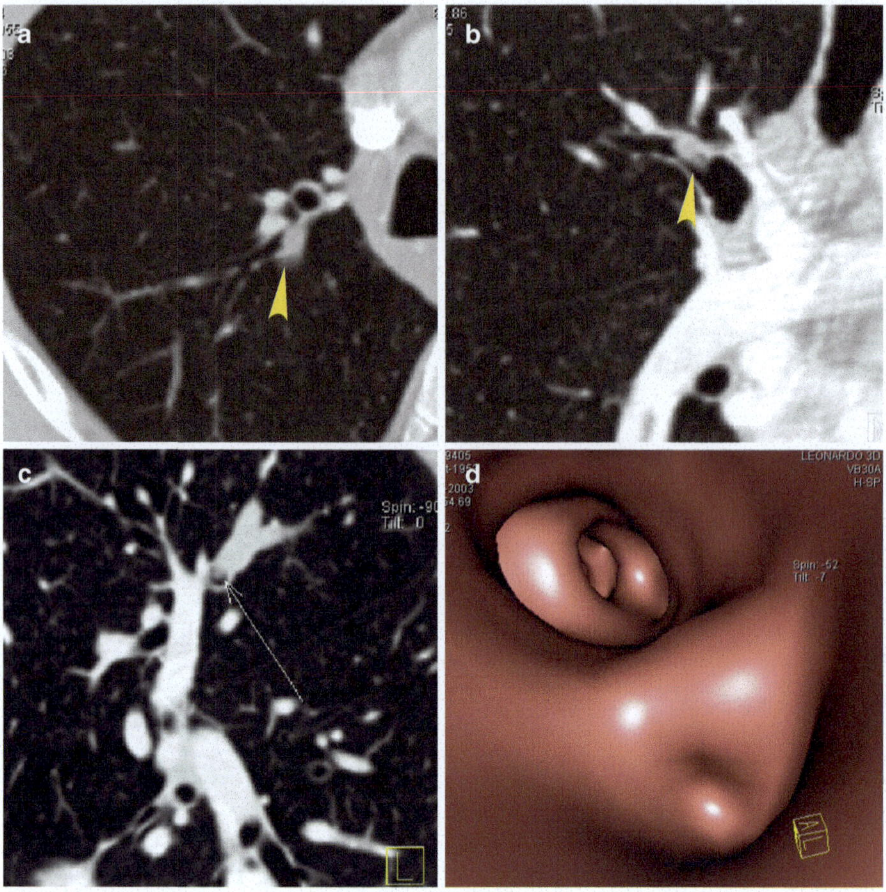

Fig. 14.4 (**a**) In the axial image, thickening of the RUL posterior segmental bronchial lumen is seen (arrowhead). (**b**) In the coronal reformation image, a nodular lesion (arrowhead) extends into the bronchial lumen. (**c**) The sagittal reformatted image and virtual endoscopy image (**d**) reveal evident stenosis (arrow) of the RUL posterior segmental bronchus

With the advance in imaging technology and bronchoscopy, the incidence of occult lung cancer dramatically decreased. The incidence of Tx lung cancer is not available. Barclay et al. reported a case of occult lung cancer in 1983. In his report, a patient exhibited several features of interest concerning occult lung cancer. The long period—more than 2 1/2 years—between the discovery of tumor cells in his sputum and location of cancer by roentgenography, for instance, does not appear to have compromised his longevity. The initial means of detecting occult cancer and its site and type are consistent with the observations that lesions detected by cytologic study are most frequently located in the major and segmental bronchi and that these tumors are usually epidermoid cancers. Widespread in situ cancer was present in the surface epithelium and also along the ducts of the subepithelial mucous-secreting glands, where there were small areas of submucous invasion, suggesting the centrifugal spread of the invasive lesion into the wall of the bronchus rather than into its lumen and thus postponement of the signs and symptoms of bronchial obstruction.

Apparently, the majority of occult lung cancer belongs to early-stage disease. However, if left untreated or inadequately treated, the early-stage disease may progress into the advanced disease with poor prognosis since a significant portion of occult lung cancer is located in the tracheal or bronchial zone. The 5-year overall survival of lung cancer patients in China was only 13%, whereas for those with stage 0 or Ia disease, the overall survival could be higher than 80%. Therefore, early detection and early treatment are the keys for improving lung cancer prognosis.

In a case of occult lung cancer, sophisticated imaging examination (CT, PET, or MRI) and post-processing are necessary to localize suspicious lesions and to guide invasive procedures, such as TBLB for pathological examination. For imaging acquisition and processing, thin slice thickness ($\leq$1.5 mm) and contrast-enhanced imaging are expected in order to collect adequate good imaging data for analysis. Tumor biomarkers, such as ProGRP, CYFRA21-1, NSE, and CEA, may also be measured for monitoring disease development.

(Guozhen Zhang, Yanqing Hua, Xiu Jin)

14.5 Case 5: Adenocarcinoma In Situ

14.5.1 Clinical History

A 51-year-old otherwise healthy female received an annual chest CT scan for routine follow-up of a small nodule in the right lower lobe. This patient had no evident clinical symptoms and tumor biomarkers were within normal range.

14.5.2 CT Findings

A well-defined part-solid small GGN is seen in RLL. A solid component is present and the nodule has heterogeneous attenuation (Fig. 14.5a–c). This GGN is suspected of AIS, and the patient was referred to a thoracic surgeon for further consultation.

14.5.3 Pathological Diagnosis

The GGN was resected via VATS-based segmentectomy. Adenocarcinoma in situ was pathologically confirmed (Fig. 14.5d).

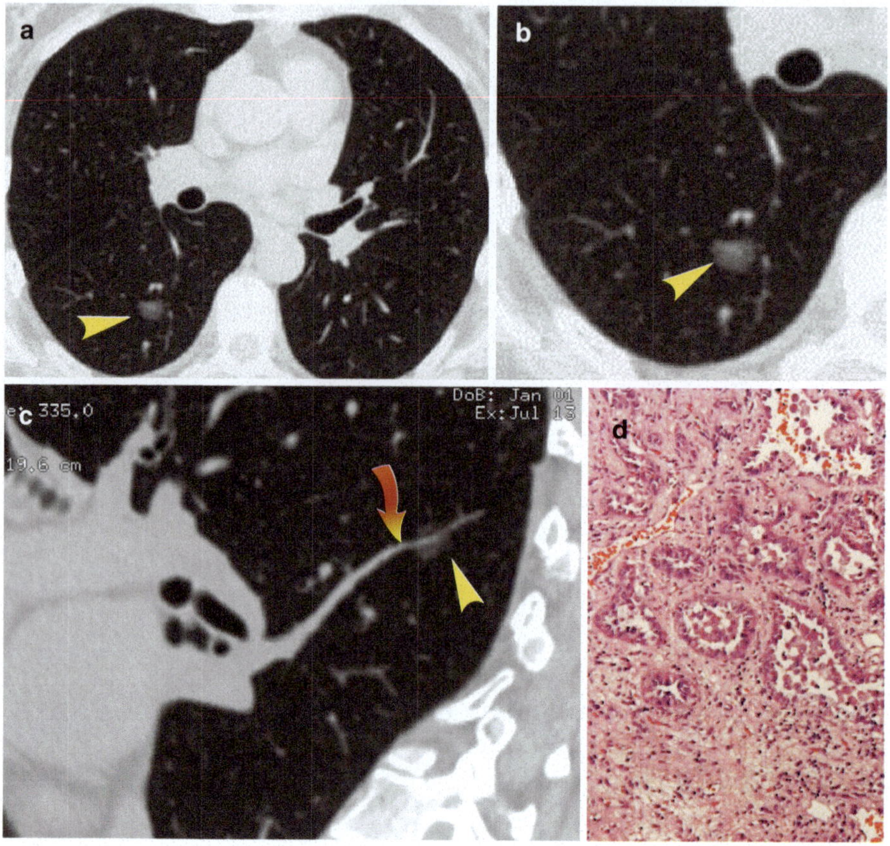

Fig. 14.5 (**a**) A well-defined part-solid nodule is seen in the right lower lobe (arrow). (**b**) The zoom view of the nodule in A. (**c**) The vascular analysis shows that the solid component within the lesion is composed of proliferating neoplastic tissue and the small blood vessel passing through the lesion (curved arrow and arrow). (**d**) H-E staining image (HE × 200)

14.5.4 Discussions and Comments

This is an AIS with typical imaging features, a part-solid GGN with well-defined margin, inhomogeneously increasing attenuation, and CTA-TA sign. In comparison with AAH, the amount and distribution of solid component increase, resulting in relatively high attenuation and clear delineation from surrounding lung tissues. MIA should be cautiously differentiated from AIS. In the former, more solid components and abnormal intravasculatures (neoangiogenesis) should be present as well as irregular tumor margin (reflecting invasive growth pattern).

As emphasized multiple times in this book, the nodule-related vascular analysis bears importance in differential diagnosis. For this purpose, axial images may not be adequate for full view of the relationship between vessels and lesions and differentiating neo-vessels from pre-existing vessels. Hence, in most cases, multiplanar reformation images (including coronal, sagittal, curved planar images and volume rendering images) could provide supplemental and valuable information for differentiation.

(Ming Li, Xiangpeng Zheng, Li Xiao)

14.6 Case 6: Adenocarcinoma In Situ

14.6.1 Clinical History

A 50-year-old female came to the clinic for a second opinion regarding an incidentally detected nodule in an annual chest CT examination. This patient was otherwise healthy without the family history of cancer.

14.6.2 CT Findings

A patchy semisolid GGO measuring 7 mm in the longest dimension is seen nearby a branch of the pulmonary artery in the left upper lobe (Fig. 14.6).

14.6.3 Pathological Diagnosis

Lobectomy via VATS was performed to remove this nodule. Pathological examination confirmed adenocarcinoma in situ.

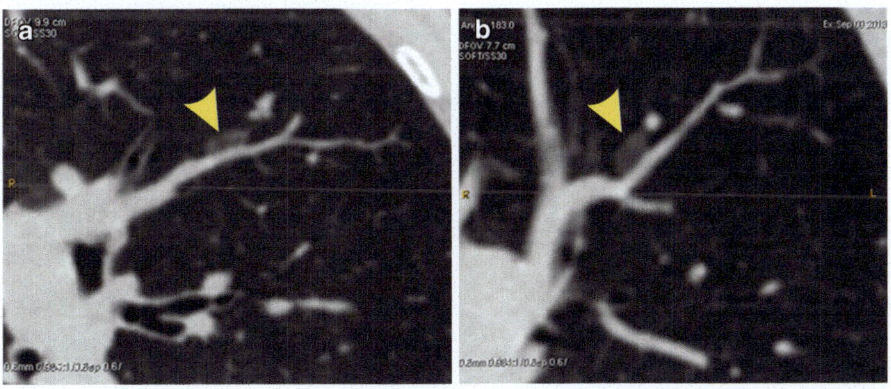

Fig. 14.6 (**a**, **b**) A semisolid GGN (arrowhead) with inhomogeneous attenuation is located along a small artery. Despite that no evident feeding vessel enters into the nodule, this lesion adjoins several pre-existing pulmonary vessels. AIS is suspected and confirmed by subsequent surgical pathology (AIS)

14.6.4 *Discussions and Comments*

The advance in medical imaging technology and increasing awareness of lung cancer screening have dramatically raised the detection rate of small pulmonary nodules. Due to limited experience in imaging features of subcentimeter nodular diseases, especially those with ground-glass attenuation, the incident that a malignant nodule is misdiagnosed as chronic inflammation or local fibrosis is not uncommon, particularly in cases with the manifestation of patchy ground-glass opacities growing along bronchus or pulmonary vessels as seen in this case. One of the key points differentiating AIS from MIA is the behavioral pattern. AIS is a dormant disease, and in follow-up imaging, the extent and density of the lesion could remain unchanged or mildly changed, whereas MIA presents as a progressive disease. Therefore, in cases with equivocal findings, routine follow-up is a good strategy to evaluate the growth pattern (e.g., volume doubling time). In this patient, the lesion could be neglected in routine 5-mm slice-thickness CT images.

(Ming Li)

14.7 Case 7: Adenocarcinoma In Situ

14.7.1 *Clinical History*

A 61-year-old male complained chronic right chest pain for 2 months. He had no fever, cough, or other pulmonary symptoms. Chest CT was ordered to evaluate his condition.

14.7.2 *CT Findings*

A subpleural, well-defined, part-solid GGN is found in the LUL. The nodule is measured 6–7 mm in diameter (Fig. 14.7).

14.7.3 *Pathological Diagnosis*

This patient received lobectomy. Adenocarcinoma in situ was pathologically confirmed.

14.7.4 *Discussions and Comments*

This case represents the typical scenario of incidentally detected lung cancer. A patient came to the clinic for nonspecific symptoms, such as chest pain in this case. Chest CT examination was ordered to evaluate the underlying causes

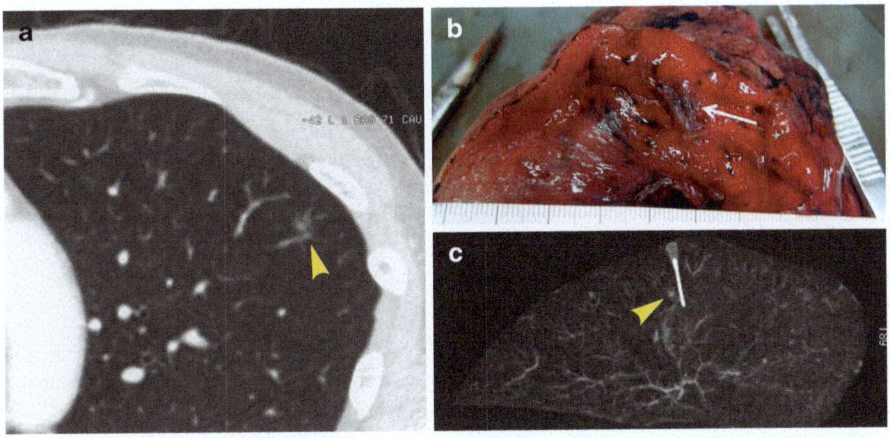

Fig. 14.7 (**a**) CT shows dotted central solid component within and three microvessels surrounding a well-defined, part-solid GGN (arrowhead). (**b**) The arrow marks the tiny GGN in the resected lung specimen. (**c**) For precise localization of the GGN in the specimen, CT-guided aerated biopsy is performed. The needle and lesion (arrowhead) are clearly visualized

related to clinical symptoms. The lung cancer or preinvasive lesion is a collateral finding since such lesion could not induce any clinical symptoms or is asymptomatic.

The combination of semisolid attenuation and CTA-TA sign is an important hint of a preinvasive AIS lesion. Despite that preoperative localization technique was utilized, postoperative aerated biopsy using CT guidance was performed to facilitate accurate pathological sampling (Fig. 14.7c).

As observed in this case and previous cases, solid components in a GGN do not necessarily reflect infiltration but probably result from the accumulation of proliferating neoplastic cells and/or reactive interstitial hyperplasia. Hence, solid components could be present in AIS as well as MIA and other invasive diseases. The imaging differential diagnosis should be based on a comprehensive imaging analysis.

(Ming Li)

14.8 Case 8: Adenocarcinoma In Situ with Tuberculosis

14.8.1 Clinical History

A 50-year-old female presents to the clinic for a second opinion on multiple pulmonary nodules detected in her annual low-dose CT lung cancer screening.

14.8.2 CT Findings

Two solid and irregular nodules are seen in the right upper lobe. In addition, the third nodule with part-solid attenuation is found in the right lower lobe. The part-solid nodule is suspected of a preinvasive lesion (AIS most likely), while nodules in RUL are probably benign (tuberculosis or granulomatous disease most likely) (Fig. 14.8).

14.8.3 Pathological Diagnosis

This patient received surgical removal of three nodular lesions. Pathological examination confirmed tuberculosis for RUL nodules and AIS for the RLL GGN.

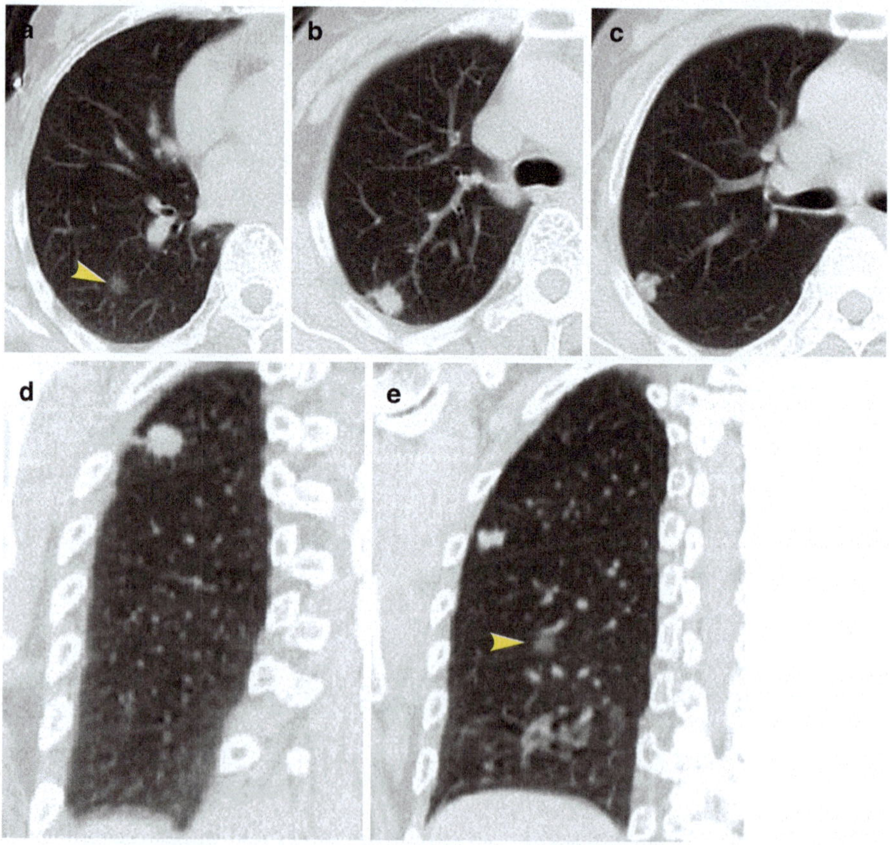

Fig. 14.8 (**a**) A part-solid GGN is located in RLL with well-defined margin (arrowhead). (**b–d**) Two irregular solid nodules are located in RUL with pleural involvement. (**d**) In this coronal image, a vessel is seen running along the GGN (arrowhead)

14.8.4 Discussions and Comments

In the initial CT report, all three nodules were considered as malignant. However, if we examine the images of three nodules carefully, they may not belong to the same category. Despite that the incidence of synchronous multiple primary lung cancer is rising, it is not the case in this patient. And considering that this patient had no previous cancer history, the likelihood of intrapulmonary metastases is slim. Both nodules in RUL tend to be multicentric or result from fusion of multiple small nodular diseases, indicative of granulomatous diseases. On the contrary, the third nodule in RLL is a classic part-solid GGN, in consistency with imaging characteristics of AIS. Hence, in our opinion, nodules in RUL were benign, while the GGN in RLL was AIS, ultimately confirmed by surgical pathology.

This case indicates that GGN could be present as a solitary lesion and also could be seen with other benign diseases. In the latter situation, imaging differentiation should be conducted with extreme caution.

(Xiaohua Zhu, Ming Li)

14.9 Case 9: Adenocarcinoma In Situ with Inflammatory Granuloma

14.9.1 Clinical History

A 46-year-old female presented to the clinic with complaints of a chronic cough. One year ago, she started an irritable cough without causative factors. With medication, the symptom improved but frequently relapsed. During the course, no bloody sputum or shortness of breath occurred. Previous chest radiography and CT reported a mass in the right middle lobe. A contrast-enhanced chest CT scan was requested for further evaluation.

14.9.2 CT Findings

Slice-thickness CT imaging reveals a part-solid GGN in the LUL and a triangle-shaped mass in the RML with a measurement of 10 mm × 20 mm (Fig. 14.9).

14.9.3 Pathological Diagnosis

Both lesions were surgically resected. Pathological examination confirmed AIS for the LUL lesion and chronic inflammatory granuloma for the mass in the RML.

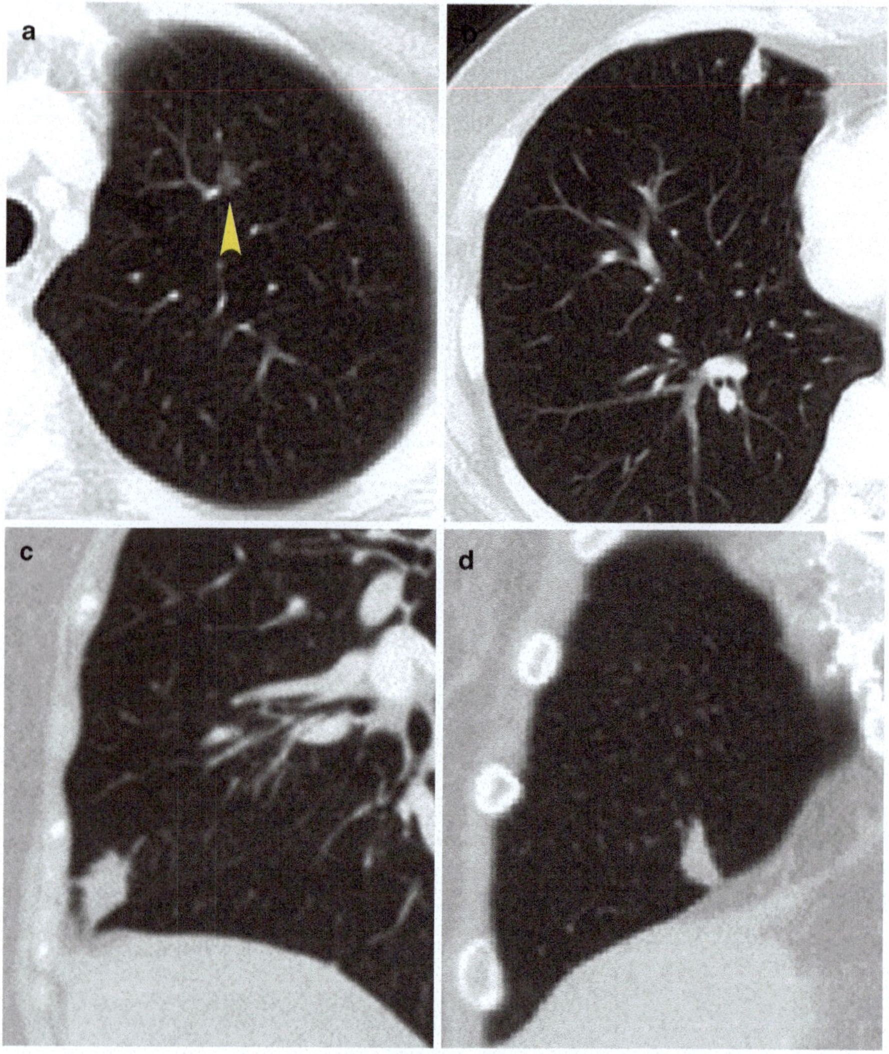

Fig. 14.9 (**a**) In LUL, a well-defined part-solid GGN (arrowhead) is seen with CTA-TA sign. (**b–d**) A mass-like opacity in a triangle shape is located in RML with evident lobulation and long spiculation. Reactive pleural thickening and attachment are observed

14.9.4 Discussions and Comments

This patient had two nodular lesions. The one in LUL was a part-solid GGN with characteristic AIS features. The second nodule was a solid mass. This mass had several benign imaging features, including long spiculation, variable shapes in different dimensions (Fig. 14.9b–d), and pleural attachment and thickening which more likely resulted from reactive pleuritis than pleural invasion due to the absence of pleural traction. The following benign pulmonary granulomatous disorders should be taken into consideration as the differential diagnosis.

1. *Discrete lung abscess*: Patients with lung abscess typically had an acute onset of pneumonia commonly from anaerobic infection. The appearance of pneumonia is usually delayed 24–72 h, at which time heterogeneous opacities are seen in dependent lung segments. Patients who delay seeking medical help for 3–4 weeks may present with a discrete lung abscess. Nearly two-thirds of these lesions occur in the apicoposterior segments of upper lobes and the superior segments of lower lobes. These may be large, ranging in size from 2 to 12 cm. Characteristically, the wall is thick and irregular.
2. *Tuberculoma*: A tuberculoma may occur in the setting of primary or postprimary tuberculosis and probably represents a localized parenchymal disease that alternately activates and heals. These 10–15 mm in diameter nodules are commonly single but may be multiple. The margins of the nodule are usually well-defined, and there may be satellite lesions nearby, though this is not a specific finding. Calcification is common. Tuberculomas frequently remain stable for years but always carry the potential risk of activation and dissemination.
3. *Fungal infection*: The most common fungal infection is cryptococcosis, caused by inhaling spores of *Cryptococcus neoformans*. The chest radiograph shows three patterns: pulmonary masses, which are usually single but may be multiple; homogeneous segmental or lobar opacifications with or without air bronchograms, cavitation, and lymphadenopathy; and diffuse nodular, occasionally miliary, or reticulonodular opacities. The masses usually have an ill-defined edge and may cavitate and range from approximately 5 mm to very large. CT reveals similar findings: some "acinar" nodules but no tree-in-bud abnormalities. In addition, laboratory fungal tests should be performed in cases of suspected fungal infection, including sputum fungal smear, Gram stain, fungal culture, and *Cryptococcus* antigen latex agglutination test.
4. *Hamartoma*: Hamartomas are tumorlike malformations composed of an abnormal mixture of mature tissues normally found in the organ in which the tumor occurs. Pulmonary hamartomas consist predominantly of masses of cartilage with clefts lined by bronchial epithelium and may contain large collections of fat. Malignant transformation is either nonexistent or extremely rare.

(Xiaohua Zhu, Ming Li)

14.10 Case 10: Minimally Invasive Adenocarcinoma

14.10.1 Clinical History

A 45-year-old male sought a second opinion on a reported nodule in his chest CT images. He was a non-smoker and otherwise healthy without a family history of any malignancy. Tumor-related biomarkers were within normal limits.

14.10.2 CT Findings

A filling-type part-solid GGN measuring 6 mm in diameter is seen in the apicoposterior segment of the left upper lobe. This nodule has a well-defined margin and a characteristic CTA-TA sign. With administration of contrast medium, the nodule is significantly enhanced with CT value increment of 24 HU in comparison with uncontrasted CT images, suggesting an angiogenic development inside. Based on these imaging features, the nodule is highly suspected of minimally invasive adenocarcinoma (MIA), and the patient is referred to a thoracic surgeon for further evaluation.

14.10.3 Pathological Diagnosis

Lobectomy was performed via VATS to remove the nodule. Pathology confirmed the diagnosis of MIA (T1N0M0, stage IA) with the invasive extent of 1 mm.

14.10.4 Discussions and Comments

The nodule was only 6 mm in diameter. However, this lesion had the characteristic triad signs of MIA, i.e., well-defined part-solid GGN, characteristic CTA-TA sign, and enhancement with contrast medium. Imaging diagnosis of MIA requires accurate recognition of these three signs.

Despite that the likelihood of a nodule being malignant increases with nodular size, there does not exist a size threshold below which the malignancy could be excluded. It has been reported that a pathologically proven lung adenocarcinoma could be as small as 4 mm in diameter. Due to the tiny size, thin-slice CT imaging (slice thickness ≤ 1 mm) and reconstruction using high-resolution setting (lung window) are the basic requirement for evaluation of a GGN lesion.

For visualization of CTA-TA sign, besides axial images, multiplanar reformation images should be referred. As in this case, the image in Fig. 14.10a displays only one vessel connecting the nodule, which is inadequate to conclude a CTA-TA sign. Luckily, the VR image in Fig. 14.10c clearly shows two vessels connecting and supporting the lesion, hence the CTA-TA sign.

Intratumoral neoangiogenesis is one of the biological events that differentiates MIA and preinvasive diseases. Neoangiogenesis could be evaluated by the extent of enhancement in lesion attenuation (i.e., increment of CT value). Besides conventional CT scanning, contrast-enhanced CT scanning should be performed in cases with part-solid nodules and CTA-TA sign. Our research showed that comparative quantitative analysis of the pre- and post-contrast images can help differentiate

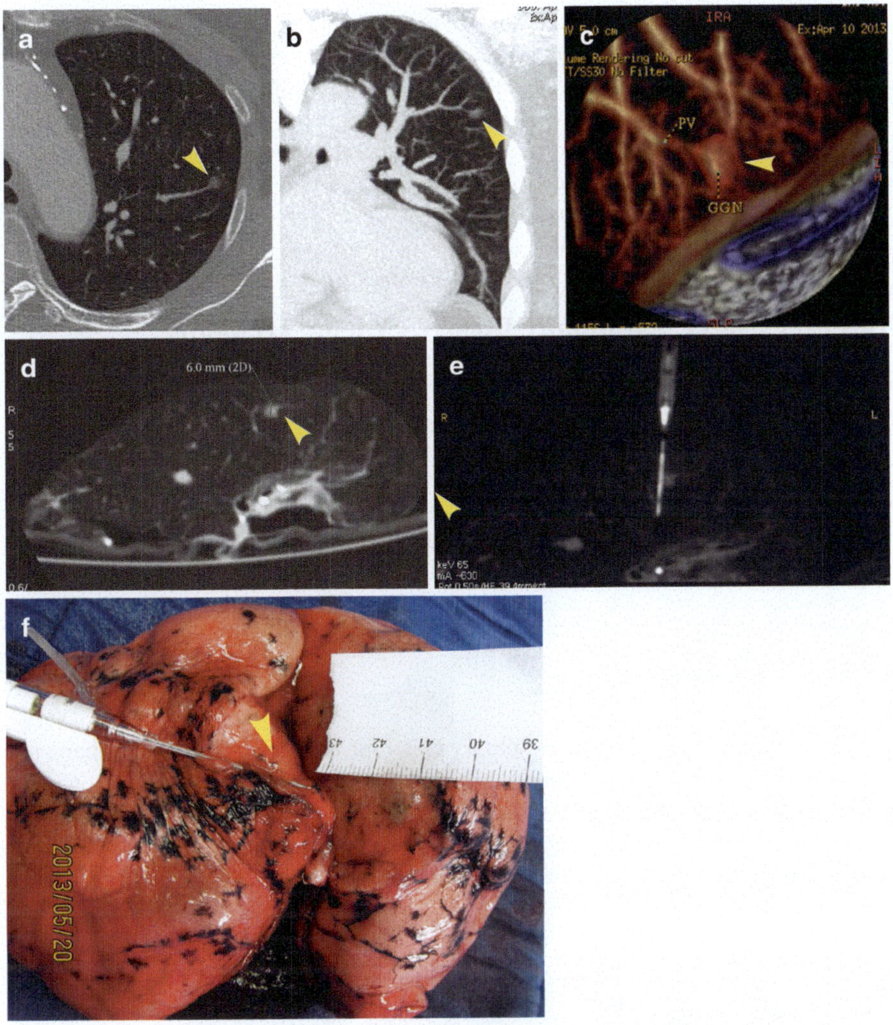

Fig. 14.10 (**a**) A part-solid 6-mm GGN is located in the LUL (arrowhead) with a feeding vessel. (**b**) MIP image provides a better visualization of relationship between the nodule (arrowhead) and surrounding pulmonary vessels. (**c**) In the volume rendering image, another vessel is seen connecting with the nodule (arrowhead). (**d**, **e**) Postoperative localization in re-aerated lung specimen under CT guidance. A needle is inserted alongside the nodule (arrowhead). (**e**) The lung specimen is incised along the needle, and a grayish lesion (arrowhead) is found with pathological confirmation of minimally invasive adenocarcinoma with the invasive extent of 1 mm

between atypical adenomatous hyperplasia (AAH), adenocarcinoma in situ (AIS), MIAs, and invasive adenocarcinomas (IACs).

In addition, the management of this patient involved multidisciplinary collaboration from radiology, thoracic surgery, and pathology. Especially, radiologists are not only involved in the preoperative diagnosis but also in the postoperative localization of the tiny lesion via CT-guided biopsy in re-aerated lung specimen (Fig. 14.9d, e), which obviously facilitates pathologists to sample the abnormal tissues accurately. In comparison with preoperative localization techniques, postoperative localization has several advantages, including facilitating preoperative preparation, avoiding anatomical interference from conventional preoperative localization procedure, and reducing intraoperative complications.

(Xiangpeng Zheng, Ming Li)

14.11 Case 11: Minimally Invasive Adenocarcinoma

14.11.1 Clinical History

A 62-year-old female came to the clinic for a second opinion on an incidentally detected pulmonary nodule in her annual chest CT scanning. This patient was otherwise healthy without clinical symptoms, smoking history, or family history of cancer. Blood tests including cell counts and tumor biomarkers were within normal limits.

14.11.2 CT Findings

In the axial image, a well-defined, solitary GGN measuring about 6 mm in diameter with few solid components is found in the right upper lobe (Fig. 14.11). However, reformatted images show connecting vessels into the lesion (CTA-TA sign). The nodule is suspected of AIS (most likely) or MIA (less likely). The patient was referred to a thoracic surgeon for a consultation.

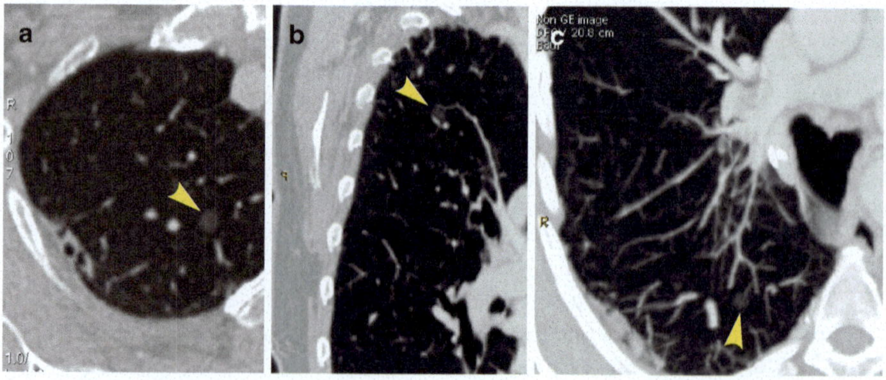

Fig. 14.11 (**a**) A 6-mm solitary GGN (arrowhead) is seen in RUL. (**b**, **c**) In curved planar reformation image and MIP image, two fine blood vessels get into the nodule (arrowhead), leading to the CTA-TA sign

14.11.3 Pathological Diagnosis

The GGN was removed with wedge resection via VATS.

Pathological examination confirmed minimally invasive adenocarcinoma.

14.11.4 Discussions and Comments

Pathologically, ground-glass opacities may have various underlying mechanisms, including the decrease of alveolar air, the increase of cellular amount, epithelial hyperplasia, alveolar septal thickening, and filling of the terminal air space with secretion or mucus. These changes produce the imaging presentations of increasing focal attenuation, elevation of CT value, and intactness or distortion of pulmonary structures. Many pulmonary entities could manifest themselves in GGOs, such as interstitial or alveolar edema or hemorrhage, focal interstitial infiltration, reactive granulomatous disease, and tumor infiltration. Therefore, a GGN can be either a benign lesion or preinvasive lesion or invasive lesion. It is crucial for radiologists to distinguish between benign and malignant GGNs.

In this case, the GGN located in RUL contained few solid components, making it more like a pure GGN than a part-solid GGN. However, the CTA-TA sign was evident. Considering both imaging features, both AIS and MIA are reasonable imaging diagnosis with more likelihood in the former. However, the pathological results confirmed the opposite, indicating that MIA may present as a pure GGN, infrequently though. Most MIAs are part-solid GGNs with solid predominance or solid nodules.

(Haiquan Liu, Ming Li)

14.12 Case 12: Minimally Invasive Adenocarcinoma

14.12.1 Clinical History

A 55-year-old female presented to the clinic complaining cough for several weeks. A chest CT was ordered for lung evaluation.

14.12.2 CT Findings

In the left lower lobe, an irregular, part-solid GGN is found with a well-defined margin and CTA-TA sign (Fig. 14.12). This nodule contains air bronchogram sign. MIA is highly suspected and referred to a thoracic surgeon.

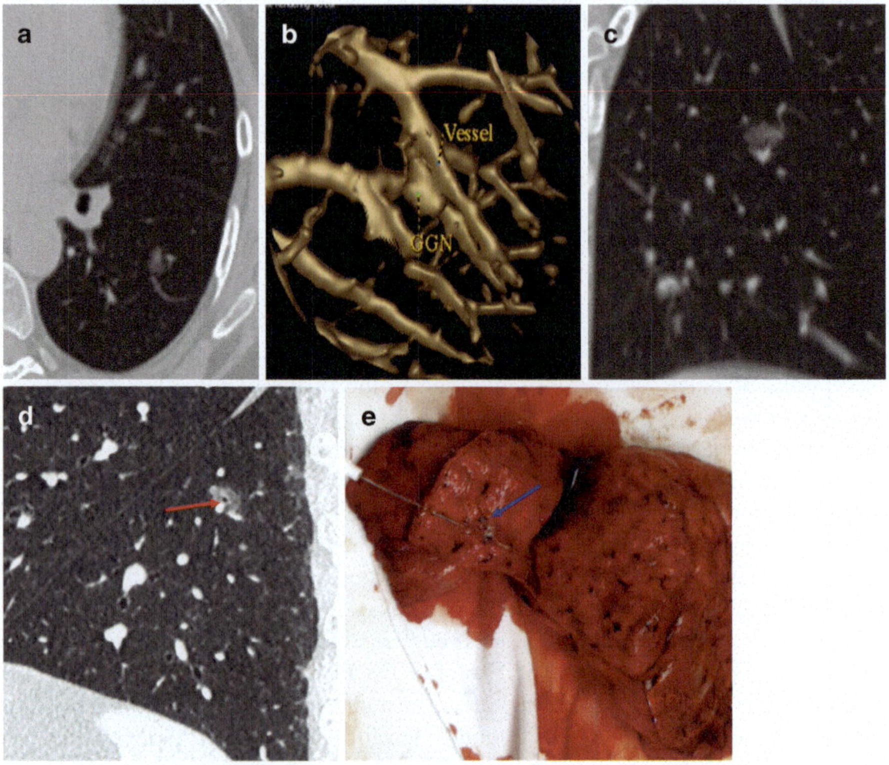

Fig. 14.12 (**a**) A 6-mm semisolid GGN with well-defined margin is seen in LLL. (**b**) In volume rendering image, the nodule is connected with several blood vessels. (**c**) In coronal image, the connecting vessels are better visualized and interconnect with intratumoral solid component, the characteristic of CTA-TA sign. (**d**) In sagittal image, a bronchus (red arrow) inside the nodule is seen with thickening walls, creating the air bronchogram sign. (**e**) Postoperative CT-guided needle-assisted localization of the nodule in re-aerated resected lung specimen

14.12.3 Pathological Diagnosis

VATS-based lobectomy was performed and pathological examination confirmed minimally invasive adenocarcinoma.

14.12.4 Discussions and Comments

The nodule in this patient has the triad sign of MIA described previously, i.e., part-solid nodule with solid component predominance, CTA-TA sign, and enhancement. In addition, air bronchogram sign, defined as air-filled bronchi seen as radiolucent, branching bands within the tumor, is present in this nodule.

The air bronchogram sign was described originally by Fleischner in 1927 and was named by Felson. This sign is nonspecific. The most common causes of an air bronchogram are consolidations of various origins and pulmonary edema. Similarly, widespread air bronchograms are seen in hyaline membrane disease. This sign is also seen in atelectatic lobes on chest radiographs when the airway is patent, notably when atelectasis is caused by pleural effusion, pneumothorax, or bronchiectasis. Additionally, this sign could be produced by lung cancers, in particular with bronchoalveolar carcinoma (currently AIS and MIA) and adenocarcinoma. The air bronchogram sign occurs when patent airways are surrounded by nonaerated lung parenchyma. The mechanism of development or the tissue that replaces the normal aerated lung is irrelevant.

In AIS and MIA, neoplastic cells partly or wholly grow along the walls of preexisting air spaces without causing destruction. The underlying mechanism for air bronchogram in both lesions is the consolidation caused by mucus secreted by the tumor or residual air space from incomplete filling with proliferating neoplastic cells. This sign is rarely seen in AAH. Therefore, the presence of air bronchogram sign marks the progression of preinvasive disease. Pathologically, the invasion is defined as (1) histological subtypes other than a lepidic pattern (i.e., acinar, papillary, micropapillary, and/or solid) or (2) myofibroblastic stroma associated with invasive tumor cells. The occurrence of invasion could cause distortion of pulmonary structures, reflected by signs such as air bronchogram in imaging.

The observation of air bronchogram sign requires multiple planar reformation images. When the reformation/reconstruction plane is vertical to the bronchus involved, it may appear as a round, oval, or cavitary lucency within a ground-glass opacity; when the imaging plane is parallel to the bronchial pathway, the characteristic tubular appearance is evident. In comparison with air bronchograms seen in benign diseases, those in lung cancers or preinvasive lesions frequently coexist with irregularly thickening bronchial walls, bronchial distortion, dilation, or even truncation.

(Xiangpeng Zheng)

14.13 Case 13: Minimally Invasive Adenocarcinoma

14.13.1 Clinical History

A 57-year-old otherwise healthy female presented for annual low-dose CT lung cancer screening due to a family history of cancer. She was a non-smoker without pulmonary symptoms. Tumor biomarkers were within normal limits.

14.13.2 CT Findings

In the right lower lobe, a part-solid GGN is located, measuring about 10 mm in diameter (Figs. 14.13 and 14.14). Other imaging features include central bubble-like lucency, CTA-TA sign, and remarkable enhancement with contrast medium.

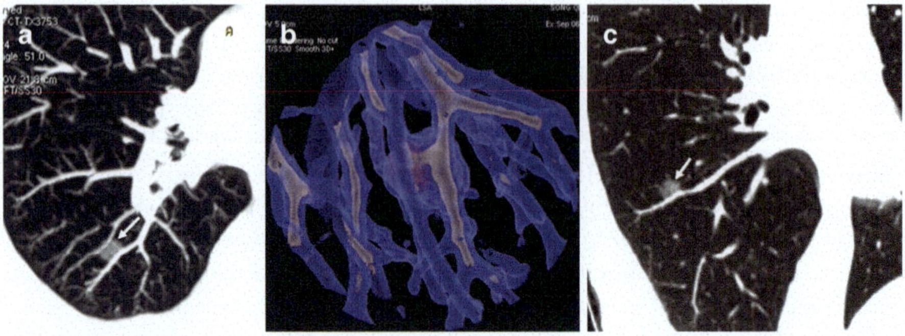

Fig. 14.13 In RLL, a well-defined part-solid GGN (arrow) is clamped by two pulmonary veins, and microvessels from veins penetrate into the lesion. (**a**) MIP image. (**b**) Volume rendering image. (**c**) CPR image

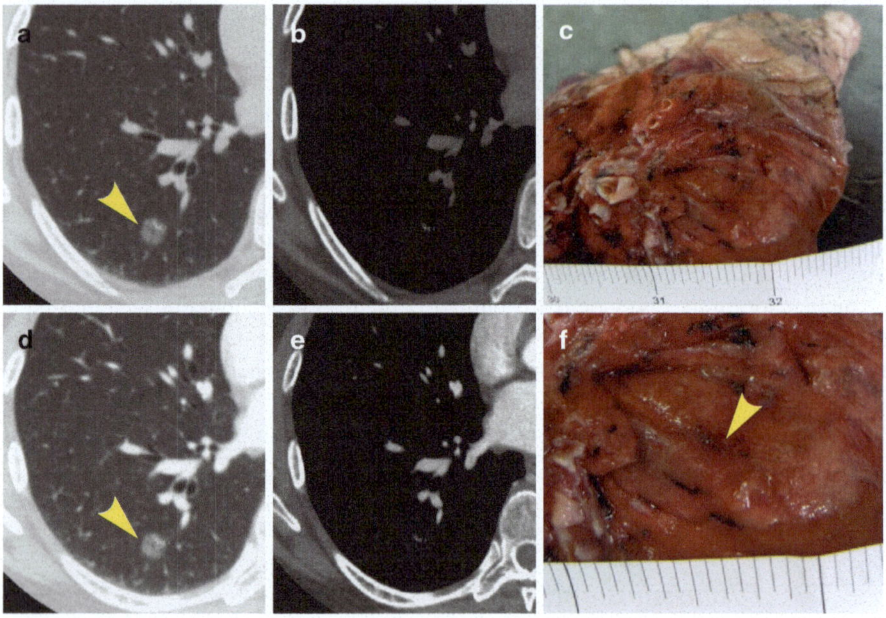

Fig. 14.14 Contrast enhancement scanning facilitates evaluation of solid component within a solid or part-solid lesion. (**a**) and (**b**) are pre-contrast CT in lung and mediastinal windows, while (**c**) and (**d**) are contrast-enhanced CT images in lung and mediastinal windows from the same scanning position. The nodule (arrowhead) is enhanced significantly with CT value increased from −316 HU (without contrast) to −210 HU (with contrast). (**e, f**) The gross specimen and zoomed view of the lesion (arrowhead). Pathological examination confirmed MIA

14.13.3 Pathological Diagnosis

The patient received RLL lobectomy via VATS.

Minimally invasive adenocarcinoma was confirmed.

14.13.4 Discussions and Comments

The nodule in this patient had characteristic imaging features of MIA. Of note are the administration of contrast enhancement scanning and the evaluation of attenuation increment. Due to the loose cellularity in GGNs, the absolute CT value of these lesions is below 0 HU, probably as low as −600 HU in AAH or AIS and −400 HU in MIA. An enhancement is evaluated by relative increment in CT value (post-contrast CT-pre-contrast CT) instead of the absolute CT value as seen in mass-like lung cancer. As in this case, despite the absolute CT value of −210 HU in contrasted CT, the relative attenuation increment is 106 HU, indicating a significant enhancement.

The display window, specifically the mediastinal window setting, has impacts on the visualization and evaluation of solid component. We conducted a study to evaluate the incremental utility of contrast enhancement in the evaluation of ground glass and mGGNs in improving diagnostic accuracy with the comparison between conventional mediastinal window (CMW, W/L = 350/50 HU) and an extended mediastinal window (EMW, W/L = 700/100 HU). Our study confirmed the incremental value of post-contrast images and utility of extension of the CT mediastinal window settings in differentiating AAHs, AISs, MIAs, and IACs. The technique is simplistic in approach and can potentially be used in downstream pathways of nodule assessment. Generally, GGNs are poorly represented on the CMW setting display, particularly when evaluating subtle contrast enhancement, which could be improved by adjusting the display window setting, i.e., using EMW. In our study, a high number of nodules manifested as an enlargement of solid portions after contrast in EMW than CMW regardless of whether the lesion was categorized as preinvasive, MIA, or IAC. In comparison with preinvasive diseases, the MIA and IAC lesions showed a remarkable enhancement due to increasing amount of solid component partly as a result of angiogenic development.

(Ming Li, Gang Shen)

14.14 Case 14: Minimally Invasive Adenocarcinoma

14.14.1 Clinical History

A 47-year-old male with a history of heavy smoking for nearly 20 years received a low-dose CT lung cancer screening. A nodule was reported in the right lower lobe. This patient had no complaints of a cough, sputum, chest pain, and other lung cancer-associated symptoms.

14.14.2 CT Findings

In the right lower lobe, a 6-mm part-solid GGN is seen nearby a segmental bronchus and pulmonary artery. Dotted solid component occurs in the central area, and multiple fine blood vessels penetrate into the lesion (Fig. 14.15).

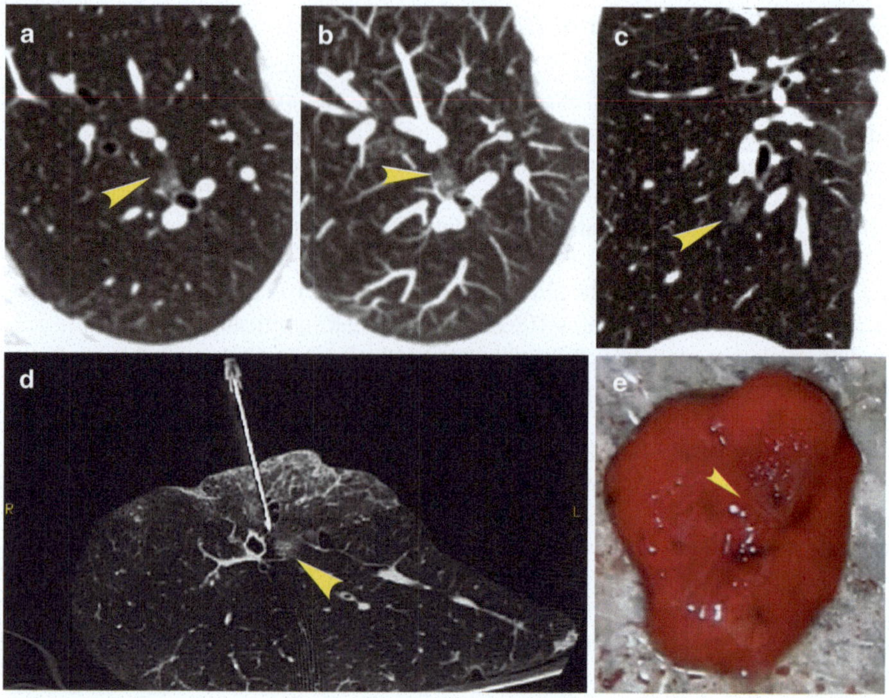

Fig. 14.15 In the axial image (**a**), MIP image (**b**), and coronary image (**c**), a poorly defined patchy GGN is visualized with dotted solid components distributed in the central area. Multiple tiny arterial vessels from the adjacent pulmonary artery enter into the nodule. This nodule is suspected of MIA and arrowheads mark the invasion front. (**d**) Postoperative localization of the lesion (arrowhead) under CT guidance in re-aerated lung specimen. (**e**) The grayish lesion is seen in the lung specimen (arrowhead)

14.14.3 Pathological Diagnosis

This patient received surgical removal of the GGN. Pathological diagnosis confirmed minimally invasive adenocarcinoma.

14.14.4 Discussions and Comments

In this case, the margin of the lesion is not as well-defined as seen in previous cases of MIA. Hence, the possibility of inflammatory or infectious nodule should be excluded before consideration of malignancy. According to NCCN guidelines on lung cancer screening and NSCLC, this patient received 2-week antibiotic treatment and multiple follow-ups. The lesion did not resolve, making it a persistent GGN with increasing likelihood of malignancy. The radiologic-pathologic correlation analysis confirmed the consistency between the fuzzy margin in imaging and micro-invasion front.

(Ming Li)

14.15 Case 15: Minimally Invasive Adenocarcinoma

14.15.1 Clinical History

A 70-year-old female presented to the clinic with complaints of a cough and fever for a week. Blood tests revealed increasing white blood cell count. An emergency chest CT was ordered and an irregular ground-glass opacity in the right upper lobe with dotted solid components reported. Initial imaging impression was most likely focal pneumonitis, but malignant disorders cannot be excluded. The patient was given antibiotics for 2 weeks. The follow-up CTs in 3 weeks later and 3 months later showed the lesion was stable without significant changes in size and attenuation. And the patient did not develop additional symptoms. Routine follow-up was advised to monitor the nodule. One year later, this patient came back for routine follow-up CT scanning. In comparison with findings in previous CT images, the nodule grew in size, and solid component increases with the occurrence of lobulation and spiculation. Malignancy was suspected, and the patient was referred to a thoracic surgeon for a further consultation. This patient was a non-smoker and had no family history of cancer. She received partial thyroidectomy for a benign adenoma and cholecystectomy for cholecystolithiasis. Tumor biomarkers, including CA199, CA125, and CA724, were within normal limits.

14.15.2 CT Findings

A mixed GGN is seen in the subpleural area with a dimension of 12 mm × 10 mm. The margin is well-defined but irregular with short spiculation and mild lobulation. The lesion has heterogeneous attenuation with mixtures of eccentric bubble-like lucencies and diffused solid components. In comparison to previous CT images, the amount of solid component increased from less than 30% of the lesion to more than 50%. Contrast-enhanced CT imaging revealed a remarkable enhancement in solid component with CT value increment of 59–86 HU. The pleural thickening and indentation are seen. Based on these imaging findings, the lesion is highly suspected of minimally invasive lung adenocarcinoma or invasive lung adenocarcinoma (Fig. 14.16).

14.15.3 Pathological Diagnosis

The patient received RUL lobectomy via VATS.

The pathological examination confirmed MIA without pleural involvement.

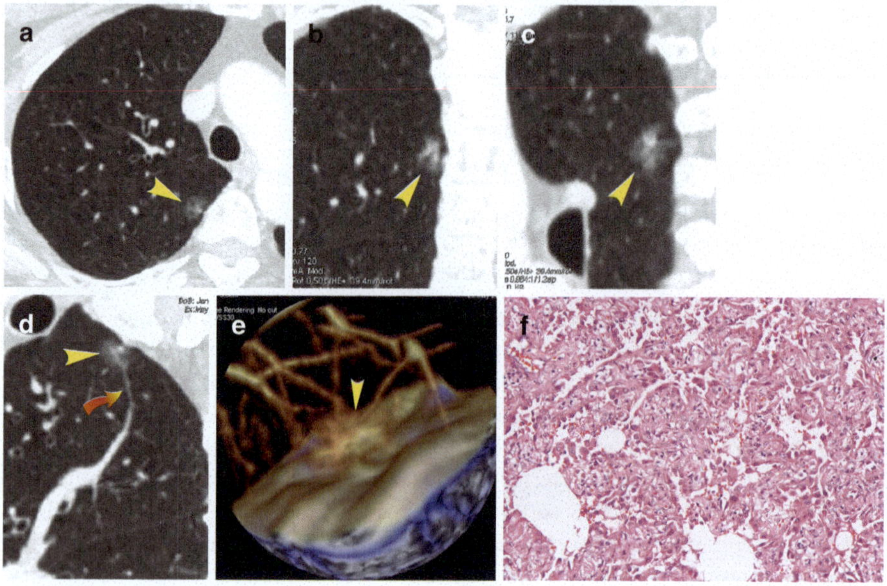

Fig. 14.16 A part-solid irregular nodule (arrowhead) is seen in the subpleural area with pleural attachment and evident CTA-TA sign. Surgical pathology confirmed MIA. (**a**), axial image; (**b**), coronal image; (**c**), sagittal image; (**d**), curved planar reformation image; (**e**), volume rendering image; (**f**), H-E stain

14.15.4 Discussions and Comments

This case described a complete workflow regarding the imaging diagnosis and management of an incidentally detected GGN in chest CT. This workflow starts from exclusion of inflammatory diseases with antibiotic usage, followed by routine monitoring to evaluate its growth pattern, and finally surgical resection if the nodule has manifestations indicative of malignancy, including increasing amount of solid component with significant enhancement with contrast medium, CTA-TA sign lobulation, spiculation, air bronchogram, bubble-like lucencies, and potential pleural involvement. The presence of these imaging features predicts increasing metastatic risks for a malignant disease. Hence, at the moment, the lesion should be progressively managed instead of continuing the "wait-and-see" strategy. Transbronchial lung biopsy or percutaneous CT-guided biopsy can be performed with the attempt to make the definitive diagnosis. However, false-negative results occur in some cases. If the malignancy probability is over 70%, definitive treatment procedures are justified to proceed, surgical resection in the majority of cases and ablation therapy (with radiation or radiofrequency) in patients unfit for surgical procedures.

(Fei Hu)

14.16 Case 16: Invasive Adenocarcinoma

14.16.1 Clinical History

A 55-year-old female complained a cough, sputum, and reduced appetite for 2 weeks. Body weight remained stable. She was a non-smoker and family history of cancer was negative. Lung cancer-associated tumor biomarkers (CA199, CA724, CA125, CA211, NSE, CEA, AFP, CA153, and SCC) were within normal limits. A chest CT was requested.

14.16.2 CT Findings

A piling-type GGN is seen in the apicoposterior segment of the right upper lobe. The lesion is measured 26 mm × 21 mm with a pile of diffused solid components. Mild lobulation, air bronchogram, and CTA-TA sign are seen (Fig. 14.17).

14.16.3 Pathological Diagnosis

This RUL lesion is highly suspected of AIS or MIA. After multidisciplinary discussions, RUL lobectomy is performed to remove the lesion.

Surgical pathological examination confirmed invasive adenocarcinoma without pleural involvement and positive hilar/mediastinal lymph nodes.

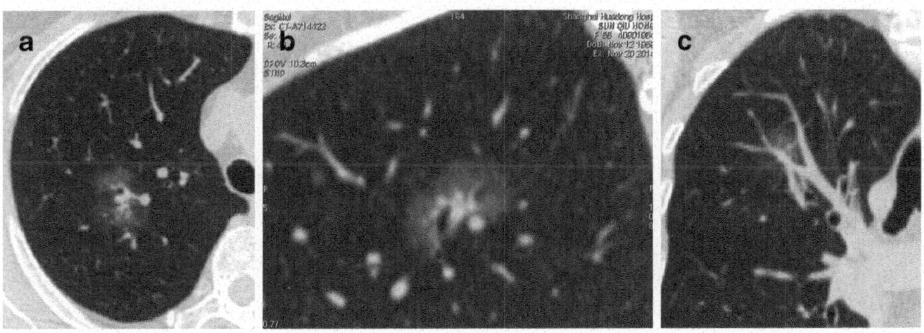

Fig. 14.17 (**a**) A part-solid GGN is located in the right upper lobe, (**b**) This zoomed view shows the solid component and air bronchogram. (**c**) Characteristic CTA-TA sign is seen in this coronal image

14.16.4 Discussions and Comments

According to the IASLC lung adenocarcinoma classification in 2011, invasive adenocarcinomas (IACs) represent more than 70–90% of surgically resected lung cases. The concept of multistep progression from AAH through AIS and MIA to invasive adenocarcinoma (IAC) has been proposed. It is generally accepted that a GGN nodule increases in size, then solid portion within the lesion tends to appear, and finally solid portion increases in extent. Regarding the size, preinvasive lesion is usually less than 5 mm in diameter, while IAC usually is more than 10 mm in diameter, and the size of MIA is between 5 and 10 mm. Of note, size is not the only criterion for differentiating these diseases, and it may vary in some cases.

Due to the step-by-step developmental biological behavioral pattern, IACs are composed of a complex heterogeneous mixture of histological subtypes with predominant subtype. Pathologically, lepidic-predominant adenocarcinoma (LPA) is the major subtype in IAC, defining a non-mucinous adenocarcinoma that has lepidic growth as its predominant component. LPA typically consists of bland pneumocytic cells (type II pneumocytes or Clara cells) growing along the surface of alveolar walls similar to the morphology in MIA and AIS, but invasive adenocarcinoma is present in at least one focus measuring more than 5 mm in greatest dimension. The diagnosis of LPA rather than MIA is made if the tumor (1) invades lymphatics, blood vessels, or pleura or (2) contains tumor necrosis. Additionally, the invasion extent in MIA and IAC is different, ≤5-mm invasion in the former and >5 mm in the latter.

Invasive adenocarcinoma is usually a solid nodule but may also be part-solid and occasionally a pure GGN (as seen in MIA). For stage IA adenocarcinoma presenting as a part-solid nodule, an extensive ground-glass component suggests a favorable prognosis. Histologically, the ground-glass component typically corresponds to a lepidic pattern and the solid component to invasive patterns.

Bubble-like or cystic lucencies in stage IA adenocarcinoma have been described as correlating with well-differentiated tumors and slow growth. An intratumoral air bronchogram usually indicates a well-differentiated tumor. The presence of notches or concave cuts on thin-section CT, more frequently seen in solid IAC, has been associated with a poor differentiation on histology and adverse outcome. Tumor growth rate may vary in different directions due to mitotic activity, physical barriers from preexisting blood vessels, fibrotic tissues, interlobar fissure, or septum, causing irregularity of the nodular shape which may manifest as lobulation or spiculation sign in imaging. Thick (≥2 mm) coarse spiculation has been associated with lymph node metastasis, vascular invasion, and decreased survival post resection. The absence of pleural retraction for stage IA adenocarcinoma is also a favorable prognostic sign. Pleural retraction is defined as a linear structure originating from the tumor and extending to the pleural surface, and the pleura was retracted toward the tumor.

IAC represents the progressive stage of adenocarcinoma from a relative dormant stage. One of the major biological changes is neoangiogenesis resulting in increasing amount of intratumoral vasculature and solid component. Hence, typical CTA-TA sign occurs in almost all IAC cases. CTA-TA should be differentiated from vascular convergence sign (VCS). VCS results from significant reactive fibrous connective tissue proliferation pulling the nearby blood vessels into the nodules. Fibrosis in the damaged lung and tumor proliferation cause destruction that leads to the collapse of the bracket structure, shrinkage, and pulling of the nearby vessels. Therefore, VCS can also be seen in benign lesions. VCS describes the impact of neoplasm on surrounding tissues, whereas CTA-TA reflects the biological behaviors of the neoplasm itself, recruiting new vessels and neoangiogenesis.

(Ping Tang)

14.17 Case 17: Invasive Adenocarcinoma

14.17.1 Clinical History

A 50-year-old male received chest CT scanning due to chest pain. Diffused pneumonia was reported in the right middle lobe. Additionally, a tiny GGN was found in the superior segment of the right lower lobe. This patient was given intravenously antibiotic treatment for 2 weeks. In the follow-up chest CT, the pneumonia resolved, but the GGN remains the same as in the initial CT. This patient had more than 10 years' history of hypertension and psoriasis vulgaris, without smoking history and family history of any cancers or genetic diseases.

14.17.2 CT Findings

A part-solid well-defined nodule is seen in the RLL with measurement of 6 mm in diameter. This nodule is ground-glass predominant with few solid components. However, mild lobulation and concave cut are seen. Typical CTA-TA sign is absent but tiny vessels are seen entering into the lesion (Fig. 14.18).

14.17.3 Pathological Diagnosis

This GGN was initially diagnosed as AIS (most likely) or MIA. The surgical pathological examination confirmed invasive adenocarcinoma, acinar predominant, without lymphatic involvement.

14.17.4 Discussions and Comments

This is an exemplary case in which the severity of the disease is underestimated. Based on the imaging features, including small size, ground-glass predominant, and absence of typical CTA-TA sign, a suspicion of AIS is reasonable. The only signs

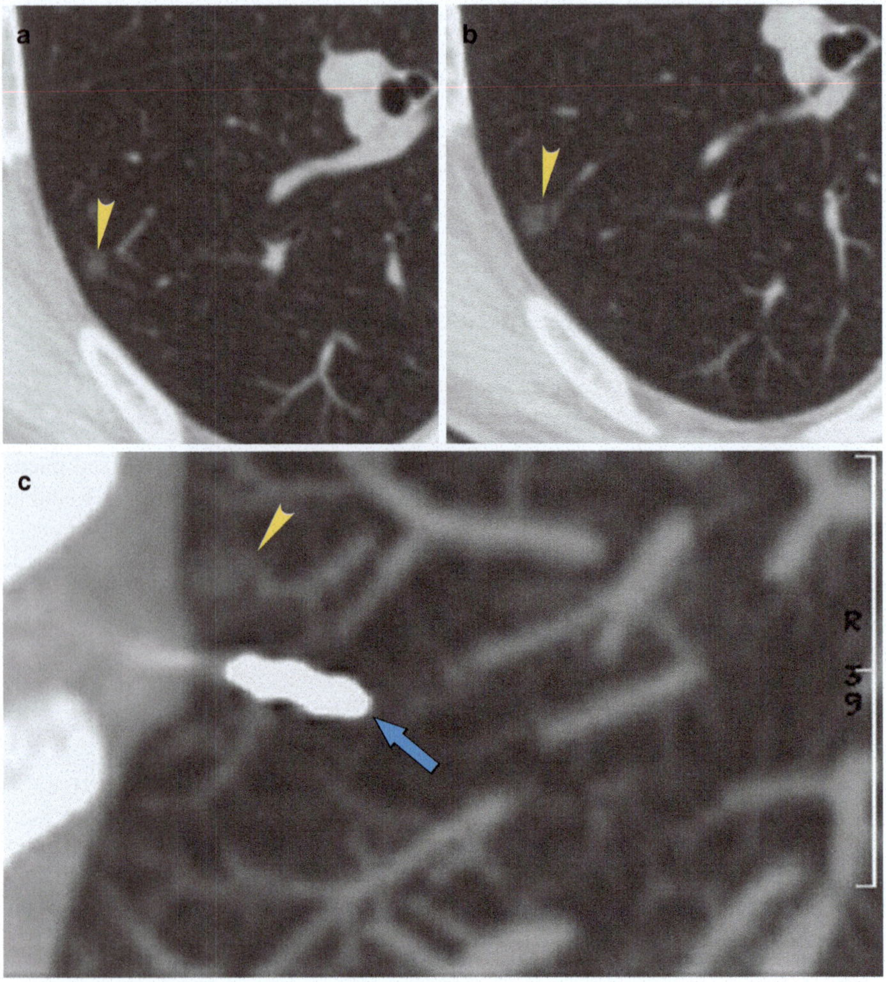

Fig. 14.18 A part-solid GGN is located in the subpleural area in RLL with mild lobulation and concave cut (arrowhead, **a**–**c**). This nodule is a wedge resected via VATS with the assistance of preoperative needle localization technique (blow arrow, **c**)

that are more frequently seen in invasive diseases instead of preinvasive lesions are the lobulation and concave cut signs. However, both signs more likely occur in solid invasive diseases or invasive diseases with solid component predominance than in ground-glass predominant lesions. This case suggests that if there exist conflicting imaging findings, radiologists should be cautious in generating a report regarding the nature of the disease.

(Fei Hu)

14.18 Case 18: Invasive Adenocarcinoma

14.18.1 Clinical History

A 40-year-old female presented to the clinic with complaints of a dry cough for several months. She was a non-smoker and did not drink alcohol. A chest radiograph revealed a cavitary lesion in the right upper lobe (RUL). A throat swab culture of *Candida albicans* was positive. This patient was prescribed antifungal medicine. One month later, a follow-up chest CT was requested for treatment outcome evaluation.

14.18.2 CT Findings

A heterogeneous lesion of 1.3 cm in diameter is seen in the right middle lobe adjoining the major fissure. The lesion contains multiple components with solid component predominance. The ground-glass component can be seen along part of the margin, creating a halo sign. A cavitary appearance occurs in the lesion. Pleural retraction, lobulation, and spiculation are visualized (Fig. 14.19).

14.18.3 Pathological Diagnosis

The patient received RML lobectomy via VATS.

Pathological examination confirmed invasive adenocarcinoma.

14.18.4 Discussions and Comments

This case presents an atypical IAC with a remarkable cavitary appearance within the lesion.

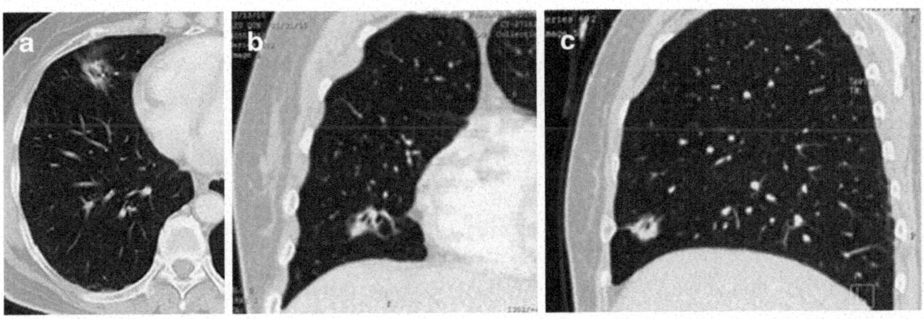

Fig. 14.19 A heterogeneous lesion is located in the RML with characteristic lobulation, spiculation, pleural retraction, and cavitary appearance

Heterogeneous central soft tissue attenuation within a pulmonary nodule is an HRCT finding predominantly associated with malignancy and correlated with (a) cavitation, (b) bubble-like pseudocavitation, (c) patent bronchi producing air bronchograms, and (d) central solid or liquefactive necrosis without overt cavitation. A cavity has been defined pathologically as "a gas-filled space within a zone of pulmonary consolidation or within a mass or nodule, produced by the expulsion of a necrotic part of the lesion via the bronchial tree" and radiologically as "a lucency within a zone of pulmonary consolidation, a mass, or a nodule." Hence, a lucent area within the lung that may or may not contain a fluid level is surrounded by a wall, usually of varied thickness. Cavities are frequent manifestations of a wide variety of pathological processes involving the lung, including suppurative necrosis (e.g., pyogenic lung abscess), caseous necrosis (e.g., tuberculosis), ischemic necrosis (e.g., pulmonary infarction), cystic dilatation of lung structures (e.g., ball valve obstruction and *Pneumocystis* pneumonia), displacement of lung tissue by cystic structures (e.g., *Echinococcus*), or malignant process because of treatment-related necrosis, internal cyst formation, or internal desquamation of tumor cells with subsequent liquefaction.

Cavitation detected by computed tomography has been reported for up to 22% of primary lung cancers; it is more frequently found among cases of squamous cell carcinomas than other histological types. Furthermore, the presence of cavitation in a lung tumor has been associated with a worse prognosis. Metastatic disease from other primary sites may also cavitate, but this occurs less frequently than in primary lung cancers: an estimated 4% of metastatic tumors have been noted to cavitate with the predominance of squamous cell origin.

Of note, cavitation in the early-stage lung adenocarcinoma (MIA and IAC) is uncommon, but the cavitation-like appearance or bubble-like lucency may be seen as in this case due to abnormal air collections in and around the tumor as results of paracicatricial emphysema, fibrosis with honeycombing, and localized bronchiectasis. Such cavitation-like appearance is named as the pseudocavitation sign to facilitate differentiation with pathological cavitations described above. Pseudocavitation was reported to be observed more frequently in bronchioloalveolar carcinoma (50%) than any other malignant lesions. This sign is uncommon but occasionally seen in non-bronchioloalveolar malignancies and benign lesions. This sign is characterized by the presence of focal areas of air attenuation peripherally or centrally within the lesion on HRCT images and corresponds either to patent small bronchi within the nodule or cystic glandular spaces formed by the tumor.

Some researchers considered bubble-like lucency equivalent to pseudocavitation, while other researchers would like to distinguish them according to the size. Bubble-like lucency is defined as a low attenuation area less than 5 mm in diameter, while pseudocavitation is larger than 5 mm with unremarkable walls. The size of air-containing space in pseudocavitation may vary during the development of diseases, either continuously increasing or shrinking as the result of alveolar collapse and central fibrosis with tumor progression (Figs. 14.20 and 14.21).

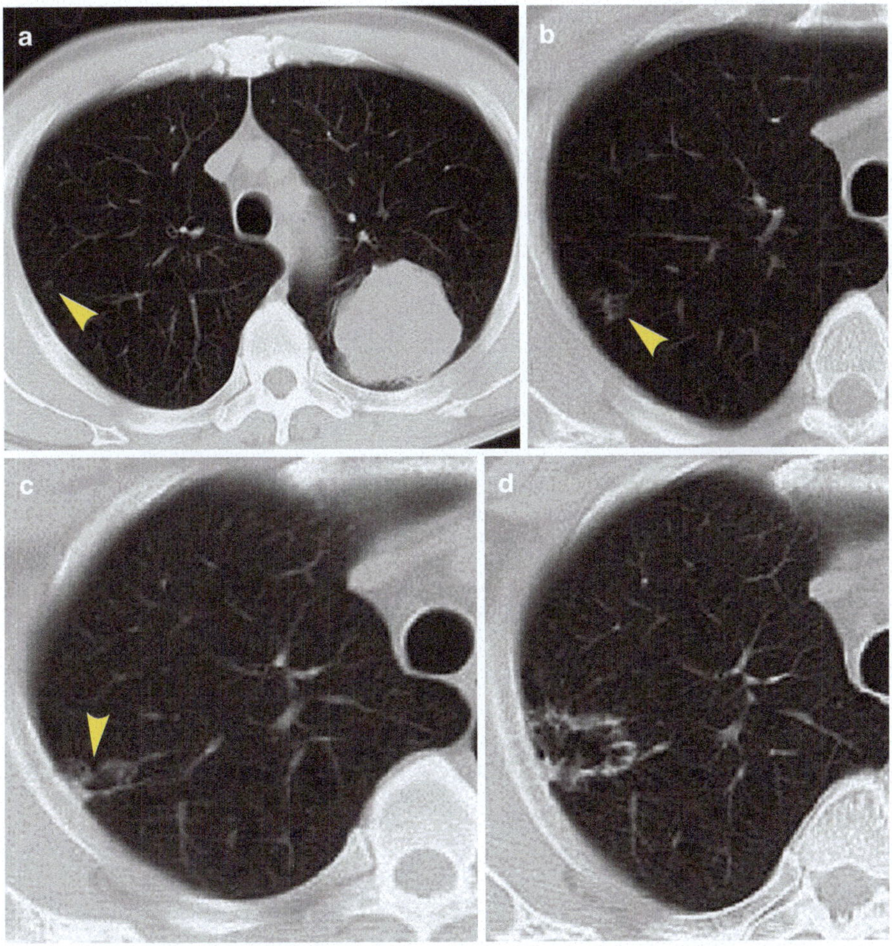

Fig. 14.20 Pseudocavitation in IAC. A 59-year-old male received surgery due to lung cancer in the left upper lobe. Preoperative chest CT revealed a tiny bubble-like lesion (arrowhead, **a**) in the right upper lobe. This lesion was advised for routine follow-up with CT imaging. In 18-month (**b**), 35-month (**c**), and 43-month CT images, the bubble-like lesion progressively develops into a pseudocavitation-predominant mass-like lesion measuring 2.5 cm in diameter. The pleural involvement was seen. This lesion did not respond to antibiotic treatment and was highly suspected of invasive adenocarcinoma. Surgical pathological examination confirmed the diagnosis

Despite that the typical features of IAC are nonspecific, the presence of a peripherally located nodule demonstrating heterogeneous attenuation, spiculated borders, and pseudocavitation is a characteristic enough to suggest the diagnosis.

(Guozhen Zhang, Xiangpeng Zheng)

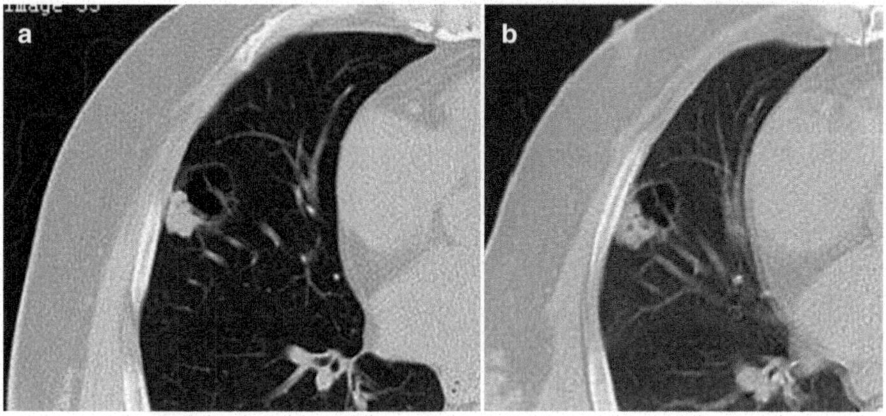

Fig. 14.21 Pseudocavitation in IAC. A heterogeneous solid nodule with an evident eccentric cavity was seen in a 69-year-old male. In the initial CT image (**a**), the cavitary area appeared larger than the solid component, whereas 3 weeks after antibiotic treatment, a follow-up CT revealed that the cavitary area shrunk in contrast to the stable solid component. Percutaneous CT-guided biopsy on the solid component confirmed invasive adenocarcinoma. Subsequent lobectomy was performed, and the pathological examination revealed that neoplastic cells accumulated only in the solid component area, and the observed cavitary area was a pseudocavitation due to fibrotic emphysema

14.19 Case 19: Scar-like Adenocarcinoma

14.19.1 Clinical History

A 56-year-old female was hospitalized for suspected tuberculosis. Chest CT showed a strip-shaped irregular lesion in the apical segment of the right upper lobe, and a TB test reported positive result. This patient received antituberculosis treatment for 6 months, and the lesion regressed to fibrotic scars. Afterward, the patient was advised to have annual chest CT to monitor the lesion. Seven years later, chest CT showed ground-glass opacity occurred around the previous TB scars. Another TB test was negative.

14.19.2 CT Findings

Reviews on consecutive follow-up CT images reveal that since the third year after anti-TB treatment, a trace amount of ground-glass opacities have occurred in previous TB scars. In subsequent CT images, ground-glass opacities continued developing in extent and attenuation, indicating cellular accumulation. Hence, scar carcinoma of the lung was suspected (Fig. 14.22).

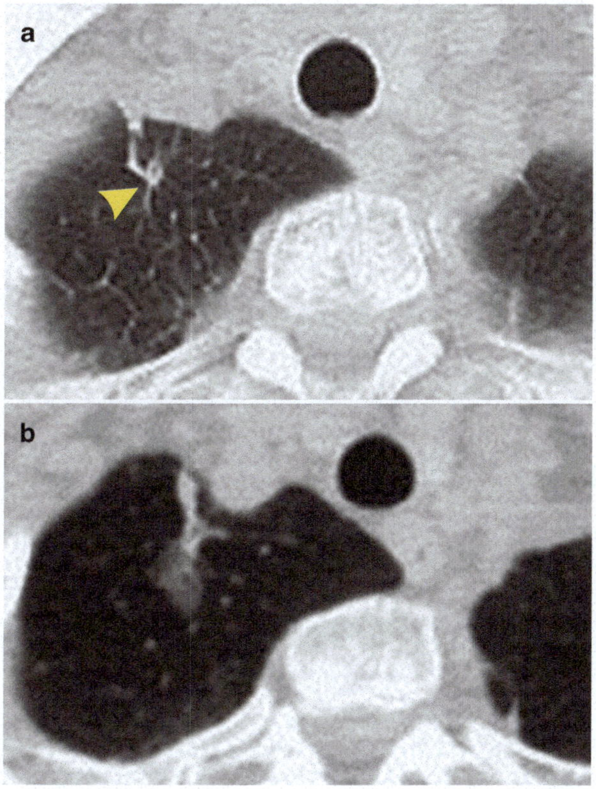

Fig. 14.22 (**a**) The arrowhead shows the fibrotic scar in a patient with previous tuberculosis. (**b**) Seven years later, the previous scar enlarges with the replacement of soft tissues, and heterogeneous ground-glass opacities are visualized in the adjacent parenchyma

14.19.3 Pathological Diagnosis

This patient received RUL lobectomy with lymph node dissection. Pathological examination confirmed a poorly differentiated adenocarcinoma arising at the edge of a dense hyalinized fibrotic tuberculous lesion with an abundance of elastic and anthracotic pigment scattered throughout the lesion and a transition from epithelial hyperplasia or metaplasia to frank carcinoma seen at the periphery of the lesion, in consistency with the imaging diagnosis of scar carcinoma of the lung (Fig. 14.23).

14.19.4 Discussions and Comments

Scar carcinoma (SC) of the lung was first described by Friedrich in 1939 as a group of lung cancers that originated around peripheral scars in the lung. SC of the lung is a histologic diagnosis and is a peripherally located tumor, with no evidence of bronchial origin, occurring in intimate relation to scar tissue. The relationship between scarring of the lung and the development of carcinoma has been a controversial issue for some time. Yu et al. [1] investigated whether localized pulmonary scarring

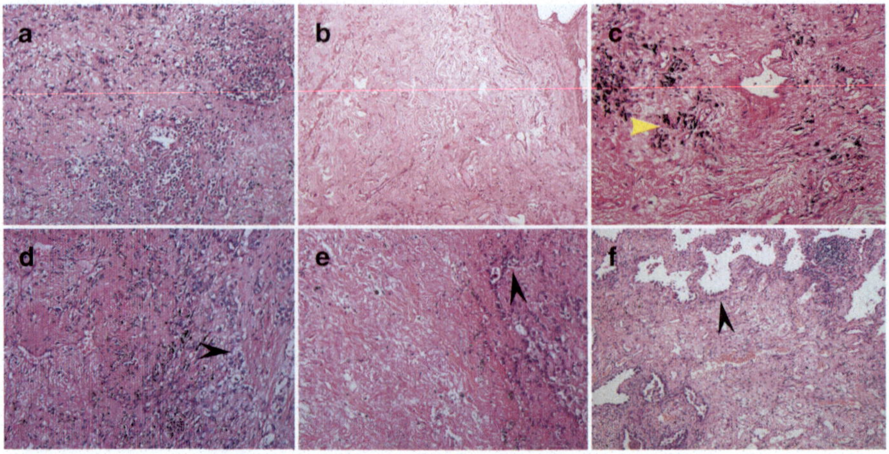

Fig. 14.23 Microscopic features of scar carcinoma in the same patient. (**a**) Infiltration of neutrophils, eosinophils, and lymphocytes was observed in patchy and focal necrotic tissues. (**b**) Within the lesion, there were fibrosis and elastosis and also foci of dense hyaline scarring. (**c**) Anthracotic pigments (arrowhead) distribute within chronic granulation tissues. (**d**) Poorly differentiated adenocarcinoma is seen along the right edge of granulation tissue (arrowhead). (**e**) Neoplastic cells (arrowhead) accumulate within fibrous scarred area. (**f**) Neoplastic cells grow in a lepidic pattern in mixture with thin and loose fibers produced by neoplastic infiltration

is associated with increased lung cancer risk based on the cohort analysis of data from the Prostate, Lung, Colorectal, and Ovarian Cancer Screening Trial, indicating that localized inflammatory processes associated with scarring promote the subsequent development of lung cancer. Even more, this disease or concept has been challenged as a separate pathological entity with the view that the presence of scars may increase the risks of developing malignancies, which have nothing different from those occurring without a scar background. Currently, SCs tend to be an imaging impression rather than a pathological diagnosis. By definition, scar formation precedes the development of the carcinoma for a variable time, years probably, which is more likely to be observed in patients with multiple follow-up CT scans.

Scarring of the lung can result from almost all of pulmonary diseases, benign or malignant, infectious or noninfectious, as their fingerprints in lungs, reflecting a history of healing or necrotic process. SCs commonly occur in the upper lobes and are usually adenocarcinomas or bronchioloalveolar variants with poor differentiation, as seen in this case. Multiple hypotheses have been proposed regarding the pathogenesis of SCs. Atypical bronchiolar epithelial proliferation may lead to SCs in pre-existing lung scars, while in some scars, the bronchiolar proliferation becomes excessive during regeneration from injury and may develop malignant change. Despite the notion of the scars produced by the tumor rather than the predecessor of tumor growth, the former cannot be strictly classified as SCs.

The typical imaging features of SCs include peripheral location with upper lobe predominance; the irregular solid component with a halo sign composed of ground-glass opacities, pleural retraction, and lobulation; progressive enlargement in multiple follow-up images; and most importantly for SCs neoplasm growing in or around fibrous scars.

According to an early study on SCs, in comparison to similar histological types without scars, SCs tend to have an increasing probability of lymph node involvement, resulting in a poor prognosis with a 5-year overall survival of 5%. One of the reasons accounting for such a poor prognosis could be the limited diagnostic capability. That is a study conducted in 1974 when CT was not clinically available for early detection of lung cancers. As in this case, due to a timely detection and surgical management, this lesion is a confirmed stage IA disease. A favorable prognosis is absolutely predictable.

Generally, scarring is considered as the last step in a series of events involved in the repair or healing process in cured or controlled disease with a good prognosis. The diagnosis of SC is a historical histologic diagnosis as well as an imaging diagnosis. The correlation between scarring and cancer remains unanswered. Traditionally, fibrous scars do not require routine follow-up or management. Based on limited reported cases of scar carcinomas, the current clinical practice pattern still works. Additional research will be necessary to determine if imaging-detected lung scarring requires clinical monitoring in the context of the development of lung cancer, when a defined set of risk factors can be identified.

(Jie Zhang, Guozhen Zhang)

14.20 Case 20: Synchronous Multiple Primary Lung Cancer

14.20.1 Clinical History

Irregular mass-like opacities were found in the left upper lobe of a 56-year-old retired otherwise healthy female staff who received her annual chest radiography. After 1-month antibiotic treatment, the opacities did not resolve. Chest CT with contrast was recommended for further evaluation. Tumor biomarkers, including CA199, CA125, CA724, CA211, and neural enolase, were reported within normal limits. The patient did not have weight loss, cough, or bloody sputum.

14.20.2 CT Findings

Multiple ground-glass opacities are seen in both lungs. The largest one is 2 cm in diameter and located in the left upper lobe with imaging features of mixed attenuation with solid component predominance, bubble-like lucencies, air bronchogram, and evident pleural retraction, indicative of invasive adenocarcinoma (IAC). Other GGN nodules are within 10 mm with the appearance of pure GGNs or part-solid GGNs. CTA-TA sign is observed in some of the part-solid GGNs (Fig. 14.24).

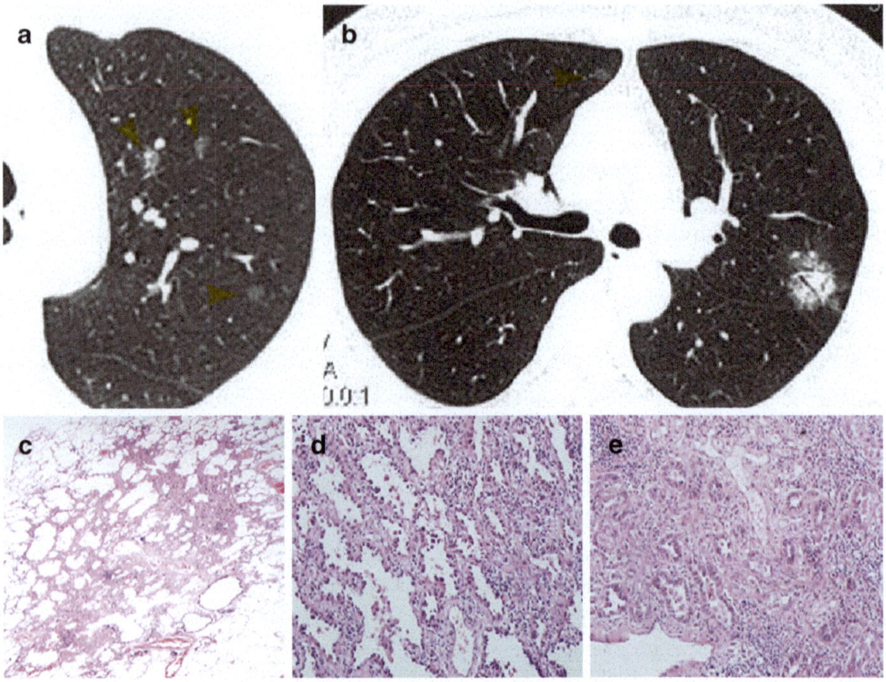

Fig. 14.24 Synchronous multiple primary lung cancer (SMPLC) . (**a**) Two mixed GGNs and one pure GGN (arrowhead) are seen in the left upper lobe with diameters ranging from 5 to 8 mm. AAH (pGGN) and AIS (mGGNs) are suspected. (**b**) A 20-mm GGN with solid component predominance is seen in the left upper lobe with signs of bubble-like lucencies, air bronchogram, and pleural retraction, characteristic of IAC; in the same image, a pure GGN (arrowhead) is seen in the right upper lobe with suspicion of AAH. (**c**) Pathological results of the pGGN in the RUL revealed mild-moderate hyperplasia of the alveolar epithelium with intact alveolar structure, in accordance with AAH. (**d**) The pathological examination of two mGGNs in the LUL confirmed AIS with lepidic growth of neoplastic cells along alveolar inner walls and without interstitial and vascular invasion. (**e**) The largest lesion was confirmed as IAC with acinar predominant

14.20.3 Pathological Diagnosis

This patient received LUL lobectomy and RUL wedge resection to remove all detected lesions via VATS.

As shown in Fig. 14.24, heterogeneous diseases were pathologically confirmed, including AAH, AIS, and IAC. Hence, synchronous multiple primary lung cancer was concluded.

14.20.4 Discussions and Comments

Multiple primary lung cancer (MPLC) describes an entity of two or more lung cancerous lesions with independent origins simultaneously or successively occurred in one patient. The pathogenesis of MPLC remains not fully understood yet. Various theories, such as field cancerization, genetic susceptibility, iatrogenic factors, and even aging, have been proposed. The diagnosis of MPLC remains challenging. Pulmonary multifocal nodules may be reflections of many entities, including infectious diseases, advanced stages of primary lung cancer (T3 or T4), and intrapulmonary metastases from other malignancies. Therefore, the diagnosis of MPLC requires a thorough review of medical history, meticulous imaging evaluations, and an exclusion strategy to rule out other possibilities. For more information, please refer to Chap. 10.

MPLC can occur in the setting of multiple AAH, AIS, and invasive adenocarcinoma, indicating that the imaging features of either sMPLC or mMPLC are the collective imaging characteristics of each independent lesion. In chest CT imaging, MPLC is commonly described as multifocal nodular opacities, and similarities or differences in attenuation may provide clues regarding the relative percentage of lepidic versus solid histologic components. Of note, subsolid nodules are very rarely metastatic.

This case presents a typical pathologically proven sMPLC with coexistence of AAH, AIS, and IAC. Each lesion has its characteristic imaging features. If occurred separately, the diagnosis is not challenging. However, when so many lesions occur simultaneously, imaging evaluation should be performed with extreme caution. After all, the sMPLC is not a common entity with reported proportion less than 10% of the whole lung cancers. Also, this case demonstrates the multistep developmental process of lung adenocarcinoma in a panoramic pattern, i.e., AAH → AIS → MIA → IAC. Preinvasive lesions, AAH and AIS, and invasive lesion coexist. It can be reasonably predicted that without proper management, those preinvasive lesions will progress into invasive diseases with increasing risks to the patient's health, life expectancy, and quality of life. The heterogeneity between different lesions of sMPLC imposes great challenge in the medical management. Despite that surgical removal remains the first choice among numerous options, it may not be unfit or short of cost-effectiveness in patients with lesions in bilateral and multi-lobe distribution. In that situation, more comprehensive management strategies should be considered, including combinations of surgery and radiotherapy, surgery and radiofrequency ablation, or surgery and systemic therapy.

(Xiangpeng Zheng)

14.21 Case 21: Synchronous Multiple Primary Lung Cancer

14.21.1 Clinical History

A 64-year-old otherwise healthy female received CT lung cancer screening in March 2013, and two ground-glass nodules were reported in each lung. Routine imaging follow-up was initiated after that. The last follow-up CT was acquired in November 2014. A comparative analysis of follow-up CT images showed that the nodule in the left lung slowly grew. Preoperative blood test on tumor biomarkers showed normal values. This patient denied smoking history and family history of any cancers.

14.21.2 CT Findings

Two GGNs are seen in this patient. A 9-mm pure GGN located in the right upper lobe has a well-defined margin with two fine blood vessels passing along the lesion. The other GGN is seen in the left upper lobe with the dotted solid component inside and evident CTA-TA sign. In comparison to the initial CT 20 months ago, the pure GGN remained unchanged, but the part-solid GGN showed increment in size and density and enhancement with the administration of contrast medium (Fig. 14.25).

14.21.3 Pathological Diagnosis

Due to progressive enlargement observed in LUL nodule, MIA is suspected and surgical removal is recommended. With multidisciplinary discussion, both nodules were surgically removed with wedge resection. Pathological examination confirmed AIS for both nodules.

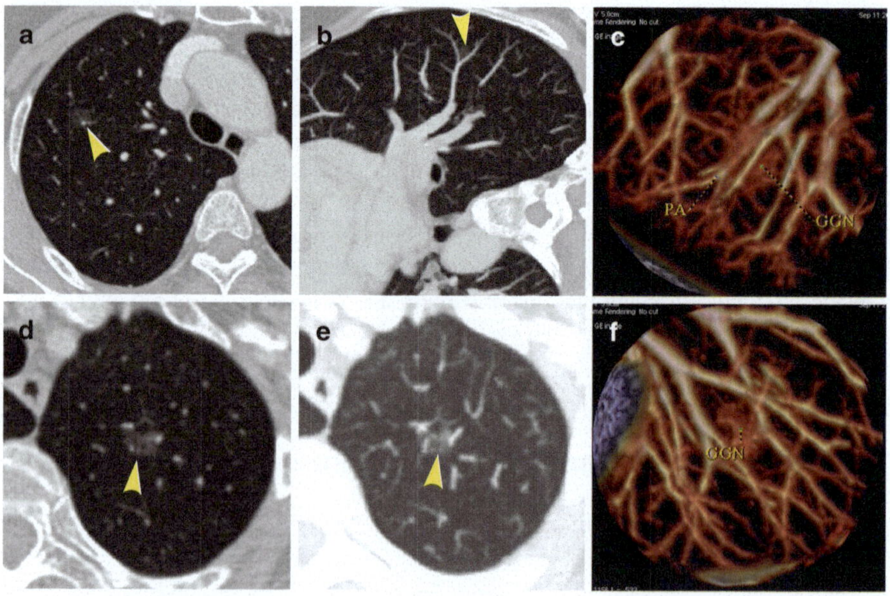

Fig. 14.25 (**a–c**) A well-defined pure GGN (arrowhead) is seen in the right upper lobe with blood vessels visualized along the margin (**a**, axial image; **b**, MIP image, **c**, volume rendering image). (**d**, **e**) An 11-mm part-solid GGN (arrowhead) is seen in the left upper lobe with characteristic CTA-TA sign (**a**, axial image; **b**, MIP image; **c**, volume rendering image)

14.21.4 Discussions and Diagnosis

MPLC could have different combinations of preinvasive and invasive diseases. In this case, two AIS lesions were confirmed. With the increasing public awareness of lung cancer and advances in medical imaging technology, the detection rate of MPLC increases. In parallel with that, the detection rate of benign nodules also rises, which certainly interferes with the diagnosis of MPLC. In contrast to MPLC reported decades ago, current MPLCs tend to be composed of early-stage and even preinvasive diseases. Hence, there exist controversies on the management. Follow-up could be a more reasonable strategy in MPLC than in solitary primary lung cancer. Follow-up evaluation will provide behavioral information to assist clinicians in making the decision of which lesion has the priority of being treated and when to initiate the treatment. This follow-up strategy is especially applicable to patients with numerous lesions (≥5 lesions in ≥3 lobes).

(Ping Tang, Dingbiao Mao)

14.22 Case 22: Synchronous Multiple Primary Lung Cancer

14.22.1 Clinical History

A 63-year-old female complained a cough and sputum for 2 weeks. Chest CT was requested with a returned report of multiple nodules in the right upper lobe. This patient was otherwise healthy, denying smoking history but admitting a family history of lung cancer.

14.22.2 CT Findings

There are three nodular lesions in the right upper lobe, two in the subpleural area and one in the central area of RUL (Fig. 14.26).

14.22.3 Pathological Diagnosis

Due to the family history of lung cancer, per the patient's request, RUL lobectomy was performed via VATS. Pathological-radiological correlation confirmed AAH for the pure GGN, AIS for the part-solid GGN, and fibrotic collagen and carbon dust accumulation for the solid nodule.

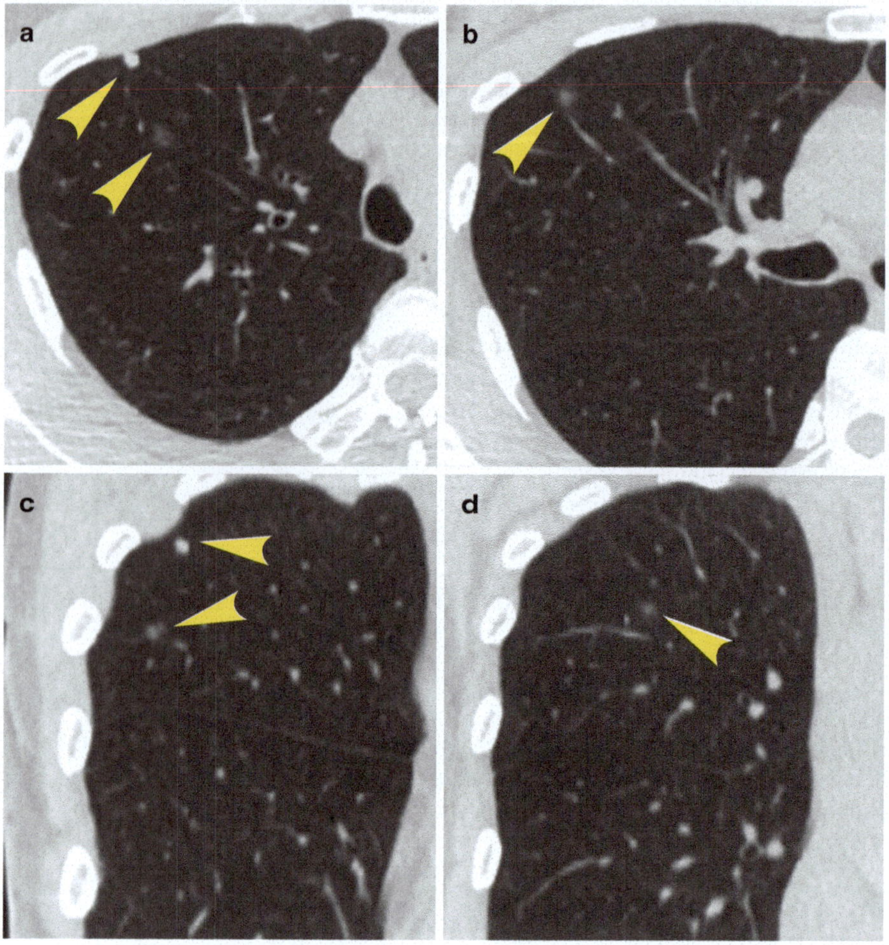

Fig. 14.26 Three nodular lesions (arrowhead) are seen in the right upper lobe: a solid nodule measuring 6 mm with attachment to the pleura, a part-solid GGN with a feeding blood vessel, and a solitary pure GGN without vascular associations. (**a**, **b**), axial images; (**c**, **d**), coronal images

14.22.4 Discussions and Comments

In this case, the surgery timing remains controversial among the multidisciplinary members. Fortunately all three nodules are located in the same lobe which enables a single lobectomy adequate for the definitive treatment. The subpleural solid nodule is a benign fibrotic scar, reminding radiologists of not taking MPLC for granted even there exist multiple malignant or premalignant lesions.

Another challenge in the management of MPLC is to find out all lesions in the surgical specimen for pathological examination. Although several preoperative localization techniques have been developed and widely utilized, failure to localize nodules in pathology occasionally occurs. Two common reasons are the small size of the nodule and excessive compression from surgical operations. In this case, considering the tiny size of GGNs (5 mm and 6 mm), besides preoperative localization technique, postoperative CT-guided needle localization in re-aerated lung specimen was performed to secure localization (Fig. 14.27). CT-guided positioning of lesions that present as GGNs on CT images using fine needles under constant,

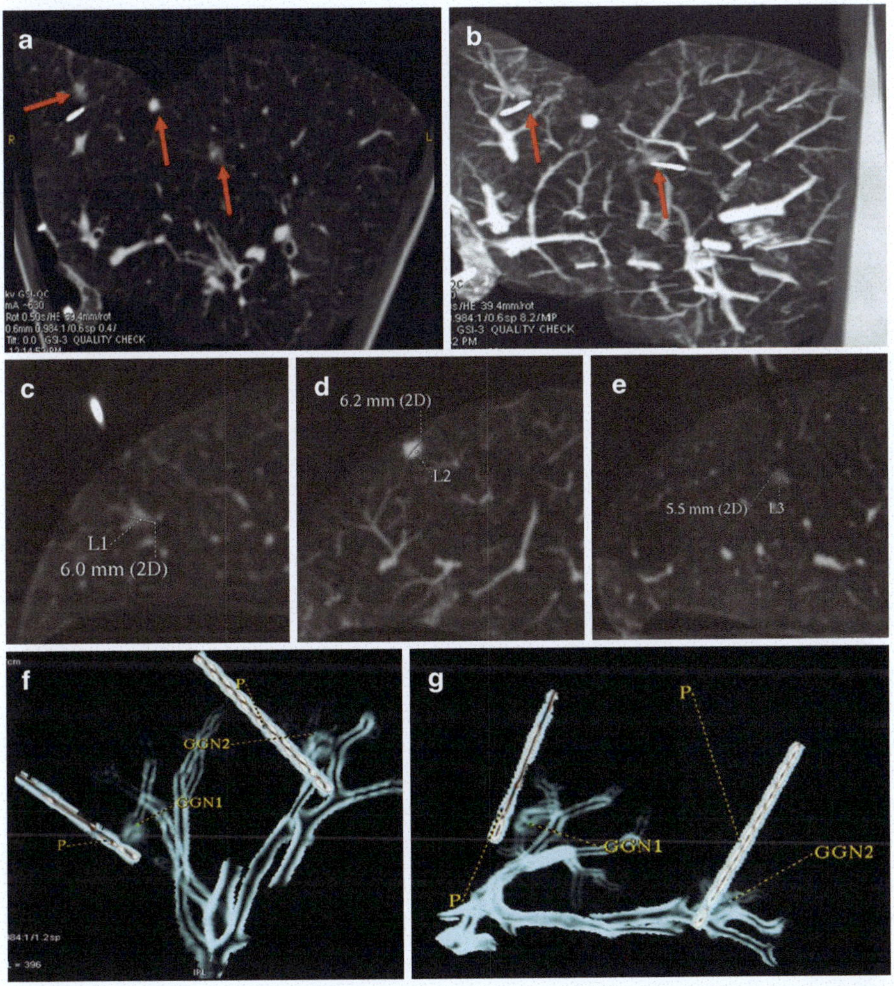

Fig. 14.27 Postoperative CT-guided needle localization in re-aerated lung specimen. Three nodular lesions (arrows) with various attenuations are seen in CT images of the re-aerated right upper lobe (**a**, axial image containing three nodules; **b**, MIP image; **c–e**, representative images corresponding to each nodular lesion with measurements). Volume rendering images (**f**, **g**) showed spatial relationships among needles, blood vessels, and nodules

moderate mechanical aeration of the specimen can increase the density of lesions relative to the surrounding lung tissue, allowing for a better access and higher quality CT images compared with the preoperative CT examination. This highly accurate method of lesion positioning allows for effective fine-needle localization of surgical specimens and avoids excessive damage to the patient. In addition, this approach is suitable for specimens resected during thoracotomy and thoracoscopic surgeries that involve either lobectomy or wedge resection.

(Ming Li, Xiangpeng Zheng)

14.23 Case 23: Small Squamous Lung Cancer

14.23.1 *Clinical History*

An 83-year-old male had a routine annual chest CT imaging due to colon cancer which had been surgically removed 4 years ago. In comparison with previous chest CT images, a nodular lesion measuring 2 mm was firstly found in the left upper lobe. This patient was a heavy smoker with a cigarette smoking history of 45 years and has been diagnosed chronic obstructive pulmonary disease since his 50s. Blood cell counts and tumor biomarkers were within normal limits.

The 6-month follow-up CT showed the nodule increased to 5 mm. Then antibiotic and supportive treatment was given. One month later, this nodule continued enlarging up to 7 mm in diameter. The subsequent FDG-PET/CT imaging revealed moderately hypermetabolic activity in the nodule, in consistency with malignancy.

14.23.2 *CT Findings*

Diffuse interstitial changes, including linear, reticular, and reticulonodular opacities, are present in both lungs. A solid nodule measuring 7 mm in diameter is firstly observed in this follow-up CT examination. The nodule has a well-defined margin with an irregular shape due to mild lobulation. Spiculation is absent. Pleural retraction is evident (Fig. 14.28).

14.23.3 *Pathological Diagnosis*

Considering the previous history of colon cancer, this nodule was initially diagnosed as oligometastasis. Multidisciplinary consultation recommended surgical removal. Consequently, wedge resection was performed. Pathological examination reported a 7-mm moderately differentiated squamous cell carcinoma.

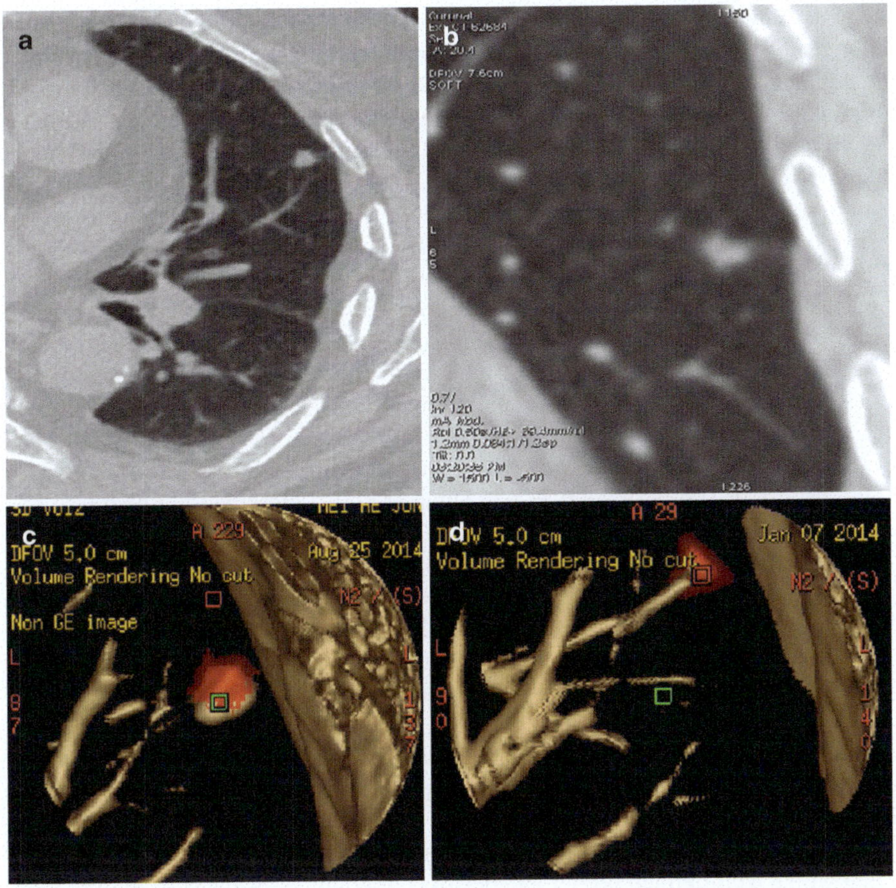

Fig. 14.28 A solid nodule is located in the left upper lobe with a progressive enlargement in follow-up imaging. (**a–c**) axial and volume rendering images in January 2014; (**b**, **d**) axial and volume rendering images of the same nodule in August 2014

14.23.4 Discussions and Comments

Peripheral squamous cell carcinoma (SCC) is not as common as central SCC. This case has several points worthwhile to be emphasized. Firstly, the possibility of oligometastasis should be considered and differentiated due to the history of colon cancer. Secondly, the quick progression of the nodule reflected a distinct entity from the common peripheral adenocarcinoma. Thirdly, a routine follow-up using imaging provides convenient and dynamic information regarding the disease.

According to the location of the primary site, squamous cell carcinoma of the lung can be divided into the central type and the peripheral type with the former predominant. The prevalence of peripheral SCCs among all SCCs has been reported to range from 15 to 30%. Smoking is an indiscriminate factor in the causation of both types of SSCs. In comparison with the common central SCCs, peripheral SSCs have some specific clinicopathologic features, including older patient population, smaller size in detection, lower prevalence of lymph node metastasis (especially in tumors ≤2 cm in diameter), less frequent squamous metaplasia, higher CK7 expression and lower CK19 expression, and relatively higher prevalence of noncancerous death. Despite that the central and peripheral SCCs have been reported to have distinct different clinicopathologic characteristics, the peripheral or central location of the tumor may not have the significant influence on the prognosis in patients with squamous cell carcinoma of the lung undergoing surgical resection.

Based on the comparative analysis of tumor growth patterns and clinicopathologic factors in 109 peripheral SCCs, Funai et al. [2] classified peripheral SCCs into three subgroups, the alveolar space-filling type, the expanding type, and the combined type with the frequency of 4.6%, 49.5%, and 45.9%, respectively. The alveolar space-filling type has a characteristic growth pattern with filling up of the alveolar space without destruction of the alveolar septal structure, similar to that observed in noninvasive small-sized adenocarcinomas of the lung. The tubular structure of nonatypical alveolar epithelium remains in alveoli that are nearly filled with cancerous tissue. The alveolar space-filling type shows neither lymphatic vessel invasion nor lymph node metastasis and has the most favorable prognosis. Hence this peripheral-type SCC may represent the early-stage or incipient disease. In the expanding type, tumors show a solid growth with no morphologic findings of alveolar space-filling characteristics within them. The tumor is lobulated with a well-defined border and destroys or compresses the surrounding lung parenchyma. Destruction of alveolar septa demonstrated by the elastic framework was prominent throughout the tumor. In the combined type, tumors demonstrate a combined growth pattern of the alveolar space-filling and the expanding types. This type of SCC is considered as an invasive carcinoma progressing from the preinvasive alveolar space-filling type, or the expanding type without any morphologic features of alveolar space filling, leading to the assumption that this type might be either an advanced phase of the alveolar space-filling type or de novo SCC.

Watanabe et al. [3–5] confirmed the ratio of alveolar space-filling (ASF) area to tumor area as a prognostic factor for small peripheral SCCs, suggesting that focally invasive tumors with ASF ratio of 70% or more might be classified as "a microinvasive carcinoma" of the peripheral SCCs and tumors with ASF ratio 100% as a noninvasive carcinoma. In another study conducted by Nagashima et al. [6] age, lymph node metastasis, and serum CEA level are considered as independent prognostic factors for small-sized peripheral SCCs.

(Xiangpeng Zheng)

14.24 Case 24: Small-Cell Lung Cancer

14.24.1 Clinical History

A 66-year-old male received annual lung cancer CT screening. A nodule was reported in the right lung. The patient had a smoking history of over 30 years. He had none of specific symptoms, such as a cough, bloody sputum, chest pain, or shortness of breath. Blood tests on cell counts and tumor-associated biomarkers were within normal limits.

14.24.2 CT Findings

A solid nodule is located in the right lower lobe. This irregular nodule had no ground-glass component (Fig. 14.29).

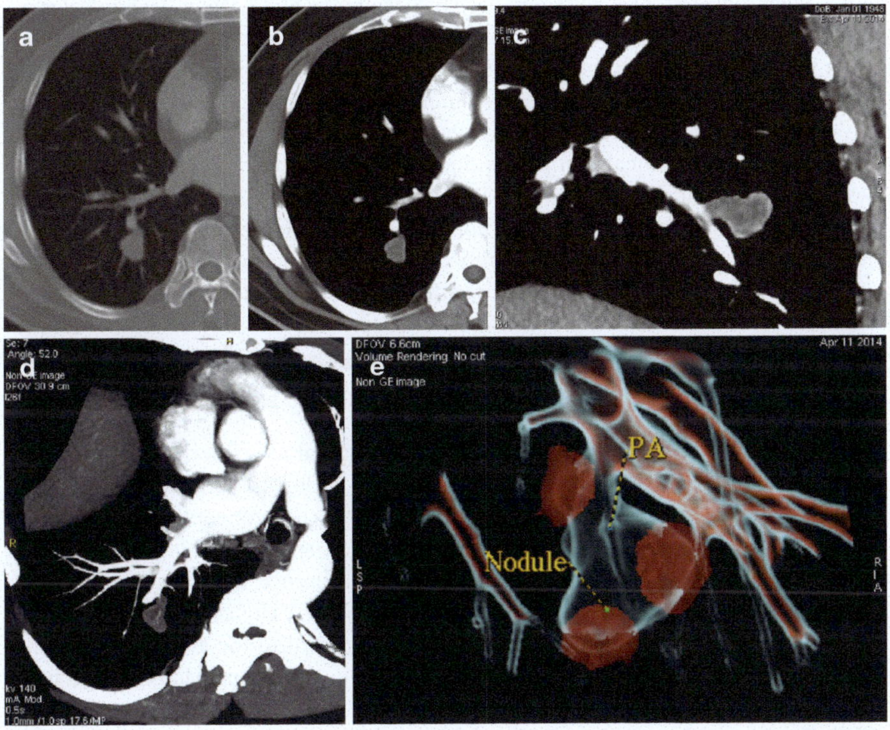

Fig. 14.29 (**a**) A homogeneous solid nodule measuring 20 mm × 17 mm is seen in the RLL with well-defined margins. Lobulation and spiculation are absent. (**b**) In the mediastinal display window, the nodule could be better visualized. (**c–e**) The sagittal (**c**), MIP (**d**), and volume rendering (**e**) images show the relationship between the nodule and pulmonary artery

14.24.3 Pathological Diagnosis

Percutaneous CT-guided needle biopsy revealed small-cell lung cancer. Due to negative findings in hilar and mediastinal lymph nodes, RUL lobectomy was performed via VATS. Surgical pathological examination confirmed small-cell lung cancer without positive lymph nodes found in hilar and mediastinal zones.

14.24.4 Discussions and Comments

Small-cell lung cancer (SCLC) can be subgrouped into central and peripheral types according to the location of the primary lesion. This case shows a peripheral SCLC. It has been long believed that the SCLC has a central predisposition in distribution and pathogenesis, with approximately two-thirds of SCLC being centrally located around the hilar area. However, recent data show an opposite trend. Several studies have reported a higher frequency of peripheral SCLC than the central type with a prevalence varying between 56 and 74%. One of the major reasons accounting for this prevalence shift is lung cancer screening program and advances in medical imaging, resulting in increasing incidental detection of nonsymptomatic early-stage SCLC. In contrast, SCLC was more frequently diagnosed in limited stage with evident clinical symptoms due to compression to central airways and involvement of hilar and/or mediastinal lymph nodes.

Radiologically, peripheral SCLCs appear as a noncalcified solid homogeneous nodule or mass without associated lymphadenopathy. The tumor margins are relatively smooth with a well-defined delineation from surrounding lung tissues. Mild lobulation and short spiculation might be seen but more frequently absent. Heterogeneous contrast enhancement in varying degrees was observed with evident imaging of intratumoral blood vessels. Occasionally, an irregular perivascular thickening adjacent to the tumor was observed.

Patients with peripheral SCLC have distinct clinical characteristics from those with central type, including a better prognosis with a longer overall survival, a high frequency of interstitial lung diseases (ILD), lower serum concentrations of tumor markers (such as cytokeratin 19 fragment and neuron-specific enolase), and higher rates of surgical treatment. However, there is no difference in response to chemotherapy and/or radiotherapy between both types of SCLC. Hence, the better prognosis associated with peripheral SCLC may be contributed to the surgical treatment, better performance status (PS), and smaller size at the detection. Many studies have reported a long-term survival after surgery and chemotherapy for early-stage SCLC. Patients with peripheral SCLC tend to have a better PS (80% of patients had a PS of 0–1) and limited disease stage, which are favorable for patients' response to, tolerance of and recovery from surgery, radiation as well as systemic therapies. Another possibility is that peripheral SCLC generally has a more slowly progressive phenotype. A relatively longer period might be permitted for detection of peripheral-type SCLC at an early stage. Additionally, the extent and severity of ILD should be imaging evaluated. Studies have reported that pre-existing ILD is associated with a shorter overall survival and a progression-free survival.

As discussed in peripheral squamous cell carcinoma, this case could be seen as a reminder that besides adenocarcinoma, squamous cell carcinoma or small-cell lung cancer should be on the list of differential entities for a peripheral solitary pulmonary nodule.

(Xiangpeng Zheng)

14.25 Case 25: Pulmonary Metastases

14.25.1 Clinical History

A 54-year-old male received surgery due to lung cancer 8 months ago. The pathological report on the resected lung cancer showed high-differentiated adenocarcinoma with bronchioloalveolar cell carcinoma and mucus secretion without lymphadenopathy (pT2N0M0). After that, this patient received four cycles of platinum-based adjuvant chemotherapy. Routine follow-up chest CT revealed multiple nodules in both lungs, which did not exist in the preoperative chest CT images. He had frequent fatigue, shortness of breath, and chest pain but no hoarseness, fever, and lymphadenopathy in the neck.

14.25.2 CT Findings

Multiple round or oval solid nodules are seen in the right middle lobe. All nodules have well-defined and smooth margins. Ground-glass appearance, lobulation, spiculation, and CTA-TA signs are absent (Fig. 14.30).

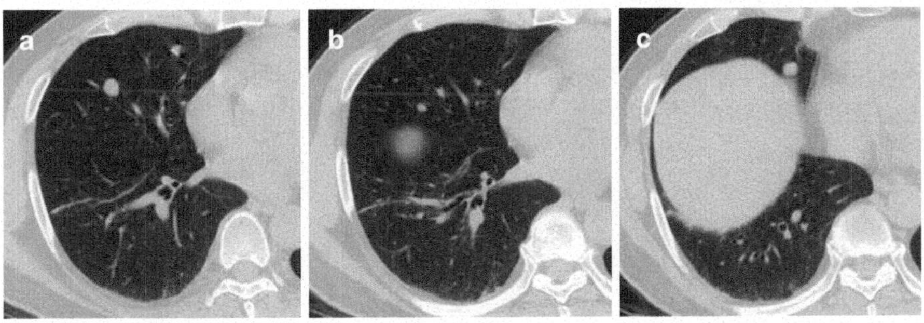

Fig. 14.30 (**a**–**c**) Three spherical solid nodules are seen in the right middle lobe. The largest one (**a**) is 7 mm in diameter. Spiculation, lobulation, satellite lesions, or pleural retraction is absent

14.25.3 Pathological Diagnosis

Due to no response to antibiotics and antifungal treatment, the largest nodule was resected via VTAS. Pathological examination confirmed adenocarcinoma, supporting the diagnosis of intrapulmonary metastases of lung cancer.

14.25.4 Discussions and Comments

This case presents an uncommon clinical situation that metastasis occurs quickly after surgical treatment in a patient with early-stage NSCLC who is supposed to have a favorable prognosis.

Pulmonary metastases could be from any malignant tumors, especially from the breast, gastrointestinal tract, kidney, and lung itself as seen in this case. The basic sign of hematogenous pulmonary metastasis is one or more discrete pulmonary nodules with the predominance of the outer portions of the lungs. The nodules are usually spherical and well-defined but can be almost any shape. Irregular-shaped metastases are more frequently seen with adenocarcinoma. Cavitation and calcification are occasionally seen in pulmonary metastases from particular types of malignancy.

Many pulmonary entities could have multiple nodular appearances, including granulomatous disease (eosinophilic granuloma and sarcoidosis), infectious disease (tuberculosis and fungal infection), alveolar microlithiasis, bronchiolitis obliterans, as well as metastases. Besides imaging findings, a full review of medical history and previous imaging materials is critically valuable for differential diagnosis.

(Xiaohua Zhu, Ming Li)

14.26 Case 26: Intrapulmonary Neuroendocrine Tumor

14.26.1 Clinical History

A female with uterine leiomyoma received preoperative chest CT. A nodule was incidentally detected. This patient had no pulmonary symptoms and denied a family history of any cancers.

14.26.2 CT Findings

A spherical nodule is seen in the left lower lobe. This nodule has a sharp, well-defined smooth margin (Fig. 14.31).

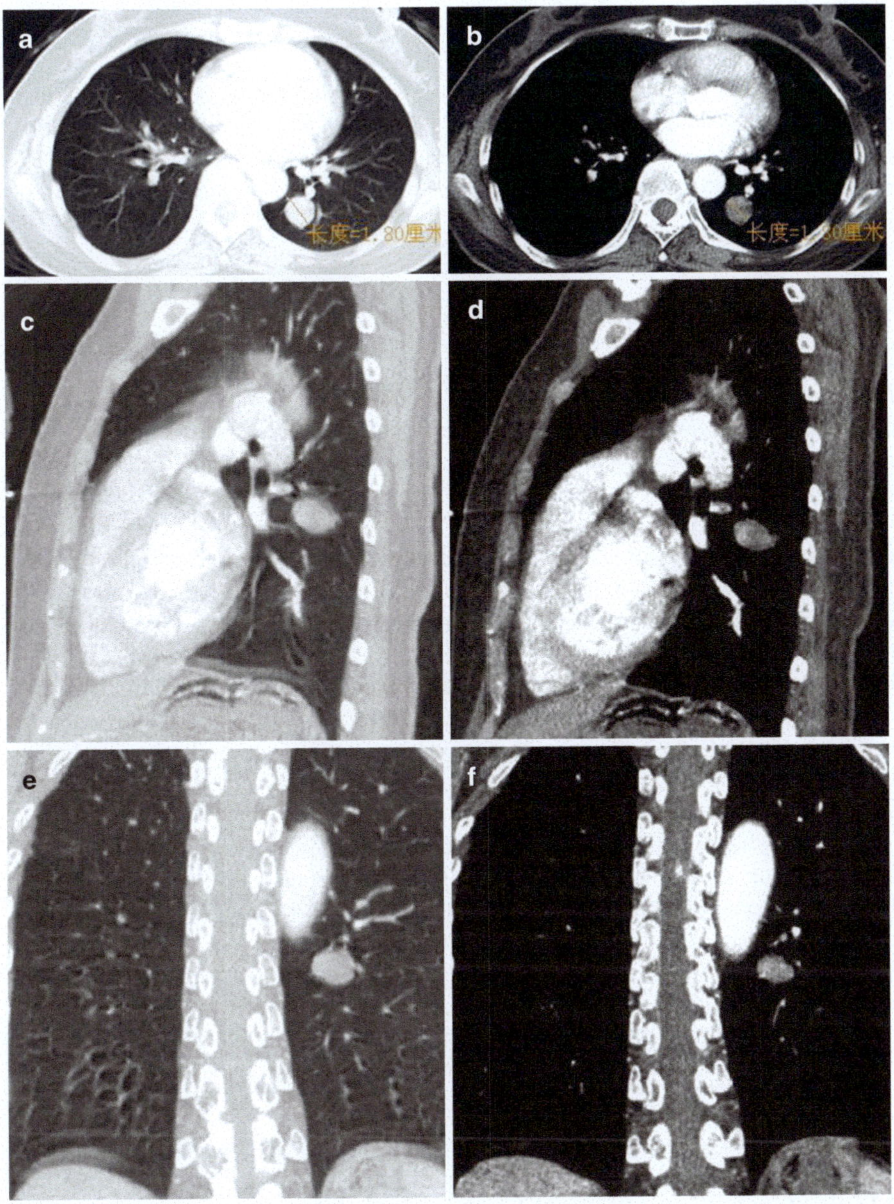

Fig. 14.31 Neuroendocrine carcinoma of the lung (paraganglioma) . A spherical nodule with a diameter of 18 mm is located in LLL. This nodule has s-shaped edge and no signs of lobulation, spiculation, and calcification. Contrast-enhanced CT scanning showed moderate homogeneous enhancement without central necrosis. No satellite lesions are seen. Pleural involvement is absent. (**a**, **c**, **e**) axial, sagittal, and coronal views in lung display window; (**b**, **d**, **f**) axial, sagittal, and coronal views in the mediastinal display window

14.26.3 Pathological Diagnosis

This nodule was surgically removed. Pathological examination confirmed a neuroendocrine tumor with immunohistochemical results of S100 (+), HMB45 (−), SMA (−), CK (−), VIM (−), KI-67 (−), P53 (less +), AFP (−), CD34 (−), SYN (−), CGA (+), PAS (−), NSE (+), NF (−), CD68 (−), and a-AT (−) and characteristic of paraganglioma.

14.26.4 Discussions and Comments

Neuroendocrine neoplasms are ubiquitous tumors found throughout the body, most commonly in the gastrointestinal tract followed by the thorax. Neuroendocrine cells normally occur in the bronchial and bronchiolar epithelium and may be solitary or may occur in clusters. Four major types of neuroendocrine neoplasms are recognized by the 2004 World Health Organization (WHO) Classification of Tumors and are grouped into three histologic grades. Typical carcinoid is characterized as a low-grade malignant neoplasm, atypical carcinoid as intermediate grade, and large-cell neuroendocrine carcinoma and SCLC as high-grade malignancies. Pulmonary neuroendocrine neoplasms constitute approximately 20–25% of all invasive primary lung cancers, and the vast majority are small-cell carcinomas. The remaining neuroendocrine neoplasms combined represent 5% of primary lung cancers. Paraganglioma is a rare neuroendocrine neoplasm that may develop at various body sites, including lungs. Most paragangliomas are either asymptomatic or present as a painless mass, frequently incidentally detected in chest CT scanning for other reasons.

Radiographically, the most characteristic imaging findings of primary neuroendocrine tumors of the lung (including paraganglioma in this case) are a peripherally located pulmonary nodule or mass without distal obstructive pneumonitis or atelectasis. Central low attenuation within the tumor at CT, a finding suggestive of necrosis or hemorrhage, is not seen. The tumor can be enhanced with intravenous contrast material with variable extents. In this case, the mass was moderately enhanced with attenuation increment of 42 HU. Calcification within the lesion is typically not present. Hilar, lower paratracheal, and subcarinal lymph node may be involved.

(Xiaohua Zhu, Ming Li)

14.27 Case 27: Carcinoid Cushing's Syndrome

14.27.1 Clinical History

A 42-year-old woman had a 10-year history of diabetes, and the blood sugar level had been maintained in a normal limit with insulin. She was admitted to the Endocrine Department with complaints of repeated attacks of lower extremity weakness for 2 months. Tumor-associated biomarker test showed increased levels of CA199 and CA125. Plasma adrenocorticotropic hormone test revealed remarkably increased ACTH and cortisol at 8 a.m. Plasma aldosterone, epinephrine, and norepinephrine were within normal limits. Whole-body PET/CT scan showed bilateral adrenal enlargement with a hypermetabolic activity and a solitary nodule in the left lower lobe without evident FDG uptake.

14.27.2 CT Findings

A solitary, spherical nodule with a diameter of about 10 mm and a clear margin is seen in the basal segment of the left lower lobe. The lesion is heterogeneous enhanced with contrast media. Abdominal CT scan showed abnormal morphology and size of bilateral adrenal glands but without evident nodular lesions. This patient received surgical removal of the LLL nodule. In the 16-month abdominal CT, bilateral adrenal glands (arrow) appear normal in both size and morphology (Fig. 14.32).

14.27.3 Pathological Diagnosis

The LLL nodule was surgically resected. Pathological examination confirmed a lung carcinoid with immunohistochemical results of CHG (+), Syn (+), NSE (+), and CK (+).

14.27.4 Discussions and Comments

Carcinoid tumors typically affect the gastrointestinal tract. The respiratory tract is the second most common location, accounting for 20–30% of carcinoids. Although pulmonary carcinoid tumors often exhibit an indolent behavior, these are malignant neoplasms with the potential to metastasize. Carcinoid tumors constitute approximately 1–2% of primary lung cancers. Most pulmonary carcinoid tumors are typical carcinoid, and approximately 10–16% are atypical carcinoid. Typical carcinoids most commonly arise in central airways. Atypical carcinoids usually occur in the lung periphery. Despite their classification as benign neoplasms, bronchial carcinoids can invade locally and may metastasize to hilar and mediastinal lymph nodes as well as to the brain, liver, and bone. The atypical carcinoids have histological and clinical features intermediate between typical bronchial carcinoid and small-cell carcinoma of the lung and have a poorer prognosis.

Typical carcinoid and atypical carcinoid have similar imaging features. Radiographic appearances vary with the location of tumors. There is no lobar predilection, and on rare occasions, carcinoids may arise in the trachea. Calcification is

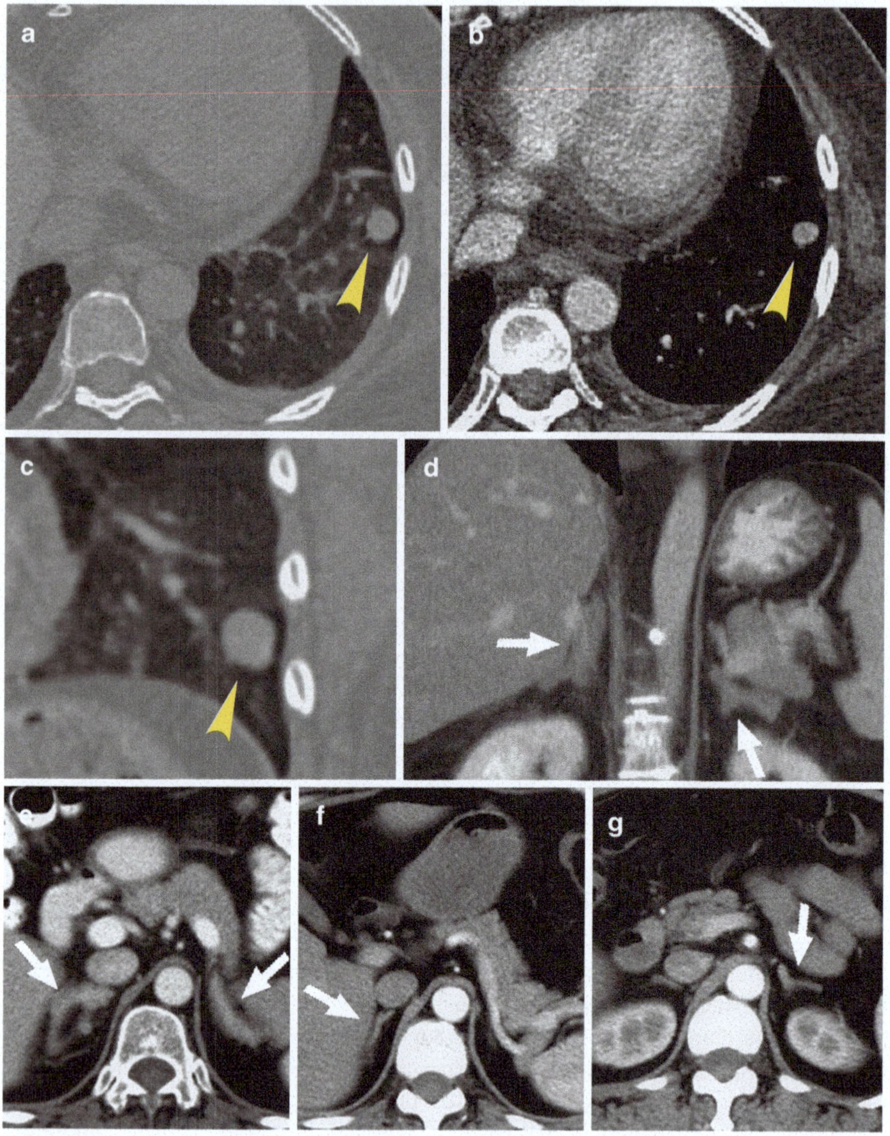

Fig. 14.32 (**a**–**c**) A solitary solid nodule with a diameter of 10 mm (arrowhead) is seen in the left lower lobe. This nodule is spherical, smooth with a sharp edge, and inhomogeneously enhanced with contrast media. Lobulation, spiculation, and calcification are absent. (**d**, **e**) Abdominal CT reveals enlarged, homogeneous contrast adrenal glands (arrow) without evident nodular lesions. (**f**, **g**) This patient received surgical removal of the LLL nodule. In the 16-month abdominal CT, bilateral adrenal glands (arrow) appear normal in both size and morphology

seen on CT in up to one-third of cases. Marked contrast enhancement may be seen on CT. Peripheral lesions (10–20% of carcinoids) present as solitary spherical or lobular nodules, 2–4 cm in diameter, with a well-defined smooth edge. Noncalcified peripheral bronchial carcinoid tumors closely resemble bronchial carcinomas, both radiologically and cytologically, and are therefore frequently removed surgically in the belief that they are carcinomas. Recent reports document increased detection of peripheral carcinoid tumors, which might be attributed to increasingly widespread use of chest CT.

Carcinoid may present with wheeze, pneumonia, or hemoptysis. Even when small, tumors may secrete adrenocorticotropic hormone (ACTH) in sufficient quantities to cause Cushing's syndrome. It is characterized by acute onset, a high concentration of ACTH, and hypokalemia. Carcinoid syndrome is caused by circulating serotonin and tachykinins produced by some carcinoids. Typically, platelets take up and store circulating serotonin. However, excess serotonin is inactivated by the liver, lung, or brain and transformed to 5-hydroxyindoleacetic acid (5-HIAA). Patients with liver metastases may develop carcinoid syndrome because vasoactive substances escape hepatic degradation and enter the systemic circulation. Carcinoid syndrome is characterized by skin flushing, bronchoconstriction, intractable diarrhea, and right-sided heart disease, and it is associated with hepatic metastases. Carcinoid syndrome is very rare if a tumor is confined to the lung (only about 0.7%). However, 2%–5% of patients with pulmonary carcinoid (typically those with metastatic disease to the liver) may develop carcinoid syndrome during the follow-up period. Therefore, the complete and thorough inquiry of medical history and physical examinations are helpful in the differentiation of carcinoid from other diseases.

(Fei Hu, Yanli Yang, Guozhen Zhang)

14.28 Case 28: Alveolar Hemorrhage

14.28.1 Clinical History

A 60-year-old female came to the clinic for a second opinion on an incidentally detected nodule in her annual chest CT lung cancer screening. She had no specific symptoms, such as a cough, bloody sputum, chest pain, or rales. Laboratory tests reported negative sputum culture and tuberculosis PPD tests (−).

14.28.2 CT Findings

A pure ground-glass opacity is seen in the left lower lobe with homogeneous attenuation. This nodule has a poorly defined margin. Other signs, such as lobulation, spiculation, and air bronchogram, are absent (Fig. 14.33).

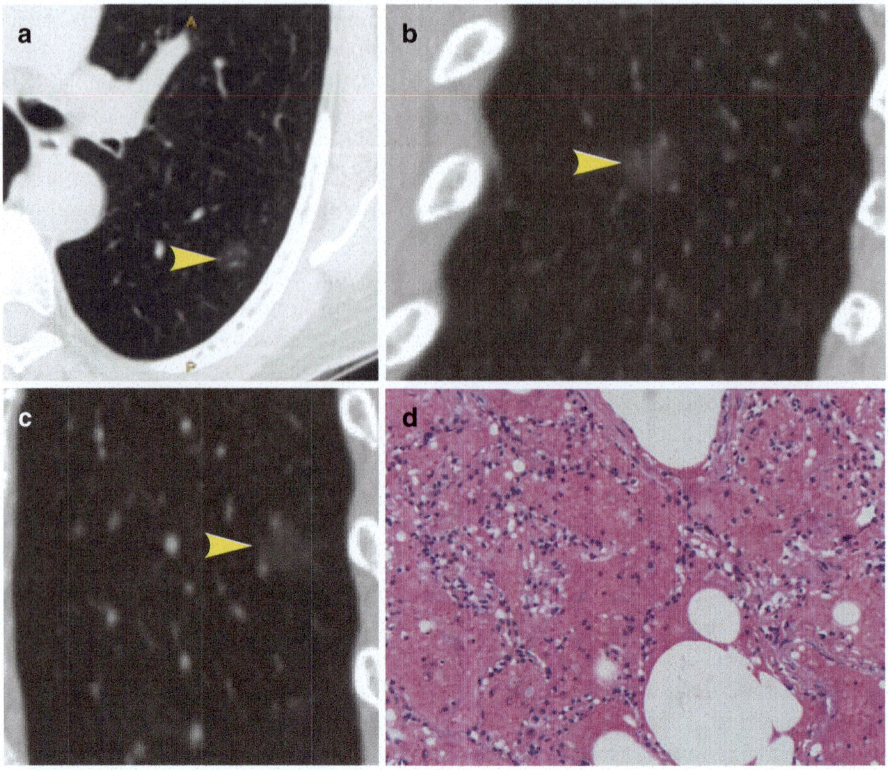

Fig. 14.33 Alveolar hemorrhage. A typical pure ground-glass opacity (arrowhead) is located in the subpleural area of the posterior segment, LLL. This lesion is about 8 mm in diameter with ill-defined margins. No solid component is seen. This lesion is overlapping with the lung parenchyma but not obscuring focal pulmonary structures. No abnormal vasculature is observed (negative CTA-TA sign). **a**–**c** are representative axial, coronal, and sagittal CT images. Per patient's request, this lesion was surgically removed, and microscopic examination revealed alveolar space filled with blood cells and mildly thickening alveolar septa (**d**)

14.28.3 Pathological Diagnosis

Despite that the nodule was considered benign with a high probability, the routine follow-up was recommended. The patient was extremely concerned and requested surgical resection. Wedge resection was performed to remove the lesion. In the pathological examination, no neoplastic cells were observed. The alveolar structures remained intact, but the alveolar cavities were filled with blood cells and plasma components. The septa were mildly thickening due to edema and capillary dilatation. Alveolar hemorrhage was confirmed with unknown reasons.

14.28.4 *Discussions and Comments*

The lesion in this case is a typical pure ground-glass opacity or nodule with characteristic features, including an ill-defined margin, an intact alveolar structure, and the absence of infiltration-associated signs (for instance, solid component, abnormal blood vessels, lobulation, spiculation).

Alveolar hemorrhage (AH) results from injury to the alveolar microcirculation. According to the hemorrhagic extent, AH could be divided into two subgroups, diffuse AH and focal AH. The former has the predominance, while the latter is an occasional event as seen in this patient. The underlying histopathology includes the presence of intra-alveolar red blood cells and fibrin and the eventual accumulation of hemosiderin-laden macrophages, which may take up to 48–72 h to accumulate. Dozens of entities can cause AH or with or without extrapulmonary involvement, including pulmonary capillaritis-related (such as granulomatous vasculitis, microscopic polyangiitis, etc.), bland pulmonary hemorrhage-related (such as Goodpasture syndrome, idiopathic pulmonary hemosiderosis, etc.), and diffuse alveolar damage-related (such as radiation therapy, systemic lupus erythematosus, etc.). In this case, the underlying hemorrhagic etiology is unknown.

Both diffuse and focal AHs have similar imaging features except the involved extent. On chest CT, AH presents with ground-glass or consolidation opacities in the acute phases, often with sparing of the subpleural and apical areas. In milder forms or the subacute phase, slight pseudonodular opacities without a preferential distribution may be associated with ground-glass findings; finally, a crazy-paving pattern characterized by ground-glass opacities over a thin reticular pattern may be observed. CT, in particular high-resolution CT (HRCT), is more sensitive than standard X-ray in identifying focal AH, especially with ground-glass patterns as in this case. However, the confirmation of AH requires bronchoscopy with bronchioloalveolar lavage with demonstrations of red blood cells and plasma components in airspaces and alveolar cavities in the absence of neoplastic cells.

Typically, AHs including focal AHs do not require surgical intervention. Etiological treatment should be initiated as soon as the underlying etiology is determined. For those focal AHs with unknown etiology, routine follow-up may be the proper management. With the absorption or organization of blood cells and plasma components, the detected ground-glass opacity or consolidation may resolve or turn into fibrotic scars.

(Xiaodan Ye, Huiqun Chen, Lei Zhu)

14.29 Case 29: Alveolar Hemorrhage

14.29.1 *Clinical History*

A 53-year-old male received a chest CT scan due to frequent right chest pain. A nodule was reported in the right lung with suspicion of malignancy. This patient had no other symptoms, such as bloody sputum, wheezing, and fever.

14.29.2 CT Findings

A spherical heterogeneous nodule is seen in the right middle lobe. The nodule is 10 mm in diameter with a well-circumscribed margin and an eccentric solid component. Lobulation, spiculation, bubble-like lucency, and CTA-TA signs are absent. The nodule is attached to the major fissure but pleural retraction is not seen (Fig. 14.34).

14.29.3 Pathological Diagnosis

Due to the probability of malignancy, this nodule was surgically removed. Pathological examination showed vascular congestion and accumulation of blood components within subpleural interstitium and intact alveolar cavities filled with red blood cells and fibrins without neoplastic cells, indicative of interstitial and alveolar hemorrhage.

14.29.4 Discussions and Comments

The imaging features of focal AH in this case are distinct from the previous case. In this case, the lesion has an appearance of mixed GGN, resembling those in AIS or MIA. Suspicion of malignancy is reasonable. The pure GGN seen in the previous

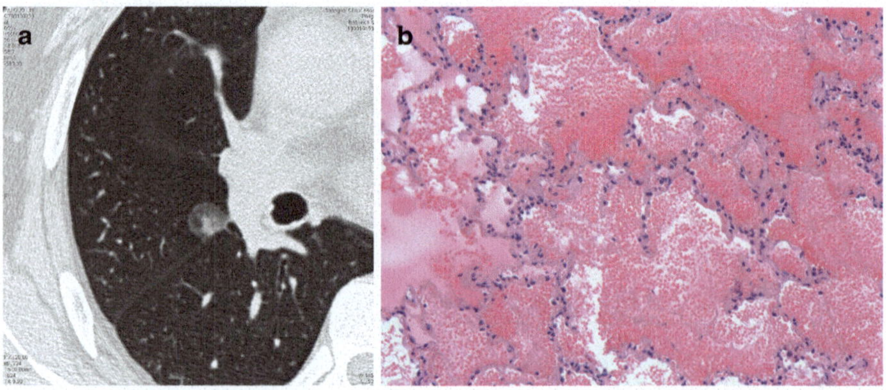

Fig. 14.34 High-resolution CT reveals a 10-mm mixed ground-glass nodule with a spherical shape and a well-defined margin in the right middle lobe. The nodule is attached to the major fissure but pleural retraction is not seen (**a**). This nodule was surgically removed, and pathological examination showed intact alveolar cavities filled with red blood cells and fibrin without neoplastic cells, indicative of alveolar hemorrhage (**b**)

case may be the manifestation of the acute stage of alveolar hemorrhage, whereas the mixed GGN in this case probably reflects a subacute or delayed stage, in which part of hemorrhagic components has liquefied or organized leading to heterogeneous density from a mixture of necrotic materials and fibrotic hyperplasia. Fibrotic hyperplasia and interstitial congestion account for the occurrence of solid components.

Reversed halo sign is observed with this lesion. A reversed halo sign is defined as the presence of central annular ground-glass opacity surrounded by a peripheral rim of consolidation. Although initially described in patients with cryptogenic organizing pneumonia, it has been described with several other noninfectious and infectious diseases, including fungal infections. Radiologic-pathologic correlation studies based on cryptogenic organizing pneumonia revealed that the central ground-glass opacity was due to alveolar septal inflammation with intact alveolar air spaces and the denser rim was due to inflammation/granulation tissue within the air space itself. In invasive fungal infections, this sign is attributed to infarct, with a greater hemorrhage at the periphery than in the center. However, this sign was composed of central necrotic islands surrounded by a peripheral ringlike hemorrhagic band in a case of tumor emboli, in which the pulmonary vasculature and lymphatics near the hemorrhagic band were occluded by tumor emboli. Therefore, this sign could be one of the imaging manifestations of various pulmonary entities. The interpretation of this sign should be based on information from the patient's history, clinical examination, and other radiologic findings.

As a summary to both cases, focal alveolar hemorrhage should be suspected when the following features are present: (1) a well-defined ground-glass opacity, with or without a solid component; (2) the absence of infiltration-related imaging finding, such as lobulation, spiculation, pleural retraction, and air bronchogram; (3) the absence of CTA-TA sign, even in a mixed/part-solid nodule; and (4) a reversed halo sign. Indeed, the definitive diagnosis requires pathological examination through percutaneous or transbronchial lung biopsy or even surgical resection in rare cases indistinguishable from malignant tumors as in this case.

(Huiqun Chen, Lingming Yu, Lei Zhu)

14.30 Case 30: Intrapulmonary Lymph Nodes

14.30.1 Clinical History

A 63-year-old male received chest CT for lung cancer screening, and multiple nodules were found in the right lung. After that, routine follow-up with CT was initiated. Fifteen months later, one of the nodules significantly enlarged with increasing amounts of solid components, while the other two nodules remained stable. The patient was referred to a thoracic surgeon for a further consultation. This patient had a cigarette smoking history of more than 30 years (15 pack-years). He denied tuberculosis and a family history of any cancers.

14.30.2 CT Findings

Three nodular lesions are seen in the right upper, middle, and lower lobes, respectively. The lesion in the anterior segment of the right upper lobe (Fig. 14.35a) is a mixed GGN, with a well-defined margin. Centrally located predominant solid component and peripheral ground-glass opacities create a halo sign. This whole lesion is approximately 12 mm in diameter. Multiple fine blood vessels are connecting with the lesion, characteristic of CTA-TA sign. The nodule in the middle lobe is solid, 5 mm in diameter, well-circumscribed, and smoothly spherical. No CTA-TA sign, lobulation, and spiculation are seen (Fig. 14.35b). In the lower lobe, a pure GGN with a diameter of 5 mm is seen. The margin is ill-defined, and CTA-TA sign is absent (Fig. 14.35c).

14.30.3 Pathological Diagnosis

Radiologically, the RUL semisolid GGN was highly suspected of malignancy, specifically an invasive adenocarcinoma, while the others were considered benign or preinvasive. The patient received lobectomy for the RUL nodule and wedge resection for the other two nodules. Pathological examination confirmed a highly differentiated adenocarcinoma for the RUL nodule, an intrapulmonary lymph node for the RML nodule, and an atypical adenomatous hyperplasia for the RLL nodule.

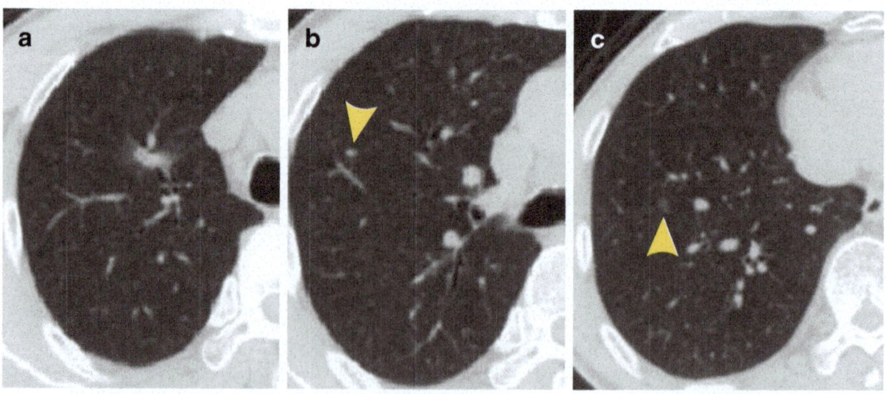

Fig. 14.35 Three nodules are found in the right lung, including a semisolid GGN in the upper lobe (**a**), a solid nodule in the middle lobe (**b**, arrowhead), and a pure GGN in the lower lobe (**c**, arrowhead)

14.30.4 Discussions and Comments

Nodules in the upper and lower lobes have typical imaging features characteristic of invasive adenocarcinoma and AAH, respectively, which are finally pathologically proven. By the definition of multiple primary lung cancer, this patient could be diagnosed with synchronous MPLC. In this case, the surgical removal of the intrapulmonary lymph node may be necessary for differential diagnosis. As a solid nodule in imaging, intrapulmonary lymph node (IPLN) is worthwhile to be further discussed in the context that the utilization of high-resolution CT has dramatically increased the detection opportunity.

Pulmonary lymph nodes can be divided into two categories depending on their location, peribronchial lymph nodes and lung parenchyma lymph nodes or IPLN. The former is mainly distributed proximal to the fourth bronchial bifurcation. In contrast, those lymph nodes distal to the fourth branching point within the lung parenchyma are designated as IPLNs. The finding of a benign IPLN on the pathologic study is not rare. However, the diagnosis of IPLN is often not considered when a pulmonary nodule is detected on CT scanning. Radiologic accounts of benign IPLNs can be dated back to 1964. Lymphoid tissue is often recognized in the peripheral lung parenchyma. Pulmonary lymphatics are known to increase with aging. It is reported that lymph nodes could be found in the lung periphery in approximately 7% of the population. Besides advances in medical imaging technology, two hypotheses have been proposed to account for the increased detection of IPLNs, (1) hyperplastic lymphoid nodules related to the inhalation of irritant dust and the attendant distortion of local lymphatic vessels and (2) supply by peripheral nodes of lymphoid tissue insufficiency in proximal lymph nodes.

Radiologically, most IPLNs are uncalcified, well-circumscribed, and less than 10 mm in diameter. Most of the IPLNs are subpleurally located (at a distance of less than 10 mm from the pleura) and are more frequently found in the right lower lobes than in other locations. A predilection for men older than 50 years is observed, which seems to be correlated with the patients' smoking habits. In approximately one-third of cases, multiple IPLNs are observed. Due to the overlap between their CT appearance and their location on both CT and pathologic studies, specific prospective identification is believed not possible. A more specific lymphatic distribution is a septal one, where 70% of the benign intrapulmonary lymph nodes are located on the pathologic study. Hence linear densities are considered the most useful characteristic of IPLNs. With a thin-section CT technique, such as collimation of 1–3 mm, nodes may be more accurately identified as having a vascular connection and a lymphatic distribution or being associated with a septum (Fig. 14.36). In contrast CT scanning, IPLNs may be enhanced in variable degrees in a homogeneous or inhomogeneous pattern.

The presence of a small, oval-shaped pulmonary nodule with sharply defined borders and subpleural locations or in a lymphatic distribution on CT scan is the characteristic CT finding for the IPLNs. Considering that the radiographic

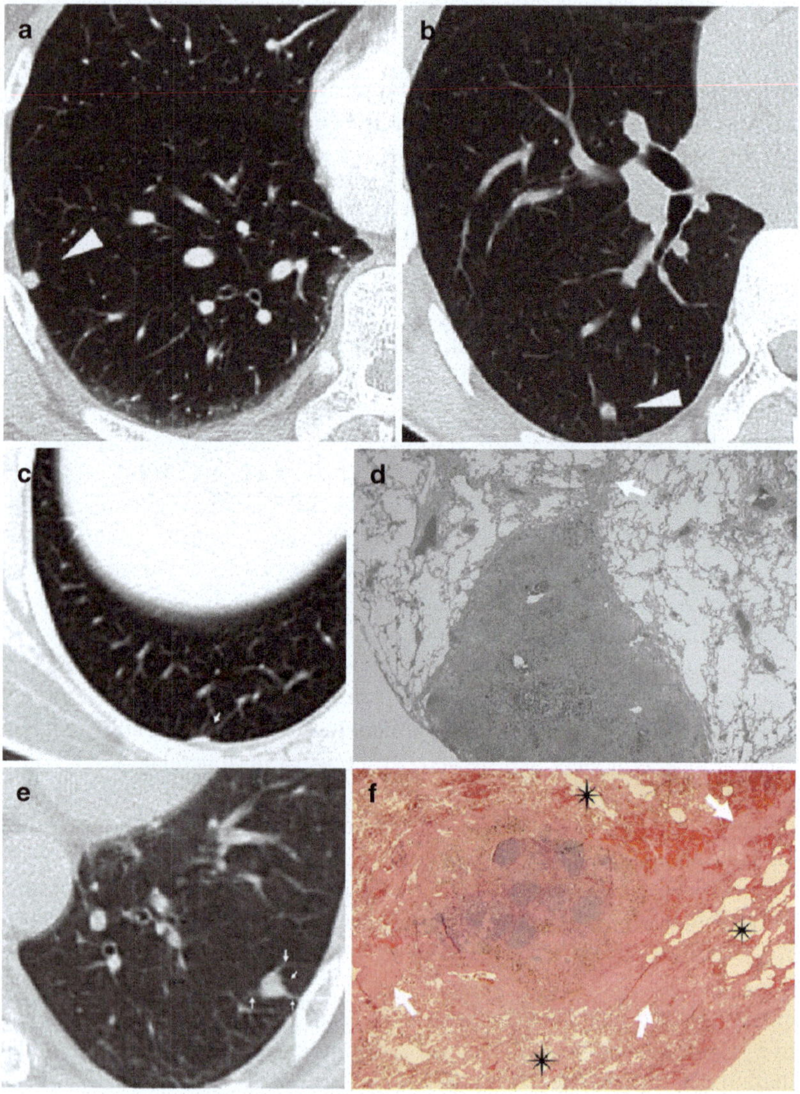

Fig. 14.36 Intrapulmonary lymph nodes. (**a**) Chest computed tomography revealed a small, round nodule in the lower lobe. (**b**) An angular and partly spiculated nodule is seen in the lower lobe. (**c**, **d**) A 53-year-old woman with an intrapulmonary lymph node found together with an aspergilloma. (**e**, **f**) A 52-year-old man with an intrapulmonary lymph node found incidentally during a health exam. The HRCT scan showed a well-circumscribed, solid, and angular-shaped nodule, which was separate from the pleura. Four linear opacities (white arrows) that extended from the nodule were identified (**e**). The histological examination revealed an intrapulmonary lymph node. Three interlobular septa (white arrows) were found to extend from the nodule. The intrapulmonary lymph node was located at the junction of three adjacent lung lobules (stars). The linear opacities on the CT scan were correlated with the interlobular septa under microscopy. (**a**, **b** from reference Takenaka et al. *Asian J Surg. 2013;36:69–73*. Reprinted with permission; **c**–**f** from reference Wang et al. *Clin Imaging. 2013;37:487–92*. Reprinted with permission)

appearance of IPLN mimics several other common conditions, particularly the early lung cancer or lymphohematogenous metastases, it should be well-differentiated from solid malignant tumors, including peripheral lung cancer and metastatic diseases. For this reason, the differential diagnosis may be challenging by CT finding alone. In such cases, a surgical biopsy or resection should be readily employed for diagnostic purposes.

(Xiangpeng Zheng)

14.31 Case 31: Hamartoma

14.31.1 Clinical History

A 66-year-old male received a chest CT to follow up a nodule in the right lung. This nodule had been annually monitored for consecutive 5 years. No specific symptoms were reported.

14.31.2 CT Findings

A solitary spherical nodule with a diameter of about 9 mm is seen in the right middle lobe (Fig. 14.37). This nodule is well-circumscribed with a smooth edge and mild lobulation. Internal attenuation is inhomogeneous with CT values

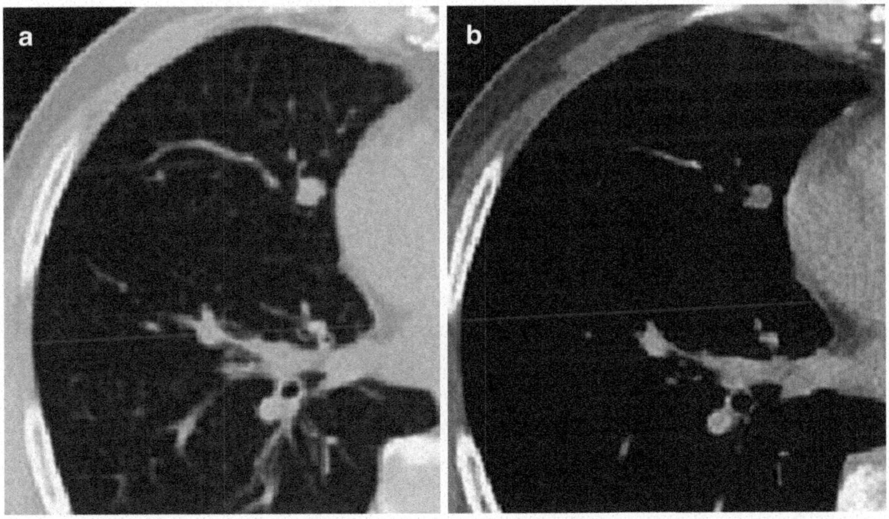

Fig. 14.37 A solid nodule with a smooth and well-circumscribed margin is located in the subpleural area nearby mediastinum (**a**). In the mediastinal view, heterogeneous attenuation is seen within the lesion (**b**)

ranging from −16 to 63 HU. In contrast-enhanced CT, the lesion is barely enhanced.

14.31.3 Pathological Diagnosis

This nodule was surgically removed via VATS. Pathological examination revealed a grayish nodule with the cartilage, adipose tissue, and respiratory epithelium, confirming the diagnosis of pulmonary hamartoma.

14.31.4 Discussions and Comments

Hamartomas are tumorlike malformations, containing an abnormal mixture of mature tissues normally found in the organ in which the tumor occurs. Hamartoma is one of the common benign pulmonary tumors, accounting for 7–10% of benign tumors. Pulmonary hamartomas consist predominantly of masses of cartilage with clefts lined by bronchial epithelium and may contain large collections of fat. Hamartoma could be encountered in all ages with a reported peak in the seventh decade. Most hamartomas are asymptomatic and incidentally detected as collateral findings in chest CT scans due to irrelevant reasons, such as lung cancer screening or CT cardiac imaging. The majority of pulmonary hamartoma is benign, and malignant transformation is extremely rare. In most cases, hamartomas present as a solitary nodule or mass, and multiple hamartoma is an uncommon incidence.

Radiologically, 90% of hamartomas present as a peripheral solitary pulmonary nodule, while only 10% arise within a major bronchus which could lead to major airway obstruction, causing evident respiratory symptoms such as wheezing, shortness of breath, and occasionally bloody sputum. Due to indolent biological behavior, hamartoma frequently manifests as a spherical or slightly lobulated, well-defined nodule, usually less than 4 cm in size, with the normal surrounding lung. Some hamartomas contain calcification, and the frequency of calcification increases significantly with the size of the lesion. The calcification may be a nonspecific spotty or linear formation. Of note, irregular popcorn-like calcification has been regarded as the characteristic of hamartoma with association with calcification in the cartilage (Fig. 14.38). If present, it is virtually diagnostic of a hamartoma. However, this feature less likely occurs in tumors less than 30 mm in diameter. Central fat density on CT is another important finding as seen in this patient. Similar to popcorn calcification, if central fat is detected, the diagnosis of hamartoma could be established with confidence. Typically, hamartoma is not or mildly enhanced (CT value increment <15 HU) following an intravenous bolus of contrast medium, also indicative of benignity.

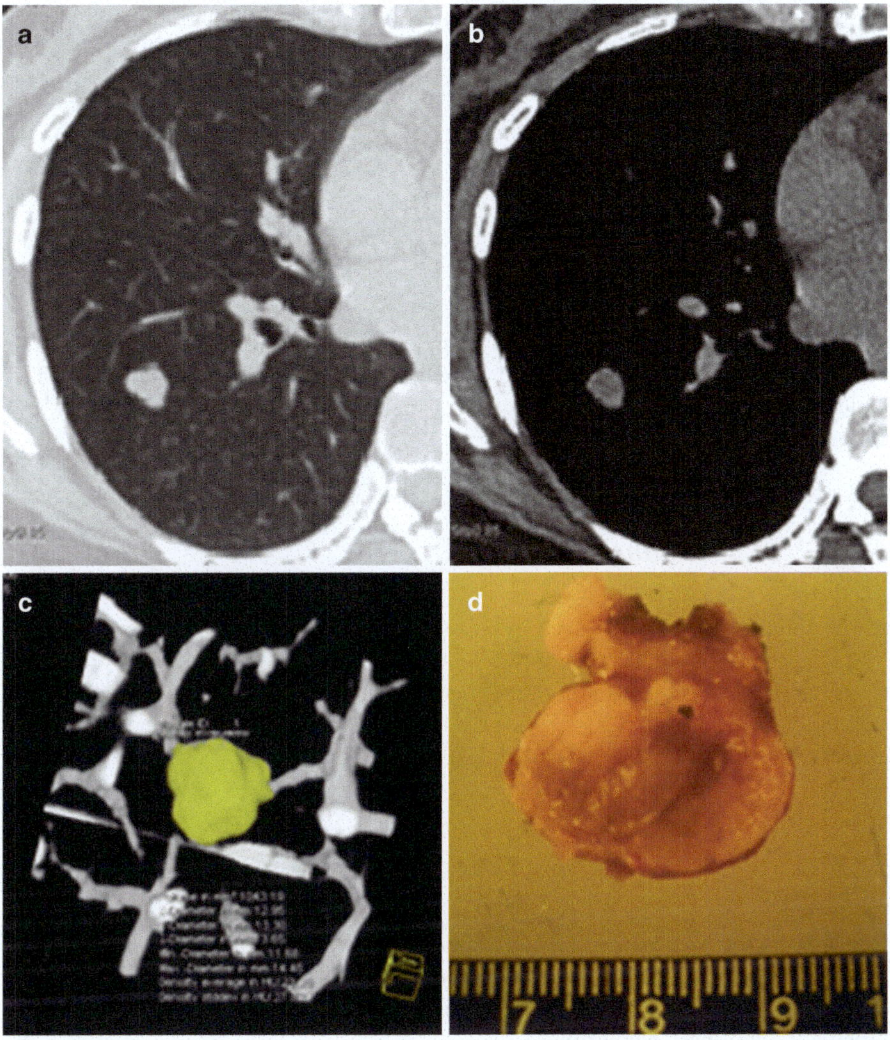

Fig. 14.38 Pulmonary hamartoma. (**a**–**c**) A spherical, well-defined, solid nodule is seen in the right lower lobe. The nodule is measured 12 mm in diameter with mild lobulation. Internal spotty calcification is evident. This nodule should be differentiated with peripheral adenocarcinoma and pulmonary metastasis. Besides morphological features, contrast CT scan could provide more information for differentiation. (**d**) Surgical pathological examination confirmed a hamartoma

In this case, the nodule has a typical imaging and clinical features of hamartoma, including slow growth, smooth and spherical shape, solid nodule with central fat density, and absence of infiltration-related signs. Hamartoma is always among the top list of differential diagnosis of a solitary pulmonary nodule. Those with characteristic findings are readily diagnosed or differentiated. However, for those with atypical presentations, the differentiation may be challenging. In such cases, biopsy or surgical resection should be recommended for a definitive diagnosis.

(Feng Zhu, Xiangpeng Zheng)

14.32 Case 32: Hamartoma

14.32.1 Clinical History

A 57-year-old female presented with complaints of occasional pains in chest and back. A chest CT was ordered, and a nodule was reported in the left lung. The patient denied other symptoms, history of malignancy, and family history of any cancers.

14.32.2 CT Findings

An irregular solid nodule is seen in the subpleural area in the left lower lobe. The longest dimension is 10 mm. Mild lobulation is evident with a smooth edge. Conventional CT scan reveals inhomogeneous internal density with a fine granular calcification. Spiculation and pleural retraction are absent. No enhancement is observed in contrast-enhanced imaging (Fig. 14.39).

14.32.3 Pathological Diagnosis

Considering the irregularity and subpleural location, this nodule was removed with wedge resection. Pathological examination revealed a capsulated grayish lesion containing mixtures of dark blue stained cartilage, fat, and calcified tissues, characteristic of pulmonary hamartoma.

14.32.4 Discussions and Comments

As the third commonest cause of a solitary pulmonary nodule, hamartomas originate in fibrous connective tissue beneath the mucous membrane of the bronchial wall. These lesions contain mixtures of myxomatous connective tissue, cartilage, epithelial-lined clefts, and variable amounts of fat, smooth muscle, marrow, and bone. As discussed in the previous case, hamartomas could be diagnosed with the presence of CT manifestation of fat-containing, or calcification (especially popcorn-like), and smooth contour and sharp outline. It is worth emphasizing that, despite

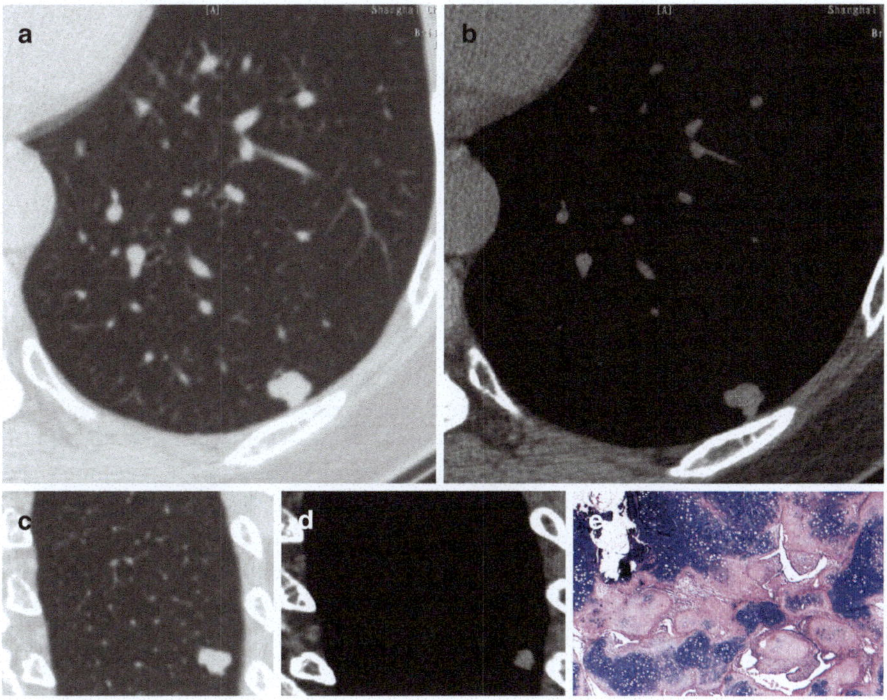

Fig. 14.39 Hamartoma. (**a**–**d**) A subpleural solid nodule is located in the left lower lobe with mild lobulation. High-density granular calcification is detected within the lesion. The nodule has an attachment to the pleura but pleural retraction is not seen. (**e**) Surgical pathological examination confirmed the diagnosis of hamartoma containing mixtures of dark blue stained cartilage, fat, and calcified tissues

their benign nature, hamartomas grow, albeit slowly. In one study of 11 cases that exhibited enlargement, recognizable changes were present only in those studied for at least 3 years.

Those hamartomas without typical imaging features should be differentiated with several pulmonary entities as the following:

1. *Peripheral lung cancers*: Lung cancers presenting as solitary solid pulmonary nodules may have a series of signs, including deep lobulation, short and coarse spiculation, bubble-like lucencies or air bronchogram, and pleural retraction. However, fat is rarely seen. Calcification may be observed but frequently in a fine and diffuse pattern. Popcorn-like calcification and cartilage tissue are absent.
2. *Tuberculoma*: A tuberculoma may occur in the setting of primary or postprimary tuberculosis and probably represents localized parenchymal disease that alternately activates and heals. The margins of the nodule are usually well-defined, and there may be satellite lesions nearby, though this is not a specific finding.

Calcification is common. Tuberculomas frequently remain stable for years but always carry the potential risk of activation and dissemination.

3. *Inflammatory pseudotumor*: Inflammatory pseudotumor is the most common primary lung mass seen in children with a peak prevalence in the second decade of life. On radiographs, pulmonary inflammatory pseudotumor typically appears as a solitary, peripheral, sharply circumscribed, lobulated mass with an anatomic bias for the lower lobes. On CT scans, inflammatory pseudotumors have a variable and nonspecific appearance, but most commonly they appear with heterogeneous attenuation and enhancement. Calcification within the lesion occurs more frequently in children than in adults. The calcification pattern ranges from an amorphous, mixed, or fine fleck-like pattern to heavy mineralization.

Histopathologically, hamartoma can be divided into three subgroups, chondromatous (more common), leiomyomatous, or a mixture. These tumors grow slowly and malignant transformation is extremely rare. Occasionally, multiple hamartomas are encountered without a particular clinical relevance. A small peripheral hamartoma with no atypical features can be safely left alone, with an infrequent follow-up to exclude growth. In atypical cases, or in cases of endobronchial hamartomas causing distal complications, surgical resection is curative. Rigid transbronchial resection is most frequently employed in the latter.

(Jianding Ye, Qunhui Chen, Lei Zhu)

14.33 Case 33: Pulmonary Leiomyoma

14.33.1 Clinical History

A 45-year-old female came to the clinic for a chest CT scan due to a suspected nodule found in annual lung cancer screening using radiograph. She was otherwise healthy without a family history of any cancers. Six years ago, she had received uterine myomectomy.

14.33.2 CT Findings

Multiple spherical, solid nodules are found in subpleural areas of bilateral lungs (Fig. 14.40). These nodules have various sizes ranging from 5 to 15 mm. Each nodule is well-circumscribed from surrounding lung tissues. Internal density is homogeneous. Mild lobulation is visualized. Calcification, spiculation, air bronchogram, and pleural retraction are absent. No hilar or mediastinal lymphadenopathy is found. Contrast CT scan reveals a significant enhancement with a CT value increment of 80 HU.

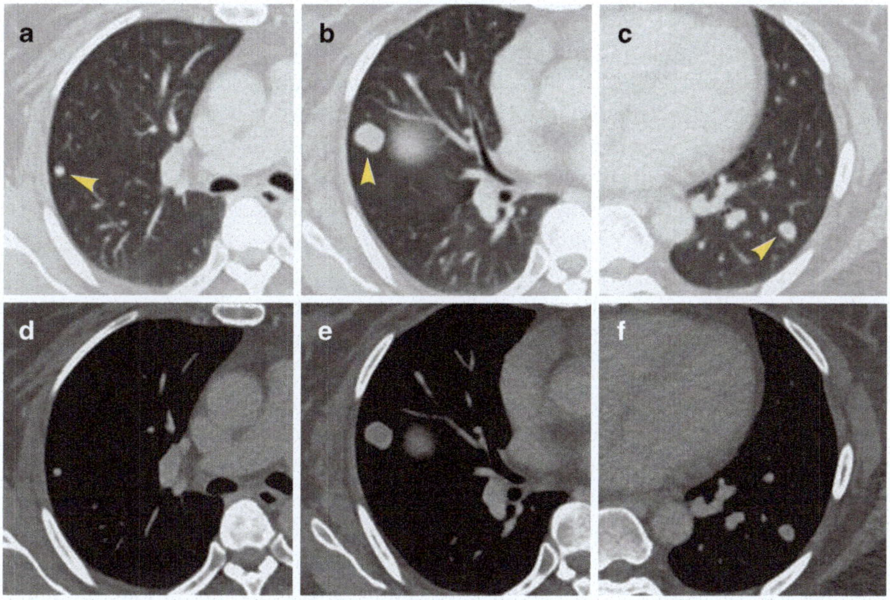

Fig. 14.40 Leiomyoma. Multiple solid nodules (arrowhead) are visualized in lungs with various sizes, sharp margins, mild lobulation, homogeneous attenuation, and subpleural distribution. **a**–c, Representative views in lung window; **d**, **e**, the corresponding views in the mediastinal window

14.33.3 Pathological Diagnosis

A comprehensive evaluation excluded extrapulmonary primary malignancies. For the definitive diagnosis, the largest nodule in the right middle lobe (Fig. 14.40b, d) was surgically resected. Pathological examination revealed clusters of spindle cells with positive SMA, estrogen receptors, and progesterone receptors. Taking this woman's history of uterine myomectomy, benign metastasizing leiomyoma was established.

14.33.4 Discussions and Comments

This case presents a rare pulmonary entity, benign metastasizing leiomyoma (BML). BML describes a rare neoplastic process in which leiomyomas of the uterus metastasize to distant sites, the most common of which are the lungs. Other sites include the skin, bone, mediastinum, lymph node, muscle, heart, and retroperitoneum. This disease affects women of reproductive age with a surgical history of uterine leiomyoma several years previously. BML has an indolent biological behavior and could remain the same size for an extended period. Patients with BML are usually asymptomatic, and the diagnosis is based on incidental imaging findings of multiple discrete pulmonary nodules.

The term metastasizing fibroleiomyoma of the uterus was introduced by Steiner in 1939 to describe multiple nodules of proliferating smooth muscle cells in the lung of women with a history of hysterectomy. Different mechanisms of spread of uterine leiomyomas have been proposed. It has been suggested that smooth muscle cells spread to the lungs after uterine extension into pelvic venous channels, that tumors gain venous access from surgical trauma during a hysterectomy, and that the lesions represent metastatic foci arising from low-grade leiomyosarcomas. The occurrence of pulmonary metastases could be 3–240 months after hysterectomy or even before the procedure.

Radiologically, pulmonary nodules can vary in size from millimeters to centimeters and be randomly distributed in the lung parenchyma. BML may be a solitary lesion but extremely rare, radiographically indistinguishable from the other benign connective tissue neoplasms. Pulmonary nodules do not calcify and cavitate. They can remain unchanged or even regress spontaneously. Atelectasis or post-obstructive pneumonia is uncommon. In contrast-enhanced CT, they usually show moderately to highly homogeneous contrast enhancement.

Characteristic pathological features include the proliferation of well-differentiated, benign-appearing spindle cells with an eosinophilic cytoplasm, moderate degree of vascularization, insignificant nuclear atypia, mitotic activity, anaplasia, necrosis, vascular invasion, or inflammatory host tissue response. The presence of estrogen receptors and progesterone receptors constitutes evidence that BML originates from uterine smooth muscle instead of extrauterine leiomyomas with uniformly negative estrogen receptor.

Besides BML, primary leiomyoma (PL) could occur in lungs. However, it is extremely rare with an incidence of 0.34%, and only 108 cases were included in a 2009 literature review. The majority (51%) of lung leiomyomas are localized in the parenchyma and 33% in the bronchial tree, and the remaining 16% affect the trachea. In comparison to BML, PL can occur at any age but mainly in young adults with an average age of 35 years for bronchial and parenchymal lesions and 40 years for tracheal lesions and with a slight female predominance. Immune deficiency and concomitant infection with Epstein-Barr virus have been implicated as a predisposing factor for the proliferation of benign and malignant smooth muscle tumors. The clinical presentation varies according to the seat and size of the lesion. The imaging features are similar to BML except for the solitary nature, which makes impossible to distinguish PL from solitary BML on imaging.

(Weilan Wu)

14.34 Case 34: Pulmonary Capillary Hemangioma

14.34.1 Clinical History

A 58-year-old male came to the clinic for a second opinion on a pulmonary nodule found on chest high-resolution CT.

14.34.2 CT Findings

In the subpleural area of the left lower lobe, an oval mixed GGN 7 mm in diameter is found with a solid component predominance. The nodule is well-defined with an irregular margin. No calcification, pleural tag, or vascular convergence is found (Fig. 14.41).

14.34.3 Pathological Feature

The nodule was surgically resected with segmentectomy via VATS. Pathological examination confirmed the diagnosis of pulmonary capillary hemangioma.

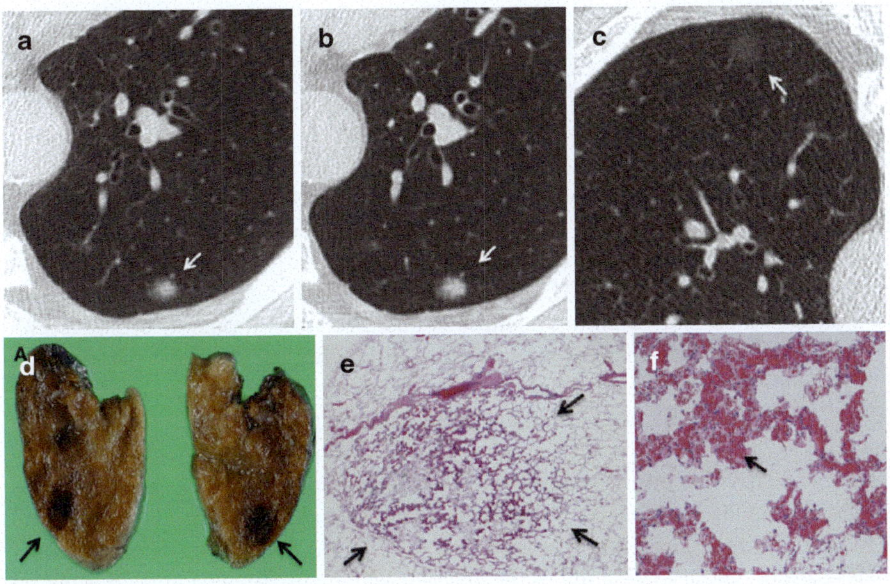

Fig. 14.41 Pulmonary capillary hemangioma. (**a**) HRCT image taken with the patient in the supine position 5 years before the operation. A solid component-predominant GGN 7 mm in size is seen in the left lower lobe (arrow). (**b**) On CT 2 months before the operation, the size is unchanged, but the density has increased slightly over the 5-year period (arrow). (**c**) In the prone CT, the mixed GGN becomes a pure GGN (arrow); due to the suspicion of early-stage lung cancer, left lower segmentectomy was performed to remove the lesion. (**d**) A cut surface of the lung reveals an ill-defined, dark-brown, nodular lesion (arrow). (**e**) An area of thickened alveolar septa (arrow) is vaguely demarcated from the surrounding lung tissue. (**f**) A thick alveolar wall with an accumulation of capillaries containing red blood cells (RBC) (arrows) is present (From Matsushita et al. *Jpn J Radiol. 2012;30:772–6*. Reprinted with permission)

14.34.4 Discussions and Comments

Solitary pulmonary capillary hemangioma (SPCH) is a rare benign pulmonary tumor; only about ten cases are reported so far. Literature reviews showed that SPCH may present as a ground-glass nodule with or without a solid component, making it a potential differential diagnosis in solitary pulmonary GGN, albeit rare incidence. In our practice, SPCH has not been encountered. This case cited the report from Matsushita et al. and discussion is literature-based [7].

SPCH is a localized pathological change resulting in pulmonary capillary hemangiomatosis (PCH). PCH has been described as multiple nodules in the lung parenchyma or bronchovascular walls that are composed of infiltrating thin-walled capillary blood vessels and cause pulmonary hypertension. In contrast to the poor prognosis associated with PCH, SPCH is reported as a good prognosis, but the long-term follow-up data had never been reported due to limited data available. Typically, patients with SPCH are asymptomatic and lesions are incidentally detected in a medical checkup. The underlying etiology of SPCH and PCH remains unknown, but evidence of increased expression of vascular endothelial growth factor and platelet-derived growth factor activity in patients with PCH has been reported.

Radiologically, SPCH could manifest as a pure GGN or mixed GGN with a solid component and a poorly defined margin. The amounts of solid portions are related to the extent of capillary proliferation and interlobular septal thickening. Of note, the pattern of ground-glass opacity is subject to the gravitational position, i.e., dependent on prone or supine scanning position, which might be related to the redistribution of blood flow in the dilated capillaries under the influence of gravity. As seen in this case, CT density dramatically changed from a mixed GGN to a pure GGN as the scanning position is changed from supine to prone, a phenomenon not reported in other pulmonary nodular entities. Hence, it may be used to differentiate SPCH from other malignancies with a GGN appearance, such as AAH, AIS, and MIA. According to Matsushita et al. no SPCH lesions were detected as pure GGO patterns in the supine position. Nodules with mixed patterns can be divided into two subtypes, GGO-dominant and solid-dominant, based on the dominant appearance. Whether the GGO or solid pattern is dominant on HRCT, the histological findings for these lesions are almost consistent with the GGO pattern: slight thickening of the alveolar walls with dilated capillaries but no secondary changes such as hyaline degeneration, inflammatory processes, or alveoli collapses.

In sum, SPCH is a very rare entity with nonspecific imaging features except the possible characteristic position-dependent density change. Due to its resemblance to preinvasive diseases or MIA, surgical removal should be considered if the lesion persistently exists or enlarges in follow-up CT.

(Xiangpeng Zheng)

14.35 Case 35: Pulmonary Sclerosing Hemangioma

14.35.1 Clinical History

A 42-year-old otherwise healthy female received low-dose CT lung cancer screening due to a family history of lung cancer. A nodule was reported in the right upper lobe.

14.35.2 CT Findings

Chest CT shows a semisolid GGN 6 mm in diameter in the right upper lobe with a central lower density. The lesion is poorly circumscribed from the surrounding lung tissues. A large blood vessel is close to the lesion, but no feeding vessels are connected with the lesion, hence negative CTA-TA sign. The lesion is not enhanced with the intravenous administration of contrast medium (Fig. 14.42).

This patient received antibiotics for 2 weeks. Two months later, a follow-up CT was performed and the lesion did not show any change. This nodule was suspected of a preinvasive disease, maybe in a transition from AAH to AIS. According to NCCN guideline on mixed GGN, a routine follow-up was recommended. However, this patient requested immediate surgical removal due to her family history of lung cancer.

14.35.3 Pathologic Features

This nodule was removed with segmentectomy via VATS. Pathological examination confirmed the pulmonary sclerosing hemangioma.

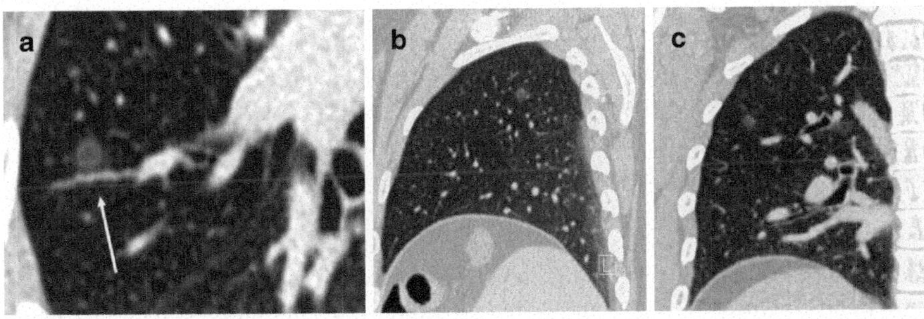

Fig. 14.42 Pulmonary sclerosing hemangioma. A circular semisolid 6-mm GGN is located in the right upper lobe with a poorly defined margin. CTA-TA sign is absent (**a**), axial view; (**b**), sagittal view; (**c**), coronal view

14.35.4 Discussion and Comments

Pulmonary sclerosing hemangioma (PSH) is an uncommon lung tumor and firstly described by Liebow and Hubbell in 1956 [8]. Although multiple theories have been proposed regarding its pathogenesis, modern immunohistochemical and molecular results suggest that sclerosing hemangioma originates from primitive respiratory epithelium. The name sclerosing hemangioma reflects two common histological features, sclerosis and vascular proliferation, that are now thought to represent secondary changes in an essentially epithelial neoplasm.

PSH typically occurs in middle-aged adults, with a female predominance. Most patients are asymptomatic with tumors identified incidentally on screening chest radiograph as seen in this case. Symptomatic patients most commonly present with hemoptysis, chronic cough, or chest pain. Generally, PSH has an indolent biological behavior with a volume doubling time up to 2–3 years. PSH may have a variable size, ranging from 1 to 11 cm in diameter, with a mean of approximately 3 cm. The smallest PSH reported is as small as 2.3 mm in diameter, incidentally detected on the close histopathological examination of lung sections but not detectable in CT.

On chest CT, PSH typically presents as a round to oval nodule or mass with a smooth, well-defined margin. The nodule has a peripheral location but without a predilection for a particular lobe (or with a predilection for the right lower lobe). It has a homogeneous attenuation. Calcification is seldom seen and, if present, may be punctate or eccentric. Cavitation does not occur. The lesion can be moderately to highly homogeneously enhanced with contrast medium. These imaging characteristics are not specific for sclerosing hemangioma but suggest a benign process. However, PSH with atypical imaging features, including smaller size and nonsolid appearance as seen in this case, may impose a challenge for differentiation with malignant disease. Several specific signs have been reported in PSH, including marginal pseudocapsule sign, air meniscus sign, halo sign, reversed halo sign, tail sign, and overlay vessel sign.

The marginal pseudocapsule sign, defined as adjacent compressed lung parenchyma next to a lesion mimicking a capsule, is reported to be seen in 50% of PSH cases. It is a correlated focal compressed parenchyma next to tumor, which is the most common sign. The air meniscus sign, also known as air trapping, air chamber, air cap, air crescent, and periparasitic emphysema, is characterized by a crescent-shaped radiolucent shadow at the periphery of a mass lesion of the lung. This sign could be seen in some lung conditions, including infection, tumors, as well as PSH. Two possible mechanisms are proposed for the production of an air meniscus in sclerosing hemangioma. First, proliferation and hyalinization of undifferentiated alveolar mesenchymal cells may wrap around the bronchus and lead to distension of the distal air spaces, with the extent and shape determined by the physical characteristics of the tumor tissues. Thus, the meniscus may be small and slit-like in a tumor with advanced hyalinization or have a prominent rim in a relatively cellular tumor. The other possibility is that the air meniscus is the result of disparate rates of contraction of the capsule and tumor, particularly when the tumor is highly cellular and hemorrhagic.

The halo sign is defined as a ringlike or semicircular region of GGO around a lesion, reported to be seen in 17.1% of PSH cases. It may be caused by the shrinkage at different speeds of the coating membrane and the tumors, causing bleeding via the gas channel and in turn potentially causing GGOs. Therefore, such a surrounding GGO could be an important indicator of PSP among benign tumors, indicating that the lepidic growth of the tumor results from not having a capsule. This sign may expand in extent in patients with hemoptysis while decrease and even disappear when the patient's symptoms relieved. A reversed halo sign is defined as the presence of central low attenuation surrounded by a peripheral rim of high attenuation, as seen in this case, probably due to hemorrhagic reaction in the periphery. Overlying vessel sign is defined as the considerable tortuous engorgement of the feeding vessel adjacent to the lesion, with a reported incidence of 26.3%. It is correlated with the mass effect of the nodule pushing or squeezing peripheral vessels. A tail sign is defined as the presence of a taillike projection from the tumor. It has been reported to be the most common sign related to PSH with an incidence of 67%.

Again, PSH is a benign tumor with a good prognosis. No tumor-related deaths have been reported, even in the rare instances of multifocal tumors or intrathoracic lymph node metastases. Surgical excision alone is curative.

(Xiangpeng Zheng)

14.36 Case 36: Pulmonary Sclerosing Hemangioma

14.36.1 Clinical History

A 47-year-old otherwise healthy craftswoman received a chest radiography for lung cancer screening. A nodular opacity was reported in the right lung. She received antibiotic treatment for 2 weeks. A follow-up chest CT with contrast medium was ordered to evaluate the pulmonary lesion. She denied histories of tuberculosis and malignancies, as well as family history of any cancers.

14.36.2 CT Findings

An irregular solid nodule with a size of 1.8 × 1.5 cm is located in the right middle lobe. The nodule is well-circumscribed from surrounding tissues with a smooth margin. The lesion has the heterogeneous internal attenuation with central punctate calcifications, but fat density is not detected. Contrast CT shows a heterogeneous

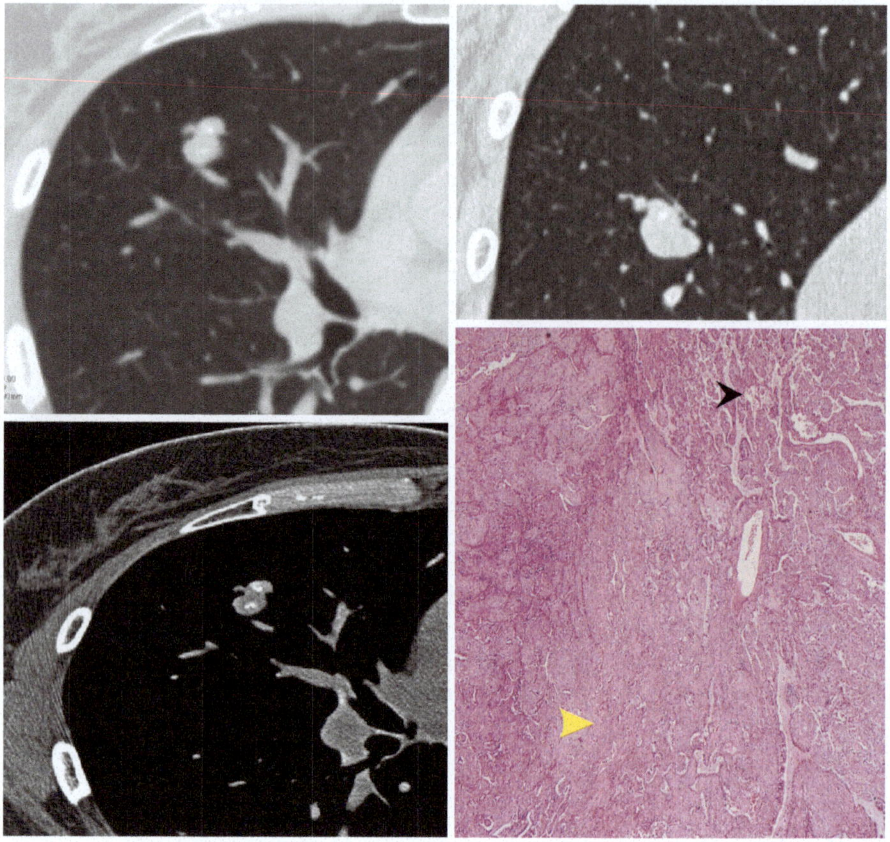

Fig. 14.43 Pulmonary sclerosing hemangioma. (**a**, **b**) A lobulated nodule (1.8 cm) is located in the right middle lobe with a central punctate calcification, a smooth edge, and a tail sign. (**c**) In the coronal view, eccentric calcification is seen. (**d**) The nodule was resected with segmentectomy. The pathologic image shows an area of the solid (yellow arrowhead) and papillary (dark arrowhead) components

enhancement at a moderate degree. Deep lobulation is evident (Fig. 14.43). Spiculation and air bronchogram are absent. This is a benign nodule with a high probability.

14.36.3 Pathological Diagnosis

Segmentectomy via VATS was performed to remove the nodule. Pathological examination revealed a solid grayish-reddish well-defined nodule with immunohistochemical staining of CK (+), VIM (+), EMA (+), TTF-1 (+), SPA (slightly +), ER (−), PR (+), and CK5/6 (slightly +), confirming the diagnosis of pulmonary sclerosing hemangioma.

14.36.4 Discussion and Comments

In contrast to the previous case, this case presents a typical PSH with a solid appearance, well-defined margin, lobulation, tail sign, and calcification in punctate and eccentric formation. The top differential diagnosis is hamartoma.

Despite the presence of calcification, the characteristic appearance is popcorn-like in hamartoma, whereas punctate and eccentric calcification is nonspecific, probably more likely seen in hemangioma than hamartoma. Internal fat density, a feature diagnostic of hamartoma, is not detected in this patient. The enhancement pattern supports PSH instead of hamartoma. With administration of contrast medium, PSH typically has a moderately homogeneous or inhomogeneous enhancement, whereas no or mild enhancement occurs in cases of hamartoma. Additionally, PSH has a series of relatively specific signs, such as air meniscus, halo sign, overlying vessel sign, and tail sign. In a single case, these signs may not be present simultaneously. In this case, a tail sign is evident, in favor of PSH instead of hamartoma.

(Jianding Ye, Qunhui Chen, Lei Zhu)

14.37 Case 37: Vaccination-Associated Pulmonary Nodules

14.37.1 Clinical History

A 70-year-old breast cancer female received breast-conserving surgery 4 years ago. The surgical pathology confirmed invasive ductal carcinoma in the right breast, WHO grades I–II with a mixture of WHO grade I–II intraductal carcinoma with a negative surgical margin and negative findings in sentinel lymph nodes. The patient received adjuvant radiation therapy and chemotherapy, followed by hormone therapy due to positive ER and PR. The patient was recommended for routine follow-up using chest CT. In previous multiple chest CT scans, none of the specific suspicious findings were detected. In the recent chest CT, multiple GGNs, pure and mixed, were found in bilateral lungs. However, this patient had no pulmonary symptoms. Her weight and appetite were unchanged. No chest pain, back pain, or headache was experienced. Blood tests including blood cell counts and tumor biomarkers were within normal limits. The patient reported that she received influenza vaccination 2 months before chest CT. After that, she experienced a fever for approximately 1 week, which relieved by using OTC nonsteroidal anti-inflammatory drug (NSAID).

14.37.2 CT Findings

Multiple (six as detected) irregular GGNs with a heterogeneous attenuation are seen in bilateral lungs with a seeming predilection for upper lobes. Pure GGNs and mixed GGNs with various amounts of solid components coexist. The largest lesion

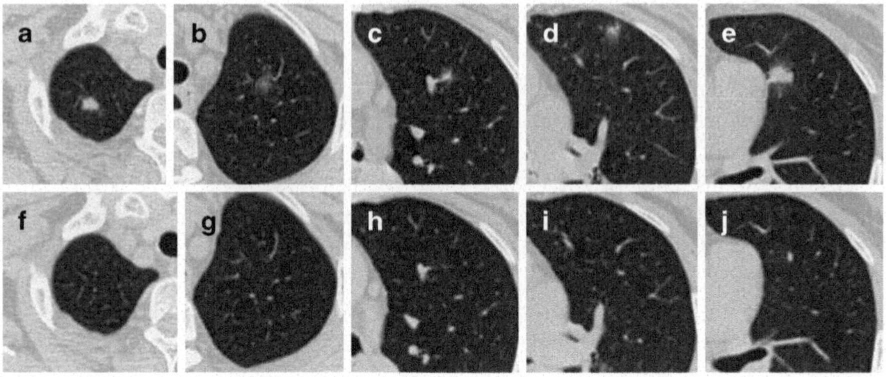

Fig. 14.44 Multiple heterogeneous ill-defined GGNs are seen in bilateral upper lobes (**a**–**e**). Three months later with antibiotic treatment, those previous GGNs completely disappear without any residual signs (**f**–**j**, the corresponding images to **a**–**e**)

has a size of 12 mm in diameter. Ill-defined margins and halo signs are seen in all nodules, not limited to pure GGNs but also mixed GGNs. Some lesions are located in the subpleural area with the attachment to the adjacent pleura, but pleural retraction is not observed. Air bronchogram and CTA-TA sign are absent (Fig. 14.44a–e). Three months later with antibiotic treatment using a Chinese herbal medicine with anti-inflammatory effects, chest CT shows that all GGNs completely disappear (Fig. 14.44f–j).

14.37.3 Pathological Features

The lesions completely resolved as a response to antibiotic treatment. Hence, the pathological evidence is not available. Based on the imaging features and the medical history, especially the history of using influenza vaccination prior to the occurrence of pulmonary lesions, the vaccination-associated pulmonary change was highly suspected.

14.37.4 Discussion and Comments

Considering the history of breast cancer, the presence of multiple pulmonary nodules should be reasonably suspected of metastasis. This patient had been diagnosed with multiple pulmonary metastases and recommended for systemic chemotherapy before coming us for a second opinion.

In adults, pulmonary metastases are usually from the breast, gastrointestinal tract, kidney, and other malignancies. The basic sign of hematogenous pulmonary metastasis is one or more discrete pulmonary nodules, usually in the outer portions or subpleural areas of the lungs. The nodules are usually solid, spherical, and well-defined. Occasionally, they may have irregular shapes, particularly with metastases from adenocarcinomas. Cavitation, calcification, and ground-glass appearance are uncommon. The rate of growth of metastases is highly variable; in some choriocarcinomas and osteosarcomas, it may be explosive and double the volume of the lesions in less than 30 days. In most cases, metastases can remain unchanged in size for a long time. Based on these features, metastases are less likely in this patient.

According to the NCCN guidelines on pulmonary GGNs, if unknown etiology, the proper management is an empirical treatment with antibiotics. And this patient had a good response to antibiotics and all GGNs resolved. Taking the medical history, especially influenza vaccination, and imaging findings together, a vaccination-associated pulmonary change is highly suspected. Vaccination-associated pulmonary change, or specifically vaccination-associated hypersensitivity pneumonitis (HP) or allergic alveolitis, has been reported sporadically.

Influenza is a serious disease that can spread around the world in seasonal epidemics. Those population at high risk of influenza-related complication or hospitalization are typically recommended for annual influenza vaccination, including the elderly over 65 years of age and adults with cardiac or pulmonary disorders (including chronic obstructive pulmonary disease, bronchopulmonary dysplasia, cystic fibrosis, and asthma), cancers, immune-compromising conditions (due to underlying disease and/or therapy), renal disease, and other severe comorbidities. The influenza vaccine is safe in general, and the most common side effects, such as injection site reaction, pain, fever, myalgia, and headache, are not important clinically. Besides influenza vaccine, anthrax vaccination has also been reported to cause HP.

Influenza vaccine-induced pulmonary change is rare, and very few studies (less than ten cases with the definitive diagnosis) have focused on the disease. Despite that the underlying mechanism remains not understood yet, two mechanisms have been proposed: cytotoxic lung injury and immune-mediated lung injury. Exposure to viral antigens could be the major triggering factor. Immunologically, HP is characterized by an early, neutrophil-type response and a later Th1-type granulomatous response to antigen. Pathological diagnosis is based on the lymphocytic alveolitis in the BAL fluid and TBLB, efficacy of corticosteroid, and a positive drug lymphocyte stimulation test.

The findings of chest CT scans are bilateral ground-glass opacities and/or patchy infiltration as seen in this case. In Rashid et al.'s report, radiographic manifestations include ground-glass opacities or diffusely increased radiodensities in the acute phase of the disease. As the disease progresses, diffuse micronodules, ground-glass attenuation, focal air trapping, and fibrotic changes are observed. In Pornsuriyasak et al.'s report, chest CT revealed multifocal areas of airspace consolidation involving the bilateral lower lobes and the right middle lobe, with a large area of ground-glass opacity with superimposed interlobular septal thickening in the right upper lobe [9].

Of note, the temporal relationship between influenza vaccination and clinical symptoms argued strongly for a causative role of this agent. Typically, pulmonary manifestations occur immediately or 2–6 weeks after vaccination. Influenza vaccination may cause a serious adverse effect in patients especially those with pre-existing chronic respiratory diseases. Clinicians should be aware of pulmonary changes induced by influenza vaccine to facilitate proper management. It may become serious without treatment, but the early detection and treatment lead to a complete remission. Careful clinical history and examination are needed in any vaccinated patients with an unexplained fever and/or dyspnea.

(Xiangpeng Zheng)

14.38 Case 38: Pulmonary Tuberculoma

14.38.1 Clinical History

A 36-year-old male received a chest CT and a nodule was reported in the right lower lobe. Tuberculosis- and fungus-related tests revealed negative PPD skin test, latex agglutination test, G test, and GM test. Antibiotic treatment was given for 2 weeks. The follow-up CT showed no change. After that, a routine follow-up was recommended. Five months later, a chest CT was performed to evaluate the nodule (Fig. 14.45).

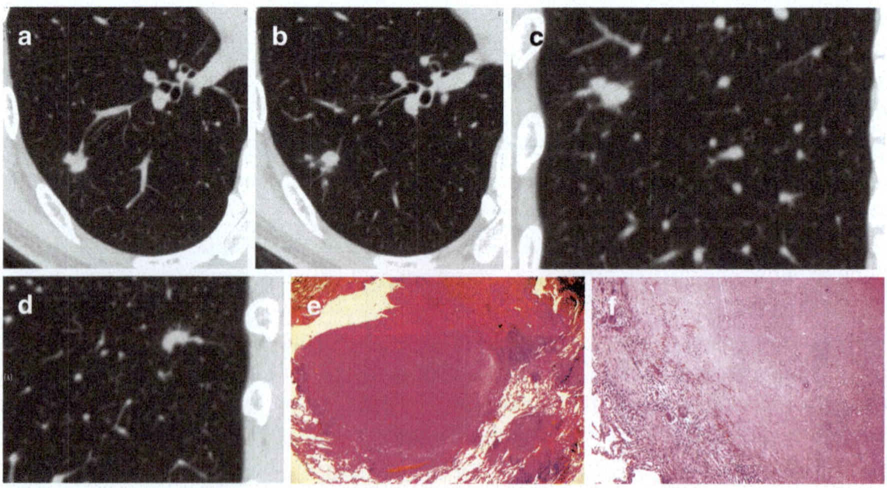

Fig. 14.45 Pulmonary tuberculoma. (**a**–**d**) A solid, well-defined nodule is located in the right lower lobe, with deep lobulation, coarse spiculation, internal punctate calcification, and satellite micronodules in adjacent lung tissues. (**e**–**f**) Surgical pathologic images reveal central caseous necrosis containing neutralized pathogens and debris from macrophages surrounded by a solid wall of bactericidal macrophages (epithelioid cells). In the periphery, fibrotic proliferation and infiltration of lymphocytes, histiocytes, and macrophages are visualized

14.38.2 CT Findings

A 10-mm solid nodule is seen in the right lower lobe. This nodule is well-circumscribed with deep lobulation and coarse spiculation. Punctate calcification is seen. In the surrounding lung tissues, satellite micronodules are observed. CTA-TA sign and air bronchogram are absent (Fig. 14.45).

14.38.3 Pathological Diagnosis

A wedge resection was performed to remove the nodule via VATS. Pathological examination confirmed pulmonary tuberculoma (Fig. 14.45e, f).

14.38.4 Discussion and Comments

Tuberculoma, as known as tuberculous granuloma, is defined as a focal mass that results from repeated episodes of arrest and progression of *Mycobacterium tuberculosis* infection. Pathologically, it is a well-circumscribed granuloma consisting of epithelioid cells with central caseous necrosis and an outer layer of lymphocytic cells.

A tuberculoma may occur in the setting of primary or postprimary tuberculosis and probably represents localized parenchymal disease that alternately activates and heals. Most tuberculomas are 3 cm in diameter, although lesions up to 5 cm have been reported. They commonly present as a single nodule but may be multiple. The margins of the nodule are usually well-defined, and there may be satellite lesions nearby, though this is not a specific finding. Calcification is common and cavitation or cystic change is occasionally seen. The characteristics of tuberculoma in contrast-enhanced CT are variable, including peripheral rim enhancement, peripheral rim or central curvilinear enhancement, partial enhancement, and homogeneous enhancement.

Most tuberculomas are inactive with abovementioned imaging features, while active tuberculoma may be encountered. Since active tuberculomas have the potential to shed bacilli into the sputum and the patient must be kept in isolation if in such a condition, it is thus very important to discriminate active and inactive tuberculomas. In contrast to inactive tuberculoma, active tuberculoma is characterized by the centrilobular lesions (nodules or branching linear opacities) and poorly marginated nodules. Other findings consist of patchy or confluent consolidation, ill-defined nodules, and cavities that commonly involve the apical and posterior segments of the upper lobes. Dynamic contrast-enhanced CTs have been suggested to be valuable in differentiation by measuring the peak height (PH) and relative flow (RF). Both PH and RF in active tuberculoma are significantly higher than those in inactive tuberculoma.

Tuberculomas frequently remain stable for years but always carry the potential risk of activation and dissemination. Patients with these tuberculomas are generally asymptomatic, and the lesions are excised because of the radiographic suspicion of malignancy.

(Lingming Yu, Lei Zhu)

14.39 Case 39: Pulmonary Cryptococcosis

14.39.1 Clinical History

A 44-year-old otherwise healthy male with an incidentally detected nodule in his right lobe came to the clinic for further consultation.

14.39.2 CT Findings

A solid nodule with central cavitation is seen in the right lower lobe. This nodule is well-defined and short spiculations are seen along the edge. Pleural attachment is seen but without pleural retraction. Calcification and lobulation are absent (Fig. 14.46).

14.39.3 Pathological Diagnosis

This nodule was surgically resected. Pathological examination confirmed a fungal granuloma from *Cryptococcus neoformans* infection.

14.39.4 Discussion and Comments

Cryptococcosis is caused by inhaling spores of *Cryptococcus neoformans*, a fungus of worldwide distribution which is found in soil and bird droppings. The fungus most commonly infects patients with human immunodeficiency virus (HIV) and other causes of reduced immunity, and it less frequently infects immunocompetent patients. Many patients have no symptoms, and the pulmonary lesions heal spontaneously, but in some, the disease may spread to many organs, meningoencephalitis being the most serious consequence. Approximately half the cases of symptomatic infection are associated with immunodeficiency.

Radiographic presentations of pulmonary cryptococcosis are varied. According to a report from Yamakawa et al., the most frequent radiologic abnormalities on chest CT scans are well-defined or ill-defined solitary or multiple solid nodules (87.5%), ground-glass nodules (37.5%), and consolidations (18.8%), with a distribution predilection for the lower lobe [10]. Other less common imaging patterns are

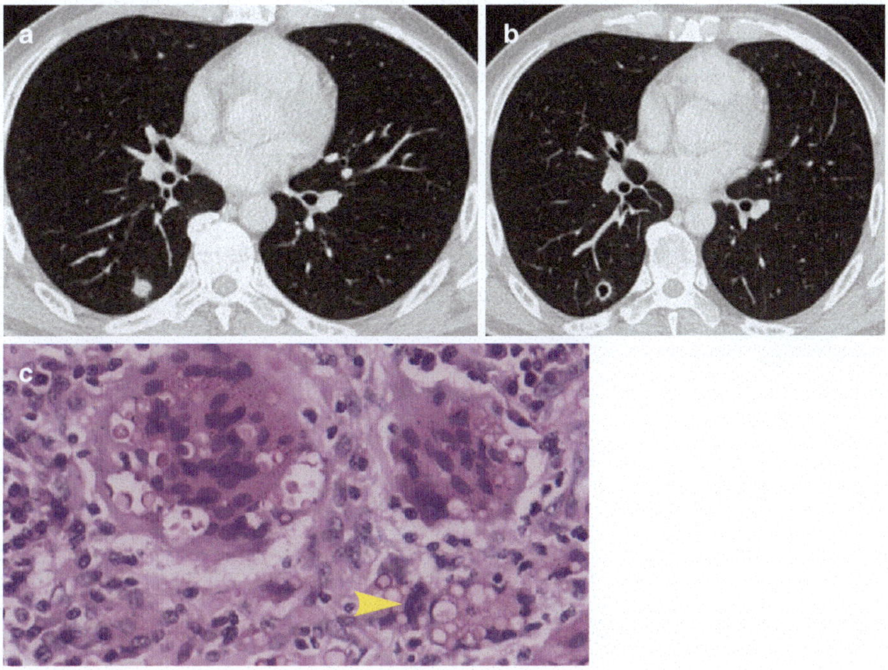

Fig. 14.46 Pulmonary cryptococcosis. (**a, b**) A 15-mm solid nodule with cavitation is seen in the right lower lobe, with well-defined margin and short spiculation. The wall of the cavity is smoothly thickening without mural nodules. (**c**) Pathologic image reveals slightly basophilic organisms under hematoxylin and eosin stain and purplish red organisms (arrowhead) in a periodic acid-Schiff reaction

homogeneous segmental or lobar opacifications with or without air bronchograms, cavitation, and lymphadenopathy and diffuse nodular, occasionally miliary, or reticulonodular opacities. Cavitation within nodules and parenchymal consolidation are more common in immunocompromised than in immunocompetent patients. Pleural effusion and calcification may be seen.

The diagnosis of pulmonary cryptococcosis is based on serological, etiological, and histological results. Lung tissue biopsies and pathological examinations are the primary methods used to confirm the diagnosis.

(Guozhen Zhang, Jie Zhang)

14.40 Case 40: Pulmonary Fungal Granuloma

14.40.1 Clinical History

A 59-year-old male came to the clinic for an incidentally detected pulmonary nodule in the right lower lobe 3 months ago, receiving antibiotic treatment for 2 weeks. A follow-up chest CT showed that the nodule remained the same as in previous CT without response to antibiotics, indicative of a possibility of malignancy. This patient was a heavy smoker with a smoking history of more than 20 years. He had frequent dry coughs. Currently, no fever or bloody sputum or coarseness was experienced.

14.40.2 CT Findings

An irregular nodule with a size of 1.6 cm × 1.8 cm is located in the right lower lobe. The lesion has a heterogeneous attenuation with a solid component predominant, and few ground-glass opacities are seen along part of the margin, causing an ill-defined edge. Deep lobulation and coarse spiculation are present but without calcification. The pleural retraction is observed with focal pleural thickening (Fig. 14.47).

14.40.3 Pathological Diagnosis

This nodule was surgically resected with wedge resection. Pathological examination showed the transparent fungal spores inside macrophages under H-E stain and positive periodic acid-Schiff stain, with positive immunohistochemical

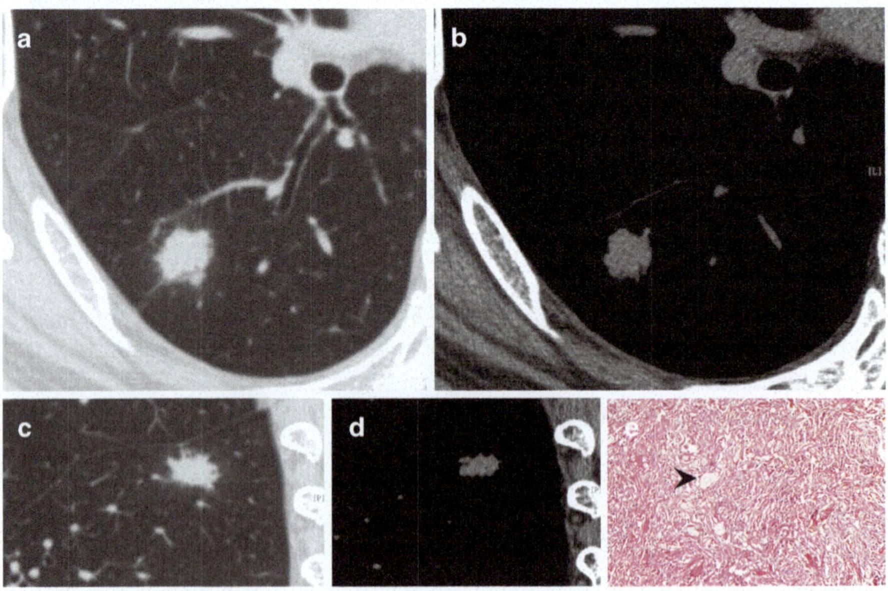

Fig. 14.47 A nodule (size, 1.6 cm × 1.8 cm) with deep lobulation, coarse spiculation, partly ill-defined margin (halo sign), and pleural retraction is seen in the right lower lobe (**a**–**d**). (**e**) Pathologic image reveals slightly basophilic organisms under hematoxylin and eosin stain (arrowhead)

results of CK (epithelia+), CD3 (lymphocytes+), Bcl-2 (lymphocytes+), KP1 (histiocytes+), and LCA (lymphocytes+), confirming the diagnosis of fungal granuloma.

14.40.4 Conclusion and Comments

In lungs, fungal infections, especially resultant granuloma, can mimic a pulmonary malignancy. The common causative pathogens include coccidioidomycosis, histoplasmosis, aspergillosis, North American blastomycosis, and cryptococcosis. Pulmonary fungal infection mimicking lung cancer is a rare entity with few series described in the literature.

Guimarães et al. [11] evaluated the clinical and radiological features of 27 patients with fungal infection mimicking thoracic malignancy determined by two inclusion criteria, (1) the presence of pulmonary lesion with CT characteristics suggestive of malignancy and (2) histological confirmation of pulmonary fungal infection. In their study, the CT findings (from more frequent to less frequent) were solid nodules, solid masses, or both. The margins could be lobulated, ill-defined, spiculated, or smooth. Additional findings included consolidation, cavitation, and pleural effusion. Lymphadenopathy was seen in nearly half of patients. However, these imaging features are nonspecific and insufficient for differentiation with lung adenocarcinoma.

Despite that solid nodule is the common finding, most fungal nodules are ill-defined due to a halo sign around lesions, as seen in this patient. The halo sign is defined as a discrete nodule surrounded by a circular margin of ground-glass attenuation. Usually representing hemorrhage surrounding a focal infarct, this sign has proved useful in the proper clinical situation as an early indication of invasive pulmonary aspergillosis (IPA). When identified in immunocompromised patients, detection of the halo sign has proved sufficiently characteristic of fungal infection to warrant empirical therapy. The halo sign is most useful in the early course of infection. In a study of 38 neutropenic patients presenting with radiographic evidence of nodular lung disease, a halo sign was noted in 16 of 22 patients evaluated within the first 7 days with documented IPA, with no false-positive studies. In distinction, a halo sign could be identified in only 3 of 13 patients with a proved invasive aspergillosis evaluated only after 10 days. Hence, the presence of the halo sign marks the ongoing development of suspected infection. Besides IPA, the halo sign may occur in fungal granulomas from other fungal pathogens.

Fungal infection should be considered in suspicious lesions negative for malignancy or when treatment for typical lung infections yields a poor response. Positive blood tests including latex agglutination test, G test, and GM test are suggestive of fungal infection. The definitive diagnosis of fungal infections is established by biopsy, either percutaneous CT-guided or transbronchial or surgical.

(Xiaodan Ye, Huiqun Chen, Lei Zhu)

14.41 Case 41: Inflammatory Pseudotumor

14.41.1 Clinical History

A 42-year-old female had a calcified lesion for over 10 years with the routine chest CT follow-up. The patient had none specific symptoms till 7 months ago. She came to the clinic with complaints of hemoptysis with the dark-reddish blood in small amounts. A chest CT was ordered for lung evaluation. An evident cavitary nodule was seen in the right lower lobe with an irregular calcification. Interstitial infiltrates were found. Hence, antibiotics were administered. Two weeks later, the hemoptysis disappeared with occasional bloody sputum. This patient was concerned and came in for a second opinion on the management of the pulmonary lesion. She denied a family history of any cancers. Blood tests on cell counts and tumor biomarkers were reported within normal limits.

14.41.2 CT Findings

An irregular heterogeneous lesion measuring 13 mm in the longest dimension is seen in the right lower lobe (Fig. 14.48). This lesion contains central angular calcification, cavitation, long and coarse spiculation, and deep lobulation. Pleura retraction is seen.

14.41.3 Pathological Diagnosis

Despite that the lesion was considered benign, the possibility of concurrent malignancy (i.e., scan carcinoma) could not be excluded in the context of the medical history of hemoptysis. The lesion was surgically resected. Pathological examination confirmed the diagnosis of pulmonary inflammatory pseudotumor based on the fibroblast proliferation and collagen accumulation within chronic inflammatory tissues in mixture with focal necrosis and calcification.

14.41.4 Conclusion and Comments

Pulmonary inflammatory pseudotumor (IP) was first described by Brunn in 1939 and named by Umiker et al. in 1954 because of its propensity to clinically and radiologically mimic a malignant process. Due to the complexity and variable histologic characteristics and behavior of this entity, many names besides IP have been used to describe this disorder, such as inflammatory myofibroblastic tumor, histiocytoma,

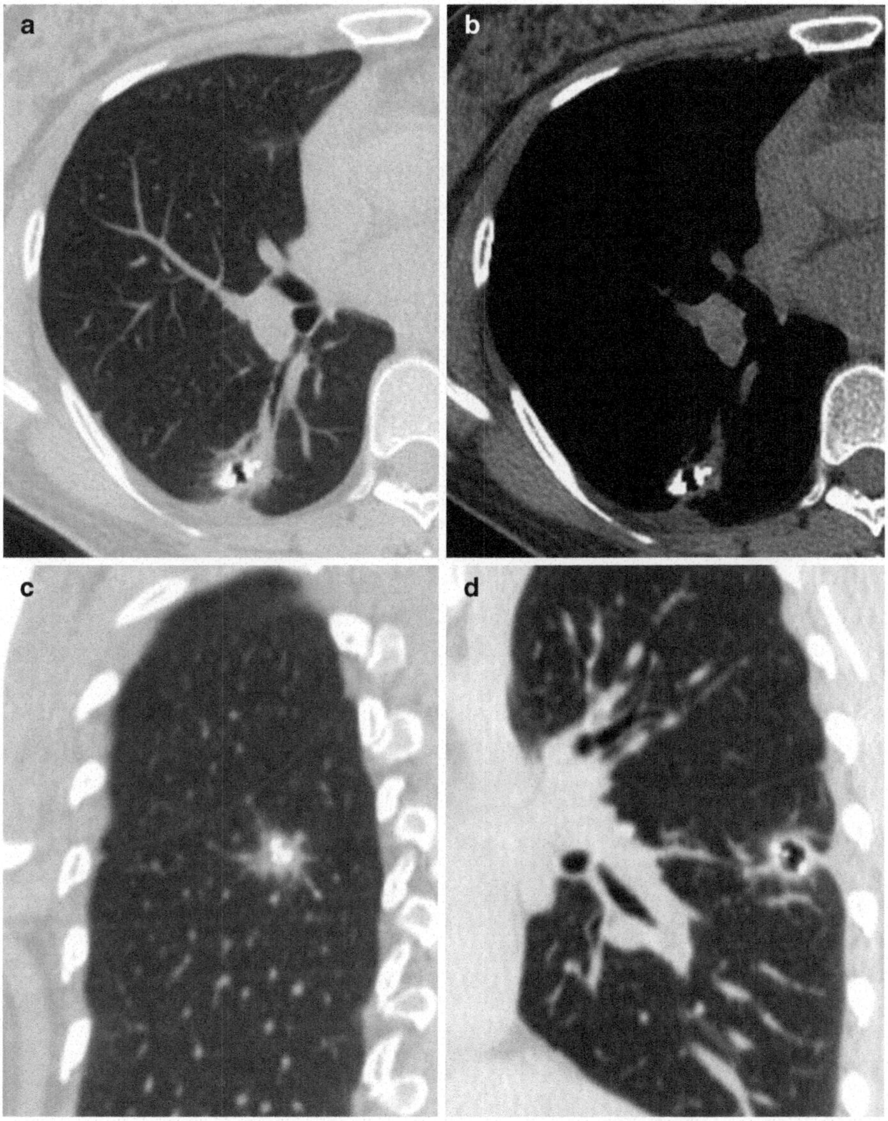

Fig. 14.48 An irregular lesion with cavitation and calcification is seen in the right lower lobe. Deep lobulation, coarse spiculation, and pleural retraction are evident, suggestive of a benign disease

fibrous xanthoma, or plasma cell-histiocytoma complex. As suggested by the name, IP is a quasi-neoplastic lesion consisting of inflammatory cells and myofibroblastic spindle cells. IP could occur in every anatomical site. Lungs are one of the most frequently involved organs, and IP is the most common primary lung mass seen in children, approximately 50% of benign intrapulmonary tumors.

The causes of inflammatory pseudotumor remain unknown. Several mechanisms have been proposed, including (1) the pulmonary presentation of a low-grade fibrosarcoma with inflammatory (lymphomatous) cells, or (2) resulting from inflammation following minor trauma or surgery or to be associated with other malignancy, or (3) a consequence secondary to pulmonary infections. Clinically, up to 70% of patients with pulmonary IPs are asymptomatic, but in symptomatic cases, cough, fever, dyspnea, and hemoptysis are the usual complaints.

Radiologically, pulmonary IP may have a variable and nonspecific appearance but typically appears as a solitary, peripheral, well-circumscribed, lobulated mass with an anatomic predilection for lower lobes. Multiple lesions are seen in 5% of cases. The lesion has a heterogeneous attenuation and can be variably enhanced with intravenous contrast medium. Internal calcification occurs more frequently in children than in adults with various patterns ranging from an amorphous, mixed, or fine fleck-like pattern to heavy mineralization. Cavitation and lymphadenopathy less likely occur. In most cases, the lesion could remain stable and be safely followed up for a long period of years. In occasional cases, a rapid growth pattern could be observed, which may reflect its origination from organizing pneumonia. Cells in "organizing pneumonia type" phase might be active and grow rapidly and then transform to inactive cells in the "fibrous histiocytoma type" or "lymphoplasmacytic type," which could remain unchanged for a longer time.

Inflammatory pseudotumor presenting as a solitary pulmonary nodule should be radiologically differentiated with primary or secondary neoplasm, hamartoma, chondroma, hemangioma, granuloma, and pulmonary sequestration. Delay in diagnosis and treatment may result in encroachment on hilar and mediastinal structures, causing severe consequences. Occasionally, pulmonary PT may show an aggressive behavior with local invasion and metastasis even without actual "malignant transformation." In cases with equivocal imaging features and potential possibility of malignancy, surgical resection may be the choice of definitive diagnosis and the treatment.

(Xiaohua Zhu, Ming Li)

14.42 Case 42: Inflammatory Granuloma

14.42.1 Clinical History

A 48-year-old female with a reported mass in the right lung presented for further assessment. She had been hospitalized for pneumonia 1 year ago and recovered with intravenous antibiotic administration. She denied cigarette smoking and family history of any cancers. A chest CT was ordered.

14.42.2 CT Findings

A nodular lesion measuring 1.5 cm × 1.4 cm is seen in the right upper lobe with an ill-defined margin. The lesion has a heterogeneous attenuation with evident air bronchogram. Deep lobulation and coarse spiculation are present. The lesion touched the minor fissure with a wide base with pleural retraction. Patchy satellite micro-lesions are seen in surrounding lung tissues. Pleural effusion is absent. Calcified lymph nodes are found in the right hilum and mediastinum (Fig. 14.49).

14.42.3 Pathological Diagnosis

Due to the suspicion of malignancy, surgical resection was performed via VATS. Pathological examination confirmed a chronic inflammatory granuloma without neoplastic findings (Fig. 14.49f).

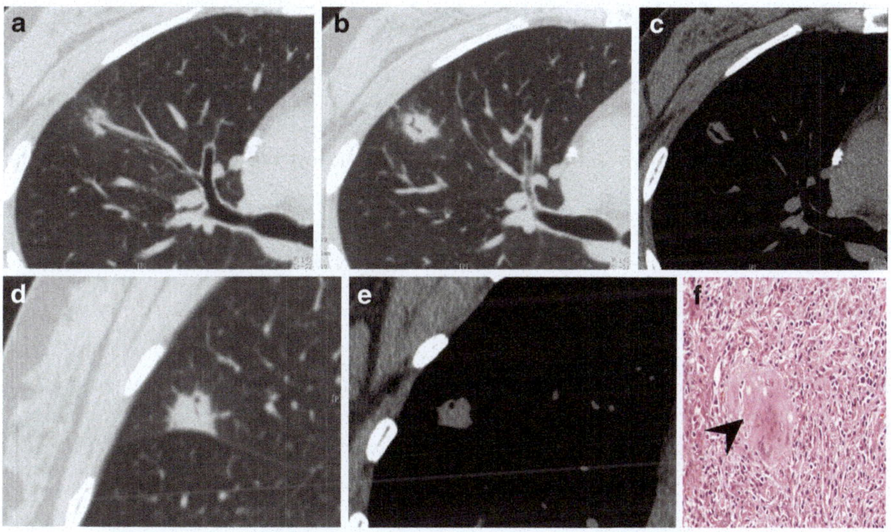

Fig. 14.49 An ill-defined solid nodular lesion is located in the right upper lobe with evident air bronchogram. Deep lobulation, spiculation, and satellite micro-lesions are present. The lesion contacts with the minor fissure with a wide base and pleural retraction is observed (**a**–**e**). The lesion was surgically removed. The pathologic image reveals chronic granulomatous reaction with mild necrosis. In the periphery, a large quantity of macrophages (arrowhead), fibroblasts, and epithelioid giant cells are seen (**f**)

14.42.4 Discussion and Comments

Various granulomatous diseases could occur in lungs, including sarcoidal granuloma, tubercular granuloma, rheumatic or rheumatoid granuloma, and infection- or tumor-associated granuloma. Pathologically, the focal concentration of cells of the macrophage system involved in forming the granuloma (macrophages, epithelioid cells, and multinucleated giant cells) varies among individual inflammations. As a result, a granuloma may be sharply demarcated or diffuse and ill-defined. The cellular composition of a granuloma depends on several factors, including the state of the body's immune system, the antigenic character of the irritant, the relative quantities of antigen and antibodies in the immune reaction, the efficiency of neutrophils, and the reactivity of the T cells.

The imaging features of inflection granuloma are similar to inflammatory pseudotumor, reflecting the chronic process and reactive pneumonitis. The distinction between inflammatory granuloma and inflammatory pseudotumor is the clinical history. In some occasions, inflammatory pseudotumor and inflammatory granuloma are considered as the same entity.

(Xiaodan Ye, Huiqun Chen, Lei Zhu)

14.43 Case 43: Inflammatory Nodules

14.43.1 Clinical History

A 55-year-old female presented for a second opinion on a nodule incidentally detected in her routine physical examination.

14.43.2 CT Findings

A solitary mixed nodule with a central solid component and evident peripheral ground-glass opacities is seen in the left lower lobe. The nodule is 16 mm in diameter, ill-defined, and abutting a blood vessel but without CTA-TA sign. Calcification and pleural retraction are absent (Fig. 14.50).

14.43.3 Pathological Diagnosis

The nodule in this patient disappeared with antibiotic treatment, in favor of an inflammatory disease.

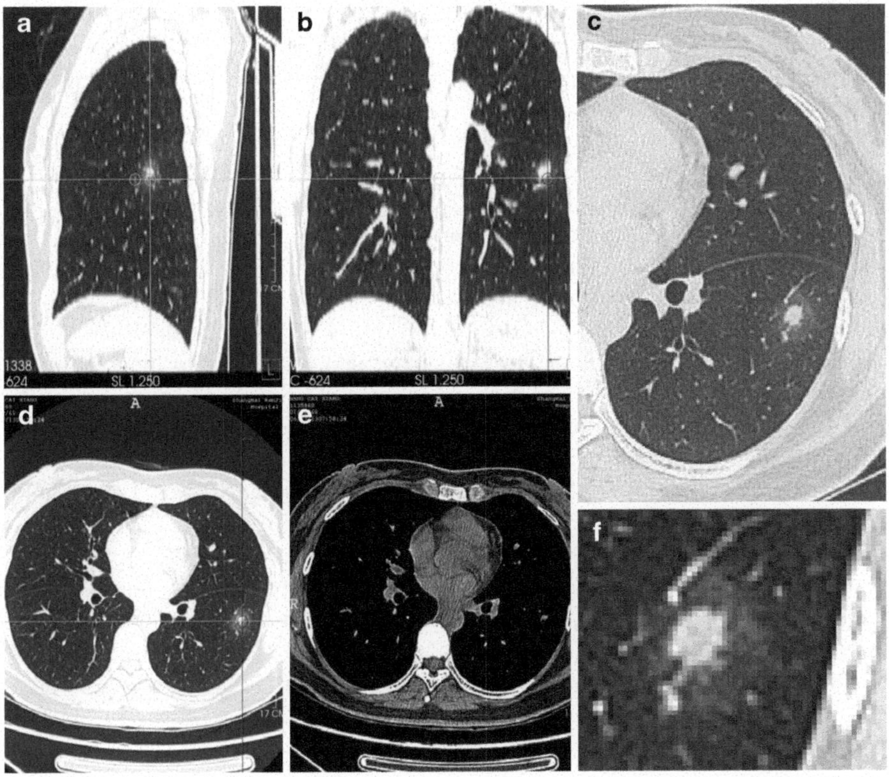

Fig. 14.50 A mixed 16-mm nodule is located in the left lower lobe. The halo sign is remarkable. The whole lesion is ill-defined, whereas the solid component is sharply circumscribed. The lesion resolved after administration of antibiotics

14.43.4 Conclusion and Comments

In this case, a mixed GGN was incidentally detected. Regarding the evaluation and management of mGGN, multiple international and domestic organizations have published a series of guidelines. If occult infection or inflammation is a possibility, a course of a broad-spectrum antibiotic with the anaerobic coverage is a choice of treatment, followed by follow-up CT in 1–3 months. Despite that the antibiotic treatment is deleted from the latest NCCN guideline on lung cancer screening, clinically anti-inflammatory medicine is still frequently used especially in those patients with severe anxiety. For them, a simple "wait-and-see" strategy is not adequate and justified. Pulmonary infections occasionally present as solitary or multiple nodular lesions with clinical and radiological features that are indistinguishable from thoracic malignancy, which remains a diagnostic challenge and may delay or misguide treatment significantly. The infectious processes of several agents, such as bacteria (*Fusobacterium*, *Pseudomonas*, *Streptococcus*), mycobacteria (*Mycobacterium tuberculosis*, *M. kansasii*), parasites (*Dirofilaria*), fungi, and, rarely, viruses (*Cytomegalovirus*), can mimic cancer.

Radiologically, inflammatory nodules, especially those in the acute phase, have characteristic CT halo sign, which could be used to distinguish inflammatory nodules from malignancies. The CT halo sign, also known as the halo sign, indicates the ground-glass attenuation surrounding a pulmonary nodule on thin-section CT. The presence of a halo of ground-glass attenuation is usually associated with hemorrhagic nodules, and the mechanism of the hemorrhage may include hemorrhagic infarction, vasculitis, fragility of neovascular tissue, bronchoarterial fistula, or necrosis. The halo may also be caused by neoplastic or inflammatory infiltration of the lung parenchyma. The most common condition with CT halo sign in immunocompetent patients is reported to be the former bronchioloalveolar carcinoma (or early-stage lung cancer) and in immunocompromised patients the aspergillosis. Table 14.1 lists pulmonary diseases with halo sign reported.

The frequency of the halo sign in patients with the invasive aspergillosis is relatively high in the early stages of the disease but alters with time and becomes progressively less frequent. Although usually regarded as an indication of hemorrhagic nodules, the halo sign may also be present when tumor develops in a lepidic pattern characterized by cells spreading along the alveolar walls without

Table 14.1 List of diseases showing the CT halo sign

Classification	Diseases
Infectious diseases	• Fungus: Aspergillosis, mucormycosis, candidiasis, coccidioidomycosis, cryptococcosis • Virus: Herpes simplex virus, varicella-zoster virus, cytomegalovirus, myxovirus • Septic embolism • Mycobacteria: Tuberculosis, *Mycobacterium avium* Complex • *Rickettsia*, *Coxiella burnetii*
Neoplastic diseases	• Primary tumors: Squamous cell carcinoma, Kaposi sarcoma, bronchioloalveolar carcinoma, adenocarcinoma • Metastatic tumors: Angiosarcoma, choriocarcinoma, osteosarcoma, melanoma, hydatidiform mole, metastatic tumors from gastrointestinal malignancies • Lymphoproliferative disorders
Nonneoplastic, noninfectious, inflammatory diseases	• Wegener's granulomatosis • Eosinophilic lung disease: Parasitic infestation (schistosomiasis), simple pulmonary eosinophilia, hypereosinophilic syndrome • Pulmonary endometriosis • Organizing pneumonia • Hypersensitivity pneumonitis • Iatrogenic injury: Transbronchial lung biopsy, catheter-induced pulmonary pseudoaneurysm

affecting the intactness of the underlying architecture. The distinct underlying mechanisms accounted for the subtle difference between inflammatory and malignant halo signs. In the former, the halo sign has an ill-defined margin with surrounding lung tissues but well-circumscribed from the internal solid components and a large ratio of GGO/solid component (greater than 1). In contrast, in most malignant conditions, the halo sign has a well-defined margin with surrounding lung tissues and undetectable border between GGO and solid component, as well as a small ratio of GGO/solid component (less than 1). In summary, the CT halo sign may be seen with a wide spectrum of pulmonary diseases; it is most commonly associated with hemorrhagic nodules and is more rarely associated with tumor cell infiltrate. Nonetheless, in the appropriate clinical setting, the halo sign is considered early evidence of pulmonary aspergillosis even before serologic tests become positive, and it warrants the administration of systemic antifungal therapy.

Besides the CT halo sign, other imaging features should be consulted in the differential diagnosis, as well as the clinical information. For those with a possibility of inflammation, a short course of diagnostic treatment with empirical antibiotics would be proper and convenient, as shown in this case. Radiologists should be aware that a mixed GGN with a halo sign does not necessarily reflect malignancies, but more likely results from neoplastic disorders. Only in those persistent mixed GGNs with a well-defined halo sign, the possibility of malignancy is high.

(Ming Li Xiangpeng Zheng)

14.44 Case 44: Chronic Alveolitis

14.44.1 Clinical History

A 52-year-old female received a chest CT scan due to complaints of a cough and sputum for 2 weeks. A nodule was found in the right lung. Empirical antibiotic treatment was given, but the lesion remained unchanged in the follow-up CT (Fig. 14.51).

14.44.2 CT Findings

In axial images, a spherical mixed GGN is seen in the right lower lobe with a poorly defined margin and linear solid components. Bubble-like lucency and central low attenuation are seen. A small blood vessel is linked to the lesion. However, in the coronal and sagittal views, the lesion appears tubular instead of nodular, dramatically distinct from the morphology in axial images (Fig. 14.51). A benign disease, specifically chronic fibrotic proliferation, is suspected.

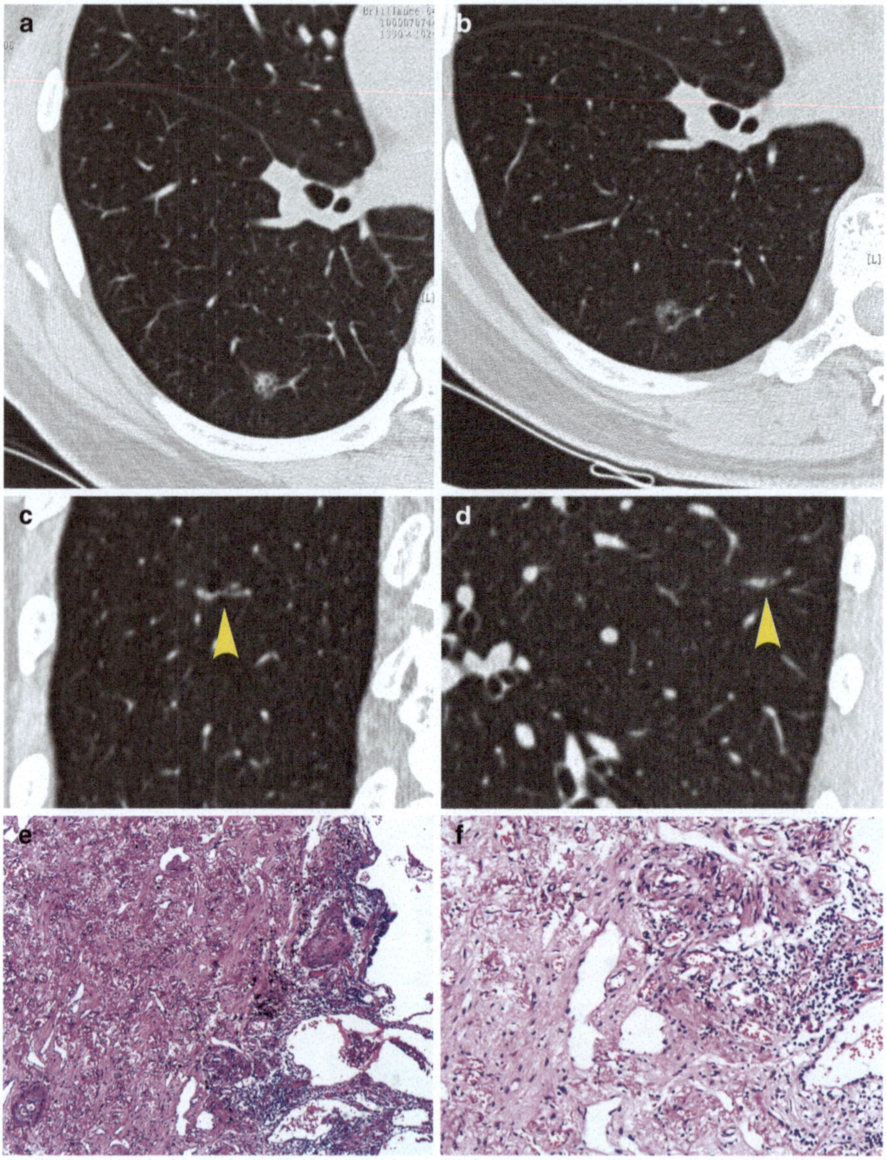

Fig. 14.51 In axial images, a mixed GGN with a size of 8 mm × 8 mm is located in the right lower lobe. In consecutive levels (**a**, **b**), the lesion appears spherical and ill-defined, containing a linear solid component and bubble lucencies. In the coronal (**c**) and sagittal (**d**) views, the lesion is in a tubular pattern. Bronchiectasis is seen nearby (arrowhead). This lesion was surgically resected. The pathologic image reveals septal thickening with focal infiltration of lymphocytes and irregular residual airspaces, diagnostic of chronic alveolitis

14.44.3 Pathological Diagnosis

Per the patient's request, this lesion was removed with wedge resection via VATS. Surgical pathological examination confirmed chronic alveolitis without neoplastic findings (Fig. 14.51e, f).

14.44.4 Conclusion and Comments

In a retrospective study, Takashima et al. [12] investigated reliable high-resolution CT features of benign lesions. The features suggestive of benign nodules with a high specificity include calcification (diffuse, popcorn, central, and laminated), internal fat, polygonal (all surfaces are concave or straight unless in contact with a pleural surface), ovoid (coffee bean-shaped)/flat/tubular pattern, and clustering of subcentimeter nodules in an isolated lung segment. Additionally, features, such as solid with no ground-glass components, subpleural distribution, and punctate calcification, are considered low specificity.

In this case, the great variation of dimension and morphology between axial view and coronal/sagittal views is highly suggestive of a benign process. The dimensional variation can be quantified using the ratio of the maximum transverse dimension to the maximum perpendicular length [three-dimensional (3D) ratio]. A large ratio is more frequently seen in benign nodules than in malignant nodules.

The case reemphasizes the value of multiplanar reformation imaging in the assessment of lung nodules. In the axial image, the nodule resembles a malignant semisolid GGN. We conducted a self-assessment within our department using this case. Only provided with axial images, our colleagues considered this nodule malignant with a confidence level of over 75%; however, when given the coronal and sagittal images, the confidence level immediately dropped to 0. And a large 3D ratio as seen in this case is suggestive of nonspecific chronic inflammation or fibrotic proliferation more likely than other benign entities, such as hamartoma and hemangioma.

(Huiqun Chen, Lei Zhu)

14.45 Case 45: Organizing Pneumonia

14.45.1 Clinical History

A 52-year-old female had high fever, cough, sputum, and chest pain for a month, with the increasing white blood cell count and plasma C-reactive protein level. Pneumonia was clinically diagnosed, and antibiotics were given for 2 weeks. Clinical symptoms were relieved. Follow-up chest CT reported a mixed ground-glass nodule in the right lung (Fig. 14.52). This patient was recommended for the

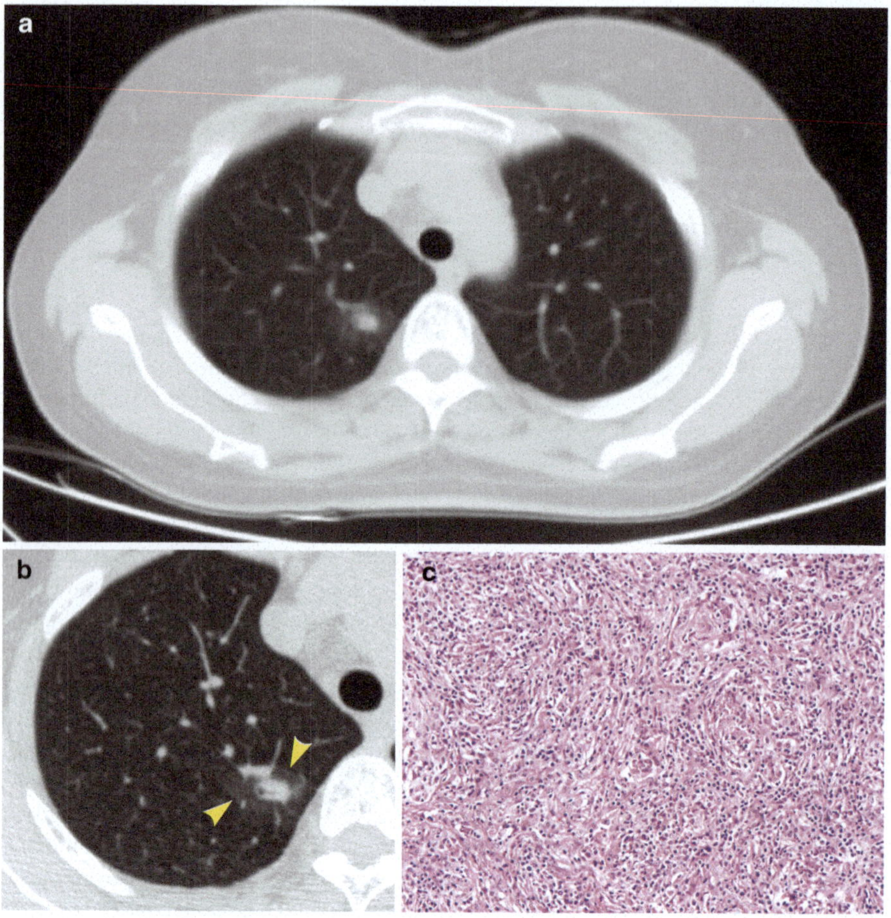

Fig. 14.52 An irregular 10-mm mixed GGN is located in the apical segment of the right upper lobe (**a**). The lesion contains centrally located sharply circumscribed solid components with the high attenuation and a peripheral poorly defined ground-glass opacity (**b**, arrowhead). The surgical pathologic image revealed a marked proliferation of type II pneumocytes and histiocytes, infiltration of lymphocytes and plasmocyte, and accumulation of fibrin and focal organizing tissues (**c**)

continuing antibiotic treatment and routine follow-up. She declined the recommendation due to the family history of lung cancer and requested surgical resection.

14.45.2 CT Findings

An irregular mixed GGN is seen in the right upper lobe with a central high-density solid component and a poorly defined peripheral ground-glass opacity (the halo sign). A slit-like low attenuation is seen within the solid component. Lobulation, spiculation, and abnormal vasculature are not absent. Pleural retraction is not seen.

14.45.3 Pathological Diagnosis

This lesion was wedge resected via VATS. The pathological examination confirmed organizing pneumonia (Fig. 14.52c).

14.45.4 Conclusion and Comments

Organizing pneumonia could present as a solitary nodular opacity on chest CT imaging, which should be distinguished from lung cancer. Most cases of focal OP are cryptogenic (COP), and the infection is identified in a minority of cases. Focal OP is often difficult to distinguish from bronchogenic carcinoma and requires surgical resection.

OP is a nonspecific inflammatory lesion composed of intraluminal organizing polyps in the peripheral airways and the alveoli associated with the chronic inflammatory infiltrate in alveolar septa and preserved alveolar structure, with clinical presentations of unresolved or chronic pneumonia. OP could be a discrete pulmonary entity, referring to unresolved/chronic pneumonia and delayed resolution of bacterial pneumonia or abscess. Sometimes, it occurs as a collateral pathological finding associated with other primary diseases, such as infectious diseases, granulomatous diseases, or even lung cancer. In the last situation, the presence of OP should not only be distinguished from the malignancy but also should not obscure the coexisting malignancy.

Variable imaging features have been described in OP. Four patterns were summarized by Elper et al. as the following: (1) diffuse, patchy "ground glass"; (2) both patchy and diffuse opacities; (3) irregular and linear; and (4) rounded and nodular. Later, a more concise three-pattern classification system was proposed by Cordier et al. [5] (1) multiple patchy pulmonary involvement of the pneumonia type; (2) solitary pulmonary involvement of the pneumonia type, usually involving an upper lobe (as seen in this case); and (3) diffuse pulmonary involvement of the interstitial lung disease type. In most cases, OP represents a mixed pattern. The major feature is bilateral, non-segmental, and patchy consolidation with subpleural or peribronchovascular in distribution; other changes consist of a ground-glass pattern and nodules.

Focal or nodular pattern is reported to be present in 30% of OP patients and usually had well-defined smooth margins and may have a predilection for subpleural distribution or bronchocentric distribution, making contact with the pleural surface and their shapes varying from wedge-shaped to round or spiculated nodules. In the majority, multiple nodules are seen. A solitary pulmonary nodule without accompanying findings is rare. Internal cavitation may be seen but not a common finding (less than 5%), if present, in an irregular and slit-like shape, distinct from the cavitation seen in lung cancer and tuberculoma. Bronchial dilatation, mediastinal lymphadenopathy, and pleural effusions were commonly seen.

Zhao et al. [13] investigated the CT characteristics of solitary focal OP. No surrounding vessels abrupt interruption, the sign of "loose composition" (defined as a lesion with an incompact structure with inhomogeneous density besides air bronchogram or small bubble-like lucency), and the presence of satellite ground-glass opacity may suggest the diagnosis of nodular OP. Furthermore, imaging differentiation between lung cancer and large OP (>3 cm) is much easier than small OP (≤3 cm). Large OP tend to have a polygon shape, irregular border, and inhomogeneous density, with a contraction or convergence of surrounding pulmonary vessels and in broad contact with the pleural surface without pleural effusion, while small OP may have a round-shaped and irregular border, resembling lung cancer.

The reversed halo sign has been reported as a characteristic imaging feature of OP. This sign is defined as a focal, rounded area of ground-glass opacity surrounded by a nearly complete ring of consolidation positivity on contrast-enhanced CT study. It was first described by Voloudaki et al. [14] as a crescent- or ring-shaped opacity surrounding areas of ground-glass attenuation in patients with cryptogenic organizing pneumonia (COP). However, this sign has been reported in a wide spectrum of diseases, including tuberculosis and invasive fungal infections. The morphologic characteristics of the reversed halos included nodular walls detected in all the active tuberculosis cases and nodules observed inside the reversed halos in most cases, which also are present in cases of sarcoidosis but absent in OP cases. The presence of reticulation inside the sign, outer rim thickness >1 cm, and associated pleural effusion is suggestive of invasive fungal infections instead of OP. Still, OP remains the most frequent cause of the reversed halo sign, and radiologists should be well aware of this sign.

(Xiaodan Ye, Lei Zhu, Xiangpeng Zheng)

14.46 Case 46: Chronic Organizing Pneumonia with Granuloma

14.46.1 Clinical History

A 70-year-old cigarette smoking male came to the clinic with complaints of a low fever and cough for 2 weeks. Laboratory tests showed no abnormalities. A chest CT was ordered for lung assessment.

14.46.2 CT Findings

A heterogeneous lesion is located in the right upper lobe with a diameter of 21 mm. The centrally located solid component is surrounding with a large amount of ground-glass opacity which creates a reversed halo sign and a "loose composition" sign. Air bronchogram and bubble-like lucencies are seen. The margin is

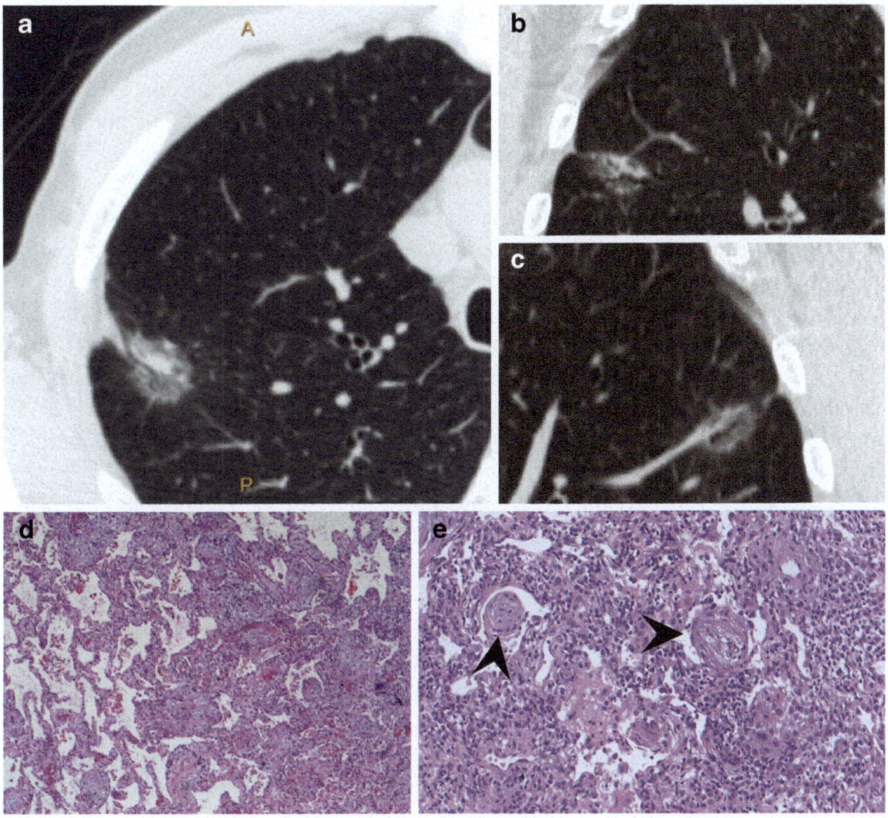

Fig. 14.53 An ovoid heterogeneous lesion with well-defined irregular border is seen in the right upper lobe. The central solid component is surrounded with remarkable low-density ground-glass opacity. Air bronchogram and bubble-like lucencies are seen in the lesion. Coarse spiculation is seen in the margin. A pulmonary vessel penetrated smoothly through the lesion. Pleural retraction and pleural thickening are evident (**a**–**c**). The lesion was surgically removed. Pathological images revealed polypoid plugs of granulation tissue (Masson body) in alveolar space (black arrowheads) and the infiltrated inflammatory cells and fibrotic hyperplasia in alveolar cavity and septa (**d**–**e**).

well-circumscribed with coarse spiculation. Pulmonary blood vessels are pulled toward and penetrating through the lesion. Pleural retraction and thickening are present (Fig. 14.53).

14.46.3 Pathological Diagnosis

The lesion is suspicious of a peripheral adenocarcinoma. Lobectomy was performed via VATS. Pathological examination confirmed chronic organizing pneumonia with granuloma (Fig. 14.53d, e).

14.46.4 Discussion and Comments

This is a case of organizing pneumonia mimicking peripheral lung cancer. Chronic organizing pneumonia with granuloma, or granulomatous organizing pneumonia (GOP), is believed to be a similar histopathological entity where non-necrotizing granulomata are intimately associated with the organizing connective tissue. In contrast, cryptogenic organizing pneumonia (COP) discussed in the previous case is a recognized common pattern of organizing pneumonia (OP), a condition that resembles pneumonia but is not caused by infection.

The granulomatous process in GOP that is intimately associated with the OP implies that they are part of the same process. Microorganisms are typically not found within the granulomatous inflammation in GOP patients, suggesting that the granulomata may be associated with an allergic or immunologic response. GOP shares some common imaging findings generally seen in OP but may have distinct characteristics due to distinct pathological features.

Feinstein et al. [15] conducted a comparative study of the pathological, clinical, and radiographical features between COP and GOP. In general, in the spectrum of demographic data, symptoms and radiographs are similar. In comparison with COP, GOP patients have fewer symptoms, require less treatment, and are consequently less severely ill, which might be associated with immune pathogenesis. Radiologically, nodules/masses are the most common abnormality, significantly more commonly among GOP patients than those with COP, in consistent with the findings that GOP patients were more likely to have moderate lymphoplasmacytic infiltrate. Consolidation and air bronchogram are less common, seen in less than one-third of patients, and then followed by ground-glass opacities (less than 20%). Honeycombing, bronchiectasis, thoracic adenopathy, and pleural effusions were uncommon, each occurring among less than 15% of patients. Cavitation is rare in COP and absent in GOP.

GOP is a newly described variant of OP, characterized by a pattern of OP in close association with small poorly formed non-necrotizing granulomata that must be confined to the same peribronchiolar location and within the OP pattern. As a particular entity of OP, GOP has relatively distinct clinical presentations and prognosis and hence should be distinguished from other subgroups in OP. And considering that GOP patients are more likely to present with nodules and masses mimicking malignancy, it should be included in the differential diagnosis under evaluation of lung nodules and/or masses.

(Xiaodan Ye, Huiqun Chen, Jianding Ye, Jie Zhang)

14.47 Case 47: Focal Fibrosis

14.47.1 Clinical History

A 36-year-old otherwise healthy female came to the clinic for a second opinion on an incidentally detected nodule in the right lung. She had a family history of cancer. She denied bloody sputum, chest pain, and weight loss.

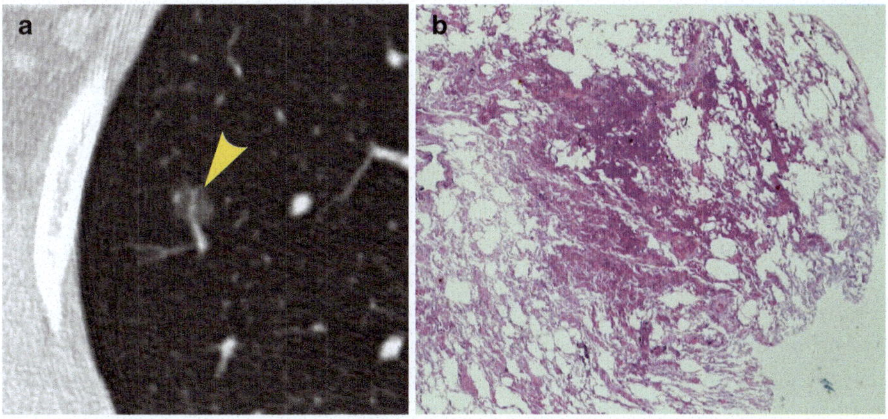

Fig. 14.54 (**a**) A mixed poorly defined GGN (arrowhead) is located in the right upper lobe without CTA-TA sign, lobulation, or spiculation. (**b**) The pathologic image shows collapsed alveoli and distorted structure due to moderate to severe fibrous hyperplasia within alveoli and septa. No neoplastic features are found

14.47.2 CT Findings

A mixed GGN is seen in the right upper lobe with poorly defined margin. The nodule is 7 mm × 6 mm in size. No lobulation, spiculation, calcification, or bubble-like lucency is present. A blood vessel is seen traversing the lesion with rigid appearance (Fig. 14.54).

14.47.3 Pathological Diagnosis

Despite that this patient was recommended for follow-up in 3 months, she declined and requested immediate surgical removal of the nodule. Considering the possibility of a preinvasive disease, the lesion was wedge resected via VATS. Pathological examination confirmed focal interstitial fibrosis (Fig. 14.54b).

14.47.4 Discussion and Comments

A GGN due to acute inflammation or bleeding may disappear during a follow-up period of several months. However, a persistent GGN (either no change or an increase in diameter for ≧1 month) may represent AAH, BAC, or focal fibrosis. Therefore, focal fibrosis is an indispensable differential diagnosis for a persistent GGN, especially mixed GGN, as in this case. However, those due to focal fibrosis remain stable and even have a potential of slow growth. In those cases, surgical resection is necessary for the establishment of a definitive diagnosis. These lesions were histologically confirmed as focal interstitial fibrosis with fibroblast and type II pneumocyte proliferation and collection of alveolar macrophages. The pathogenesis of focal fibrosis remains not well understood. It may reflect a focal tissue response to local lung injury due to infection or radiation, drug, or physical pressure.

Focal fibrosis is a relatively rare disease entity constituting 15–21% of persistent focal GGO. In a report from Nakajima et al. [16] among the 20 resected localized pure GGNs, 15% were from fibrosis, and the remaining were preinvasive diseases or invasive adenocarcinoma. In another report from Lee et al. [17] the prevalence of focal fibrosis was 8.3% in pure persistent GGN ≤10 mm, in comparison to 40% in those >10 mm. Radiologically, focal fibrosis is a sharply demarcated nodular GGO, especially pure GGO, with a maximal diameter of less than 2 cm on thin-section CT. The size can vary, and the possibility of focal fibrosis increases with the increasing size of persistent GGN. Mixed or solid GGNs are less frequent than pure GGN. Solid components pathologically may correspond to compact fibrotic foci or alveolar collapse. One possible characteristic imaging feature for discriminating focal fibrosis from lung cancer is that focal fibrosis does not increase in size over a considerable period, but this requires a significantly long period of follow-up which may not be well complied by patients as seen in this case. Other ancillary findings in focal fibrosis may be retracted bronchiectasis, dilated vasculatures, satellite lesions, or thickening of the interlobular septa, reflecting an inflammatory background.

In sum, focal fibrosis represents a chronic pulmonary benign process with imaging features of a persistent pure GGN predominantly which may mimic preinvasive diseases. Follow-up may be a proper strategy for differentiation. Due to the potential of slow growth, in cases with equivocal findings, surgical removal is the choice of diagnosis and treatment.

(Huiqun Chen, Lei Zhu)

14.48 Case 48: Focal Fibrosis

14.48.1 Clinical History

A 57-year-old female presented to the clinic with complaints of a cough and sputum for 2 months. Two weeks ago, antibiotic treatment was initiated. Clinical symptoms were improved. She denied shortness of breath, coarseness, night sweating, and family history of any cancers.

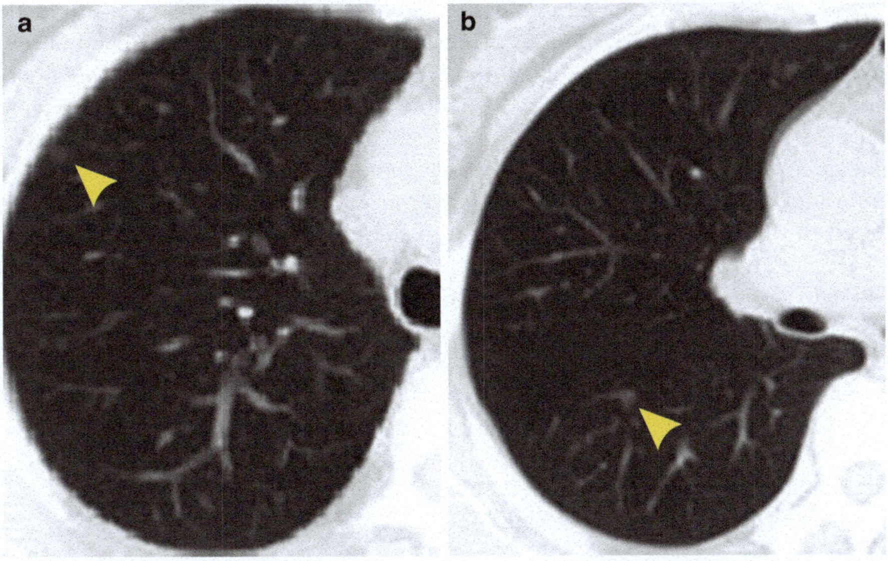

Fig. 14.55 Two ill-defined pure GGNs (arrowhead) in the subpleural area are seen in the right upper and lower lobes. A small blood vessel is penetrating through the nodule in the right lower lobe, but CTA-TA sign is not visualized

14.48.2 CT Findings

Chest CT shows two pure ground-glass nodules in the subpleural area in the right upper and lower lobes, respectively. Both nodules are measuring approximately 5 mm in diameter with ill-defined margin. Lobulation, spiculation, and pleural retraction are absent (Fig. 14.55).

14.48.3 Pathological Diagnosis

Per patient's request, both nodules were resected via VATS. Pathological examinations revealed interstitial fibrotic hyperplasia with inflammatory cell infiltration without neoplastic findings.

14.48.4 Discussion and Comments

Focal interstitial fibrosis (FIF) could present as a GGN mimicking a pulmonary malignancy and be a challenge in differential diagnosis. In this case, two pure GGNs are seen and pathologically diagnosed as FIF, much more in consistent with the common imaging pattern discussed in the previous case.

Si et al. [18] conducted a radiologic-pathologic comparison between FIF and AAH/AIS/MIA with presentations of pure GGN. FIF showed a predilection for male and smokers, while the others occurred more frequently in female and non-smokers. All FIF and most of the MIA nodules demonstrated a polygonal or irregular shape with obvious lobulation and/or spiculation. In FIF, an irregular shape and spiculated margin are caused by a large amount of stromal fibers with dense infiltration of inflammatory cells. However, a concave margin was only manifested in FIF resulting from contraction of the fibers with a high prevalence of 85.7%. No significant differences were seen in age, malignant history, attenuation value, location, and presence of bubble-like lucency between FIF and AAH/AIS/MIA.

Taken together, a ground-glass nodule should be suspicious of FIF if the following imaging features are seen: (1) stable and unchanged in size, attenuation, and morphology during multiple follow-ups; (2) a concave margin; (3) if a pure GGN, larger size (>10 mm) has a higher possibility; (4) if a mixed GGN, irregular shape and spiculated margin in favor of FIF; and (5) absence of CTA-TA sign.

(Xiangpeng Zheng, Xiaohua Zhu, Ming Li)

14.49 Case 49: SABR in Early-Stage Lung Cancer

14.49.1 Clinical History

A 79-year-old female presented with complaints of a dry cough for a month, without fever and other symptoms. Chest CT revealed a 3-cm diameter mass in the right upper lung (Fig. 14.56a). This mass was first seen in CT 4 years ago with less than 10 mm. Annual follow-up showed continuous growth with an acceleration in the past 10 months, from 1.9 cm to current 3 cm. The mass was well-circumscribed, deeply lobulated with short spiculation. No satellite lesion, calcification, or cavitation was seen. The major fissure was involved. No evident hilar or mediastinal lymphadenopathy was found. Based on CT findings, this mass was highly suspected of a lung cancer, specifically a peripheral adenocarcinoma. For further evaluation, FDG-PET/CT was performed, and heterogeneous hypermetabolic activity was seen within the mass with an average SUV of about 8.4, in favor of the suspected diagnosis of lung cancer. No lymphadenopathy or suspicious metastases were found in PET/CT images. After that, a multidisciplinary discussion on this case was convened. Considering her unfavorable pulmonary function tests, including base FEV1 <40% predicted, postoperative FEV1 <30% predicted, and pulmonary diffusing capacity decreased significantly (<40% predictive value), this patient was deemed as unfit for surgical treatment due to predicted high risk of perioperative mortality. SABR was recommended for this limited suspected pulmonary mass. Percutaneous CT-guided needle biopsy or transbronchial lung biopsy was suggested for definitive diagnosis but declined by the patient and her family members. The probability of

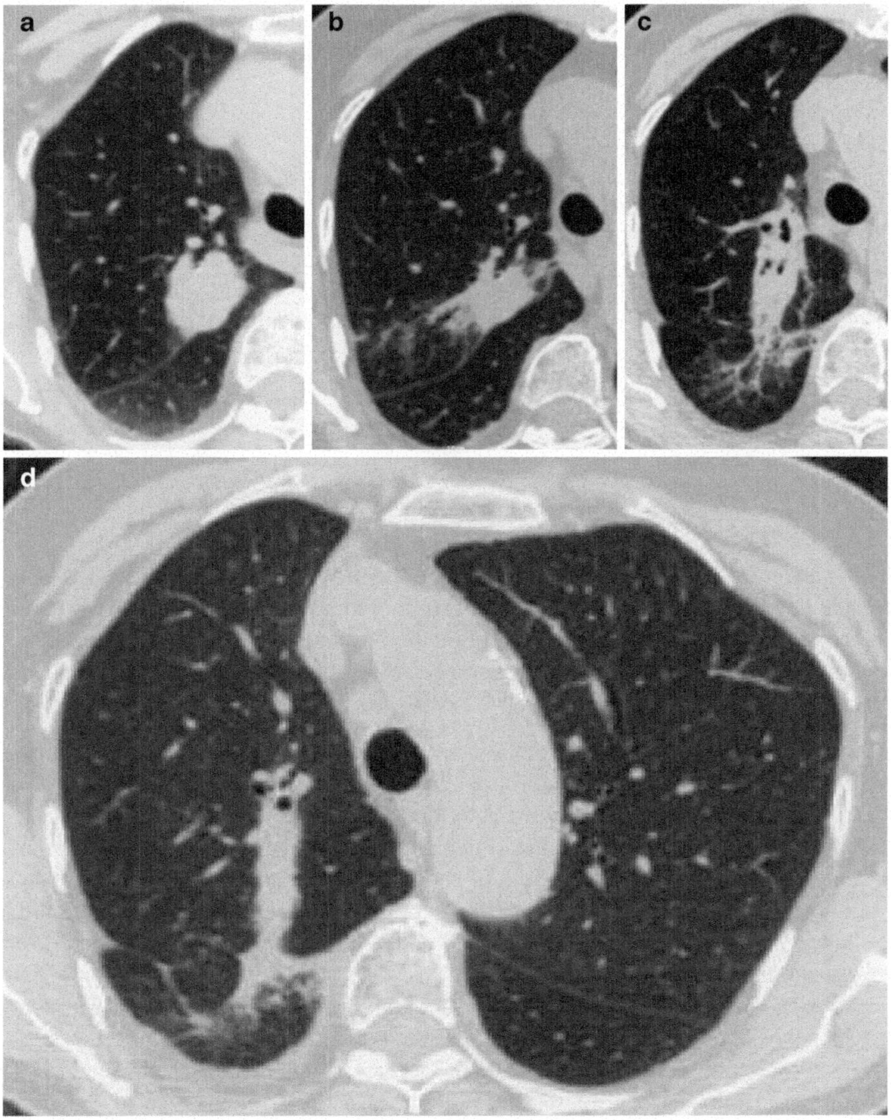

Fig. 14.56 SABR in early-stage lung cancer. (**a**) In the pretreatment CT image, a lobulated mass 30 mm × 24 mm in size is located in the right upper lobe with pleural involvement. This mass progressively grew in the past 4 years, suspected of a lung cancer. (**b**) One month after treatment, CT shows the mass regressed significantly by over 30% in the longest dimension and a partial response was achieved; mild radiation-induced pneumonitis with a ground-glass pattern is seen in the adjacent lung tissues, particularly distal to the mass. (**c**) Six months later, the mass completely disappeared and replaced by fibrotic tissues, corresponding to the late changes of radiation pneumonitis. A complete response was achieved. (**d**) Twenty-two months later, no recurrence is observed, and focal fibrotic consolidation remains the same to the findings in previous follow-ups. Annual CT follow-up is recommended

malignancy was estimated over 85% based on information from CT, PET/CT, and clinical history. The tumor board finally approved the SABR treatment for the RUL mass in this patient.

14.49.2 Pathological Diagnosis

Due to the decline for invasive biopsy procedures from the patient and family members, a pathological diagnosis was not available. The clinical diagnosis of lung cancer, most likely adenocarcinoma, was based on comprehensive evaluation of imaging findings and medical history by our multidisciplinary team.

14.49.3 SABR Procedure

This patient with a clinical lung cancer (cT1bN0M0, stage cIA) received SABR treatment with a signed written consent form for radiation therapy. The SABR treatment is a specialized technique in radiation therapy, and strict procedures should be followed for quality control and assurance. More detailed information could be found in Chap. 12. For this patient, the SABR procedure is described below.

1. *Position immobilization*: A combination of vacuum body cushion and thermoplastic body mask was utilized for position immobilization. Patient was coached to lay comfortably on a vacuum body cushion with both arms extending overhead with hands gripping the position bar. The vacuum cushion provided support and immobilization from the bottom and sides. In the meanwhile, thermoplastic body mask applied pressure from the anterior direction to strengthen immobilization and inhibit the respiratory amplitude with functioning similar to abdominal compression to some extent.
2. *CT simulation and respiratory movement management*: CT simulation was conducted using a three-phase scanning protocol on a specialized big-bore CT scanner (Somatom Definition AS, Siemens). Three series of non-enhancement CT imaging from the level of the thyroid cartilage to the upper pole of the right kidney were acquired with a slice thickness of 5 mm at free breathing, end of expiration, and end of inspiration, respectively. Afterward, reconstructed images with 2-mm slice thickness were transferred to TPS workstation for target delineation and treatment planning.
3. *Treatment planning and validation*: On the TPS workstation (Eclipse 8.5, Varian Co.), end-of-inspiration and end-of-expiration CT imaging series were fused with the free-breathing CT imaging series used as the planning reference imaging, respectively. Gross tumor volume (GTV) was contoured on three CT imaging series with lung window setting. On the fused imaging, GTVs from three CT series were combined ("or" in the Boolean calculation) to produce the ITV (internal target volume) on the planning reference imaging. Planning target volume (PTV)

included the ITV plus a 3-mm margin in posteroanterior and lateral directions (x- and y-axis) and a 5-mm margin in the craniocaudal direction (z-axis). Afterward, structures and organs at risk, including the lungs, trachea, main bronchus, ribs, esophagus, heart, spinal cord, and brachial plexus (in cases with tumors located in the lung apex), were delineated on the reference imaging. Based on patient's physical condition and tumor location, individualized dose prescription was administrated with ≥90% of PTV being encompassed by ≥90% of the prescription dose at the premise of biologically effective dose (BED) not less than 90 Gy, unless in cases with special discretion. The biologic effective dose was calculated based on the linear quadratic equation: $BED = nd\,[1 + d/(\alpha/\beta)]$, where n represents the number of fractions, d is the dose per fraction, and α/β is 10 for lung cancer. SABR plans were evaluated according to RTOG 0813 using parameters such as the ratio of prescription isodose volume to the PTV volume (R100%), the ratio of 50% prescription isodose volume to the PTV volume (R50%), and maximum dose at 2 cm from PTV in any direction (D2 cm). Each SABR plan should respect all critical organ dose-volume constraints: for the lung, V20 Gy < 10% and V12.5 Gy < 15%; for the esophagus, V 35 Gy < 0.1 cm^3; for the trachea and main bronchus, V32 Gy < 0.1 cm^3; for ribs in the fields, V30 Gy < 30 cm^3; and for the spinal cord, V32 Gy < 0.1 cm^3 (Fig. 14.57). Prior to approval for implementation, all plans were validated with the Octavius 4D system (PTW, Freiburg, Germany) with a pass rate of 95% using a gamma index acceptance criteria of 3%/3 mm (dose difference of 3% and distance to the agreement of 3 mm).

4. *Image guidance treatment delivery*: The treatment was delivered using a linear accelerator (Trilogy®. Varian Medical Systems, Inc.). Treatment course was completed within 2 weeks with 1-day off after every two treatments. Each treatment was image-guided with cone-beam CT (CBCT), including pretreatment, intrafractional, and posttreatment acquisition. All imaging was online real-time evaluated to validate the tumor position, and positional errors over 3 mm at any direction were corrected. For prevention of acute radiation-induced pulmonary toxicity, patients were given dexamethasone (3 mg, qd) orally unless contraindicated from 1 day before treatment to the end of the treatment.
5. *Follow-up evaluation*: For assessment of treatment outcomes and adverse events, the patient was followed routinely every 3 months in the first year. Chest CT (with contrast media, if possible) was acquired at each follow-up visit. If tumor shrank and no recurrence were suspected, the follow-up frequency could be extended to every 6 months from the second year. In case of suspicion of disease recurrence, ^{18}FDG-PET scans were obtained for diagnostic differentiation from organizing pneumonitis and assessment of the feasibility for salvage treatment. As the most common radiation-related toxicity, the incidence and severity of radiation-induced pneumonitis (RP) were recorded following the guidelines of the NCI Common Terminology Criteria for Adverse Events 4.0 (CTCAE 4.0): grade I RP, nonsymptomatic or mild symptomatic without medication requirement; grade II RP, symptomatic and required oral dexamethasone; grade III RP, required hospitalization and intravenous hormonal treatment and oxygen; grade IV RP, needs mechanical ventilation; and grade V RP, irreversible fatal pneumonitis.

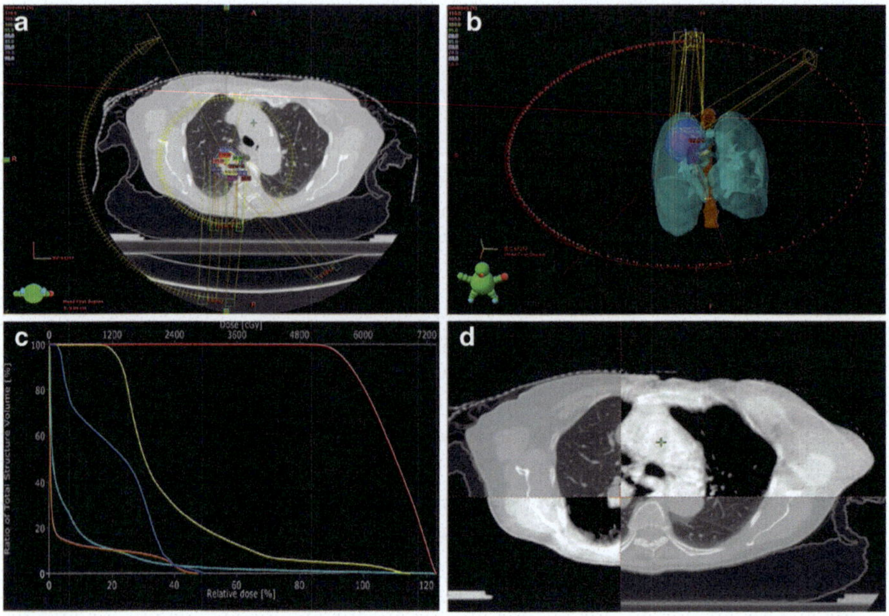

Fig. 14.57 The radiotherapy planning and image guidance during SABR treatment. (**a**, **b**) Beam arrangement in the treatment planning. One full arc and one partial arc are used to deliver the prescribed dose (total dose 60 Gy given in eight fractions ×7.5 Gy) to the tumor target. (**c**) The dose-volume histogram (DVH) is used to evaluate dose distribution in the tumor target and interested normal organs or tissues. (**d**) Image guidance for treatment delivery. For each treatment, CBCT images (upper left and lower right) are acquired to match the simulated CT images (upper right and lower left). If there are significant anatomical variations (>5 mm), the error should be real-time corrected by adjusting treatment couch for precise treatment

14.49.4 Discussion and Comments

Lung cancer remains the leading cause of cancer mortality worldwide and poses a much graver challenge in China than other countries due to the huge population and developing economy. According to the latest cancer statistics from the National Central Cancer Registry (NCCR) of China, estimated 733,300 new lung cancer cases and 610,200 deaths would occur in China in 2015. Among them, 30–50% of patients are aged over 75 years, just second to the age group of 60–74 years. With the society aging, it is reasonable to predict that the incidence and prevalence of lung cancer in the elderly population continuously increase. Thus, the management of lung cancer in this particular population demands more attention and research. Surgical resection is the standard management of early-stage non-small-cell lung cancer (NSCLC). However, considering high prevalence of comorbidities, including limited pulmonary function due to chronic obstructive pulmonary diseases and cardiovascular risks, the percentage of elderly early-stage NSCLC patients unsuitable for surgery would be higher than that in younger patients (70% vs. 29%). To provide definitive treatment with good local tumor control rather than conventional palliative treatment to those fragile elderly patients seems challenging but is worthwhile to be investigated for the maintenance of quality of life and relatively healthy aging.

Mounting evidence has shown that hypofractionated stereotactic ablative radiotherapy (SABR) can achieve comparable treatment outcomes, regarding local control and overall survival, in both operable and inoperable early-stage lung cancer patients in comparison to surgical approaches. Our meta-analysis validated that patient age could influence the treatment outcomes from either SABR or surgery. So far, clinical data of SABR in elderly patients are limited but have shown promising results.

According to a meta-analysis, medium (83.2–106 Gy) or medium to high (106–146 Gy) BED SABR regimens could produce a better outcome than low (<83.2 Gy) or high (106–146 Gy) BED regimens in stage I NSCLC. This patient received a medium BED (105 Gy), which may account for the mild pulmonary toxicity, i.e., radiation pneumonitis. Prophylactic administration of dexamethasone during treatment course could be another favorable factor. Evidence has shown that dexamethasone could reduce the incidence or severity of RP and the efficacy of a smaller dosage (3 mg per day) is comparable to a larger dosage (10 mg per day) but with less adverse effects.

Currently, no consistent predictive biomarkers for RP were identified. TNF-α, interleukin (IL)-1β, IL-6, IL-8, and IL-18 have been shown among the promising predictive biomarkers for acute lung injury. Our analysis on hematological parameters revealed that plasma D-dimer level was correlated with the RP incidence, which could be explained by radiation-induced endothelial injury and intravascular coagulation. It has been reported elevated levels of plasma D-dimer predict a worse treatment outcome in many cancer patients, such as nasopharyngeal carcinoma.

Given the tumor biological behavior and fragile physical condition in elderly patients, SABR treatment planning and delivery should be cautious with individualized optimization to assure both the treatment outcome and the protection of the quality of life since radiation-induced pulmonary toxicity in elderly patients may more severe and require more time to recovery. For optimization, multiple factors should be taken into consideration. First of all, dose regimen has impacts on treatment outcomes as well as adverse effects. Multiple studies and the National Comprehensive Cancer Network have published SABR treatment guidelines, including total dose and fractional dose as well as dose constraints of critical organs. In our clinical practice, we gradually modified the dose regimen by reducing fractional dose on the premise of maintaining total BED over 90 Gy and treatment course within 2 weeks to minimize the incidence of acute pulmonary adverse events. Approximately 50% of elderly patients received 60 Gy/8 fractions. In comparison to regimens with higher fractional dose (10 Gy or 12 Gy), this fractionation caused a lower incidence of symptomatic radiation pneumonitis (grade II or above), and local tumor control was not compromised.

Patient selection carries more significance in elderly patients than the younger. Each patient was through strict assessment regarding position robustness, tumor movement, and compliance on the couch. Due to the treatment complexity and high fractional dose, SABR demands high-quality and robust patient position immobilization and efficient control of respiration-related tumor movement. Several movement management strategies such as abdominal compression and respiration-gating technique are currently clinically available. However, the complex and time-consuming process leads to unsatisfactory compliance in elderly patients. To ensure the treatment compliance and patient comfort during treatment delivery, we utilized thermoplastic body mask for compression and vacuum cushion for immobilization in combination with online CBCT validation.

A well-designed treatment plan correlates with the efficiency of treatment delivery. The fractional dose in SABR is four to six times higher than in conventional radiotherapy. As a direct consequence, the beam-on time in SABR is longer. The noncoplanar conformal technique could use 15 fields to achieve the required dose distribution for SABR and may take at least 7 min to complete the treatment plan. When taking the position correction and online imaging guidance into consideration, the on-couch time could be six to eight times longer than in conventional radiotherapy, which is unfavorable for elderly patients. Rotational radiation techniques, RapidArc and VMAT, have proven advantages over conventional technique, including improved dose distribution without noncoplanar beam alignment and increased implementation efficiency benefiting from continuous irradiation. Technically, a two-arc treatment plan was applied in 85% of cases, each arc delivering half of fractional dose and between arcs, and intrafractional CBCT was acquired for tumor position validation. In comparison to conformal radiotherapy, arc technique saved 30% of the on-couch time (8 min vs. 6 min). Also, due to the reduction of on-couch time, the possibility of uncertainties from the involuntary movement of patients on the couch decreased. Considering the simplicity of immobilization and movement management maneuver used in elderly patients, it is critically important to conduct image guidance and online real-time position validation and correction in the course of treatment delivery. In our study, each patient received three series of CBCT, pretreatment, intrafractional, and posttreatment, for tumor position validation and quality assurance.

(Xiangpeng Zheng, Zi Tan, Jianjian Qiu)

14.50 Case 50: Radiofrequency Ablation Therapy in Early-Stage Lung Cancer

14.50.1 Clinical History

Male, 79 years old. Chest CT showed an 18 mm in diameter solid nodule in the right upper lobe. This nodule had well-defined margin with deep lobulation and short spiculation. Bubble lucencies were seen inside. Multiple blood vessels were penetrating into the lesion. The pleural retraction was present. Hilar and mediastinal lymphadenopathy was not found. Peripheral lung adenocarcinoma was highly suspected (Fig. 14.58a, b).

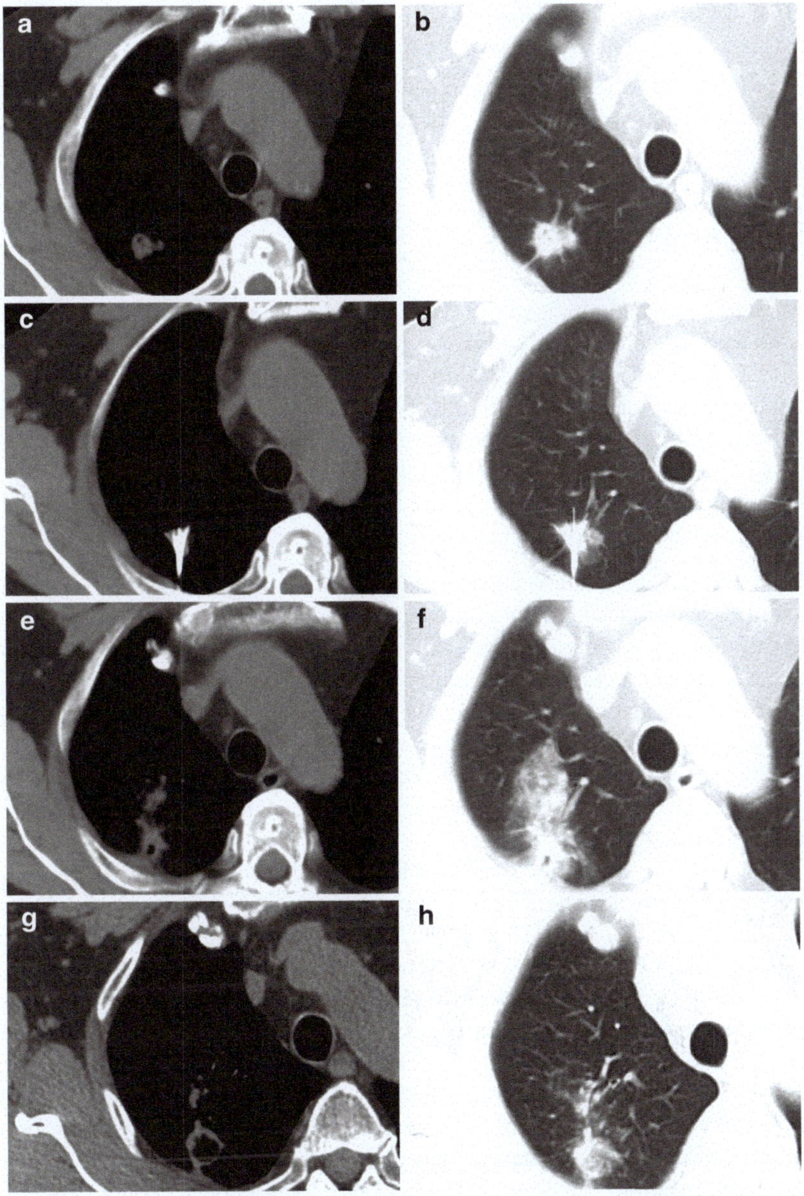

Fig. 14.58 Radiofrequency ablation (RFA) therapy in peripheral lung adenocarcinoma. (**a**, **b**) In pretreatment CT images, a heterogeneous well-defined nodule is located in the apical segment of the right upper lobe, with lobulation, spiculation, and pleural retraction, diagnostic of peripheral adenocarcinoma. (**c**, **d**) Intra-RFA CT shows deployed RF tines in the deepest part of the tumor. (**e**, **f**) Immediate after RFA, CT images show cavitation with the lesion and a large area of ground-glass opacity encompassing the ablation zone. (**g**, **h**) One month after RFA, follow-up CT shows that tumor is partly absorbed, the cavitation expands, and treatment-induced ground-glass opacity barely disappears with residual fibrotic tissues

14.50.2 Pathological Diagnosis

For a definitive diagnosis, a percutaneous CT-guided needle biopsy was performed. Pathological examination confirmed adenocarcinoma.

14.50.3 RFA Procedure

This patient had a pathologically proven lung adenocarcinoma (pT1aN0M0, stage pIa) with a performance status score of 1. Pulmonary function tests showed lowered FEV1 (1.31 L, 76.2% of predicted) and lowered FVC (1.54 L, 66.9% of predicted), confirming the presence of restriction with obstructive small airways. A comprehensive evaluation by the multidisciplinary team concluded that this patient was not a candidate for surgery, and nonsurgical treatment should be considered. Finally, the patient agreed to receive radiofrequency ablation for the tumor. Briefly, the RFA was conducted as the following protocol.

1. *Preparation*: The patient was prone positioned on the CT table, so the RF electrode can be introduced along a line that represents the shortest distance from the skin to the targeted tumor. Consecutive CT images with 5-mm slice thickness were acquired to determine the tumor location, the anticipated skin entry site, and the distance from the tumor center to the entry site. The skin entry site was prepared with antiseptic solutions and surrounded with sterile towels and drapes. Local anesthesia with lidocaine was administered with a small-bore hypodermic needle. This hypodermic needle was left in place along the projected access for possible further use.
2. *Electrode deployment*: The deployment of RF electrodes is similar to percutaneous needle biopsy. The RF electrodes used were 14-gauge multitine expandable electrodes that were 15 cm long, with a 2.0-, 3.0-, 3.5-, or 4.0-cm array diameter when fully expanded. Electrode sizes were always chosen to be at least 15 mm larger than the largest tumor diameter. Multiple CT scanning was performed to guide the deployment and adjust the tine to cover the entire tumor (Fig. 14.58c, d).
3. *The tumor ablation*: To perform ablation, two grounding pads were applied to the back of the patient. The tip of the electrode was advanced with the prongs retracted, to the desired location, and then the prongs were partially deployed. There was an automated program that will slowly raise the generator power from 25 W to peak within 1–1.5 min. At the target temperature (90 °C), the tumor was ablated for 10 min. Afterward, full deployment of the prongs was performed, and the target temperature was maintained for ablation for another 15 min. After completion of the ablation cycle, the temperature reading from the central electrode must be >65 °C for at least 30 s. The needle tract was ablated with a tract ablation program, maintaining the temperature over 70 °C while removing the needle.

4. *Immediate assessment*: A complete chest CT study was obtained immediately after the end of the treatment for assessment of ablation effects and possible complications. CT section of lung windows obtained immediately after the RF electrode was removed shows that perilesional opacities are present, indicating probable complete tumor ablation. No pneumothorax was found (Fig. 14.58e, f). After the treatment, patients complained about chest pain. Intramuscular meperidine 50 mg was given. The patient safely returned to the ward without other symptoms.
5. *Follow-up*: CT images with and without contrast agent enhancement are commonly obtained at 1, 3, 6, 9, and 12 months and yearly thereafter to assess for disease progression or regression. In the 1-month CT, the tumor was partly absorbed with the formation of a central cavitary zone with low attenuation, and treatment-induced ground-glass opacity barely disappears with residual fibrotic tissues.

14.50.4 Discussion and Comments

As a promising nonsurgical therapeutic alternative for small, peripheral tumors, RFA could be performed percutaneously, under conscious sedation and image guidance, and as an outpatient procedure or with a short hospital stay. The use of RFA to treat lung malignancies in human was first reported in 2000. The largest prospective, multicenter trial of RFA for lung tumors was the RAPTURE study published in 2008, which enrolled 106 inoperable patients with 183 lung tumors, including 33 primary NSCLC patients. A 75% 2-year OS has been shown in patients with stage INSCLC, and a confirmed complete response lasting at least 1 year was 88%. Radiofrequency ablation treatment was well tolerated. Major complications were symptomatic pneumothorax needing drainage and pleural effusion needing drainage. Minor complications were pneumothorax or pleural effusion not needing treatment and self-limiting intrapulmonary hemorrhage. However, the majority of RFA studies in early-stage NSCLC are small case series, and the reported LCRs ranged greatly from 58 to 95%.

A strong correlation between the sizes of the targeted tumors and the RFA treatment results has been reported. Higher rates of relapse were noted in tumors larger than 2–4 cm. A recent study including 55 ablations in 45 patients with stage I NSCLC reported more local failures in tumors >3 cm (80%), compared with lesions <3 cm (29%), implying that those patients with larger tumors should be more frequently followed up and provided adjuvant therapy if necessary or immediately after RFA.

PET/CT in the preoperative positioning and during the radiofrequency ablation is believed to be better than CT, especially on the lung disease with atelectasis, obstructive pneumonia, and other complex patients. PET/CT has the capabilities of revealing the relationship between the lesion and surrounding lung tissue and detecting the areas with hypermetabolic activity for precise ablation. However, the radiation exposure and cost are the major limitations.

Regarding outcome assessment, routine chest CT with and without contrast agent enhancement is recommended at 1, 3, 6, 9, and 12 months and yearly thereafter. The expected findings immediate after RFA treatment would be the absence of the previously radiointense focus of tumor and presence of a larger diameter, less radiointense ring representing surrounding inflammatory granulation tissue at the interface of necrotic tissue and viable tissue. A PET/CT scan at 1 month may be useful to assess for adequacy of tumor ablation. Additionally, in cases with suspected relapse or differentiation between treatment-induced fibrotic consolidation and recurrence, PET/CT has the advantage over other imaging modalities.

(Xudong Ni, Dawei Yang, Xiangpeng Zheng)

References

1. Yu YY, Pinsky PF, Caporaso NE, Chatterjee N, Baumgarten M, Langenberg P, Furuno JP, Lan Q, Engels EA. Lung cancer risk following detection of pulmonary scarring by chest radiography in the prostate, lung, colorectal, and ovarian cancer screening trial. Arch Intern Med. 2008;168(21):2326–2332.; discussion 2332. https://doi.org/10.1001/archinte.168.21.2326.
2. Funai K, Yokose T, Ishii G, Araki K, Yoshida J, Nishimura M, Nagai K, Nishiwaki Y, Ochiai A. Clinicopathologic characteristics of peripheral squamous cell carcinoma of the lung. Am J Surg Pathol. 2003;27(7):978–84.
3. Cheung YC, Ng SH, Chang JW, Tan CF, Huang SF, Yu CT. Histopathological and CT features of pulmonary sclerosing haemangiomas. Clin Radiol. 2003;58(8):630–5.
4. Choplin RH, Kawamoto EH, Dyer RB, Geisinger KR, Mills SE, Pope TL. Atypical carcinoid of the lung: radiographic features. AJR Am J Roentgenol. 1986;146(4):665–8. https://doi.org/10.2214/ajr.146.4.665.
5. Cordier JF, Loire R, Brune J. Idiopathic bronchiolitis obliterans organizing pneumonia. Definition of characteristic clinical profiles in a series of 16 patients. Chest. 1989;96(5):999–1004.
6. Nagashima T, Sakao Y, Mun M, Ishikawa Y, Nakagawa K, Masuda M, Okumura S. A clinicopathological study of resected small-sized squamous cell carcinomas of the peripheral lung: prognostic significance of serum carcinoembryonic antigen levels. Ann Thorac Cardiovasc Surg. 2013;19(5):351–7.
7. Matsushita M, Kawakami S, Matsushita T, Sugiyama Y, Endo M, Shimojo H, Toishi M, Kadoya M. Changes in CT density of solitary capillary hemangioma of the lung upon varying patient position. Jpn J Radiol. 2012;30(9):772–6. https://doi.org/10.1007/s11604-012-0113-4.
8. Liebow AA, Hubbell DS. Sclerosing hemangioma (histiocytoma, xanthoma) of the lung. Cancer. 1956;9(1):53–75.
9. Pornsuriyasak P, Suwatanapongched T, Klaewsongkram J, Buranapraditkun S, Rotjanapan P. Acute respiratory failure secondary to eosinophilic pneumonia following influenza vaccination in an elderly man with chronic obstructive pulmonary disease. Int J Infect Dis. 2014;26:14–6. https://doi.org/10.1016/j.ijid.2014.04.019.
10. Yamakawa H, Yoshida M, Yabe M, Baba E, Okuda K, Fujimoto S, Katagi H, Ishikawa T, Takagi M, Kuwano K. Correlation between clinical characteristics and chest computed tomography findings of pulmonary cryptococcosis. Pulmonary Med. 2015;2015:703407. https://doi.org/10.1155/2015/703407.
11. Guimaraes MD, Marchiori E, Meirelles GS, Hochhegger B, Santana PR, Gross JL, Bitencourt AG, Boonsirikamchai P, Godoy MC. Fungal infection mimicking pulmonary malignancy: clinical and radiological characteristics. Lung. 2013;191(6):655–62. https://doi.org/10.1007/s00408-013-9506-0.

12. Takashima S, Sone S, Li F, Maruyama Y, Hasegawa M, Matsushita T, Takayama F, Kadoya M. Small solitary pulmonary nodules (< or =1 cm) detected at population-based CT screening for lung cancer: reliable high-resolution CT features of benign lesions. AJR Am J Roentgenol. 2003;180(4):955–64.
13. Zhao F, Yan SX, Wang GF, Wang J, PX L, Chen B, Yuan J, Zhang SZ, Wang YX. CT features of focal organizing pneumonia: an analysis of consecutive histopathologically confirmed 45 cases. Eur J Radiol. 2014;83(1):73–8. https://doi.org/10.1016/j.ejrad.2013.04.017.
14. Voloudaki AE, Bouros DE, Froudarakis ME, Datseris GE, Apostolaki EG, Gourtsoyiannis NC. Crescentic and ring-shaped opacities. CT features in two cases of bronchiolitis obliterans organizing pneumonia (BOOP). Acta Radiol. 1996;37(6):889–92. https://doi.org/10.1177/02841851960373p289.
15. Feinstein MB, DeSouza SA, Moreira AL, Stover DE, Heelan RT, Iyriboz TA, Taur Y, Travis WD. A comparison of the pathological, clinical and radiographical, features of cryptogenic organising pneumonia, acute fibrinous and organising pneumonia and granulomatous organising pneumonia. J Clin Pathol. 2015;68(6):441–7. https://doi.org/10.1136/jclinpath-2014-202626.
16. Nakajima R, Yokose T, Kakinuma R, Nagai K, Nishiwaki Y, Ochiai A. Localized pure ground-glass opacity on high-resolution CT: histologic characteristics. J Comput Assist Tomogr. 2002;26(3):323–9.
17. Lee YR, Choi YW, Lee KJ, Jeon SC, Park CK, Heo JN. CT halo sign: the spectrum of pulmonary diseases. Br J Radiol. 2005;78(933):862–5. https://doi.org/10.1259/bjr/77712845.
18. Si MJ, Tao XF, Du GY, Cai LL, Han HX, Liang XZ, Zhao JM. Thin-section computed tomography-histopathologic comparisons of pulmonary focal interstitial fibrosis, atypical adenomatous hyperplasia, adenocarcinoma in situ, and minimally invasive adenocarcinoma with pure ground-glass opacity. Eur J Radiol. 2016;85(10):1708–15. https://doi.org/10.1016/j.ejrad.2016.07.012.

Suggested Readings

1. Abramson S, Gilkeson RC, Goldstein JD, Woodard PK, Eisenberg R, Abramson N. Benign metastasizing leiomyoma: clinical, imaging, and pathologic correlation. AJR Am J Roentgenol. 2001;176(6):1409–13. https://doi.org/10.2214/ajr.176.6.1761409.
2. Allen MS. Multiple benign lung tumors. Semin Thorac Cardiovasc Surg. 2003;15(3):310–4.
3. Bahk YW, Shinn KS, Choi BS. The air meniscus sign in sclerosing hemangioma of the lung. Radiology. 1978;128(1):27–9. https://doi.org/10.1148/128.1.27.
4. Bankoff MS, McEniff NJ, Bhadelia RA, Garcia-Moliner M, Daly BD. Prevalence of pathologically proven intrapulmonary lymph nodes and their appearance on CT. AJR Am J Roentgenol. 1996;167(3):629–30. https://doi.org/10.2214/ajr.167.3.8751667.
5. Benson RE, Rosado-de-Christenson ML, Martinez-Jimenez S, Kunin JR, Pettavel PP. Spectrum of pulmonary neuroendocrine proliferations and neoplasms. Radiographics. 2013;33(6):1631–49. https://doi.org/10.1148/rg.336135506.
6. Bi N, Shedden K, Zheng X, Kong F. Comparison of the effectiveness of radiofrequency ablation with stereotactic body radiation therapy in inoperable stage I non-small cell lung cancer: a systemic review and meta-analysis. Pract Radiat Oncol. 2013;3(2 Suppl 1):S19. https://doi.org/10.1016/j.prro.2013.01.066.
7. Blum U, Windfuhr M, Buitrago-Tellez C, Sigmund G, Herbst EW, Langer M. Invasive pulmonary aspergillosis. MRI, CT, and plain radiographic findings and their contribution for early diagnosis. Chest. 1994;106(4):1156–61.
8. Bobba RK, Holly JS, Loy T, Perry MC. Scar carcinoma of the lung: a historical perspective. Clin Lung Cancer. 2011;12(3):148–54. https://doi.org/10.1016/j.cllc.2011.03.011.
9. Butt Y, Kurdowska A, Allen TC. Acute lung injury: a clinical and molecular review. Arch Pathol Lab Med. 2016;140(4):345–50. https://doi.org/10.5858/arpa.2015-0519-RA.

10. Chang JY, Senan S, Paul MA, Mehran RJ, Louie AV, Balter P, Groen HJ, McRae SE, Widder J, Feng L, van den Borne BE, Munsell MF, Hurkmans C, Berry DA, van Werkhoven E, Kresl JJ, Dingemans AM, Dawood O, Haasbeek CJ, Carpenter LS, De Jaeger K, Komaki R, Slotman BJ, Smit EF, Roth JA. Stereotactic ablative radiotherapy versus lobectomy for operable stage I non-small-cell lung cancer: a pooled analysis of two randomised trials. Lancet Oncol. 2015;16(6):630–7. https://doi.org/10.1016/s1470-2045(15)70168-3.
11. Chen W, Zheng R, Baade PD, Zhang S, Zeng H, Bray F, Jemal A, Yu XQ, He J. Cancer statistics in China, 2015. CA Cancer J Clin. 2016;66(2):115–32. https://doi.org/10.3322/caac.21338.
12. Chen WH, Tang LQ, Wang FW, Li CP, Tian XP, Huang XX, Mai SJ, Liao YJ, Deng HX, Chen QY, Liu H, Zhang L, Guo SS, Liu LT, Yan SM, Li CF, Zhang JP, Liu Q, Liu XW, Liu LZ, Mai HQ, Zeng MS, Xie D. Elevated levels of plasma D-dimer predict a worse outcome in patients with nasopharyngeal carcinoma. BMC Cancer. 2014;14:583. https://doi.org/10.1186/1471-2407-14-583.
13. Cortese G, Nicali R, Placido R, Gariazzo G, Anro P. Radiological aspects of diffuse alveolar haemorrhage. Radiol Med. 2008;113(1):16–28. https://doi.org/10.1007/s11547-008-0229-x.
14. da Silva RA, Gross JL, Haddad FJ, Toledo CA, Younes RN. Primary pulmonary paraganglioma: case report and literature review. Clinics (Sao Paulo, Brazil). 2006;61(1):83–6. doi: S1807-59322006000100015.
15. Diederich S. Pulmonary nodules: do we need a separate algorithm for non-solid lesions? Cancer Imaging. 2009;9(Special issue A):S126–8. https://doi.org/10.1102/1470-7330.2009.9046.
16. Dupuy DE, Zagoria RJ, Akerley W, Mayo-Smith WW, Kavanagh PV, Safran H. Percutaneous radiofrequency ablation of malignancies in the lung. AJR Am J Roentgenol. 2000;174(1):57–9. https://doi.org/10.2214/ajr.174.1.1740057.
17. Edey AJ, Hansell DM. Incidentally detected small pulmonary nodules on CT. Clin Radiol. 2009;64(9):872–84. https://doi.org/10.1016/j.crad.2009.03.006.
18. Epler GR, Colby TV, McLoud TC, Carrington CB, Gaensler EA. Bronchiolitis obliterans organizing pneumonia. N Engl J Med. 1985;312(3):152–8. https://doi.org/10.1056/nejm198501173120304.
19. Ettinger DS, Wood DE, Akerley W, Bazhenova LA, Borghaei H, Camidge DR, Cheney RT, Chirieac LR, D'Amico TA, Demmy TL, Dilling TJ, Dobelbower MC, Govindan R, Grannis FW Jr, Horn L, Jahan TM, Komaki R, Krug LM, Lackner RP, Lanuti M, Lilenbaum R, Lin J, Loo BW Jr, Martins R, Otterson GA, Patel JD, Pisters KM, Reckamp K, Riely GJ, Rohren E, Schild SE, Shapiro TA, Swanson SJ, Tauer K, Yang SC, Gregory K, Hughes M. Non-small cell lung cancer, version 6.2015. J Ntal Compr Canc Netw. 2015;13(5):515–24.
20. Frazier AA, Franks TJ, Mohammed TL, Ozbudak IH, Galvin JR. From the archives of the AFIP: pulmonary veno-occlusive disease and pulmonary capillary hemangiomatosis. Radiographics. 2007;27(3):867–82. https://doi.org/10.1148/rg.273065194.
21. Freant LJ, Joseph WL, Adkins PC. Scar carcinoma of the lung. Fact or fantasy? Ann Thorac Surg. 1974;17(6):531–7.
22. Glynn C, Zakowski MF, Ginsberg MS. Are there imaging characteristics associated with epidermal growth factor receptor and KRAS mutations in patients with adenocarcinoma of the lung with bronchioloalveolar features? J Thorac Oncol. 2010;5(3):344–8. https://doi.org/10.1097/JTO.0b013e3181ce9a7a.
23. Godoy MC, Naidich DP. Overview and strategic management of subsolid pulmonary nodules. J Thorac Imaging. 2012;27(4):240–8. https://doi.org/10.1097/RTI.0b013e31825d515b.
24. Goldberg SN, Gazelle GS, Mueller PR. Thermal ablation therapy for focal malignancy: a unified approach to underlying principles, techniques, and diagnostic imaging guidance. AJR Am J Roentgenol. 2000;174(2):323–31. https://doi.org/10.2214/ajr.174.2.1740323.
25. Goshima H, Tomioka H, Nishio C, Fujii H, Katsuyama E. Reversed halo sign in pulmonary infarction with tumor emboli: a case report. Respir Investig. 2014;52(3):199–202. https://doi.org/10.1016/j.resinv.2013.08.004.

26. Goto T, Maeshima A, Kato R. Microscopic sclerosing hemangioma diagnosed by histopathological examination after lung cancer surgery. Ann Thorac Cardiovasc Surg. 2011;17(5):507–10.
27. Gould MK, Donington J, Lynch WR, Mazzone PJ, Midthun DE, Naidich DP, Wiener RS. Evaluation of individuals with pulmonary nodules: when is it lung cancer? Diagnosis and management of lung cancer, 3rd ed: American College of Chest Physicians evidence-based clinical practice guidelines. Chest. 2013;143(5 Suppl):e93S–e120S. https://doi.org/10.1378/chest.12-2351.
28. Gurney JW. Determining the likelihood of malignancy in solitary pulmonary nodules with Bayesian analysis. Part I Theory. Radiology. 1993;186(2):405–13. https://doi.org/10.1148/radiology.186.2.8421743.
29. Haasbeek CJ, Lagerwaard FJ, Antonisse ME, Slotman BJ, Senan S. Stage I nonsmall cell lung cancer in patients aged > or =75 years: outcomes after stereotactic radiotherapy. Cancer. 2010;116(2):406–14. https://doi.org/10.1002/cncr.24759.
30. Hansell DM, Bankier AA, MacMahon H, McLoud TC, Muller NL, Remy J. Fleischner society: glossary of terms for thoracic imaging. Radiology. 2008;246(3):697–722. https://doi.org/10.1148/radiol.2462070712.
31. Henschke CI, Yankelevitz DF, Mirtcheva R, McGuinness G, McCauley D, Miettinen OS. CT screening for lung cancer: frequency and significance of part-solid and nonsolid nodules. AJR Am J Roentgenol. 2002;178(5):1053–7. https://doi.org/10.2214/ajr.178.5.1781053.
32. Herder GJ, van Tinteren H, Golding RP, Kostense PJ, Comans EF, Smit EF, Hoekstra OS. Clinical prediction model to characterize pulmonary nodules: validation and added value of 18F-fluorodeoxyglucose positron emission tomography. Chest. 2005;128(4):2490–6. https://doi.org/10.1378/chest.128.4.2490.
33. Hess A, Palussiere J, Goyers JF, Guth A, Auperin A, de Baere T. Pulmonary radiofrequency ablation in patients with a single lung: feasibility, efficacy, and tolerance. Radiology. 2011;258(2):635–42. https://doi.org/10.1148/radiol.10100771.
34. Hiraki T, Gobara H, Mimura H, Matsui Y, Toyooka S, Kanazawa S. Percutaneous radiofrequency ablation of clinical stage I non-small cell lung cancer. J Thorac Cardiovasc Surg. 2011;142(1):24–30. https://doi.org/10.1016/j.jtcvs.2011.02.036.
35. Honma K, Nelson G, Murray J. Intrapulmonary lymph nodes in South African miners—an autopsy survey. Am J Ind Med. 2007;50(4):261–4. https://doi.org/10.1002/ajim.20436.
36. Hyodo T, Kanazawa S, Dendo S, Kobayashi K, Hayashi H, Kouno Y, Fujishima M, Hiraki Y. Intrapulmonary lymph nodes: thin-section CT findings, pathological findings, and CT differential diagnosis from pulmonary metastatic nodules. Acta Med Okayama. 2004;58(5):235–40.
37. Jensen KG, Schiodt T. Growth conditions of hamartoma of the lung: a study based on 22 cases operated on after radiographic observation for from one to 18 years. Thorax. 1958;13(3):233–7.
38. Kaitoukov Y, Rakovich G, Trahan S, Gregoire J. Inflammatory pseudotumour of the lung. Can Respir J. 2011;18(6):315–7.
39. Kanaji N, Sakai K, Ueda Y, Miyawaki H, Ishii T, Watanabe N, Kita N, Kadota K, Kadowaki N, Bandoh S. Peripheral-type small cell lung cancer is associated with better survival and higher frequency of interstitial lung disease. Lung Cancer. 2017;108:126–33. https://doi.org/10.1016/j.lungcan.2017.03.013.
40. Kharofa J, Cohen EP, Tomic R, Xiang Q, Gore E. Decreased risk of radiation pneumonitis with incidental concurrent use of angiotensin-converting enzyme inhibitors and thoracic radiation therapy. Int J Radiat Oncol Biol Phys. 2012;84(1):238–43. https://doi.org/10.1016/j.ijrobp.2011.11.013.
41. Kradin RL, Spirn PW, Mark EJ. Intrapulmonary lymph nodes. Clinical, radiologic, and pathologic features. Chest. 1985;87(5):662–7.
42. Kroemer G, Zitvogel L. Abscopal but desirable: the contribution of immune responses to the efficacy of radiotherapy. Oncoimmunology. 2012;1(4):407–8.
43. Lanuti M, Sharma A, Willers H, Digumarthy SR, Mathisen DJ, Shepard JA. Radiofrequency ablation for stage I non-small cell lung cancer: management of locoregional recurrence.

Ann Thorac Surg. 2012;93(3):921–927.; discussion 927-988. https://doi.org/10.1016/j.athoracsur.2011.11.043.
44. Lara AR, Schwarz MI. Diffuse alveolar hemorrhage. Chest. 2010;137(5):1164–71. https://doi.org/10.1378/chest.08-2084.
45. Lencioni R, Crocetti L, Cioni R, Suh R, Glenn D, Regge D, Helmberger T, Gillams AR, Frilling A, Ambrogi M, Bartolozzi C, Mussi A. Response to radiofrequency ablation of pulmonary tumours: a prospective, intention-to-treat, multicentre clinical trial (the RAPTURE study). Lancet Oncol. 2008;9(7):621–8. https://doi.org/10.1016/s1470-2045(08)70155-4.
46. Li M, Gao F, Jagadeesan J, Gill RR, Hua Y, Zheng X. Incremental value of contrast enhanced computed tomography on diagnostic accuracy in evaluation of small pulmonary ground glass nodules. J Thorac Dis. 2015;7(9):1606–15. https://doi.org/10.3978/j.issn.2072-1439.2015.09.37.
47. Marchiori E, Marom EM, Zanetti G, Hochhegger B, Irion KL, Godoy MCB. Reversed halo sign in invasive fungal infections: criteria for differentiation from organizing pneumonia. Chest. 2012;142(6):1469–73. https://doi.org/10.1378/chest.12-0114.
48. Marchiori E, Zanetti G, Irion KL, Nobre LF, Hochhegger B, Mancano AD, Escuissato DL. Reversed halo sign in active pulmonary tuberculosis: criteria for differentiation from cryptogenic organizing pneumonia. AJR Am J Roentgenol. 2011;197(6):1324–7. https://doi.org/10.2214/ajr.11.6543.
49. Maredia R, Snyder BJ, Harvey LA, Schwartz AM. Benign metastasizing leiomyoma in the lung. Radiographics. 1998;18(3):779–82. https://doi.org/10.1148/radiographics.18.3.9599398.
50. Matsuki M, Noma S, Kuroda Y, Oida K, Shindo T, Kobashi Y. Thin-section CT features of intrapulmonary lymph nodes. J Comput Assist Tomogr. 2001;25(5):753–6.
51. Matsuo Y, Shibuya K, Nakamura M, Narabayashi M, Sakanaka K, Ueki N, Miyagi K, Norihisa Y, Mizowaki T, Nagata Y, Hiraoka M. Dose—volume metrics associated with radiation pneumonitis after stereotactic body radiation therapy for lung cancer. Int J Radiat Oncol Biol Phys. 2012;83(4):e545–9. https://doi.org/10.1016/j.ijrobp.2012.01.018.
52. Maturu VN, Agarwal R. Reversed halo sign: a systematic review. Respir Care. 2014;59(9):1440–9. https://doi.org/10.4187/respcare.03020.
53. Miyauchi E, Motoi N, Ono H, Ninomiya H, Ohyanagi F, Nishio M, Okumura S, Ichinose M, Ishikawa Y. Distinct characteristics of small cell lung cancer correlate with central or peripheral origin: subtyping based on location and expression of transcription factor TTF-1. Medicine. 2015;94(51):e2324. https://doi.org/10.1097/md.0000000000002324.
54. Murphy J, Schnyder P, Herold C, Flower C. Bronchiolitis obliterans organising pneumonia simulating bronchial carcinoma. Eur Radiol. 1998;8(7):1165–9. https://doi.org/10.1007/s003300050527.
55. Nakazono T, Sakao Y, Yamaguchi K, Imai S, Kumazoe H, Kudo S. Subtypes of peripheral adenocarcinoma of the lung: differentiation by thin-section CT. Eur Radiol. 2005;15(8):1563–8. https://doi.org/10.1007/s00330-004-2595-7.
56. Narla LD, Newman B, Spottswood SS, Narla S, Kolli R. Inflammatory pseudotumor. Radiographics. 2003;23(3):719–29. https://doi.org/10.1148/rg.233025073.
57. Nobashi T, Koyasu S, Nakamoto Y, Kubo T, Ishimori T, Kim YH, Yoshizawa A, Togashi K. Prognostic value of fluorine-18 fludeoxyglucose positron emission tomography parameters differs according to primary tumour location in small-cell lung cancer. Br J Radiol. 2016;89(1059):20150618. https://doi.org/10.1259/bjr.20150618.
58. Okuma T, Matsuoka T, Yamamoto A, Oyama Y, Hamamoto S, Toyoshima M, Nakamura K, Miki Y. Determinants of local progression after computed tomography-guided percutaneous radiofrequency ablation for unresectable lung tumors: 9-year experience in a single institution. Cardiovasc Intervent Radiol. 2010;33(4):787–93. https://doi.org/10.1007/s00270-009-9770-9.
59. Palma D, Visser O, Lagerwaard FJ, Belderbos J, Slotman B, Senan S. Treatment of stage I NSCLC in elderly patients: a population-based matched-pair comparison of stereotactic

radiotherapy versus surgery. Radiother Oncol. 2011;101(2):240–4. https://doi.org/10.1016/j.radonc.2011.06.029.
60. Palma D, Visser O, Lagerwaard FJ, Belderbos J, Slotman BJ, Senan S. Impact of introducing stereotactic lung radiotherapy for elderly patients with stage I non-small-cell lung cancer: a population-based time-trend analysis. J Clin Oncol Off J Am Soc Clin Oncol. 2010;28(35):5153–9. https://doi.org/10.1200/jco.2010.30.0731.
61. Palma DA, Tyldesley S, Sheehan F, Mohamed IG, Smith S, Wai E, Murray N, Senan S. Stage I non-small cell lung cancer (NSCLC) in patients aged 75 years and older: does age determine survival after radical treatment? J Thorac Oncol. 2010;5(6):818–24.
62. Park CM, Goo JM, Lee HJ, Lee CH, Chung DH, Chun EJ, Im JG. Focal interstitial fibrosis manifesting as nodular ground-glass opacity: thin-section CT findings. Eur Radiol. 2007;17(9):2325–31. https://doi.org/10.1007/s00330-007-0596-z.
63. Pennathur A, Luketich JD, Abbas G, Chen M, Fernando HC, Gooding WE, Schuchert MJ, Gilbert S, Christie NA, Landreneau RJ. Radiofrequency ablation for the treatment of stage I non-small cell lung cancer in high-risk patients. J Thorac Cardiovasc Surg. 2007;134(4):857–64. https://doi.org/10.1016/j.jtcvs.2007.04.060.
64. Perez N, Lhoste-Trouilloud A, Boyer L, Michel JL, Escande G, Kemeny JL. Computed tomographic appearance of three intrapulmonary lymph nodes. Eur J Radiol. 1998;28(2):147–9.
65. Pinto PS. The CT halo sign. Radiology. 2004;230(1):109–10. https://doi.org/10.1148/radiol.2301020649.
66. Raeburn C, Spencer H. A study of the origin and development of lung cancer. Thorax. 1953;8(1):1–10.
67. Rauschenbach BM, Mackowiak L, Malhotra HK. A dosimetric comparison of three-dimensional conformal radiotherapy, volumetric-modulated arc therapy, and dynamic conformal arc therapy in the treatment of non-small cell lung cancer using stereotactic body radiotherapy. J Appl Clin Med Phys. 2014;15(5):4898. https://doi.org/10.1120/jacmp.v15i5.4898.
68. Rekers NH, Troost EG, Zegers CM, Germeraad WT, Dubois LJ, Lambin P. Stereotactic ablative body radiotherapy combined with immunotherapy: present status and future perspectives. Cancer Radiother. 2014;18(5–6):391–5. https://doi.org/10.1016/j.canrad.2014.06.012.
69. Riley RS, Gilbert AR, Dalton JB, Pai S, McPherson RA. Widely used types and clinical applications of D-dimer assay. Lab Med. 2016;47(2):90–102. https://doi.org/10.1093/labmed/lmw001.
70. Saijo T, Ishii G, Nagai K, Funai K, Nitadori J, Tsuta K, Nara M, Hishida T, Ochiai A. Differences in clinicopathological and biological features between central-type and peripheral-type squamous cell carcinoma of the lung. Lung Cancer. 2006;52(1):37–45. https://doi.org/10.1016/j.lungcan.2005.12.006.
71. Sakaguchi Y, Isowa N, Tokuyasu H, Miura H. A resected case of solitary pulmonary capillary hemangioma showing pure ground glass opacity. Ann Thorac Cardiovasc Surg. 2014;20(Suppl):578–81. https://doi.org/10.5761/atcs.cr.12.02222.
72. Sakurai H, Asamura H, Watanabe S, Suzuki K, Tsuchiya R. Clinicopathologic features of peripheral squamous cell carcinoma of the lung. Ann Thorac Surg. 2004;78(1):222–7. https://doi.org/10.1016/j.athoracsur.2004.01.029.
73. Sanders BM, West KW, Gingalewski C, Engum S, Davis M, Grosfeld JL. Inflammatory pseudotumor of the alimentary tract: clinical and surgical experience. J Pediatr Surg. 2001;36(1):169–73.
74. Schneider T, Heussel CP, Herth FJ, Dienemann H. Thermal ablation of malignant lung tumors. Dtsch Arztebl Int. 2013;110(22):394–400. https://doi.org/10.3238/arztebl.2013.0394.
75. Shin SY, Kim MY, Oh SY, Lee HJ, Hong SA, Jang SJ, Kim SS. Pulmonary sclerosing pneumocytoma of the lung: CT characteristics in a large series of a tertiary referral center. Medicine. 2015;94(4):e498. https://doi.org/10.1097/md.0000000000000498.
76. Shirvani SM, Jiang J, Chang JY, Welsh J, Likhacheva A, Buchholz TA, Swisher SG, Smith BD. Lobectomy, sublobar resection, and stereotactic ablative radiotherapy for early-stage

non-small cell lung cancers in the elderly. JAMA Surg. 2014;149(12):1244–53. https://doi.org/10.1001/jamasurg.2014.556.
77. Shirvani SM, Jiang J, Chang JY, Welsh JW, Gomez DR, Swisher S, Buchholz TA, Smith BD. Comparative effectiveness of 5 treatment strategies for early-stage non-small cell lung cancer in the elderly. Int J Radiat Oncol Biol Phys. 2012;84(5):1060–70. https://doi.org/10.1016/j.ijrobp.2012.07.2354.
78. Sider L, Westcott MA. Pulmonary manifestations of cryptococcosis in patients with AIDS: CT features. J Thorac Imaging. 1994;9(2):78–84.
79. Steiner PE. Metastasizing fibroleiomyoma of the uterus: report of a case and review of the literature. Am J Pathol. 1939;15(1):89–110.117.
80. Subramanian SV, Subramani V, Swamy ST, Gandhi A, Chilukuri S, Kathirvel M. Is 5 mm MMLC suitable for VMAT-based lung SBRT? A dosimetric comparison with 2.5 mm HDMLC using RTOG-0813 treatment planning criteria for both conventional and high-dose flattening filter-free photon beams. J Appl Clin Med Phys. 2015;16(4):112–24. https://doi.org/10.1120/jacmp.v16i4.5415.
81. Sudo N, Nambu A, Yamakawa T, Kawamoto M, Fujino S, Watanabe M, Mizuguchi K, Tago M. Pulmonary focal fibrosis associated with microscopic arterio-venous fistula manifesting as focal ground-glass opacity on thin-section CT. BMC Pulm Med. 2013;13:3. https://doi.org/10.1186/1471-2466-13-3.
82. Suh RD, Wallace AB, Sheehan RE, Heinze SB, Goldin JG. Unresectable pulmonary malignancies: CT-guided percutaneous radiofrequency ablation—preliminary results. Radiology. 2003;229(3):821–9. https://doi.org/10.1148/radiol.2293021756.
83. Swarnakar R, Sinha S. Endobronchial leiomyoma: a rare and innocent tumour of the bronchial tree. Lung India. 2013;30(1):57–60. https://doi.org/10.4103/0970-2113.106175.
84. Swensen SJ, Silverstein MD, Ilstrup DM, Schleck CD, Edell ES. The probability of malignancy in solitary pulmonary nodules. Application to small radiologically indeterminate nodules. Arch Intern Med. 1997;157(8):849–55.
85. Sykes AM, Swensen SJ, Tazelaar HD, Jung SH. Computed tomography of benign intrapulmonary lymph nodes: retrospective comparison with sarcoma metastases. Mayo Clin Proc. 2002;77(4):329–33. https://doi.org/10.1016/s0025-6196(11)61785-0.
86. Takenaka M, Uramoto H, Shimokawa H, So T, Hanagiri T, Aoki T, Tanaka F. Discriminative features of thin-slice computed tomography for peripheral intrapulmonary lymph nodes. Asian J Surg. 2013;36(2):69–73. https://doi.org/10.1016/j.asjsur.2012.11.005.
87. Tateishi U, Kusumoto M, Akiyama Y, Kishi F, Nishimura M, Moriyama N. Role of contrast-enhanced dynamic CT in the diagnosis of active tuberculoma. Chest. 2002;122(4):1280–4.
88. Teixeira BC, Mahfouz K, Escuissato DL, Costa AF, Noronha L. Solitary benign metastasizing leiomyoma: imaging features and pathological findings. J Bras Pneumol. 2014;40(2):193–5.
89. Timmer SJ, Amundson DE, Malone JD. Hypersensitivity pneumonitis following anthrax vaccination. Chest. 2002;122(2):741–5.
90. Trapnell DH. Recognition and incidence of intrapulmonary lymph nodes. Thorax. 1964;19:44–50.
91. Travis WD, Brambilla E, Noguchi M, Nicholson AG, Geisinger K, Yatabe Y, Powell CA, Beer D, Riely G, Garg K, Austin JH, Rusch VW, Hirsch FR, Jett J, Yang PC, Gould M. International Association for the Study of Lung Cancer/American Thoracic Society/European Respiratory Society: international multidisciplinary classification of lung adenocarcinoma: executive summary. Proc Am Thorac Soc. 2011;8(5):381–5. https://doi.org/10.1513/pats.201107-042ST.
92. Travis WD, Colby TV, Lombard C, Carpenter HA. A clinicopathologic study of 34 cases of diffuse pulmonary hemorrhage with lung biopsy confirmation. Am J Surg Pathol. 1990;14(12):1112–25.
93. Tuddenham WJ. Glossary of terms for thoracic radiology: recommendations of the nomenclature Committee of the Fleischner Society. AJR Am J Roentgenol. 1984;143(3):509–17. https://doi.org/10.2214/ajr.143.3.509.

94. Ujita M, Renzoni EA, Veeraraghavan S, Wells AU, Hansell DM. Organizing pneumonia: perilobular pattern at thin-section CT. Radiology. 2004;232(3):757–61. https://doi.org/10.1148/radiol.2323031059.
95. Vellozzi C, Burwen DR, Dobardzic A, Ball R, Walton K, Haber P. Safety of trivalent inactivated influenza vaccines in adults: background for pandemic influenza vaccine safety monitoring. Vaccine. 2009;27(15):2114–20. https://doi.org/10.1016/j.vaccine.2009.01.125.
96. Wahba H, Truong MT, Lei X, Kontoyiannis DP, Marom EM. Reversed halo sign in invasive pulmonary fungal infections. Clin Infect Dis. 2008;46(11):1733–7. https://doi.org/10.1086/587991.
97. Wang CW, Teng YH, Huang CC, YC W, Chao YK, CT W. Intrapulmonary lymph nodes: computed tomography findings with histopathologic correlations. Clin Imaging. 2013;37(3):487–92. https://doi.org/10.1016/j.clinimag.2012.09.010.
98. Watanabe K, Harada T, Yoshida M, Shirakusa T, Iwasaki A, Yoneda S, Kikuchi M. Organizing pneumonia presenting as a solitary nodular shadow on a chest radiograph. Respiration. 2003;70(5):507–14. https://doi.org/10.1159/000074208.
99. Watanabe S, Waseda Y, Takato H, Inuzuka K, Katayama N, Kasahara K, Fujimura M. Influenza vaccine-induced interstitial lung disease. Eur Respir J. 2013;41(2):474–7. https://doi.org/10.1183/09031936.00146912.
100. Watanabe Y, Yokose T, Sakuma Y, Hasegawa C, Saito H, Yamada K, Ito H, Tsuboi M, Nakayama H, Kameda Y. Alveolar space filling ratio as a favorable prognostic factor in small peripheral squamous cell carcinoma of the lung. Lung Cancer. 2011;73(2):217–21. https://doi.org/10.1016/j.lungcan.2010.12.001.
101. Weisbrod GL, Chamberlain D, Herman SJ. Cystic change (pseudocavitation) associated with bronchioloalveolar carcinoma: a report of four patients. J Thorac Imaging. 1995;10(2):106–11.
102. Wong JS, Weisbrod GL, Chamberlain D, Herman SJ. Bronchioloalveolar carcinoma and the air bronchogram sign: a new pathologic explanation. J Thorac Imaging. 1994;9(3):141–4.
103. Yamamoto A, Nakamura K, Matsuoka T, Toyoshima M, Okuma T, Oyama Y, Ikura Y, Ueda M, Inoue Y. Radiofrequency ablation in a porcine lung model: correlation between CT and histopathologic findings. AJR Am J Roentgenol. 2005;185(5):1299–306. https://doi.org/10.2214/ajr.04.0968.
104. Yano Y, Mori M, Kagami S, Fushitani K, Sugano T, Namba Y, Yoneda T, Yokota S, Maeda H, Ueda K. Inflammatory pseudotumor of the lung with rapid growth. Intern Med. 2009;48(15):1279–82.
105. Yokomise H, Mizuno H, Ike O, Wada H, Hitomi S, Itoh H. Importance of intrapulmonary lymph nodes in the differential diagnosis of small pulmonary nodular shadows. Chest. 1998;113(3):703–6.
106. Zhang J, Yang F, Li B, Li H, Liu J, Huang W, Wang D, Yi Y, Wang J. Which is the optimal biologically effective dose of stereotactic body radiotherapy for stage I non-small-cell lung cancer? A meta-analysis. Int J Radiat Oncol Biol Phys. 2011;81(4):e305–16. https://doi.org/10.1016/j.ijrobp.2011.04.034.
107. Zheng X, Schipper M, Kidwell K, Lin J, Reddy R, Ren Y, Chang A, Lv F, Orringer M, Spring Kong FM. Survival outcome after stereotactic body radiation therapy and surgery for stage I non-small cell lung cancer: a meta-analysis. Int J Radiat Oncol Biol Phys. 2014;90(3):603–11. https://doi.org/10.1016/j.ijrobp.2014.05.055.
108. Zidane A, Elktaibi A, Benjelloun A, Arsalane A, Afandi O, Bouchentouf R. Primary leiomyoma of the lung: an exceptional localization. Asian Cardiovasc Thorac Ann. 2016;24(4):393–6. https://doi.org/10.1177/0218492316638608.
109. Zwirewich CV, Vedal S, Miller RR, Muller NL. Solitary pulmonary nodule: high-resolution CT and radiologic-pathologic correlation. Radiology. 1991;179(2):469–76. https://doi.org/10.1148/radiology.179.2.2014294.

Index

X. Zheng et al. (eds.), *Early-stage Lung Cancer*,
https://doi.org/10.1007/978-981-10-7596-4

The manufacturer's authorised representative in the EU is Springer Nature Customer Service Centre GmbH, Europaplatz 3, 69115 Heidelberg, Germany. If you have any concerns regarding our products, please contact ProductSafety@springernature.com

Printed and bound by CPI Group (UK) Ltd, Croydon, CR0 4YY
25/09/2026
02222880-0001